Ophthalmology: Diagnosis and Treatment of Eye Diseases

Ophthalmology: Diagnosis and Treatment of Eye Diseases

Editor: Anastasia Maddox

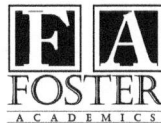

FA FOSTER
A C A D E M I C S

www.fosteracademics.com

www.fosteracademics.com

FA
FOSTER
ACADEMICS

Cataloging-in-Publication Data

Ophthalmology : diagnosis and treatment of eye diseases / edited by Anastasia Maddox.
    p. cm.
Includes bibliographical references and index.
ISBN 978-1-63242-751-9
1. Ophthalmology. 2. Eye--Diseases. 3. Eye--Diseases--Diagnosis.
4. Eye--Diseases--Treatment. I. Maddox, Anastasia.
RE46 .O54 2019
617.7--dc23

Foster Academics,
118-35 Queens Blvd., Suite 400,
Forest Hills, NY 11375, USA

ISBN 978-1-63242-751-9 (Hardback)

Contents

Permissions

List of Contributors

Index

Preface

The diagnosis and treatment of the diseases of the eye is under the scope of ophthalmology. It studies the anatomy and physiology of eyes, along with the diseases related to them. A specialist in the field of medical and surgical eye disorders is called an ophthalmologist. The tasks of an ophthalmologist include the use of medicines to treat eye disorders, performing surgery and implementing laser therapy. Cataract, glaucoma, strabismus, proptosis, macular degeneration, diabetic retinopathy, excessive tearing and eye tumors are some of the common eye diseases. Ultrasonography, optical coherence tomography and fluorescein angiography are some of the specialized diagnostic methods used to diagnose eye disorders. Ocular surgery is an effective way to cure eye disorders. This book studies, analyses and upholds the pillars of ophthalmology and its utmost significance in modern times. It aims to shed light on some of the unexplored aspects of ophthalmology and the recent researches in this field. Those in search of information to further their knowledge will be greatly assisted by this book.

This book unites the global concepts and researches in an organized manner for a comprehensive understanding of the subject. It is a ripe text for all researchers, students, scientists or anyone else who is interested in acquiring a better knowledge of this dynamic field.

I extend my sincere thanks to the contributors for such eloquent research chapters. Finally, I thank my family for being a source of support and help.

Editor

Cap-preserving SMILE Enhancement Surgery

Ahmed N. Sedky[1*], Sherine S. Wahba[2], Maged M. Roshdy[2] and Nermeen R. Ayaad[3]

Abstract

Background: Different enhancement procedures have been suggested for reduction of residual refractive errors after SMILE. The aim of this study is to evaluate an improved cap-preserving technique for enhancement after SMILE (Re-SMILE).

Methods: A retrospective case series was conducted at Eye subspecialty center, Cairo, Egypt on 9 eyes with myopia or myopic astigmatism (spherical equivalent − 8.0 and − 12.0D). undergoing SMILE procedure and needed second interference. This was either because the more myopic meridian was more than − 10.0 D and therefore planned to have two-steps procedure (six eyes) or because of under correction needing enhancement (three eyes). Assessment after the primary SMILE procedure was conducted at 1 day, 1 week, 1 month and 3 months postoperatively. Assessment after Re-SMILE was conducted at 1 day, 1 week, 1 month, 3 months, 6 months and 1 year postoperatively. The assessments included full ophthalmic examination, objective and subjective refraction, and rotating Scheimpflug camera imaging.

Results: Preoperatively, the mean refractive spherical equivalent (MRSE) values were: − 9.36 ± 0. 89. After primary SMILE it was − 2.18 ± 0.71. After Re-SMILE it was − 0.13 ± 0.68. MRSE was significantly improved after both procedures ($P < 0.01$). The safety index of primary SMILE cases was 1.65 ± 0.62 and for Re-SMILE 1.13 ± 0.34 and the efficacy index was 1.14 ± 0.24 after primary SMILE and 1.11 ± 0.26 after Re-SMILE.

Conclusion: Centered cap-preserving Re-SMILE is an effective procedure in reducing residual refractive errors after primary SMILE in high myopes.

Keywords: SMILE, SMILE enhancement, Cap-preserving SMILE enhancement, Re-SMILE

Background

Laser in-situ keratomileusis (LASIK) and photorefractive keratectomy (PRK) have been the two standard keratorefractive procedures. Small incision lenticule extraction (SMILE) was developed to reduce the corneal biomechanical compromise of LASIK and PRK. In numerous studies, the SMILE procedure was shown to be safe, predictable, and effective in treating myopia and myopic astigmatism [1–3].

As in any refractive procedure, residual refractive errors might occur. For example, Hjortdal et al. published that 20% of eyes have ≥0.5 D and 6% have ≥1.0 D of residual refractive error three months after SMILE in eyes with moderate to high myopia (mean refractive spherical equivalent (MRSE) -7.19 ± 1.30 D) [4].

Different enhancement procedures have been suggested for the reduction of residual refractive errors after SMILE.

Surface ablation, such as in PRK, causes postoperative pain and can lead to corneal haze. The Circle option, which converts the SMILE cap into a complete LASIK flap followed by excimer laser ablation similar to LASIK, has also been suggested as an enhancement procedure [5]. Another suggestion is the creation of a LASIK flap within the SMILE cap followed by ablation. However, this procedure comes with a risk of crossing the existing cap interface or creation of gas breakthrough [6].

One great benefit of SMILE is the preservation of the anterior layer of the corneal stroma and Bowman's membrane. All enhancement procedures mentioned above share the disadvantage of losing this SMILE benefit.

* Correspondence: asedky60@hotmail.com
[1]Eye Subspecialty Center, Cairo, Egypt, 18 Elkhalifa Elmamoun Street, Heliopolis, Cairo, Egypt
Full list of author information is available at the end of the article

Table 1 Showing the surgical parameters used in every patient during the SMILE Procedure

Eye	Initial central corneal thickness	Cap thickness	Planned spherical correction	Planned cylindrical correction	Lenticule central thickness	Calculated residual stromal bed
1	549	100	−8.75	− 1.25	158	291
2	554	100	−9	−1	159	295
3	552	120	−9	−1	172	270
4	533	100	−9	−0.5	139	294
5	577	100	−9	−1	160	317
6	555	120	−10	0	133	302
7	574	120	−10	0	125	329
8	534	100	−10	0	151	283
9	505	100	−6	−2.25	130	275

Recently, Donate and Thäeron published the first case report on creating a new SMILE lenticule underneath the interface of the primary SMILE procedure with the Sub-Cap-Lenticule-Extraction technique [7]. This method aims to keep the benefits associated with SMILE (i.e. preserving the anterior corneal stroma, including Bowman's membrane) and re-use the interface of the primary SMILE procedure for the Re-SMILE enhancement procedure.

Through this procedure, it is crucial to achieve a precise geometrical match between the interface of the primary SMILE procedure and the new cuts introduced by Re-SMILE to avoid difficulties associated with lenticule dissection and further subsequent complications.

In our study, our goal was to develop a protocol that provides precise centration of the Re-SMILE procedure with respect to the interface after primary SMILE. The

change in the term used in the previous study to the new term "cap-preserving SMILE enhancement surgery" is intended to reflect that the main benefits of the SMILE procedure are preserved.

Methods

A case series of consecutive 9 eyes of 7 patients was conducted in the Eye Subspecialty Center, Cairo, Egypt. The study adhered to the Tenets of the Declaration of Helsinki. Inclusion criteria were patients asking for laser vision correction with myopia or myopic astigmatism between − 8.0 and − 12.0 diopters (D) undergoing SMILE procedure and needed second interference. This was either because the more myopic meridian was more than − 10.0 D (since this is the maximum treatment allowed by our software version of the VisuMax femtosecond laser (Carl Zeiss Meditec AG, Jena, Germany)

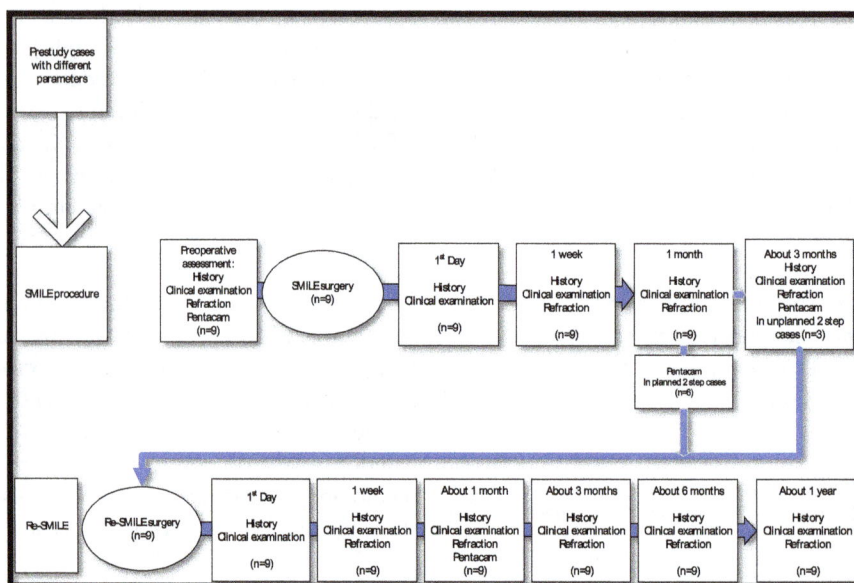

Fig. 1 Details of workflow and follow up visits

and therefore planned to have two-steps procedure (six eyes of four patients) or because of undercorrection needing enhancement (three eyes of three patients). To preserve the SMILE benefits, as less dryness induction, we went for the cap-preserving technique. Exclusion criteria were keratoconus, keratoconus suspects, insufficient corneal thickness to leave 250 μm residual stromal bed, corneal scars, and previous anterior segment surgeries. These patients were not specifically enrolled to receive this surgery for the research aim but when we reached good parameters for a centered cap-preserving Re-SMILE technique we collect and analysed the available data retrospectively.

Primary SMILE

Preoperative assessment included full ophthalmic examination, objective and subjective refraction including uncorrected distant visual acuity (UDVA) and corrected distant visual acuity (CDVA) and rotating Scheimpflug camera (Pentacam, OCULUS Optikgeräte GmbH, Wetzlar, Germany) imaging.

The primary SMILE surgery was performed using the VisuMax femtosecond laser system with the following parameters used: cap thickness of 100 to 120 μm, cap diameter of 7.5 to 7.7 mm, cap side cut angle 70°, 3 mm incision positioned at 100° and angled at 45°. The lenticule diameter (optical zone) was 6.5 mm, transition zone of 0 to 0.1, and clearance of 0.5 mm, lenticule side cut angle of 90° and edge lenticule thickness of 10 μm. Table 1 shows the other surgical parameters used in the primary SMILE procedure that varied from case to case.

At the end of the procedure, we performed good massage to the cap, evenly from the center to the periphery, to avoid any potential complications from the mismatch between the bed and the cap like mud-crack type microfolds.

Postoperative treatment included topical steroids and antibiotics 4 times per day for 10 days and tear substitutes 4 times daily for one to two months. Follow-up visits were on the first day, one week, one month and 3 months postoperatively. Follow-up visits included full ophthalmic examination, objective and subjective refraction, and rotating Scheimpflug camera imaging. In the planned two-step procedures, Pentacam was done after one month. If the refraction was consistent with the predicted one and stable since the first postoperative week the decision was to proceed to RE-SMILE after patient counseling. Figure 1 shows the details of each visit.

Re-SMILE

The eyes eligible for enhancement were those with expected mean K readings after ablation of not less than 33 D, residual stromal bed of at least 250 μm, and those with no suspicion of ectasia based on tomography.

All Re-SMILE procedures were performed using the same laser device as in the primary SMILE procedure. The Sedky SMILE Retreatment Centering Marker (Fig. 2) was utilized in the centration of the Re-SMILE procedure. Some refractive laser settings were modified with respect to the primary SMILE treatment.

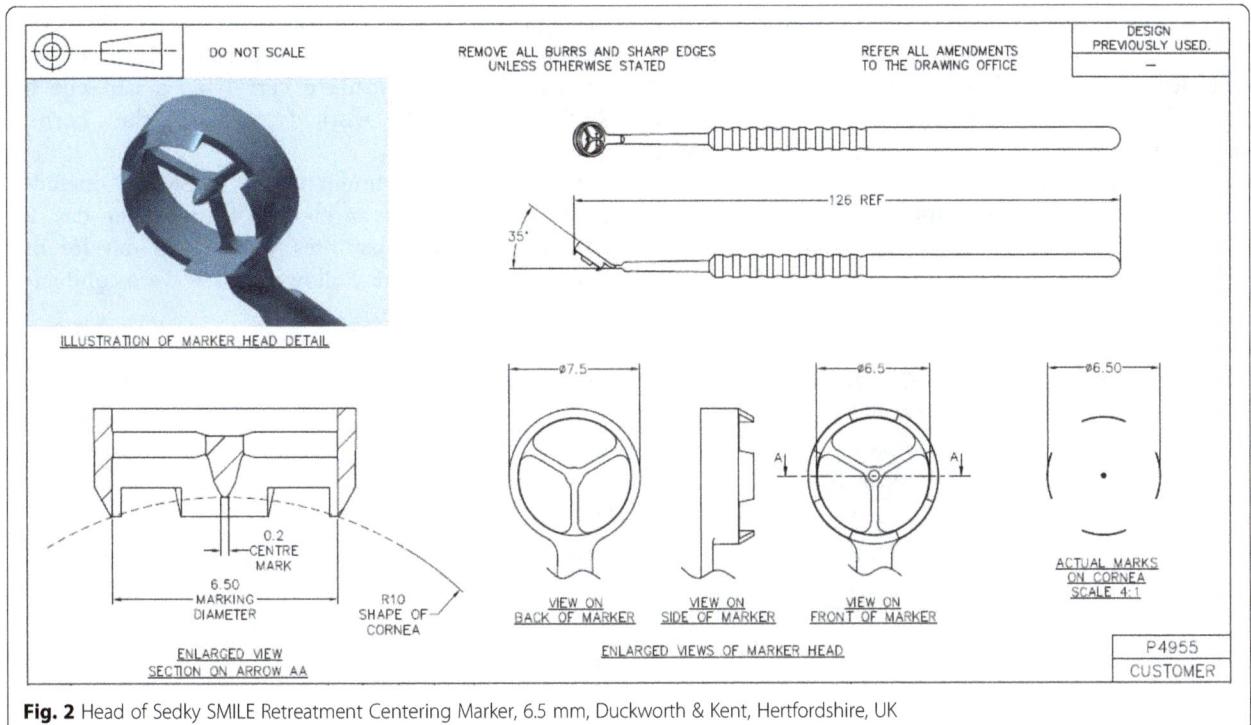

Fig. 2 Head of Sedky SMILE Retreatment Centering Marker, 6.5 mm, Duckworth & Kent, Hertfordshire, UK

Table 2 Showing the variable surgical parameters used in every patient during the Re-SMILE Procedure

Eye	Central corneal thickness before Re-SMILE	Planned spherical correction	Planned cylindrical correction	Lenticule central thickness	Calculated Residual stromal bed
1	411	−2.25	−0.5	55	256
2	414	0	−2.5	51	263
3	410	−3	0	37	253
4	433	−1.25	−0.5	50	283
5	398	−2	0	30	260
6	427	−2	−1[a]	45	257
7	449	−1.5	−1.5	60	269
8	405	−3.25	0	55	250
9	378	−1	− 0.75	25	250

[a]In the eye number 6, although the refractive cylinder was found to be − 2.75 D, only − 1 D was corrected to respect the 250 μm limit

The cap thickness was set to the value used in the primary SMILE treatment. Also, the cap thickness defines the depth of the anterior edge of the lenticule side cut. The parameter for the minimum edge thickness of the lenticule was set at greater or equal to 18 μm. Table 2 shows the variable surgical parameters used in the Re- SMILE procedure.

The programmed sum of optical zone and transitional zone diameters for the Re-SMILE procedure was found to be optimal if it is 0.2 mm less than that of the primary SMILE procedure.

Before arriving at this protocol, a Re-SMILE treatment with a lenticule diameter larger than the primary SMILE lenticule diameter was tested. This setting showed difficult dissection and postoperative intrastromal scaring due to lenticule edge overlapping. The lenticule with the same size as the primary SMILE lenticule demonstrated better postoperative outcome and less intrastromal scaring. However, difficult dissection remained, which might have been due to some mismatch between the Re-SMILE procedure and the primary SMILE.

A new centration marker (Sedky SMILE Retreatment Centering Marker, Duckworth & Kent, Hertfordshire, UK) was developed to improve the centration of the secondary treatment with respect to the primary SMILE treatment (Fig. 2).

The Sedky SMILE Retreatment Centering Marker as shown in Fig. 2 was designed to have four peripheral footplates and central marker pin. The 4 footplates are used to mark the primary cap edge and the central marker pin is used as a docking reference point for the retreatment procedure. The distal 1/3 of the marker handle is designed to have a 35-degree inclination to facilitate usage with the slit lamp at the outpatient clinic or with the built-in VisuMax slit lamp. Both footplates and central marker pin should be inked with a surgical ink (e.g. Viscot Surgical Skin Marker #1404, Viscot Medical, Hanover, NJ, USA) before using the marker. The marker is available in 2 sizes: 6.5 mm for the usage of a 6.7 mm primary lenticule diameter, and 6.3 mm for the usage of a 6.5 mm primary lenticule diameter.

Right before commencing the Re-SMILE procedure, the centration marker was used to mark the patient's cornea according to the centration of the primary SMILE. During the subsequent docking procedure, these marks were used to achieve precise positioning of the Re-SMILE treatment.

During the actual laser procedure, the surgeon aborted the automated cutting sequence immediately after the laser finished the lenticule side cut.

Then, the new lenticule was removed manually through the primary corneal incision after dissecting the inferior plane. The superior plane of the primary SMILE procedure served as a cap cut for Re-SMILE, which worked because the corneal stroma didn't heal.

Postoperative treatment after Re-SMILE included topical steroids and antibiotics 4 times per day for 10 days and tear substitutes 4 times per day for one month to two months. Follow-up visits were conducted

Table 3 MRSE, refractive cylinder, UDVA, and CDVA preoperatively, after the initial SMILE and cap-preserving RE-SMILE procedure. t = t-test statistic, p = p-value, z = Wilcoxon signed rank statistic

	MRSE(D) Mean ± SD	Cylinder(D) Mean ± SD	UDVA(logMAR) Mean ± SD	CDVA(logMAR) Mean ± SD
Preoperative	−9.36 ± 0. 89	−0.78 ± 0.74	0.93 ± 0.20	0.45 ± 0.12
Post primary SMILE	−2.18 ± 0.71	−0.75 ± 0.83	0.40 ± 0.15	0.26 ± 0.20
Significance of changes due to primary SMILE	z = − 2.67 p = 0.008	t = − 0.073 p = 0.943	z = −2.692 p = 0.007	t = 3.875 p = 0.005
Post Re-SMILE	−0.13 ± 0.68	−0.53 ± 0.34	0.22 ± 0.12	0.21 ± 0.11
Significance of changes due to Re- SMILE	t = −5.447 p = 0.001	t = − 730 p = 0.486	t = 3.568 p = 0.007	z = −1.187 p = 0.235

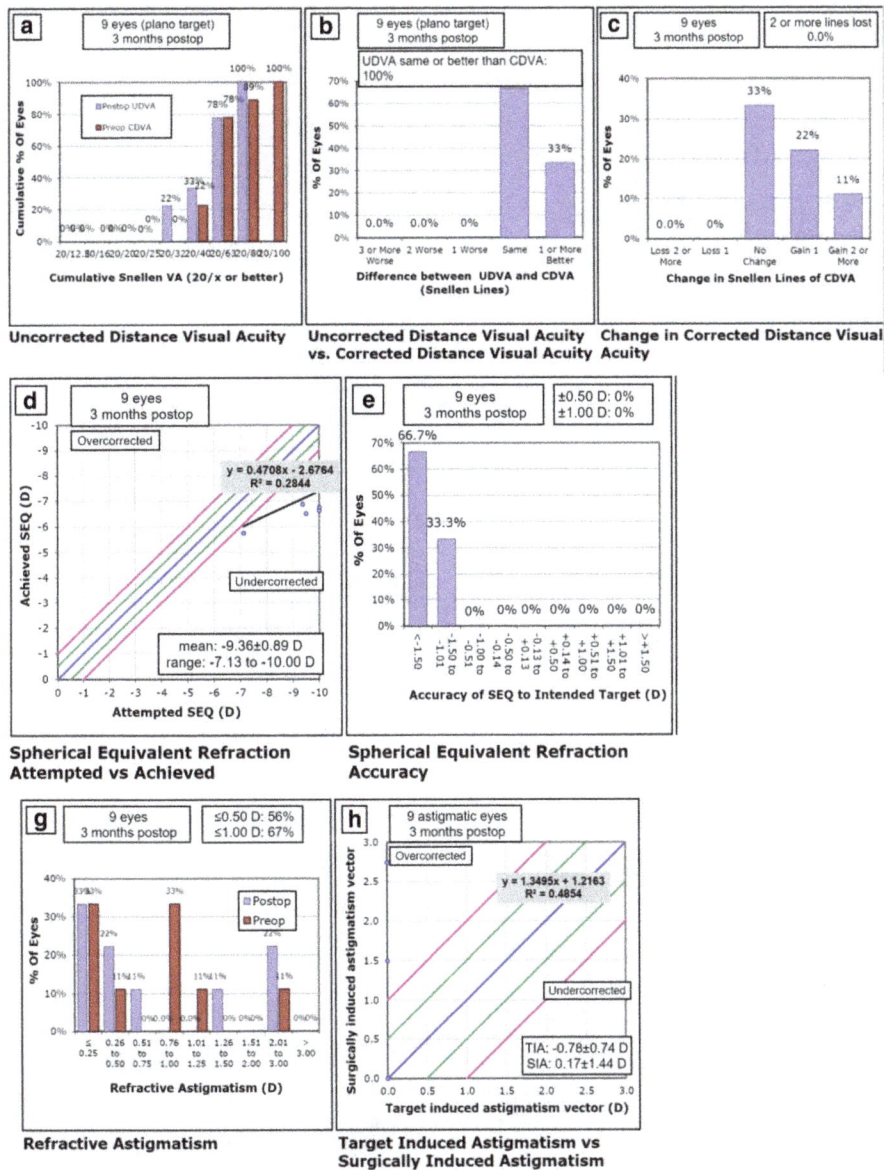

Fig. 3 Primary SMILE standardized graphs. **a** Postoperative cumulative uncorrected distance Snellen visual acuity (UDVA) versus preoperative cumulative corrected distance Snellen VISUAL acuity (CDVA). **b** Efficacy of the surgery by comparing postoperative UDVA to preoperative CDVA. **c** Safety of the procedure by comparing pre- and postoperative CDVA. **d** Accuracy of the surgery by comparing attempted versus achieved refractive spherical equivalent (SEQ) and presenting the regression formula describing the relation between them. **e** Accuracy of the surgery by showing the deviation of achieved SEQ compared to attempted SEQ in steps. **g** The residual refractive astigmatism. **h** Accuracy of the surgery by comparing attempted versus achieved refractive cylinder and presenting the regression formula describing the relation between them

on the first day, one week, one month, 3 months, 6 months and one year. The assessment included a full ophthalmic examination, objective and subjective refraction and Pentacam imaging. Figure 1 shows the details of each visit.

For each treatment case, the safety index was calculated in decimal units, as postoperative CDVA /preoperative CDVA and the efficacy index as postoperative UDVA /preoperative CDVA [8].

Data were collected, verified, and differences were calculated using Microsoft Excel 2013 (Redmond, Washington, USA). Statistical analyses were performed using MedCalc Statistics (v14.8.1; MedCalc, Belgium) and IBM SPSS Statistics (version 23, SPSS Inc., Chicago, IL, USA). The following statistical tests were performed: calculation of the mean, standard deviation (SD), paired t-test or its non-parametric equivalent Wilcoxon test according to the results of the one-

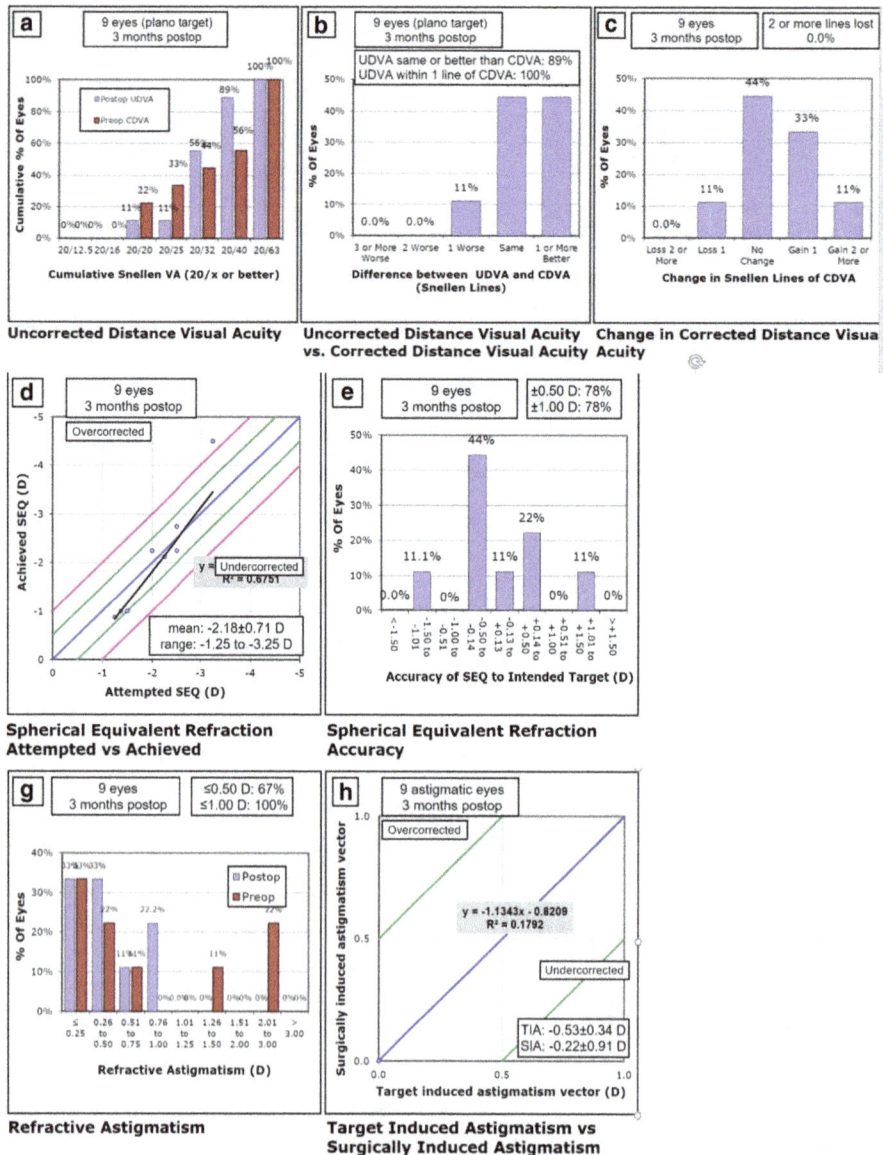

Fig. 4 Re-SMILE standardized graphs. **a** Postoperative cumulative uncorrected distance Snellen visual acuity (UDVA) versus preoperative cumulative corrected distance Snellen visual acuity (CDVA). **b** Efficacy of the surgery by comparing postoperative UDVA to preoperative CDVA. **c** Safety of the procedure by comparing pre- and postoperative CDVA. **d** Accuracy of the surgery by comparing attempted versus achieved refractive spherical equivalent (SEQ) and presenting the regression formula describing the relation between them. **e** Accuracy of the surgery by showing the deviation of achived SEQ compared to attempted SEQ in steps. **g** The residual refractive astigmatism. **h** Accuracy of the surgery by comparing attempted versus achieved refractive cylinder and presenting the regression formula describing the relation between them

sample Kolmogorov-Smirnov test with Lilliefors significance correction.

Results

The mean patient age was 28.2 ± 6.3 years (range: 19 to 42). Four eyes were of male patients and the others of female patients.

The MRSE significantly improved after primary SMILE and after Re-SMILE. The refractive cylinder change did not show the same statistical significance, neither after primary SMILE nor after the Re-SMILE procedure as shown in Table 3.

The UDVA was significantly improved after the primary SMILE and the Re-SMILE procedures. The CDVA shows statistically significant improvement after the primary SMILE but not after Re-SMILE.

The standardized graphs of the primary SMILE and of the Re-SMILE procedures presented in Figs. 3 and 4, respectively.

The safety and efficacy indices are summarized in Table 4.

The mean Keratometry (k) reading significantly flattened after the primary SMILE procedure (t = 18.725, P < 0.001) (Fig. 5). Further reduction was achieved after the Re-SMILE procedure but was not statistically significant (t = 2.245, P = 0.055). The mean central corneal thickness (CCT) significantly decreased after the primary SMILE procedure (t = 18.577, P < 0.001). Further reduction was achieved after Re-SMILE but was also not significant (t = 1.494, P = 0.173). Detailed results are shown in Table 5.

No adverse events or side effects occurred during or after primary SMILE and Re-SMILE procedures.

Discussion

In a recent meta-analysis of SMILE versus femtosecond LASIK composed of 1101 eyes, no significant difference between the two procedures was evident in terms of final MRSE (P = 0.72), MRSE within 1 D of the target values (P = 0.70), the proportion of eyes losing one or more lines of CDVA after surgery (P = 0.69), or those achieving a UDVA of 0.0 logMAR (6/6) or better (P = 0.35). However, SMILE was found to be significantly better in terms of tear break-up time (P < 0.05) and corneal sensitivity (P < 0.003) [8]. Also, SMILE demonstrated a higher predictability compared to femtosecond LASIK. Published reports suggest that with SMILE, 77% to 92% of patients obtain postoperative MRSE within 0.50 D of the intended correction in low to moderate myopic errors. The range decreases slightly for patients with high myopia (77% to 88% within 0.50 D) [1, 4, 9, 10].

A recent review of literature confirmed that SMILE may be of greater benefit in higher refractive corrections [9]. It is reported that between 37% and 98.1% (mean 68.0%) of patients achieved UDVA ≥0.0 logMAR (6/6) and that between 95% and 100% (mean 97.8%) achieved ≥0.3 logMAR (6/12) or better which

represents excellent visual outcomes in patients with significant ammetropia [9].

In our study, the time interval between primary SMILE and Re-SMILE was about three months to ensure refraction stability [11].

In our opinion, precise positioning is the key step in the Re-SMILE procedure, because crossing of the new lenticule edge into the edge step in the primary SMILE interface might lead to dissection difficulties and postoperative scarring. Therefore, we developed the Sedky SMILE Retreatment Centering Marker for better centration of the Re-SMILE lenticule with respect to the existing interface of the primary SMILE procedure.

In the study presented, a statistically significant improvement of MRSE after each of the two successive treatment steps occurred. On the other hand, a statistically significant improvement in the refractive cylinder was achieved only by both successive treatments. This may be due to that in the planned two-step surgery cases, full astigmatic correction was not intended in the primary SMILE treatment step, and the residual was reserved for the Re-SMILE treatment. In our case series of two-step treatments, we observed an under correction of cylinder components after both successive treatments. Ivarsen and Hjordal [10] also found a slight under correction of cylinder components in the correction of spherical equivalent and astigmatism in both moderate and high myopia. SMILE patients with high astigmatism (mean cylinder 3.22 ± 0.67 D) were under corrected by 16% of the amplitude of astigmatism leading to the low incidence of patients achieving UDVA of 0.0 logMAR (6/6) or greater. Optimization of personal nomograms and careful orientation control in cases of high cylinder corrections (e.g. by using an orientation marker) may ameliorate this [10].

Our current study shows that after cap-preserving SMILE enhancement surgery with our technique, 89% of enhanced eyes can achieve 0.3 logMAR (6/12) or better UDVA in comparison to only 33% after primary SMILE. Enhanced eyes after cap-preserving SMILE achieved 0.18 logMAR (6/9) or better UDVA in 56% of cases, in comparison to only 11% after primary SMILE. The residual refractive error was − 0.13 ± 0.68 D. All the enhanced eyes had a final MRSE within 1.25 D of intended correction, and 78% were within 0.5 D. All of them became within 1 D of target astigmatism, and 67% were within 0.5 D. At three months postoperatively, results by Chansue et al. were 0.3 logMAR (6/12) or better UDVA in 100% of the eyes, and 0.0 logMAR (6/6) or better in 95.8% of the 24 eyes that were corrected for distance vision [12]. Residual refractive error (spherical equivalent) averaged + 0.1 D. However, their study was conducted to enhance eyes with residual − 0.74 ± 0.80 D of MRSE and − 0.7 ± 0.34 D of refractive cylinder compared

Table 4 Safety and efficacy indices in primary SMILE and in Re-SMILE. t = t-test statistic, p = p-value, z = Wilcoxon signed rank statistic

	Mean ± SD	Range	Significance of difference between the two procedures
Primary SMILE Safety Index	1.65 ± 0.62	1.0 to 3.02	t = 1.716, p = 0.124
Re-SMILE Safety Index	1.16 ± 0.34	0.67 to 1.67	
Primary SMILE Efficacy Index	1.14 ± 0.24	1.0 to 1.67	z = −0.141, p = 0.888
Re-SMILE Efficacy Index	1.11 ± 0.26	0.67 to 1.50	

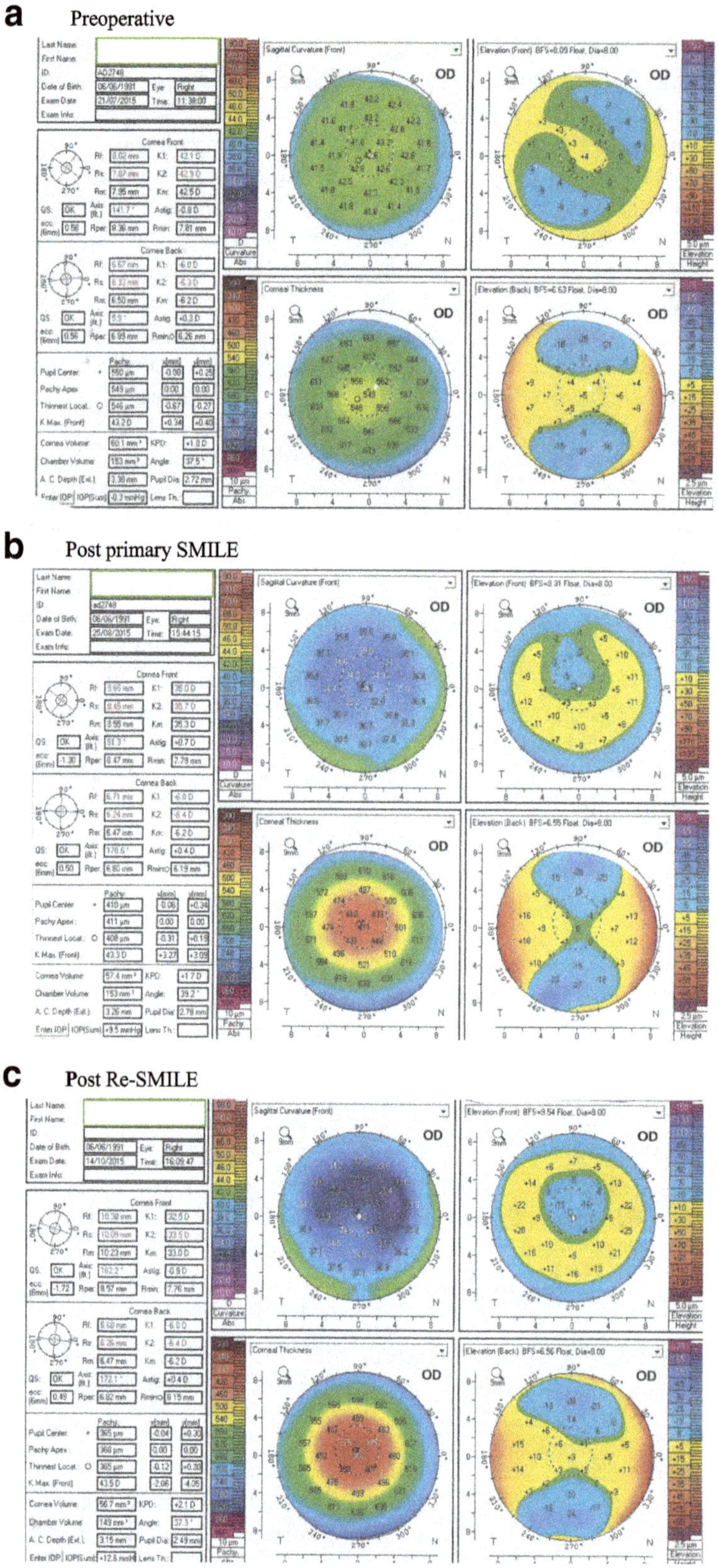

Fig. 5 Pentacam scans of one case of planned two-steps procedure: **a** Preoperative **b** Post primary SMILE **c** Post Re-SMILE

Table 5 K Readings and CCT, before and after the primary SMILE and after the Re-SMILE procedure

	K readings	CCT
	Mean ± SD	Mean ± SD
Preoperative	43.93 ± 1.54	548.11 ± 22.05
Post primary SMILE	37.31 ± 2.27	412.44 ± 21.40
Post Re-SMILE	36.51 ± 2.84	399.44 ± 17.52

to -2.18 ± 0.71 D of MRSE and -0.75 ± 0.83 D of refractive cylinder in our study, which resembled more to real life cases suffering clinically significant residual error that deserve second interference.

In our study, the CDVA of some cases improved, especially after primary SMILE correcting the majority of the refractive error. The low preoperative CDVA could be due to most patients' inexperience with high quality optical correction because of wearing inadequate glasses for a long period of time. In such thick trial set lenses, the minifications and the higher-order aberrations, such as spherical aberration, can compromise the CDVA. Patients often need months after refractive surgery to adapt to the better optical situation resulting in higher visual acuity. It is not uncommon in our practice to find significantly less preoperative CDVA than postoperative CDVA. This is much less encountered in hyperopic patients (magnification effect). However, in some cases, UDVA does not change much. This can be due to induced high-order aberrations by two successive surgeries. Unfortunately, this is not part of our study. Moreover, there is a sort of ceiling effect attained with such high myopic retinae. This also manifested as no improvement with correction post Re-SMILE; the final UDVA is equal to the final CDVA.

To the best of our knowledge, our study presents the first case series results of cap-preserving SMILE enhancements after the first single case report of Donate and Thäeron [7]. We additionally presented here the details of our technique utilizing the Sedky SMILE Retreatment Centering Marker for better centration with determination of both the safety and efficacy index for this case series and the reason for changing the term to cap-preserving SMILE enhancement.

Before reaching the final parameters set for the enhancement lenticule used during this study, we faced some minor complications or difficulties, like when we tried to make the enhancement lenticule same size or bigger than the primary one, dissection of the second lenticule was more difficult particularly over the overlapping edges. Also, during the first cases which are not included in this study, one of the enhancement edge lenticule thickness was thin enough to be torn during dissection. Therefore, we set 18 μm as the minimum enhancement edge lenticule thickness. Creating a new

lenticule within the primary lenticule cavity showed no difficulties as long as the new lenticule is well centered especially with the use of Sedky SMILE Retreatment Centering Marker.

A limitation of our study is that we did not evaluate the epithelial thickness before and after the Re-SMILE procedure. However, we accounted for the effect of epithelial thickening by increasing the minimum edge lenticule thickness to at least 18 μm. We also did not evaluate the visual quality. Comparative studies provided mixed results in terms of visual quality. Several authors have found no significant difference between the degree of induced third and fourth order aberrations [13, 14]. Other studies found low induction of HOAs [15]. Both concerns are already under study. More importantly, our technique should be evaluated using a larger sample size to ascertain its safety.

Although the presented technique is not limited to the correction of myopic residual errors in general, it is practically limited to myopic enhancements as long as the commercial indication range of SMILE does not yet allow us to apply the presented approach for hyperopic and mixed astigmatism treatments. Despite the present demand, our new technique increases the need to extend the indication range for SMILE to also include hyperopia and mixed astigmatism.

Conclusion

SMILE is an effective procedure for the correction of myopia and myopic astigmatism. Enhancement after SMILE can be done using different methods. SMILE enhancement performed using a centered cap-preserving technique (Re-SMILE) is an effective procedure, especially with the use of a special marker to center the cut.

Abbreviations
CCT: Central corneal thickness; CDVA: Corrected distance visual acuity; D: Diopters; K: Keratometry; LASIK: Laser in-situ keratomileusis; MRSE: Mean refractive spherical equivalent; PRK: Photorefractive keratectomy; SD: Standard deviation; SMILE: Small incision lenticule extraction; UDVA: Uncorrected distance visual acuity

Acknowledgements
Not applicable.

Funding
Not applicable.

Authors' contributions
ANS: Conception and design. Revising the manuscript. Final approval of the version to be published. Agreed to be accountable for all aspects of the work. SSW: Analysis and interpretation of data. Drafting and revising the manuscript. Final approval of the version to be published. Agreed to be accountable for all aspects of the work. MMR: Analysis and interpretation of data. Drafting and revising the manuscript. Final approval of the version to be published. Agreed to be accountable for all aspects of the work.

NRA: Acquisition of data. Drafting the manuscript. Final approval of the version to be published. Agreed to be accountable for all aspects of the work. All authors read and approved the final manuscript.

Competing interests
Dr. Sedky received speaker fees from Alcon Labs and travel support from Abbott Medical Optics. Dr. Roshdy received travel support from Alcon Labs, Bayer and Orchidia Pharma. Dr. Wahba and Dr. Ayaad have no financial disclosures to declare.

Author details
[1]Eye Subspecialty Center, Cairo, Egypt, 18 Elkhalifa Elmamoun Street, Heliopolis, Cairo, Egypt. [2]Ain Shams University, Al Watany Eye Hospital and Watany Research and Development Center (WRDC), Cairo, Egypt. [3]Eye Subspecialty Center, Cairo, Egypt.

References
1. Vestergaard A, Ivarsen AR, Asp S, Hjortdal JØ. Small-incision lenticule extraction for moderate to high myopia: predictability, safety, and patient satisfaction. J Cataract Refract Surg. 2012;38(11):2003–10. https://doi.org/10.1016/j.jcrs.2012.07.021. Epub 2012 Sep 14.
2. Sekundo W, Kunert KS, Blum M. Small incision corneal refractive surgery using the small incision lenticule extraction (SMILE) procedure for the correction of myopia and myopic astigmatism: results of a 6 month prospective study. Br J Ophthalmol. 2011;95(3):335–9. https://doi.org/10.1136/bjo.2009.174284. Epub 2010 Jul 3.
3. Wang Y, Bao XL, Tang X, Zuo T, Geng WL, Jin Y. Clinical study of femtosecond laser corneal small incision lenticule extraction for correction of myopia and myopic astigmatism. Zhonghua Yan Ke Za Zhi. 2013;49:292–8.
4. Hjortdal JØ, Vestergaard AH, Ivarsen A, Ragunathan S, Asp S. Predictors for the outcome of small-incision lenticule extraction for myopia. J Refract Surg. 2012;28(12):865–71. https://doi.org/10.3928/1081597X-20121115-01.
5. Riau AK, Ang HP, Lwin NC, Chaurasia SS, Tan DT, Mehta JS. Comparison of four different VisuMax circle patterns for flap creation after small incision lenticule extraction. J Refract Surg. 2013;29(4):236–44. https://doi.org/10.3928/1081597X-20130318-02.
6. Reinstein DZ. Scientific rationale for why femtorefractive keratomileusis is the future of corneal refractive surgery. In: Course IC-80: small incision lenticule extraction for myopia and astigmatism: ESCRS; 2013. http://escrs.org/amsterdam2013/programme/instructional-courses.asp?day=III.
7. Donate D, Thaëron R. Preliminary evidence of successful enhancement after a primary SMILE procedure with the sub-cap-Lenticule-extraction technique. J Refract Surg. 2015;31(10):708–10.
8. Zhang Y, Shen Q, Jia Y, Zhou D, Zhou J. Clinical outcomes of SMILE and FS-LASIK used to treat myopia: a meta-analysis. J Refract Surg. 2016;32(4):256–65.
9. Chan C, Lawless M, Sutton G, Versace P, Hodge C. Small incision lenticule extraction (SMILE) in 2015. Clin Exp Optom. 2016;99(3):204–12. https://doi.org/10.1111/cxo.12380. Epub 2016 May 7.
10. Ivarsen A, Hjortdal J. Correction of myopic astigmatism with small incision lenticule extraction. J Refract Surg. 2014;30(4):240–7. https://doi.org/10.3928/1081597X-20140320-02.
11. Shah R, Shah S, Sengupta S. Results of small incision lenticule extraction: all-in-one femtosecond laser refractive surgery. J Cataract Refract Surg. 2011;37(1):127–37. https://doi.org/10.1016/j.jcrs.2010.07.033.
12. Chansue E, Tanehsakdi M, Swasdibutra S, McAlinden C. Efficacy, predictability and safety of small incision lenticule extraction (SMILE). Eye Vis (Lond). 2015;2:14. https://doi.org/10.1186/s40662-015-0024-4. eCollection 2015.
13. Ağca A, Demirok A, Cankaya Kİ, Yaşa D, Demircan A, Yildirim Y, Ozkaya A, Yilmaz OF. Comparison of visual acuity and higher-order aberrations after femtosecond lenticule extraction and small-incision lenticule extraction. Cont Lens Anterior Eye. 2014;37(4):292–6. https://doi.org/10.1016/j.clae.2014.03.001. Epub 2014 Mar 27.
14. Vestergaard AH, Grauslund J, Ivarsen AR, Hjortdal JØ. Efficacy, safety, predictability, contrast sensitivity, and aberrations after femtosecond laser lenticule extraction. J Cataract Refract Surg. 2014;40(3):403–11. https://doi.org/10.1016/j.jcrs.2013.07.053. Epub 2014 Jan 27.
15. Lin F, Xu Y, Yang Y. Comparison of the visual results after SMILE and femtosecond laser-assisted LASIK for myopia. J Refract Surg. 2014;30(4):248–54. https://doi.org/10.3928/1081597X-20140320-03.

2

Quantification of macular perfusion using optical coherence tomography angiography: repeatability and impact of an eye-tracking system

Maged Alnawaiseh[1*†], Cristin Brand[2†], Eike Bormann[3], Cristina Sauerland[3] and Nicole Eter[1]

Abstract

Background: The aim of the study was to evaluate the impact of integration of the eye-tracking system (ET) on the repeatability of flow density measurements using optical coherence tomography (OCT) angiography.

Methods: 20 healthy subjects were included in this study. OCT-angiography was performed using RTVue XR Avanti (Optovue Inc., Fremont, California, USA). The macula was imaged using a 3×3 mm scan twice with and twice without activation of the ET. Flow density data of the macular in the superficial and deep OCT angiograms were extracted and analyzed.

Results: The difference between the flow density (whole en face) in the first session and second session with and without ET was statistically non-significant (with ET: superficial retinal OCT angiogram: $p = 0.50$; deep retinal OCT angiogram: $p = 0.89$; without ET: superficial retinal OCT angiogram: $p = 0.81$; deep retinal OCT angiogram: $p = 0.24$). There was no significant difference in the coefficients of repeatability for measurements with and without ET in the superficial retinal OCT angiogram (adjusted p-value = 0.176), whereas the difference was significant for the deep retinal OCT angiogram (adjusted p-value = 0.008).

Conclusions: Integration of the ET improved the repeatability of flow density measurements in the deep OCT angiogram; this needs to be considered when evaluating the long-term changes of flow density and when comparing data of different studies and different devices.

Keywords: Eye-tracking system, Macular perfusion, Optical coherence tomography angiography

Background

Optical coherence tomography angiography (OCT angiography) was first reported by Makita et al. using Doppler OCT [1]. OCT angiography is a novel technology allowing layer-specific visualization of normal chorioretinal vasculature and neovascularizations without the need for intravenously injected fluorescent dyes [2–5]. The visualization of normal vessels and pathological neovascularization using OCT angiography has been evaluated in different retinal or choroidal neovascular diseases such as chronic central serous chorioretinopathy, age-related macular degeneration, retinal vein occlusion, diabetic retinopathy, and retinal arterial macroaneurysms and also in different animal models. This facility of OCT angiography imaging has been described as a useful tool in the diagnosis and follow-up of such diseases [3–8].

Another promising aspect of OCT angiography, which could be very useful in clinical practice and for clinical and experimental research, is the ability to quantify blood flow. Various recent studies have evaluated flow density (FD) in normal subjects and in different retinal pathologies as well as pathologies of the optic nerve head [9–16].

In the past, OCT angiography and measurement of blood flow have usually been evaluated using the RTVue XR Avanti with AngioVue (Optovue Inc., Fremont,

* Correspondence: magedbonn@hotmail.de
†Maged Alnawaiseh and Cristin Brand contributed equally to this work.
[1]Department of Ophthalmology, University of Muenster Medical Center, Albert-Schweitzer-Campus 1, Building D15, 48149 Muenster, Germany
Full list of author information is available at the end of the article

California, USA), while split-spectrum amplitude-decorrelation angiography (SSADA) was used to extract the OCT angiography information. A new development of the RTVue XR Avanti is the integration of an eye-tracking system (ET) with OCT angiography imaging. The newly introduced software update of this device enables the ET to be activated or deactivated on imaging.

The aim of the study was to evaluate the impact of integration of the eye-tracking system on the repeatability of flow density measurements.

Methods

This prospective study included 20 eyes of 20 healthy volunteers with no history of any ocular or systemic disease or ocular surgery. Before performing OCT angiography imaging, the study protocol was explained in detail and each participant signed an informed consent form. The study followed the tenets of the Declaration of Helsinki.

After performing slit-lamp biomicroscopy and funduscopy of the macula and the optic nerve head (ONH), all participants were asked to rest for five minutes. The macula was imaged using a 3×3 mm scan twice with and twice without activation of the eye-tracking system; the sequence (with ET and without ET) was randomly defined. *Flow density data of the macula in the superficial retinal OCT angiograms* (from the inner limiting membrane with an offset of 3 μm to the inner plexiform layer with an offset of 15 μm) and deep OCT angiograms (segmented with an inner boundary at 15 μm beneath the inner plexiform layer and the outer boundary at 70 μm beneath the inner plexiform layer) were extracted and analyzed.

OCT angiography

The teleological principles of OCT-angiography have been described in detail in a number of previous studies [3–6, 13–15]. Briefly, OCT scans of a defined region of the retina or of the optic nerve head are performed several times, and the OCT images analyzed and examined for changes. Static tissue shows little or no change, whereas blood flow will result in changes between successive images [17].

In the present study OCT angiography imaging was performed using the RTVue XR Avanti with AngioVue (Optovue Inc., Fremont, California, USA). The system has an A-scan rate of 70,000 scans per second, using a light source centered on 840 nm and a bandwidth of 45 nm. Each OCT angiography volume contained 304×304 A-scans with two consecutive B-scans that were captured at each fixed position before proceeding to the next sampling location. The SSADA algorithm is used to identify blood flow and to generate the OCT angiograms [3–6].

Only one eye of each participant was randomly included in the study. OCT angiography imaging was performed

under the same setting by the same examiner in the same location, and only images with a signal strength index of ≥60 were included. In cases with significant motion artifacts or poor signal strength, the resulting OCT angiography image contains lines or gaps. Images with these artifacts were not included in the study.

Statistical analysis

Microsoft Excel 2010 was used for data management. Statistical analyses were performed using IBM SPSS® Statistics 23 for Windows (IBM Corporation, Somers, NY, USA). Data are presented as mean ± standard deviation, minimum and maximum. The mean of the two measurements before and after activation of the eye-tracking system were compared using t-tests for paired data. All *p*-values below 0.05 were considered significant.

In order to assess the repeatability between the first and second scan, the intraclass correlation coefficient (ICC(2,1)) as well as the coefficient of repeatability (CR) were calculated [18, 19]. A two-sided paired t-test was used to compare the coefficients of repeatability for measurements with and measurements without eye tracker for both the superficial and deep retinal OCT angiograms. For those two tests a Bonferroni correction was applied to adjust the *p*-values. Bland Altman plots were used to show the agreement between the two measurements for each subject. In these plots the difference of the two measurements is plotted against their mean. Since differences can be assumed to be normally distributed, one would expect 95% of the observed differences to lie within the limits of agreement (mean-1.96*SD, mean + 1.96*SD) [20].

Results

20 eyes of 20 subjects were included in the study (age = 33 ± 2.5 (20–56) years). The differences between the flow density (whole en face) in the first session and second session with and without ET were statistically non-significant (with ET: superficial retinal OCT angiogram: first session: 54.4 ± 1.9; second session: 54.2 ± 2.1; *p* = 0.50; deep retinal OCT angiogram: first session: 59.8 ± 1.5; second session: 59.9 ± 1.5; *p* = 0.89; without ET: superficial retinal OCT angiogram: first session: 54.3 ± 2.0; second session: 54.4 ± 1,8; *p* = 0.81; deep retinal OCT angiogram: first session: 58.0 ± 3.3; second session: 58.9 ± 1.6; *p* = 0.24) (Tables 1 and 2).

The flow density, the mean of the absolute difference (AD) between the first and second session, the CR and the ICC for the two sessions with and without ET are shown in Table 1 (superficial retinal OCT angiogram) and in Table 2 (deep retinal OCT angiogram). There was no significant difference in the coefficients of repeatability (CR) for measurements with and without ET in the superficial retinal OCT angiogram (adjusted *p*-value = 0.176), whereas for the deep retinal OCT angiogram, the CR for

Table 1 Mean flow density ± SD; (min- max) in the superficial OCT angiogram for each session; p Val.: P-value (paired t-test); CR: coefficients of repeatability (95% confidence intervals) and ICC: intraclass correlation coefficient (95% confidence intervals) with and without eye tracker AD: Mean of the absolute difference between the first and second session; p Val.:

		Vessel density 1 Mean ± SD (min -max)	p Value with vs. without eye tracker	Vessel density 2 Mean ± SD (min -max)	p Value with vs. without eye tracker	AD Mean ± SD	p Value density 1 vs. density 2	CR 95% CI (lower limit-upper limit)	ICC 95% CI (lower limit-upper limit)
whole en face	with eye tracker	54.4 ± 1.9 (51.3–56.8)	0.79	54.2 ± 2.1 (48.5–57.3)	0.55	1.3 ± 0.9	0.50	3.07 (1.88–4.26)	0.70 (0.37–0.87)
	without eye tracker	54.3 ± 2.0 (49.0–56.6)		54.4 ± 1.8 (51.5–58.0)		1.3 ± 1.1	0.81	3.33 (2.04–4.62)	0.62 (0.25–0.83)
fovea	with eye tracker	32.7 ± 4.1 (23.7–38.3)	0.61	32.7 ± 3.9 (21.9–39.6)	0.21	1.5 ± 1.2	0.98	3.88 (2.38–5.38)	0.88 (0.72–0.95)
	without eye tracker	33.0 ± 4.0 (22.8–41.1)		33.2 ± 3.7 (22.6–38.6)		1.4 ± 1.1	0.61	3.50 (2.15–4.86)	0.89 (0.75–0.96)
parafovea	with eye tracker	56.2 ± 2.2 (52.5–60.0)	0.72	56.1 ± 2.4 (49.7–59.7)	0.99	1.4 ± 0.9	0.74	3.37 (2.06–4.67)	0.72 (0.41–0.88)
	without eye tracker	56.1 ± 2.1 (52.0–59.1)		56.1 ± 2.1 (52.2–59.9)		1.5 ± 1.0	0.98	3.60 (2.20–4.99)	0.62 (0.25–0.83)
temporal	with eye tracker	54.5 ± 2.3 (50.8–59.1)	0.50	54.5 ± 2.7 (48.2–58.1)	.034	1.2 ± 1.1	0.97	3.31 (2.03–4.59)	0.77 (0.51–0.90)
	without eye tracker	54.8 ± 2.5 (50.1–58.2)		54.9 ± 2.4 (50.9–59.5)		1.8 ± 1.3	0.79	4.36 (2.67–6.05)	0.59 (0.22–0.82)
superior	with eye tracker	57.6 ± 2.4 (54.6–63.0)	0.36	57.6 ± 2.2 (53.5–61.0)	0.44	1.4 ± 1.1	0.88	3.53 (2.17–4.90)	0.69 (0.36–0.86)
	without eye tracker	57.2 ± 2.4 (52.0–61.0)		57.1 ± 2.9 (51.6–62.6)		1.5 ± 1.3	0.82	3.92 (2.40–5.44)	0.72 (0.41–0.88)
nasal	with eye tracker	55.1 ± 2.6 (50.3–59.9)	0.75	54.3 ± 2.4 (48.6–58.3)	0.17	1.5 ± 0.8	0.04	3.10 (1.90–4.30)	0.81 (0.57–0.92)
	without eye tracker	54.9 ± 2.8 (49.9–58.8)		55.0 ± 2.0 (51.2–59.1)		2.5 ± 1.7	0.89	6.01 (3.68–8.33)	0.18 (− 0.27–0.57)
inferior	with eye tracker	57.8 ± 2.7 (52.0–61.6)	0.47	57.5 ± 3.5 (47.3–62.0)	0.74	1.9 ± 1.4	0.69	4.65 (2.85–6.45)	0.71 (0.39–0.87)
	without eye tracker	57.5 ± 2.7 (53.2–61.6)		57.3 ± 2.9 (49.9–61.8)		2.4 ± 1.8	0.78	5.94 (8.25–3.64)	0.40 (− 0.04–0.71)

Table 2 Mean flow density ± SD; (min- max) in the deep OCT angiogram for each session; P-value: paired t-test; CR: coefficients of repeatability (95% confidence intervals) and ICC: intraclass correlation coefficient (95% confidence intervals) with and without eye tracker

		Vessel density 1 Mean ± SD (min -max)	p Value with vs. without eye tracker	Vessel density 2 Mean ± SD (min -max)	p Value with vs. without eye tracker	AD Mean ± SD	p Value density 1 vs. density 2	CR 95% CI (lower limit-upper limit)	ICC 95% CI (lower limit-upper limit)
whole en face	with eye tracker	59.8 ± 1.5 (56.8–62.5)	0.02	59.9 ± 1.5 (57.7–62.8)	0.01	1.4 ± 1.0	0.89	3.51 (2.15–4.86)	0.3 (−0.15–0.65)
	without eye tracker	58.0 ± 3.3 (48.2–62.2)		58.9 ± 1.6 (54.6–61.3)		2.1 ± 3.0	0.24	6.92 (4.24–9.60)	0.07 (−0.37–0.49)
fovea	with eye tracker	31.1 ± 5.8 (20.9–43.7)	0.74	31.4 ± 5.2 (22.1–45.2)	0.90	1.6 ± 1.1	0.49	3.79 (2.32–5.26)	0.94 (0.85–0.98)
	without eye tracker	31.3 ± 5.5 (21.7–44.2)		31.3 ± 5.9 (18.7–45.6)		2.6 ± 2.1	0.98	6.59 (4.04–9.15)	0.83 (0.61–0.93)
parafovea	with eye tracker	62.6 ± 1.6 (60.1–65.8)	0.01	62.5 ± 2.0 (58.6–65.4)	0.02	1.4 ± 1.1	0.81	3.56 (2.18–4.94)	0.50 (0.08–0.77)
	without eye tracker	60.7 ± 3.3 (53.4–65.6)		61.6 ± 2.1 (56.9–64.5)		2.2 ± 2.3	0.22	6.07 (3.72–8.42)	0.37 (−0.08–0.69)
temporal	with eye tracker	60.7 ± 2.3 (55.5–64.5)	0.35	60.8 ± 2.2 (57.1–65.6)	0.82	2.0 ± 1.6	0.86	5.11 (7.09–3.13)	0.33 (−0.12–0.67)
	without eye tracker	59.9 ± 3.1 (52.4–65.1)		60.9 ± 2.3 (57.1–64.8)		2.3 ± 2.4	0.18	6.20 (3.80–8.60)	0.35 (−0.10–0.68)
superior	with eye tracker	64.0 ± 1.8 (60.6–69.0)	0.01	64.4 ± 1.8 (60.0–67.6)	< 0.01	1.7 ± 1.2	0.48	4.13 (2.53–5.73)	0.49 (0.08–0.76)
	without eye tracker	62.0 ± 3.7 (54.4–68.0)		62.5 ± 2.6 (56.9–66.1)		1.9 ± 2.2	0.43	5.74 (3.52–7.97)	0.57 (0.19–0.81)
nasal	with eye tracker	61.6 ± 1.6 (58.2–63.4)	0.01	61.0 ± 2.1 (56.9–63.9)	0.53	1.5 ± 1.1	0.14	3.43 (2.10–4.76)	0.55 (0.16–0.80)
	without eye tracker	59.2 ± 4.2 (50.7–65.0)		60.6 ± 3.0 (53.9–67.6)		3.6 ± 3.3	0.19	9.22 (5.65–12.79)	0.16 (−0.29–0.55)
inferior	with eye tracker	64.2 ± 1.8 (60.5–67.9)	0.05	64.2 ± 2.6 (57.8–67.9)	0.01	1.8 ± 1.6	0.99	4.71 (2.88–6.53)	0.41 (−0.03–0.72)
	without eye tracker	61.9 ± 5.3 (45.0–69.4)		62.4 ± 2.8 (53.6–66.4)		3.6 ± 4.3	0.68	11.07 (6.78–15.35)	0.11 (0.34–0.52)

measurements with ET was significantly lower than for measurements without ET (adjusted p-value = 0.008).

Bland-Altman plots for the superficial (Fig. 1) and the deep (Fig. 2) retinal OCT angiograms demonstrate the agreement between the two sessions for measurements with and without eye tracker.

Discussion

OCT angiography is a noninvasive imaging technique that enables visualization of retinal vessels in the superficial and deep vascular plexuses without intravenously injected dye. A very interesting feature of OCT angiography is the possibility of blood flow quantification in the different retinal layers. The quantification of retinal or choroidal blood flow and the analysis of repeatability and reproducibility of blood flow measurements have attracted increasing interest over the last two years. The new approach has been described, using various OCT angiography devices, in healthy subjects and in patients with different ocular and systemic diseases [9–16, 21].

The split-spectrum amplitude-decorrelation angiography (SSADA) algorithm is used by the RTVue XR Avanti to extract the OCT angiography information. This device is used to visualize retinal or choroidal vessels and to quantify blood flow in the macula and in the optic nerve head without using an eye-tracking system, and a number of studies in the literature have evaluated its utility [9, 10, 12–17]. New software provided with the device enables activation of an ET. In the study presented here, we evaluated the repeatability of flow density measurements and the impact of the eye-tracking system on the repeatability of FD measurements in the different retinal layers. Especially in the deep OCT angiogram, integration of the ET in the RTVue XR Avanti device while performing OCT angiography imaging has improved the repeatability of quantification of blood flow measurements.

Coscas et al. evaluated the repeatability and reproducibility of FD measurements using the Optovue device. In this study, evaluation of the FD measurements of 135 eyes of 70 subjects (aged 19–66 years) demonstrated high inter- and intra-examiner repeatability and interexaminer reproducibility. The ICCs of FD measurements were not statistically significantly different between the two sessions or between the two examiners in either the deep or superficial capillary plexuses [9]. Al-Sheikh et al. presented a study with a similar design on 41 eyes of 21 healthy subjects (age: between 18 and 90 years old) for the NIDEK RS-3000 Advance device [11]. The CR and CV measurements in these studies are comparable to our findings, although the ICCs measured by Al-Sheik et al., especially in the deep OCT angiogram, were higher than those obtained by us. The ICC is the ratio of the intersubject component of the variance to the total variance. The higher the ratio, the better the

repeatability; the variability of measurements is primarily the result of interindividual differences [22]. The differences in ICCs between these studies may be explained by the different numbers of subjects, the differences in subject age or by the inclusion of both eyes of the same subject in the evaluations reported by Al-Sheikh et al. and Coscas et al. Analysis of the Bland-Altman plots and CR readings in these studies are comparable to our results and demonstrate good repeatability of vessel density measurements with OCT angiography in healthy subjects [9, 11].

Our study was also designed to evaluate the impact of the eye-tracking system on the repeatability of the flow density measurements. On examining the Bland-Altman plots with and without eye-tracking, a considerable improvement in repeatability is apparent in the deep OCT angiogram and would be of importance when evaluating flow density in a specific sector. The difference in the CR between measurements with and without eye tracking was also only significant for the deep retinal OCT angiogram.

Different studies in the literature show that the repeatability of FD measurements in the superficial retinal OCT angiogram was higher compared with the deep OCT angiogram [11, 23]. This finding might be related to the higher resolution and image quality of the superficial plexus compared to the deep plexus. Fenner et al. found that different factors affected repeatability of FD in the deep retinal OCT angiogram including low visibility of fine vessels or the presence of motion artefact [23]. The ET technology offers an improved image quality in OCT-A imaging regarding presence of motion artifacts [24]. This would explain the more pronounced improvement in the repeatability of FD described in our study.

The FD in the deep retinal OCT angiogram was found to be altered in different ocular diseases such as glaucoma, adult-onset foveomacular vitelliform dystrophy or in patients with retinitis pigmentosa [25–27]. The OCTA technology is still in its infancy; improved repeatability of OCTA metrics would encourage ophthalmologists to evaluate this metrics in different diseases and to use them in daily clinical practice.

As our study was carried out on healthy subjects with high quality images, the impact of the eye-tracking system on the repeatability of flow density measurements in patients with different retinal diseases remain to be evaluated in further studies. The eye-tracking system will be even more valuable in such cases, due to the challenges related to poor patient fixation and motion artifacts [17].

OCT angiography technology is still under development and the integration of the eye-tracking system has an impact on the repeatability of the blood flow measurements. This needs to be considered when comparing data of different studies using the same device or comparing

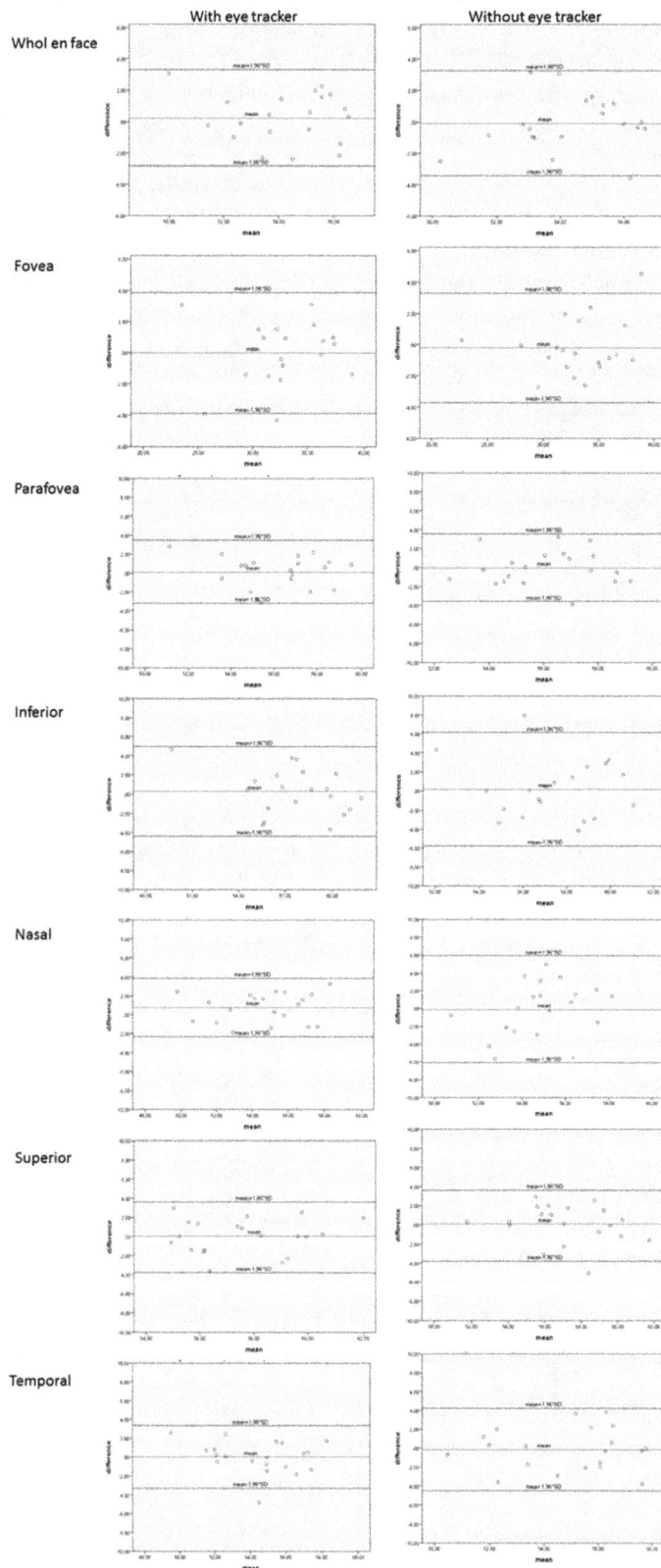

Fig. 1 Bland-Altman plots showing the level of agreement for the superficial retinal layer with and without eye tracker. Blue line represents the mean difference; black lines represent the limits of agreement

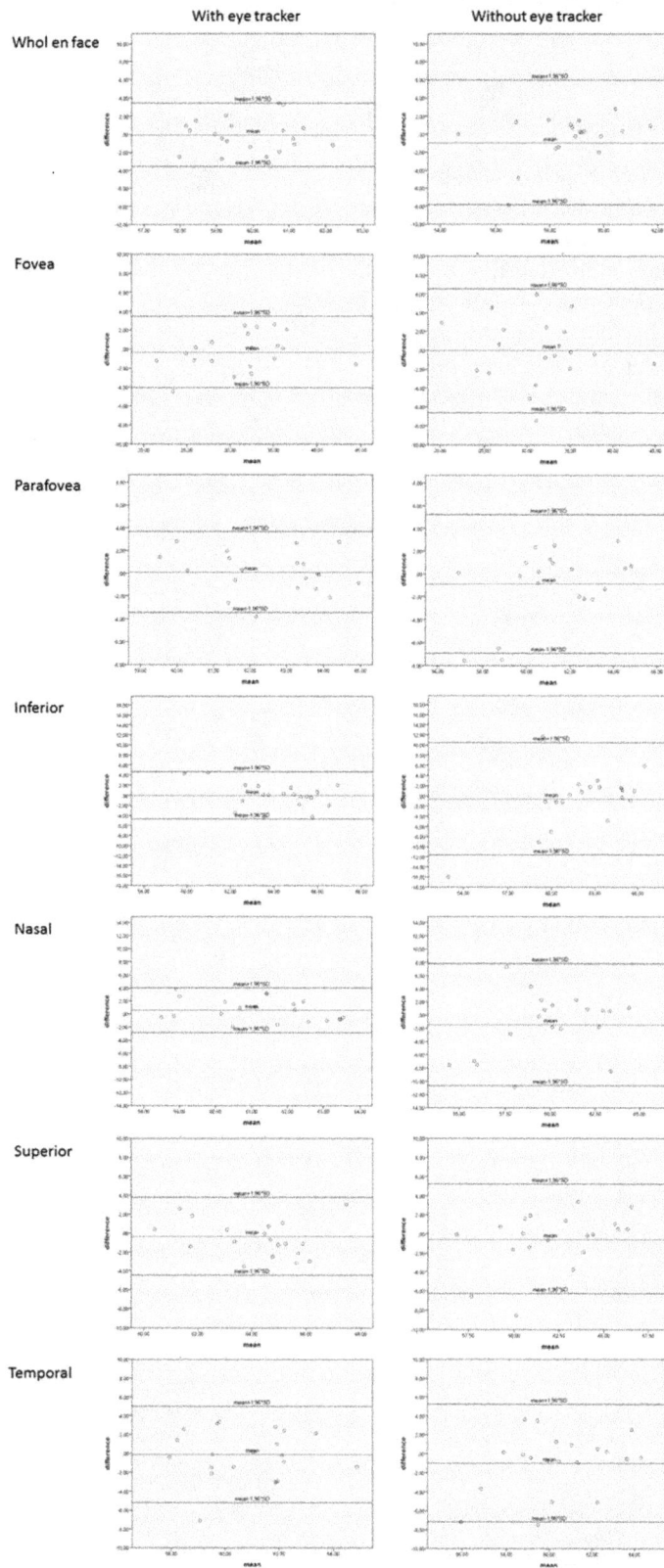

Fig. 2 Bland-Altman plots showing the level of agreement for the deep OCT angiogram with and without eye tracker. Blue line represents the mean difference; black lines represent the limits of agreement

measurements obtained with different OCT angiography equipment.

Conclusions

In conclusion, the integration of the eye-tracking system improved the repeatability of flow density measurements especially in the deep OCT angiogram. This should be taken into consideration when evaluating the long-term changes of flow density and comparing data from different studies and different devices. In evaluation of the long-term changes of flow density measurements in the deep OCT angiogram, it is advisable to activate the eye-tracking system.

Abbreviations

CR: Coefficient of repeatability; ET: Eye-tracking system; FD: Flow density; ICC: Intraclass correlation coefficient; OCT: Optical coherence tomography; SSADA: Split-spectrum amplitude-decorrelation angiography

Authors' contributions

Concept and design: MA, CB; Data acquisition: MA, CB; Data analysis / interpretation: MA, CB, EB, CS, NE; Drafting manuscript: MA; Critical revision of manuscript: MA, CB, EB, CS, NE; Supervision: NE. All authors read and approved the final manuscript.

Competing interests

The authors declare that they have no competing interests.

Author details

[1]Department of Ophthalmology, University of Muenster Medical Center, Albert-Schweitzer-Campus 1, Building D15, 48149 Muenster, Germany. [2]Centre of Reproductive Medicine and Andrology, University of Muenster, Muenster, Germany. [3]Institute of Biostatistics and Clinical Research, University of Muenster, Muenster, Germany.

References

1. Makita S, Hong Y, Yamanari M, Yatagai T, Yasuno Y. Optical coherence angiography. Opt Express. 2006;14(17):7821–40.
2. Leitgeb RA, Werkmeister RM1, Blatter C, Schmetterer L. Doppler optical coherence tomography. Prog Retin Eye Res. 2014;41:26–43.
3. Quaranta-El Maftouhi M, El Maftouhi A, Eandi CM. Chronic central serous Chorioretinopathy imaged by optical coherence tomographic angiography. Am J Ophthalmol. 2015;160(3):581–7.
4. Jia Y, Bailey ST, Wilson DJ, et al. Quantitative optical coherence tomography angiography of choroidal neovascularization in age-related macular degeneration. Ophthalmology. 2014;121(7):1435–44.
5. Powner MB, Sim DA, Zhu M, Nobre-Cardoso J, et al. Evaluation of nonperfused retinal vessels in ischemic retinopathy. Invest Ophthalmol Vis Sci. 2016;57(11):5031–7.
6. Ishibazawa A, Nagaoka T, Takahashi A, et al. Optical coherence tomography angiography in diabetic retinopathy: a prospective pilot study. Am J Ophthalmol. 2015;160(1):35–44.e1.
7. Alnawaiseh M, Schubert F, Nelis P, et al. Optical coherence tomography (OCT) angiography findings in retinal arterial macroaneurysms. BMC Ophthalmol. 2016;16:120.
8. Alnawaiseh M, Rosentreter A, Hillmann A, et al. OCT angiography in the mouse: a novel evaluation method for vascular pathologies of the mouse retina. Exp Eye Res. 2016;145:417–23.
9. Coscas F, Sellam A, Glacet-Bernard A, et al. Normative data for vascular density in superficial and deep capillary plexuses of healthy adults assessed by optical coherence tomography angiography. Invest Ophthalmol Vis Sci. 2016;57(9):OCT211–23.
10. Lupidi M, Coscas F, Cagini C, et al. Automated quantitative analysis of retinal microvasculature in normal eyes on optical coherence tomography angiography. Am J Ophthalmol. 2016;169:9–23.
11. Al-Sheikh M, Tepelus TC, Nazikyan T, Sadda SR. Repeatability of automated vessel density measurements using optical coherence tomography angiography. Br J Ophthalmol. 2016;101(4):449–52.
12. Wang X, Kong X, Jiang C, et al. Is the peripapillary retinal perfusion related to myopia in healthy eyes? A prospective comparative study. BMJ Open. 2016;6(3):e010791.
13. Liu L, Jia Y, Takusagawa HL, et al. Optical coherence tomography angiography of the Peripapillary retina in Glaucoma. JAMA Ophthalmol. 2015;133(9):1045–52.
14. Jia Y, Wei E, Wang X, et al. Optical coherence tomography angiography of optic disc perfusion in glaucoma. Ophthalmology. 2014;121(7):1322–32.
15. Wang X, Jiang C, Ko T, et al. Correlation between optic disc perfusion and glaucomatous severity in patients with open-angle glaucoma: an optical coherence tomography angiography study. Graefes Arch Clin Exp Ophthalmol. 2015;253(9):1557–64.
16. Li J, Yang YQ, Yang DY, et al. Reproducibility of perfusion parameters of optic disc and macula in rhesus monkeys by optical coherence tomography angiography. Chin Med J. 2016;129(9):1087–90.
17. Spaide RF, Fujimoto JG, Waheed NK. Image artifacts in optical coherence tomography angiography. Retina. 2015;35:2163–80.
18. Shrout PE, Fleiss JL. Intraclass correlations: uses in assessing rater reliability. Psychol Bull. 1979;86(2):420–8.
19. Bland JM, Altman DG. Applying the right statistics: analyses of measurement studies. Ultrasound Obstet Gynecol. 2003;22:85–93.
20. Bland JM, Altman DG. Measuring agreement in method comparison studies. Stat Methods Med Res. 1999;8(2):135–60.
21. Wang X, Jia Y, Spain R, Potsaid B, et al. Optical coherence tomography angiography of optic nerve head and parafovea in multiple sclerosis. Br J Ophthalmol. 2014;98(10):1368–73.
22. Carpineto P, Mastropasqua R, Marchini G, et al. Reproducibility and repeatability of foveal avascular zone measurements in healthy subjects by optical coherence tomography angiography. Br J Ophthalmol. 2016;100(5):671–6.
23. Fenner BJ, Tan GSW, Tan ACS, et al. Identification of imaging features that determine quality and repeatability of retinal capillary plexus density measurements in OCT angiography. Br J Ophthalmol Apr. 2018;102(4):509–14.
24. Lauermann JL, Treder M, Heiduschka P, et al. Impact of eye-tracking technology on OCT-angiography imaging quality in age-related macular degeneration. Graefes Arch Clin Exp Ophthalmol. 2017;255(8):1535–42.
25. Alnawaiseh M, Schubert F, Heiduschka P, Eter N. Optical coherence tomography angiography in patients with retinitis PIGMENTOSA. Retina. 2017; https://doi.org/10.1097/IAE.0000000000001904. [Epub ahead of print]
26. Alnawaiseh M, Lahme L, Müller V, et al. Correlation of flow density, as measured using optical coherence tomography angiography, with structural and functional parameters in glaucoma patients. Graefes Arch Clin Exp Ophthalmol. 2018;256(3):589–97.
27. Treder M, Lauermann JL, Alnawaiseh M, et al. Quantitative changes in flow density in patients with adult-onset foveomacular vitelliform dystrophy: an OCT angiography study. Graefes Arch Clin Exp Ophthalmol. 2018;256(1):23–8.

3

A white membrane beneath the inner limiting membrane of the retina in a 4-year-old child with ultrastructural evidence

Wenyi Tang[1], Ruiping Gu[1], Ting Zhang[1] and Gezhi Xu[1,2]*

Abstract

Background: Epiretinal membranes (ERMs), secondary to retinal cell proliferation on the retinal surface, usually affect patients over 50 years of age but occur rarely in children. Here we report the case of a 4-year-old patient with a unilateral sub-inner limiting membrane (sub-ILM) membrane mimicking epiretinal membrane with notable ultrastructural features indicating its possible origin from old sub-ILM hemorrhage.

Case presentation: A 4-year-old boy was admitted with the complaint of poor vision in his right eye, which had been detected at school vision screening performed 6 months earlier. Fundal examination showed a feather-shaped white membrane in the macula of the right eye, and optical coherence tomography (OCT) revealed a thickened retina with a hyper-reflective band on the retinal nerve fiber layer. We suspected epiretinal membrane in the right eye, and pars plana vitrectomy with membrane peeling was performed to improve the patient's vision. Surprisingly, the membrane was found intraoperatively to be located beneath the intact ILM; it was lifted carefully from the underlying retina as it was strongly adhered to a retinal artery of the superotemporal arcade. Postoperative scanning electron microscopy showed that the membrane consisted of hemosiderin, collagenous fibre and fibrinoid deposits. At follow-up visits, fundal examination and OCT revealed improvement in the retinal structure with disappearance of the hyper-reflective band and reduced retinal thickness. The patient's visual acuity in the right eye was stable at 20/100 at 1 year post operation.

Conclusions: The white membrane presented here was found to lie between the intact ILM and the rest of the retina, adhering firmly to the superotemporal vessel arch. Given the ultrastructural findings of the membrane and the medical history, we speculate that the sub-ILM membrane probably developed secondary to a sub-ILM hemorrhage.

Keywords: Sub-inner limiting membrane membrane, Children, Ultrastructural pathology, Sub-inner limiting membrane hemorrhage, Vitrectomy, Case report

Background

Epiretinal membrane (ERM) is a nonvascular fibrocellular proliferation that occurs on the surface of the retina and causes retinal thickening and wrinkling, leading to visual impairment and metamorphopsia. ERMs are usually idiopathic and occur predominantly in patients over 50 years of age [1, 2]. In children and adolescents, however, an ERM is a very rare condition often associated with an underlying etiology such as trauma, ocular inflammation, retinal vascular disease or combined hamartoma of the retina and retinal pigment epithelium [3].

Here we report a case of a unilateral ERM-like membrane with a unique location, just beneath the inner limiting membrane (ILM), in a 4-year-old child. Scanning electron microscopy revealed hemosiderin and collagenous fibres as the main components of the membrane.

* Correspondence: xugezhi@sohu.com
[1]Department of Ophthalmology, Eye and ENT Hospital of Fudan University, 83 Fenyang Road, Shanghai 200031, China
[2]Shanghai Key Laboratory of Visual Impairment and Restoration, Fudan University, Shanghai 200031, China

Case presentation

A 4-year-old boy was admitted to our centre with the complaint of poor vision in his right eye, which had been detected at school vision screening performed 6 months earlier. There was no pain, redness or any other discomfort in either eye. The patient was born at full term via uncomplicated vaginal delivery. His ocular, medication, traumatic and familial histories were unremarkable. A general physical examination was normal. An ocular examination revealed a best-corrected visual acuity (BCVA) of 20/100 in the right eye and 20/20 in the left eye. There was no evidence of strabismus. Intraocular pressure and the anterior segment of both eyes were normal. Fundal examination showed a glistening light reflex from a feather-shaped white membrane in the macular region of the right eye (Fig. 1a). The left eye was normal (Fig. 1b). The membrane of about 1.5-papilla disc size was located near the superotemporal arcade vessels, and caused radial wrinkling of the central macula and vascular distortion. The vitreous was clear, and posterior vitreous detachment (PVD) was not evident. The optic disc was unremarkable. Optical coherence tomography (OCT) revealed a hyper-reflective band on the retinal nerve fibre layer (RNFL) in the thickened retina (Fig. 2a, b). The surface of the retina was nearly smooth and uninterrupted.

We suspected that the decreased vision was caused by the membrane in the right eye. The patient was treated by pars plana vitrectomy using a 25 G vitrector with membrane dissection under general anaesthesia. Surprisingly, the surgeon found intraoperatively that the ILM was intact and the white membrane was located just beneath the ILM. The surgeon first peeled away the ILM following indocyanine green staining. The edge of the membrane was then lifted using forceps to separate the membrane from the underlying retina, despite its strong adhesion to a retinal artery of the superotemporal arcade (Fig. 3). There was no obvious retinal bleeding or tears. Air tamponade was used at the end of surgery. Vision training was performed 1 month after the operation. At postoperative follow-up visits, fundus photography and OCT showed successful removal of the membrane and improvement in the retinal structure with disappearance of the hyper-reflective band and reduced retinal thickness, respectively (Figs. 1c, d and 2c–f). One year later, the patient's BCVA in the right eye was stable at 20/100. Postoperative scanning electron microscopy revealed that the membrane was composed of collagenous fibre, fibrinoid deposits and cell debris containing clusters of dense iron particles (hemosiderin) (Fig. 4). Combined with the ultrastructural results and the sub-ILM location, we speculated that the organized membrane was caused by sub-ILM haemorrhage.

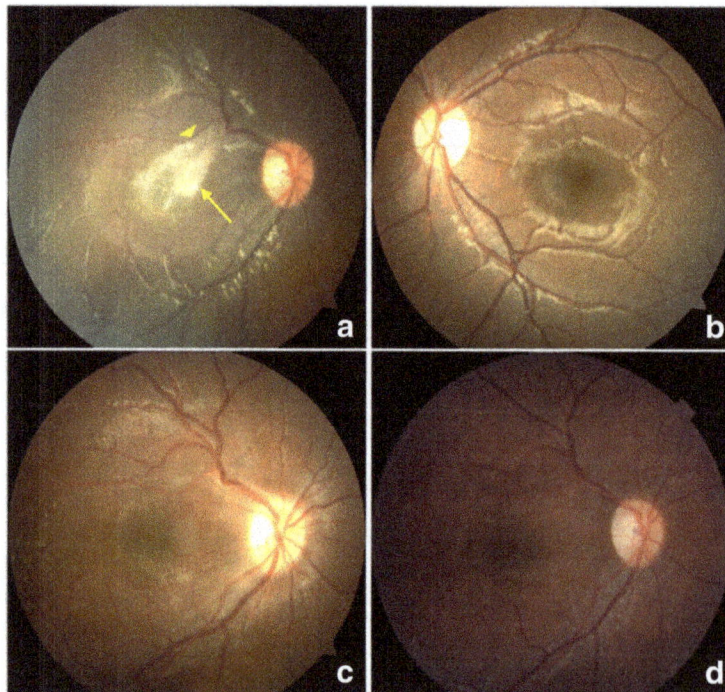

Fig. 1 Fundus photography showing changes in the eye of a 4-year-old patient with a white membrane. **a** Preoperative fundus photography reveals a feather-shaped opaque white membrane of an approximately 1.5-papilla disc size with radial wrinkling of the retina and distorted retinal vessels in the macular region (*arrow*). The upper edge of the membrane was close to the superotemporal vessel arch (*triangle*). **b** Fundus photography of the normal left eye. **c** Fundus photography on postoperative day 1 shows the disappearance of the white membrane. **d** Fundus photography at postoperative year 1 reveals alleviation of the vessel distortion

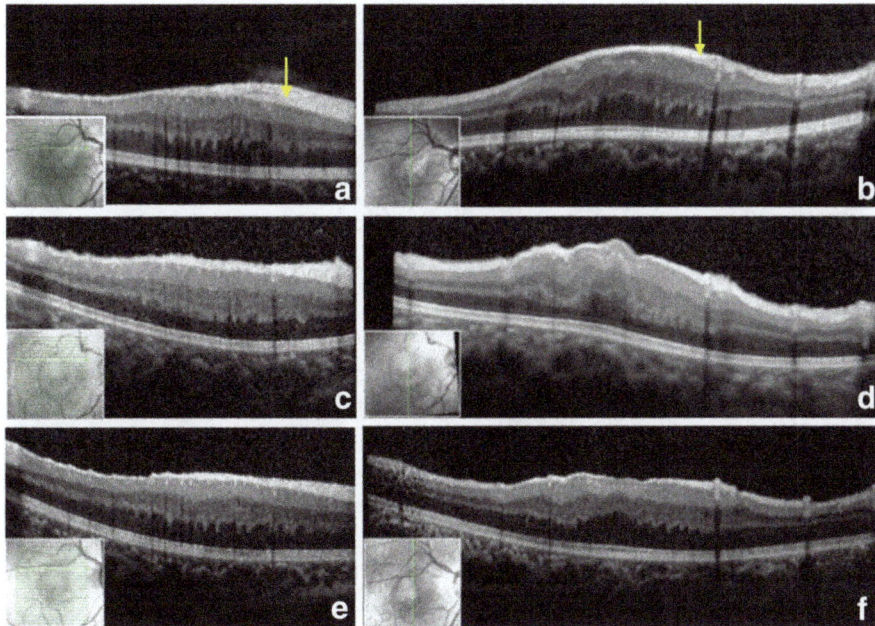

Fig. 2 Optical coherence tomography (OCT) reveals changes in the retinal structure of the eye of a 4-year-old patient exhibiting a white membrane. **a, b** Preoperative horizontal and vertical OCT scans of the membrane show retinal thickening with a hyper-reflective band on the retinal nerve fibre layer (RNFL) (*arrow*) and disappearance of the fovea. **c, d** OCT on postoperative day 1 shows disappearance of the hyper-reflective band on the RNFL. **e, f** OCT at postoperative year 1 shows a reduction in retinal thickness

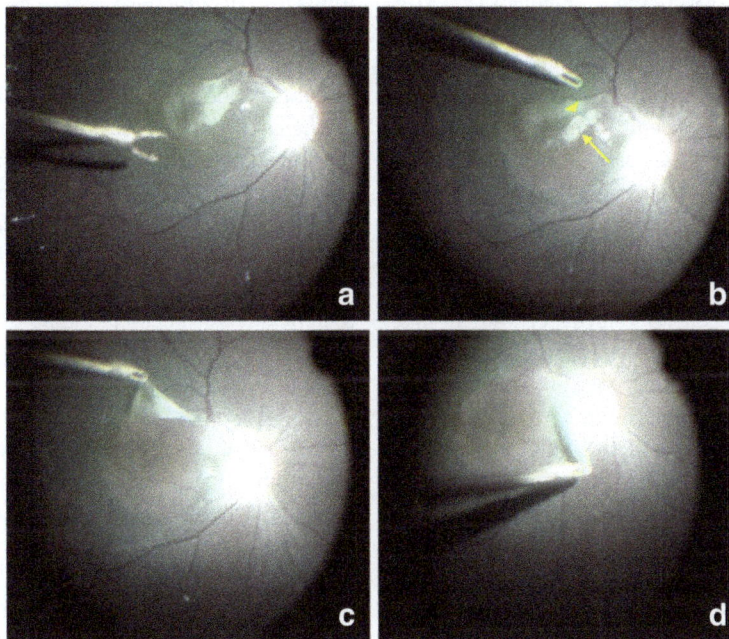

Fig. 3 Typical video images of the surgical process. **a** Indocyanine green was used to stain the inner limiting membrane (ILM). **b** The opaque white membrane (*arrow*) was located beneath the ILM (*triangle*). **c** The thick membrane was peeled away from the rest of the retina. **d** The membrane, which was tightly adhered to the superotemporal arcade vessels, was then completely dissected from the retinal artery

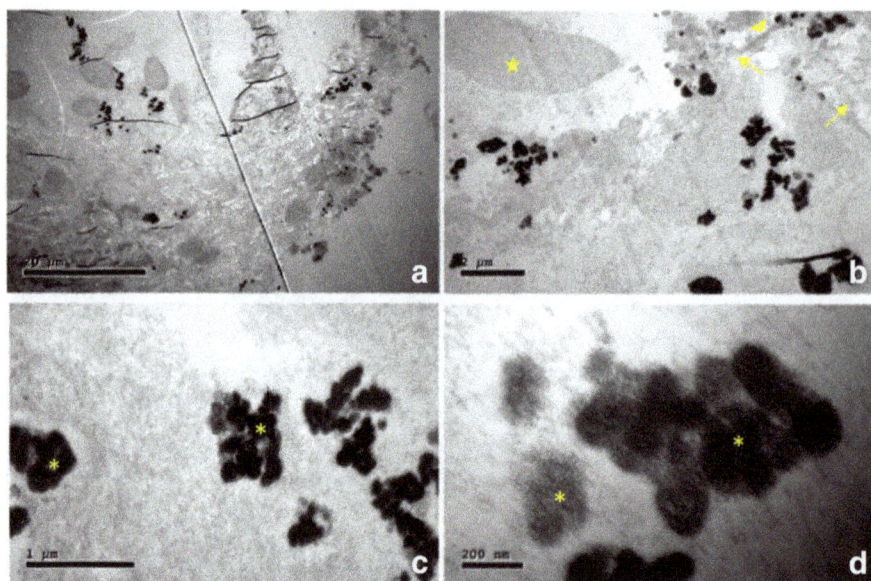

Fig. 4 Postoperative scanning electron microscopic images of the white membrane. **a** Overview of a segment of the membrane. **b** The membrane was made up of collagenous fibres (*arrows*), fibrinoid deposits (*triangle*) and cell debris (broken nuclei, *star*). **b–d** The membrane contained abundant hemosiderin (*asterisks*)

Discussion

An ERM arises secondary to the proliferation of cells along the ILM on the retinal surface. ERMs have been well characterized in adults: they are mostly idiopathic, associated with PVD and a defective ILM, and are found mainly in the elderly [1]. They are rare in adolescents and even rarer in children, as PVD is not likely to occur in these populations. The estimated incidence of ERM is 0.54 per 100,000 patients aged < 19 years [4]. The most commonly reported aetiologies are trauma (39%), uveitis (20%) and rare causes such as combined hamartoma of the retina and retinal pigment epithelium (11%); 30% of cases are idiopathic [4]. Other causes such as ocular toxocariasis, retinopathy of prematurity and Coats' disease can also lead to secondary ERM in children [2]. However, none of these conditions were found in the case presented here.

In adult patients, ERMs generally have a cellophane-like appearance. In the present case, the fibrotic membrane was white, thick, and opaque enough to obscure the underlying retina. Preoperative OCT images depicted the membrane as a smooth hyper-reflective band located just above the RNFL, without severe involvement of the inner retinal layers, which is different to the appearance of the ERMs commonly seen in elderly patients. The widely-accepted theory of ERM formation is related to cellular proliferation and phenotypic transition on remnants of the vitreous cortex after anomalous PVD [5–7]. However, in this 4-year-old patient, the retinal surface was almost continuous and PVD was not identified. Furthermore, the membrane was located between the relatively intact ILM and the rest of the retina. As a result of this unexpected finding, we analysed the structure and composition of the membrane using scanning electron microscopy, a powerful magnification tool that revealed abundant hemosiderin deposits within the membrane. Hemosiderin is an iron-storage complex found most often in macrophages after phagocytosis of red blood cells and is especially abundant following haemorrhage [8]. Hemosiderin is hardly observed in idiopathic ERMs; previous histological studies on surgically excised ERMs have revealed the main components to be retinal glial or myoblastic retinal pigment epithelial cells [9]. Although some fibrovascular ERMs present in eyes with extensive retinal ischemia may have a primarily vascular composition, such as blood vessels with hemocytes lined by endothelial cells [10], the unremarkable retinal vasculature and medical history of this patient's vascular disease make this case very unlikely. Taken together, it is speculated that the membrane developed after retinal sub-ILM haemorrhage and the gradual absorption and organization of the haemorrhage.

The possible causes of sub-ILM haemorrhage in children are Terson's syndrome, shaken-baby syndrome, Valsalva maculopathy and birth-canal compression [11, 12]. However, the patient's parents reported no history of baby-shaking, Valsalva maneuver or birth-canal compression. Nevertheless, we cannot rule out the possibility of trauma due to an accidental craniocerebral injury that could have occurred without the parents noticing. The retinal vessels of babies are not fully developed, and a surge in pressure in the intraocular veins, secondary to increased intracranial pressure during a craniocerebral injury, can cause spontaneous rupture of retinal capillaries [13]. This also partially explains the location of the membrane adjacent to the retinal vessels.

Conservative management with observation may be suitable for young patients with idiopathic ERMs, while surgical treatment may be indicated for eyes with symptomatic vision disturbances or significant anatomical changes on OCT [14, 15]. In our case, pars plana vitrectomy was performed without any complications. The BCVA, although not progressive, remained stable at 1 year postoperatively. The patient is still undergoing visual training, and the final results will be revealed at future follow-ups.

Conclusions

To our knowledge, this case is the first report of sub-ILM haemorrhage in a child without evident retinal diseases. In contrast to the commonly seen idiopathic or secondary ERMs in terms of location and components, in this child the white membrane was composed of abundant hemosiderin deposits and located beneath the intact ILM. Therefore, we speculate that the white membrane probably developed secondary to the sub-ILM haemorrhage.

Abbreviations
BCVA: Best-corrected visual acuity; ERM: Epiretinal membrane; ILM: Inner limiting membrane; OCT: Optical coherence tomography; PVD: Posterior vitreous detachment; RNFL: Retinal nerve fiber layer

Acknowledgements
Not applicable.

Funding
This work was supported by research grants from the National Key Basic Research Program of China (2013CB967503), the National Natural Science Foundation of China (81570854), and Science and Technology Commission of Shanghai Municipality (16411953700). The funding organisations had no role in collection, analysis or interpretation of data or in writing of the manuscript.

Authors' contributions
WYT was a major contributor in acquisition of the data, literature search and manuscript draft. RPG contributed to analysis of the data and preparation of the manuscript. TZ provided conception and critical revision of the manuscript. GZX did the surgery and participated in design of the study and revision of the manuscript. All authors read and approved the final manuscript.

Competing interests
The authors declare that they have no competing interests.

References
1. Appiah AP, Hirose T, Kado M. A review of 324 cases of idiopathic premacular gliosis. Am J Ophthalmol. 1988;106(5):533–5.
2. Kimmel AS, Weingeist TA, Blodi CF, Wells KK. Idiopathic premacular gliosis in children and adolescents. Am J Ophthalmol. 1989;108(5):578–81.
3. Benhamou N, Massin P, Spolaore R, Paques M, Gaudric A. Surgical management of epiretinal membrane in young patients. Am J Ophthalmol. 2002;133(3):358–64.
4. Khaja HA, McCannel CA, Diehl NN, Mohney BG. Incidence and clinical characteristics of epiretinal membranes in children. Arch Ophthalmol. 2008; 126(5):632–6.
5. Sebag J. Anomalous posterior vitreous detachment: a unifying concept in vitreo-retinal disease. Graefes Arch Clin Exp Ophthalmol. 2004;242(8):690–8.
6. Sommer F, Pollinger K, Brandl F, Weiser B, Tessmar J, Blunk T, Gopferich A. Hyalocyte proliferation and ECM accumulation modulated by bFGF and TGF-beta1. Graefes Arch Clin Exp Ophthalmol. 2008;246(9):1275–84.
7. Bu SC, Kuijer R, Li XR, Hooymans JM, Los LI. Idiopathic epiretinal membrane. Retina. 2014;34(12):2317–35.
8. Fischbach FA, Gregory DW, Harrison PM, Hoy TG, Williams JM. On the structure of hemosiderin and its relationship to ferritin. J Ultrastruct Res. 1971;37(5):495–503.
9. Smiddy WE, Michels RG, Gilbert HD, Green WR. Clinicopathologic study of idiopathic macular pucker in children and young adults. Retina. 1992;12(3): 232–6.
10. Glazer LC, Maguire A, Blumenkranz MS, Trese MT, Green WR. Improved surgical treatment of familial exudative vitreoretinopathy in children. Am J Ophthalmol. 1995;120(4):471–9.
11. Meier P, Schmitz F, Wiedemann P. Vitrectomy for pre-macular hemorrhagic cyst in children and young adults. Graefes Arch Clin Exp Ophthalmol. 2005; 243(8):824–8.
12. De Maeyer K, Van Ginderdeuren R, Postelmans L, Stalmans P, Van Calster J. Sub-inner limiting membrane haemorrhage: causes and treatment with vitrectomy. Br J Ophthalmol. 2007;91(7):869–72.
13. Medele RJ, Stummer W, Mueller AJ, Steiger HJ, Reulen HJ. Terson's syndrome in subarachnoid hemorrhage and severe brain injury accompanied by acutely raised intracranial pressure. J Neurosurg. 1998;88(5): 851–4.
14. Meyer CH, Rodrigues EB, Mennel S, Schmidt JC, Kroll P. Spontaneous separation of epiretinal membrane in young subjects: personal observations and review of the literature. Graefes Arch Clin Exp Ophthalmol. 2004; 242(12):977–85.
15. Banach MJ, Hassan TS, Cox MS, Margherio RR, Williams GA, Garretson BR, Trese MT. Clinical course and surgical treatment of macular epiretinal membranes in young subjects. Ophthalmology. 2001;108(1):23–6.

4

Central retinal artery occlusion – rethinking retinal survival time

Stephan Tobalem[1], James S. Schutz[1] and Argyrios Chronopoulos[1,2]*

Abstract

Background: The critical time from onset of complete occlusion of the central retinal artery (CRA) to functionally significant inner retinal infarction represents a window of opportunity for treatment and also has medical-legal implications, particularly when central retinal artery occlusion (CRAO) complicates therapeutic interventions. Here, we review the evidence for time to infarction from complete CRAO and discuss the implications of our findings.

Methods: A Medline search was performed using each of the terms "central retinal artery occlusion", "retinal infarction", "retinal ischemia", and "cherry red spot" from 1970 to the present including articles in French and German. All retrieved references as well as their reference lists were screened for relevance. An Internet search using these terms was also performed to look for additional references.

Results: We find that the experimental evidence showing that inner retinal infarction occurs after 90–240 min of total CRAO, which is the interval generally accepted in the medical literature and practice guidelines, is flawed in important ways. Moreover, the retinal ganglion cells, supplied by the CRA, are part of the central nervous system which undergoes infarction after non-perfusion of 12–15 min or less.

Conclusions: Retinal infarction is most likely to occur after only 12–15 min of complete CRAO. This helps to explain why therapeutic maneuvers for CRAO are often ineffective. Nevertheless, many CRAOs are incomplete and may benefit from therapy after longer intervals. To try to avoid retinal infarcton from inadvertent ocular compression by a headrest during prone anesthesia, the eyes should be checked at intervals of less than 15'.

Keywords: Central retinal artery occlusion, Retinal infarction, Retinal stroke, Choroidal infarction, Post-operative visual loss, Cherry red spot

Background

Central retinal artery occlusion (CRAO) of sufficient duration causes a stroke, infarction of the inner retina including the retinal ganglion cells and their axons which form the optic nerve, central nervous system tissue [1, 2]. The retinal ganglion cell layer is critically dependent on oxygen supplied by the end-artery circulation of the central retinal artery (CRA) [3, 4].

Retinal stroke from CRAO typically presents as acute, catastrophic, permanent visual loss in one eye, about 80% of the time with a visual acuity of 20/400 or worse, an afferent pupillary defect, a classic retinal cherry red spot on ophthalmoscopy from opacification of the infarcted ganglion cell layer surrounding the fovea, and sometimes a visible CRA embolus or other retinal arterial emboli [1, 3, 5]. Sometimes, segmentation of retinal blood columns (box-carring) with stagnation of retinal arterial flow may be present, indicating complete CRAO [1, 3]. Areas of inner retina supplied by cilioretinal arteries, which are common and not branches of the CRA, survive with visual function; if a cilioretinal artery supplies the macula despite surrounding infarction from CRAO, central vision may remain normal [4, 6]. Infarction of the retinal ganglion cell somata is followed by progressive axonal degeneration with pale optic atrophy evident after some weeks [3]. The outer retina including the photoreceptors and underlying retinal pigment epithelium is supplied with oxygen by the lush choroidal circulation derived from the long and short posterior

* Correspondence: aris_c@web.de
[1]Department of Ophthalmology, University Hospitals and School of Medicine, Geneva, Switzerland
[2]Department of Ophthalmology, Addenbrooke's Hospital, Cambridge University Hospital NHS Foundation Trust, Box 41, Hills Road, Cambridge CB2 0QQ, UK

ciliary arteries and is not infarcted in pure CRAO [3]. Nevertheless, conduction of visual information centrally is blocked by the loss of retinal ganglion cell function.

The critical time from onset of complete CRA occlusion to inner retinal infarction represents a window of opportunity for emergency treatment to try to prevent catastrophic visual loss. We examined the experimental evidence for the interval between complete CRA occlusion and subsequent retinal ganglion cell infarction. Therapeutic implications for emergency treatment as well as medical-legal considerations are discussed.

Methods

Medline was systematically searched using the terms "retinal stroke", "central retinal artery occlusion", "retinal infarction", "retinal ischemia", and "cherry red spot" from 1970 to the present including articles in English, French, and German literature. These terms were connected with "or". An Internet search using these search terms was also performed to look for additional references with no year restriction. All retrieved references as well as their reference lists were screened for evidence relevant to determination of the time to infarction of complete CRAO as well as articles relevant to the physiology of retinal stroke.

Eligible criteria

All publications obtained from Internet-based searches were screened by the above predefined selection criteria. Eligible studies were all studies reporting on the time to retinal infarction from complete CRAO as well as articles relevant to the physiology of retinal stroke. Two reviewers (S.T. and S.J) completed the assessment of search results to identify included studies.

Results

It is generally accepted that the human ganglion cell layer will survive without infarction and with preservation of vision if CRA circulation is restored after up to 90 to 240 min of complete non-perfusion from CRAO [3, 7–15]. We find that this clinically important time limit for inner retinal non-perfusion has been greatly overestimated for several reasons.

First, it is based on a series of experiments on non-human primates by Hayreh and coworkers [11, 12, 14] which are inappropriate for extrapolation to human CRAO because:

a) The experiments were performed on barbiturate anesthetized monkeys. Barbiturate anesthesia has an important neuro-protective effect which prolongs neuronal survival during ischemia [16–20].
b) The experiments were not controlled for the presence of hypothermia in the experimental animals which was likely to have had an additional

neuro-protective effect prolonging retinal ganglion cell survival [17].
c) Clamping of the CRA just before its entrance into the optic nerve sheath was performed in all the monkey experiments but is not an appropriate model for complete CRAO because there is collateral circulation to the CRA distal to the clamp in the monkey (and in the human eye) derived mostly from posterior ciliary artery branches of the ophthalmic artery [4, 21]. Persistent CRA perfusion was demonstrated in most of the experimental animals by fluorescein angiography with CRA filling in as little as 4 s; this was caused by either incomplete clamping of the CRA or collateral circulation distal to the clamping [11, 12]. Collateral circulation distal to the clamped CRA at its dural entry into the optic nerve sheath may very much delay or prevent inner retinal ischemia and infarction from CRAO; consequently, proper determination of the interval to inner retinal infarction after complete CRAO should be predicated on actual complete CRAO with no flow to the inner retina.
d) While it has been suggested that the site of CRA occlusion in humans is at the dural entry of the CRA into the optic nerve [13, 22–24], careful review of the references cited as evidence do not support this assertion nor can we find substantiation for this anywhere else in the peer reviewed literature. CRAO sometimes occurs at the posterior surface of the lamina cribrosa [1, 25]. There is good clinical evidence that human CRA occlusion is often on the optic nerve head where the CRA narrows suddenly, branching into its major subdivisions, much more distal than the entrance of the CRA into the optic nerve dura [9]; the CRA at this point on the surface of the optic nerve head is normally an end-artery with no collateral circulation [4]. Complete CRAO with no flow through the CRA, whether embolic or thrombotic, is well documented and would not occur if occlusion were present at the entry of the CRA into the optic nerve dural sheath because there would be residual flow and filling of the CRA from variable fine arterial collaterals along the course of the CRA within the optic nerve and collaterals in the area of the scleral wall from the circle of Zinn-Haller [4, 26].

Second, the retinal ganglion cells are central nervous system tissue. The central nervous system undergoes progressive significant infarction after 12–15′ of non-perfusion [5, 27, 28]. Brain tissue is particularly vulnerable with neuronal death reported to begin after only 5 min of ischemia [29]. Patients undergoing temporary arterial occlusion during intracranial aneurysm surgery for more than 14 min are prone to secondary stroke [30] and a subsequent study found less than 10 min of occlusion generally safe [20]. New neurological deficit from temporary arterial clipping during aneurysm surgery was reported in 30.7% in cases with less than 8 min of clipping but 80.9% with clipping over 8 min [21]. Retinal tissue oxygen consumption per gram is even higher than brain which is one of the most energy consuming organs and it has been suggested the retina is equally or even more vulnerable to oxygen deprivation than brain [31–37]. Cerebral oxygen consumption is about 3.5 ml/100 g/min compared to about 3.8 ml/100 g/min for inner cat retina and between 8 and 13 ml/100 g/min for human retina, the highest in the body [38–41].

Third, oxygenation of the ganglion cells from the vitreous or choroid is clinically insufficient when breathing room air and cannot compensate for complete CRAO by prolonging inner retinal survival time [42, 43].

Consequently, it is most likely that complete CRAO in the human will cause progressive, significant, irreversible retinal ganglion cell death after 12–15 min.

Discussion

The time to inner retinal infarction from complete CRAO has clinical treatment implications for emergency treatment as well as medical-legal significance.

a) *Time to emergency CRAO treatment – the window of opportunity*

If complete CRAO is confirmed by observation of segmentation and stagnation of retinal arterial blood flow for longer than 15 min on successive fundus examinations, treatment is likely to be futile because of inner retinal infarction. However, it is not possible to be certain of the prior duration of a complete CRAO observed on a single fundus examination and a variable degree of reperfusion may occur at any time and intermittently. Even a cherry red spot is not a reliable sign of complete occlusion with retinal infarction because it may occur from inner retinal ischemia without infarction [44]. CRAO is most often incomplete or complete but temporary with subsequent intermittent or permanent degrees of reperfusion resulting from transient arterial spasm or break up of embolus or thrombus [24]. Residual circulation is present demonstrated on fluorescein angiography in most CRAO patients and even a modest level of perfusion may prolong inner retinal survival [45]. Consequently, patients presenting with CRAO usually are offered treatment even if the time from onset of occlusion is believed to be many hours when there is uncertainty regarding completeness and duration of the occlusion. Patients with incomplete occlusions are more

likely to benefit from therapy [45] although, unfortunately, no strong evidence based treatment has been shown to be effective for CRAO [1, 3, 6, 9, 46].

Treatments for CRAO include:

- hyperbaric oxygen [47, 48].
- anticoagulation [1, 3].
- vasodilation by retrobulbar injection tolazoline or local anesthetic, sublingual isosorbide dinitrate, oral pentoxifylline, breathing elevated levels of carbon dioxide [1, 3, 7, 49, 50].
- topical ocular hypotensive agents, intravenous mannitol and acetazolamide to decrease extramural arterial tissue pressure by lowering IOP [1, 3, 49].
- paracentesis with release of aqueous from the anterior chamber to lower IOP and restore perfusion or dislodge CRA embolus, an effective method of acute dramatic IOP lowering [1, 50–53].
- ocular massage to lower IOP or dislodge CRA embolus or thrombus [1, 3, 6, 49, 54].
- fibrnolyitic therapy, intravenous or selective intra-arterial thrombolysis most oftenwith tissue plasminogen activator (tPA), popular in some centers but with complications reported in up to 37% of cases [3, 55–67]. Recently, a small uncontrolled series using tPA by intra-retinal arterial micro-cannulation has been reported with limited success [68].

CRAO treatments commonly offered at present are listed in Table 1; however, it is important to note that there is no generally accepted consensus with respect to CRAO treatment and treatment offered at different locations varies greatly according to local protocols and physician experience.

After ophthalmic examination and treatment of retinal stroke from CRAO, further urgent evaluation is indicated to search for a cause of occlusion or the source of a visible embolus because CRAO patients are at elevated risk for other cerebral or myocardial infarction [1, 3, 6].

b) *Medical-legal implications*

Retinal survival time after complete CRAO may have important medical legal implications when a treating doctor is alleged not to have diagnosed or treated in a timely fashion, particularly when CRAO is iatrogenic, for example the result of acute retrobulbar hemorrhage following retrobulbar injection, blepharoplasty, orbital surgery, sinus surgery entering the orbit, and facial injections causing CRA embolization. In such cases, it is very important to recognize that there is no generally accepted, effective treatment for CRAO and also that inner retinal infarction occurs rapidly, within about 15 min if CRAO is complete.

Table 1 Common Emergency CRAO Treatment Options

Treatment	Action
Sublingual isosorbide dinitrate	Vasodilation
Oral pentoxifylline	Vasodilation
Carbogen inhalation	Cerebral vasodilation and increased oxygen
Retrobulbar alpha adenergic blocker (tolazoline) or local anesthetic	Vasodilation
Hyperbaric oxygen	Increased oxygen
Ocular massage	Attempt to dislodge emboli or thrombus
Systemic anticoagulation	Limit thrombosis
Intravenous acetazolamide and mannitol	Reduce IOP to increase perfusion pressure
Aqueous humor removal by paracentesis	Reduce IOP to increase perfusion pressure
Thrombolysis, intra-arterial or systemic	Dissolve thrombus

Combined CRAO and choroidal occlusion, sometimes iatrogenic, may be caused by acute, severe, intraocular pressure (IOP) elevation causing infarction of both inner and outer retina as well as optic nerve head with complete permanent loss of retinal function if occlusion is sufficiently prolonged. Such acute IOP elevation has two typical mechanisms:

1. Internal – severe IOP elevation can arise from acute internal ocular volume increase from intraocular injection or intraocular gas expansion following intraocular surgery resulting from too high gas concentration, nitrous oxide anesthesia, or reduced atmospheric pressure during flight or high altitude mountain ascent [69–71].
2. External – acute ocular pressure elevation can result from external pressure on the globe, for example by a head rest during prone general anesthesia, pre-operative ocular compression for intraocular surgery, acute retrobulbar hemorrhage, orbital infection with severe edema, acute large scleral buckle, orbital emphysema, as well as from a variety of objects pressing on the eye [72–82].

Retinal infarction in cases of combined CRAO and choroidal vascular occlusion from acute, highly elevated IOP will occur after only 12–15′ of complete CRAO. Consequently, the eyes of a prone patient positioned on a head rest during general anesthesia should be checked at intervals of 15 min or less.

Conclusion

Complete CRAO of more than 12–15 min duration is likely to be sufficient to cause stroke of the retinal ganglion cells which form the optic nerve. This may be one reason why no strong evidence based therapy exists for CRAO. If multiple serial fundus examinations show no retinal arterial flow as evidenced by segmentation and stagnation of the arterial blood columns for more than about 15′, treatment is likely to be futile. Otherwise, emergency treatment is offered after much longer intervals in most cases because it is usually not possible to be sure that CRAO has been complete from the onset of symptoms to the time of diagnosis. Retinal stroke from CRAO requires further urgent evaluation, after ophthalmic examination and treatment, to search for a cause of occlusion because CRAO patients are at elevated risk for other cerebral or myocardial infarction. To try to avoid CRAO from inadvertent ocular compression by a headrest during prone anesthesia, the eyes should be checked at intervals of less than 15′.

Abbreviations
CRA: Central retinal artery; CRAO: Central retinal artery occlusion; IOP: Intraocular pressure

Funding
The study was not funded.

Authors' contributions
ST, JSS and AC have contributed equally in the conception, writing and editing of the manuscript. All authors have read and approved the manuscript.

Competing interests
The authors declare that they have no competing interests.

References
1. Cugati S, Varma DD, Chen CS, Lee AW. Treatment options for central retinal artery occlusion. Curr Treat Options Neurol. 2013;1:63–77.
2. Monro TK. Optic nerve as part of the central nervous system. J Anat Physiol. 1895;Pt 1:45–8.
3. Varma DD, Cugati S, Lee AW, Chen CS. A review of central retinal artery occlusion: clinical presentation and management. Eye (London, England). 2013;6:688–97.
4. Michalinos A, Zogana S, Kotsiomitis E, Mazarakis A, Troupis T. Anatomy of the ophthalmic artery: a review concerning its modern surgical and clinical applications. Anat Res Int. 2015:591961. https://doi.org/10.1155/2015/591961.
5. Astrup J, Siesjö BK, Symon L. Thresholds in cerebral ischemia - the ischemic penumbra. Stroke. 1981;6:723–5.
6. Olsen TW, Pulido JS, Folk JC, Hyman L, Flaxel CJ, Adelman RA. Retinal and ophthalmic artery occlusions preferred practice pattern(R). Ophthalmology. 2017;2:P120–43.
7. Sharma S, Brown GC. In: Ryan SJ, editor. Retinal artery obstruction in: section 5, chapter 69, retina. Philadelphia: Mosby; 2006. 978–0–323-02598-0 978–0–323-04091-4 978–0–323-04323-6.

8.   Hayreh SS, Zimmerman MB, Kimura A, Sanon A. Central retinal artery occlusion. Retinal survival time. Exp Eye Res. 2004;3:723–36.

9.   McCannel CA. In: Basic and Clinical Science Course, editor. Retina and vitreous in basic and clinical science course; 2016. 133.978–1–61525-739-3.

10. Hayreh SS, Kolder HE, Weingeist TA. Central retinal artery occlusion and retinal tolerance time. Ophthalmology. 1980;1:75–8.

11. Hayreh SS, Weingeist TA. Experimental occlusion of the central artery of the retina. I. Ophthalmoscopic and fluorescein fundus angiographic studies. Br J Ophthalmol. 1980;12:896–912.

12. Hayreh SS, Weingeist TA. Experimental occlusion of the central artery of the retina. IV: retinal tolerance time to acute ischaemia. Br J Ophthalmol. 1980;11:818–25.

13. Hayreh SS. Prevalent misconceptions about acute retinal vascular occlusive disorders. Prog Retin Eye Res. 2005;4:493–519.

14. Hayreh SS, Jonas JB. Optic disk and retinal nerve fiber layer damage after transient central retinal artery occlusion: an experimental study in rhesus monkeys. Am J Ophthalmol. 2000;6:786–95.

15. Murphy-Lavoie H, Butler F and Hagan C. Central retinal artery occlusion treated with oxygen: a literature review and treatment algorithm. Undersea & Hyperbaric Medicine: Journal of the Undersea and Hyperbaric Medical Society, Inc. 2012;39:943–53.

16. Kawaguchi M, Furuya H, Patel PM. Neuroprotective effects of anesthetic agents. J Anesth. 2005;2:150–6.

17. Steen PA, Michenfelder JD. Cerebral protection with barbiturates: relation to anesthetic effect. Stroke. 1978;2:140–2.

18. Steen PA, Michenfelder JD. Barbiturate protection in tolerant and nontolerant hypoxic mice: comparison with hypothermic protection. Anesthesiology. 1979;5:404–8.

19. Almaas R, Saugstad OD, Pleasure D, Rootwelt T. Effect of barbiturates on hydroxyl radicals, lipid peroxidation, and hypoxic cell death in human NT2-N neurons. Anesthesiology. 2000;3:764–74.

20. Lavine SD, Masri LS, Levy ML, Giannotta SL. Temporary occlusion of the middle cerebral artery in intracranial aneurysm surgery: time limitation and advantage of brain protection. J Neurosurg. 1997;6:817–24.

21. Tanabe J, Ishikawa T, Moroi J, Suzuki A. Preliminary study on safe thresholds for temporary internal carotid artery occlusion in aneurysm surgery based on motor-evoked potential monitoring. Surg Neurol Int. 2014;5:47.

22. Hayreh SS. Pathogenesis of occlusion of the central retinal vessels. Am J Ophthalmol. 1971;5:998–1011.

23. Singh S, Dass R. The central artery of the retina. II. A study of its distribution and anastomoses. Br J Ophthalmol. 1960;44:280–99.

24. Singh S, Dass R. The central artery of the retina. I. Origin and course. Br J Ophthalmol. 1960;44:193–212.

25. Foroozan R, Savino PJ, Sergott RC. Embolic central retinal artery occlusion detected by orbital color Doppler imaging. Ophthalmology. 2002;4:744–7. discussion 747-748

26. Bron AJ, Tripathi RC, Tripathi BJ, Wolff E. Wolff's anatomy of the eye and orbit. London: Chapman & Hall Medical; 1997. 978–0–412-41010-9

27. Raichle ME. The pathophysiology of brain ischemia. Ann Neurol. 1983;1:2–10.

28. Patterson JT, Hanbali F, Franklin RL, HWJ N. Ch 72 neurosurgery in Sabiston textbook of surgery, 18th edn. Philadelphia: Saunders Elsevier; 2008.

29. Lee JM, Grabb MC, Zipfel GJ, Choi DW. Brain tissue responses to ischemia. J Clin Invest. 2000;6:723–31.

30. Samson D, Batjer HH, Bowman G, Mootz L, Krippner WJ Jr, Meyer YJ, et al. A clinical study of the parameters and effects of temporary arterial occlusion in the management of intracranial aneurysms. Neurosurgery. 1994;1:22–8. discussion 28-29

31. Alder VA, Ben-Nun J, Cringle SJ. PO2 profiles and oxygen consumption in cat retina with an occluded retinal circulation. Invest Ophthalmol Vis Sci. 1990;6:1029–34.

32. Ames A 3rd. Earliest irreversible changes during ischemia. Am J Emerg Med. 1983;2:139–46.

33. Ames A 3rd, Nesbett FB. Pathophysiology of ischemic cell death: I. Time of onset of irreversible damage; importance of the different components of the ischemic insult. Stroke. 1983;2:219–26.

34. Pournaras CJ, Riva CE, Tsacopoulos M, Strommer K. Diffusion of O2 in the retina of anesthetized miniature pigs in normoxia and hyperoxia. Exp Eye Res. 1989;3:347–60.

35. Pournaras CJ, Tsacopoulos M, Bovet J, Roth A. Diffusion of O2 in the normal and the ischemic retina of miniature pigs. Ophtalmologie. 1990;1:17–9.

36. Wangsa-Wirawan ND, Linsenmeier RA. Retinal oxygen: fundamental and clinical aspects. Arch Ophthalmol. 2003;4:547–57.

37. Yu DY, Cringle SJ. Oxygen distribution and consumption within the retina in vascularised and avascular retinas and in animal models of retinal disease. Prog Retin Eye Res. 2001;2:175–208.

38. Braun RD, Linsenmeier RA, Goldstick TK. Oxygen consumption in the inner and outer retina of the cat. Invest Ophthalmol Vis Sci. 1995;3:542–54.

39. Braun RD, Linsenmeier RA. Retinal oxygen tension and the electroretinogram during arterial occlusion in the cat. Invest Ophthalmol Vis Sci. 1995;3:523–41.

40. Hadanny A, Maliar A, Fishlev G, Bechor Y, Bergan J, Friedman M, Avni I, Efrati. Reversibility of retinal ischemia due to central retinal artery occlusion by hyperbaric oxygen. Clin Ophthalmol. 2017;11:115–25. https://doi.org/10.2147/OPTH.S121307.

41. Gabrielli A, Layon AJ, Yu M. Civetta, Taylor and Kirby's critical care. New York: WW Norton; 2008.

42. Yu DY, Cringle SJ. Oxygen distribution and consumption within the retina in vascularised and avascular retinas and in animal models of retinal disease. Prog Retin Eye Res. 2001;20:175–208.

43. Yu DY, Cringle SJ, Yu PK, Su EN. Intraretinal oxygen distribution and consumption during retinal artery occlusion and graded hyperoxic ventilation in the rat. Invest Ophthalmol Vis Sci. 2007;5:2290–6.

44. Terelak-Borys B, Skonieczna K, Grabska-Liberek I. Ocular ischemic syndrome - a systematic review. Med Sci Monit. 2012;8:RA138–44.

45. McLeod D, Beatty S. Evidence for an enduring ischaemic penumbra following central retinal artery occlusion, with implications for fibrinolytic therapy. Prog Retin Eye Res. 2015;49:82–119.

46. Youn TS, Lavin P, Patrylo M, Schindler J, Kirshner H, Greer DM, Schrag M. Current treatment of central retinal artery occlusion: a national survey. J Neurol. 2018;265(2):330–35. https://doi.org/10.1007/s00415-017-8702-x.

47. Beatty S, Au Eong KG. Acute occlusion of the retinal arteries: current concepts and recent advances in diagnosis and management. J Accid Emerg Med. 2000;5:324–9.

48. Deutsch TA, Read JS, Ernest JT, Goldstick TK. Effects of oxygen and carbon dioxide on the retinal vasculature in humans. Arch Ophthalmol. 1983;8:1278–80.

49. Rumelt S, Dorenboim Y, Rehany U. Aggressive systematic treatment for central retinal artery occlusion. Am J Ophthalmol. 1999;6:733–8.

50. Atebara NH, Brown GC, Cater J. Efficacy of anterior chamber paracentesis and Carbogen in treating acute nonarteritic central retinal artery occlusion. Ophthalmology. 1995;12:2029–34. discussion 2034-2025

51. Hwang CK, Kolomeyer AM, Brucker AJ. Optical coherence tomography angiography of a central retinal artery occlusion before and after anterior chamber paracentesis. Ophthalmology. 2017;5:608.

52. Fiess A, Cal O, Kehrein S, Halstenberg S, Frisch I, Steinhorst UH. Anterior chamber paracentesis after central retinal artery occlusion: a tenable therapy? BMC Ophthalmol. 2014;14:28.

53. Trivedi D, Denniston AK, Murray PI. Safety profile of anterior chamber paracentesis performed at the slit lamp. Clin Exp Ophthalmol. 2011;8:725–8.

54. Ffytche TJ. A rationalization of treatment of central retinal artery occlusion. Trans Ophthalmol Soc U K. 1974;2:468–79.

55. Schrag M, Youn T, Schindler J, Kirshner H, Greer D. Intravenous fibrinolytic therapy in central retinal artery occlusion: a patient-level meta-analysis. JAMA Neurol. 2015;72(10):1148–54. https://doi.org/10.1001/jamaneurol.2015.1578.

56. Hazin R, Dixon JA, Bhatti MT. Thrombolytic therapy in central retinal artery occlusion: cutting edge therapy, standard of care therapy, or impractical therapy? Curr Opin Ophthalmol. 2009;3:210–8.

57. Mehta N, Marco RD, Goldhardt R, Modi Y. Central retinal artery occlusion: acute management and treatment. Curr Ophthalmol Rep. 2017;5(2):149–59. https://doi.org/10.1007/s40135-017-0135-2.

58. Agarwal N, Gala NB, Baumrind B, Hansberry DR, Thabet AM, Gandhi CD, Prestigiacomo CJ. Endovascular management of central retinal arterial occlusion. Vasc Endovasc Surg. 2016;50(8):579–81. https://doi.org/10.1177/1538574416682158.

59. Schumacher M, Schmidt D, Jurklies B, Gall C, Wanke I, Schmoor C, Maier-Lenz H, Solymosi L, Brueckmann H, Neubauer AS, Wolf A, Feltgen N, EAGLE-Study Group. Central retinal artery occlusion: local intra-arterial fibrinolysis versus conservative treatment, a multicenter randomized trial. Ophthalmology. 2010; 117(7):1367–75.e1. https://doi.org/10.1016/j.ophtha.2010.03.061.

60. Schumacher M, Schmidt D, Wakhloo AK. Intra-arterial fibrinolytic therapy in central retinal artery occlusion. Neuroradiology. 1993;8:600–5.

61. Gilbert AL, Choi C, Lessell S. Acute Management of Central Retinal Artery Occlusion. Int Ophthalmol Clin. 2015;55(4):157–66. https://doi.org/10.1097/IIO.0000000000000087.

62. Arnold M, Koerner U, Remonda L, Nedeltchev K, Mattle HP, Schroth G, et al. Comparison of intra-arterial thrombolysis with conventional treatment in patients with acute central retinal artery occlusion. J Neurol Neurosurg Psychiatry. 2005;2:196–9.

63. Aldrich EM, Lee AW, Chen CS, Gottesman RF, Bahouth MN, Gailloud P, et al. Local intraarterial fibrinolysis administered in aliquots for the treatment of central retinal artery occlusion: the Johns Hopkins Hospital experience. Stroke. 2008;6:1746–50.

64. Richard G, Lerche RC, Knospe V, Zeumer H. Treatment of retinal arterial occlusion with local fibrinolysis using recombinant tissue plasminogen activator. Ophthalmology. 1999;4:768–73.

65. Weber J, Remonda L, Mattle HP, Koerner U, Baumgartner RW, Sturzenegger M, et al. Selective intra-arterial fibrinolysis of acute central retinal artery occlusion. Stroke. 1998;10:2076–9.

66. Padolecchia R, Puglioli M, Ragone MC, Romani A, Collavoli PL. Superselective intraarterial fibrinolysis in central retinal artery occlusion. AJNR Am J Neuroradiol. 1999;4:565–7.

67. Hattenbach LO, Kuhli-Hattenbach C, Scharrer I, Baatz H. Intravenous thrombolysis with low-dose recombinant tissue plasminogen activator in central retinal artery occlusion. Am J Ophthalmol. 2008;5:700–6.

68. Kadonosono K, Yamane S, Inoue M, Yamakawa T, Uchio E. Intra-retinal arterial cannulation using a microneedle for central retinal artery occlusion. Sci Rep. 2018;1:1360.

69. Fang IM, Huang JS. Central retinal artery occlusion caused by expansion of intraocular gas at high altitude. Am J Ophthalmol. 2002;4:603–5.

70. Baath J, Ells AL, Crichton A, Kherani A, Williams RG. Safety profile of intravitreal triamcinolone acetonide. Journal of ocular pharmacology and therapeutics: the official journal of the Association for Ocular. Pharmacol Ther. 2007;3:304–10.

71. Fu AD, McDonald HR, Eliott D, Fuller DG, Halperin LS, Ramsay RC, et al. Complications of general anesthesia using nitrous oxide in eyes with preexisting gas bubbles. Retina. 2002;5:569–74.

72. Morgan CM, Schatz H, Vine AK, Cantrill HL, Davidorf FH, Gitter KA, et al. Ocular complications associated with retrobulbar injections. Ophthalmology. 1988;5:660–5.

73. Epstein NE. Perioperative visual loss following prone spinal surgery: a review. Surg Neurol Int. 2016;Suppl 13:S347–60.

74. Leibovitch I, Casson R, Laforest C, Selva D. Ischemic orbital compartment syndrome as a complication of spinal surgery in the prone position. Ophthalmology. 2006;1:105–8.

75. Brown GC, Magargal LE, Sergott R. Acute obstruction of the retinal and choroidal circulations. Ophthalmology. 1986;11:1373–82.

76. Walkup HE, Murphy JD. Retinal ischemia with unilateral blindness–a complication occurring during pulmonary resection in the prone position; report of two cases. J Thorac Surg. 1952;2:174–5.

77. Hoski JJ, Eismont FJ, Green BA. Blindness as a complication of intraoperative positioning. A case report. J Bone Joint Surg Am. 1993;8:1231–2.

78. Grossman W, Ward WT. Central retinal artery occlusion after scoliosis surgery with a horseshoe headrest. Case report and literature review. Spine. 1993;9:1226–8.

79. Wolfe SW, Lospinuso MF, Burke SW. Unilateral blindness as a complication of patient positioning for spinal surgery. A case report. Spine. 1992;5:600–5.

80. Jampol LM, Goldbaum M, Rosenberg M, Bahr R. Ischemia of ciliary arterial circulation from ocular compression. Arch Ophthalmol. 1975;12:1311–7.

81. Newman NJ. Perioperative visual loss after nonocular surgeries. Am J Ophthalmol. 2008;4:604–10.

82. American Society of Anesthesiologists Task Force on Perioperative Visual L. Practice advisory for perioperative visual loss associated with spine surgery: an updated report by the American Society of Anesthesiologists Task Force on perioperative visual loss. Anesthesiology. 2012;2:274–85.

5

Prevalence and clinical characteristics of dry eye disease in community-based type 2 diabetic patients: the Beixinjing eye study

Xinrong Zou[1,5], Lina Lu[2], Yi Xu[2], Jianfeng Zhu[2], Jiangnan He[2], Bo Zhang[2] and Haidong Zou[1,2,3,4*]

Abstract

Background: This study was performed to evaluate the prevalence and clinical characteristics of dry eye disease (DED) in community-based type 2 diabetic patients and to identify the associated factors related with DED.

Methods: A total of 1360 type 2 diabetic patients in the Beixinjing community were randomly selected. All participants were given a questionnaire that assessed basic information and subjective symptoms.DED was diagnosed using the revised Japanese DED diagnostic criteria. All subjects underwent a routine ophthalmic examination, corneal sensitivity test, tear film break-up time(BUT) test, Schirmer I test, fluorescein and lissamine green staining(FL) and fundus photography. Diabetic retinopathy (DR) was graded according to the International severity scale of diabetic retinopathy and diabetic macular edema.

Results: Of the 1360 subjects, 238 (17.5%) were diagnosed with DED. There was a significant association between the presence of DED and higher blood glucose ($P < 0.001$, OR1.240) as well as higher levels of glycosylated hemoglobin HbA1c ($P < 0.001$, OR1.108). Corneal sensitivity was negatively correlated with the prevalence of DED ($P = 0.02$, OR0.973).

Conclusions: The prevalence of DED in this community-based study was 17.5%, which was lower than that observed in hospital-based studies. Diabetic patients with poor metabolic control were more likely to present with DED. A dry eye examination should be added to the routine screening of diabetes.

Keywords: Prevalence, Dry eye disease, Community-based, Type 2 diabetic patients

Background

Diabetes mellitus is a serious public health problem in many countries. Over the last three decades, the number of diabetic patients worldwide has more than doubled [1]. Diabetes mellitus is a systemic disease that can cause a variety of ocular complications, including diabetic retinopathy, cataracts, glaucoma, keratopathy, and dry eye disease (DED). According to the international dry eye workshop, DED is defined as an abnormality in the quality or quantity of tears or in tear dynamics due to any cause, resulting in ocular discomfort, visual disturbance, decreased tear film stability, and potential damage to the ocular surface [2]. Previous studies have reported an increased prevalence of DED in diabetic patients compared with healthy subjects. Moreover, dry eye symptoms, such as itching, burning, and foreign body sensation, are frequently encountered among diabetic patients [3]. For example, Jin et al. found that type 2 diabetic patients were more likely to suffer from tear film dysfunction [4]. Manaviat et al. reported that the prevalence of DED was 54.3% in type 2 diabetic patients and that the morbidity rate was much higher than that in non-diabetic subjects [5]. They also found that DED was significantly associated with age, sex, duration of diabetes, and diabetic retinopathy. Najafi et al. showed that the prevalence of DED was 27.7% in diabetic patients and that DED showed a significant correlation with glycosylated hemoglobin (HbA1c) [6].

* Correspondence: zouhaidong@hotmail.com

[1]Shanghai General Hospital, Nanjing Medical University, No. 100, Haining Road, Hongkou District, Shanghai 200080, China

[2]Department of Preventative Ophthalmology, Shanghai Eye Disease Prevention and Treatment Center, No. 380, Kangding Road, Jingan, Shanghai 200040, China

Full list of author information is available at the end of the article

However, all of the published epidemiological studies on DED in type 2 diabetic patients are hospital-based. DED risk factors may differ between hospital-based and community-based populations. Among studies of diabetic patients, hospital-based studies enrolled patients who were in a more serious condition, such as those with a long duration of diabetes and higher level of HbA1C. Until now, it was unknown whether DED was also prevalent in community-based populations. In the present study, we examined the prevalence and clinical characteristics of DED in community-based type 2 diabetic patients in Shanghai, China, and explored the risk factors associated with DED in this group.

Methods

The study was carried out following the tenets of the Declaration of Helsinki. The Medical Ethics Committee of the Shanghai General Hospital, Shanghai Jiaotong University approved this study protocol, and informed written consent was obtained from all subjects.

Study design

This community-based cross-sectional study focused on DED among type 2 diabetic patients in the Beixinjing community of Shanghai. The Beixinjing community is in the northwest region of Shanghai and exhibits nationally representative demographic and socioeconomic characteristics. A series of epidemiological investigations have been carried out in this community because of its relatively stable population (43,839 in the 2010 census, of which 11,312 were aged 60 years or older).The social and economic demographics in the Beixinjing community are representative of the middle class in China: the average per capita annual income among urban households is 43,185 yuan(6170 US dollars) [7].

Diagnostic criteria

Since there is no international diagnostic standard for DED, this study used the revised Japanese DED diagnostic criteria:(1) the presence of dry eye symptoms; (2) presence of either a quantitative or qualitative disturbance of the tear film (BUT ≤5 s or SchirmerItest ≤5 mm); and (3) presence of conjunctivo-corneal epithelial damage (fluorescein staining score ≥ 3 points, Rose Bengal staining score ≥ 3points, or lissamine green staining score ≥ 3 points). A definitive diagnosis of DED was established only if all three criteria were present. Subjects with 0–1 positive criteria were diagnosed as normal [8].

Diabetic retinopathy (DR)

The DR for each subject was graded based on the worse eye. The grading was performed using the International severity scale of diabetic retinopathy and diabetic macular edema [9].

Diabetic nephropathy

The urine sample was collected from every subjects to measure urine albumin and creatinine. Microalbuminuria was diagnosed if the albumin/creatinine ratio was greater than 30μg/ mg. And if the ratio was greater than 300 μg/mg, then the subject was identified as macroalbuminuria [6].

Sampling and exclusion criteria

The reported DED prevalence rate of Chinese adults varied from 7.99 to 21% [10–12]. The formula $n = Z^2(p) (1-p)/B^2$ was adopted to calculate the required sample size via simple random sampling, where $Z = 1.96$ (with a 95% confidence interval), p is the estimated prevalence, and B is the presupposition error. If it is assumed that $p = 7.99\%$, $B = 7.99\% \times 0.25$(with a 25% error bound) $= 0.019975$, and $Z = 1.96$, then $n = 708$. Using a sample effect coefficient of 1.1 for this study, the estimated response rate was 90%. The calculated number of samples was 865.

From April to September 2016, a community-based study of the prevalence of dry eye in type 2 diabetic patients was performed in the Beixinjing community of Shanghai. Random cluster sampling was used to select the samples used in this study. The clusters were defined geographically based on residential registration data. According to the chronic disease records of the Beixinjing Community Health Service Center, 1503 T2DM residents lived in the 10 randomly selected geographical clusters from total 34 clusters. Type 2 diabetes mellitus was diagnosed according to the criteria of the World Health Organization [13]. The healthy group was aslo selected using random cluster sampling.

Patients with the following ocular disorders that can affect tear production or quality were excluded from the study: (1) eyelid disease: ectropion, entropion, trichiasis, ptosis,eyelid movement disorder caused by facial paralysis; (2) diseases of the conjunctiva: conjunctivochalasis, pterygium; (3)ocular surgeries within 6 months, refractive surgeries within 2 years, history of ocular chemical injury, or use of ocular medications or nutritional tear supplements; and (4) systemic diseases:autoimmune disease:such as Sjogren's, rheumatoid arthrits,systemic lupus erythematosus. Other systemic diseases: Grave's disease,Parkinson's disease.

Study procedures

At the beginning of the investigation, all participants answered a subjective symptoms questionnaire. The subjective complaints that were assessed included dry eye, itching, burning, foreign body sensation, eye fatigue, lacrimation, and photophobia. If the individual presented with two or more of these symptoms, the subject was classified as having subjective complaints [11, 13]. Next, the participants completed a detailed interview assessing basic information (such as age, gender, nationality, marital status, degree of education, working situation) and past medical histories of systemic diseases (including diabetes, hypertension, rheumatoid arthritis, and cardio-cerebrovascular illnesses). The duration of illnesses and medications were noted. The subjects' height, weight and blood pressure were assessed, then the blood samples and urine samples were collected for the measurement of glucose, glycosylated hemoglobin (HbA1C), serum lipids, and urine albumin and creatinine. The subjects also underwent the following ophthalmological examinations: automatic refractor testing, visual acuity testing(if visual acuity was worse than 0.7, the best-corrected visual acuity was measured), corneal sensitivity testing using a Cochet-Bonnet aesthesiometer (Luneau Ophthalmology, Paris, France), tear-film breakup time (BUT) testing, fluorescein and lissamine greenstaining(FL), SchirmerItest without anesthesia, and slit-lamp examination. In addition, two digital photographs of the fundus were obtained for each eye using a digital 45-μ non-mydriatic retinal camera (non-mydriatic retinal camera; Topcon, Tokyo, Japan). One fundus photograph was centered on the optic nerve head, and the other was centered on the macula.

A Cochet-Bonnet aesthesiometer was used to measure corneal sensitivity The central region of the cornea was tested. An aesthesiometer with a 60 mm long monofilament was placed perpendicularly to the participant's cornea. The subject was asked whether this touch could be felt when the monofilament was slightly bent. The length of monofilament was recorded as the corneal sensitivity if the subject had felt this touch, and if not, the length of was decreased by 5.0 mm each time until the subject could feel the touch. Three measurements were performed at each monofilament length, and the average length was considered to be the corneal sensitivity at the tested region.

To determine the BUT, a fluorescein strip was placed in the inferior fornix of the subject. Then, the patient was asked to blink several times to distribute the fluorescein across the entire cornea. A cobalt blue filter was used in slit lamp biomicroscopy to record the interval between the last blink and first appearance of a dry spot on the cornea. This measurement was repeated three times, and the average value was calculated. Values shorter than 5 s are diagnostic for DED.

For the Schirmer I test, a Schirmer strip was inserted into the inferior fornix beneath the temporal lid margin without anesthesia. After 5 min, the Schirmer strip was removed and the scale of wetness was measured. Patients were informed not to rotate their eyes. Values lower than 5 mm imply a diagnosis of DED.

To evaluate the FL of the ocular surface, the eye was divided into three equal compartments: the cornea, the nasal conjunctiva and the temporal conjunctiva. The maximum staining score for each area was 3points, and the maximum overall staining score was 9 points [8].

Statistical methods

IBM-SPSS version 23 was used for statistical analysis. The chi-square test, independent paired t test and Pearson correlation analyses were performed. A P value < 0.05 was accepted as statistically significant.

A binary logistic regression analysis was performed using the presence of DED as the dependent parameter. The independent variables included those parameters that were significantly associated with DED in univariate analysis.

Results

The Diabetes Group was well matched with the Healthy Group in terms of age and sex. The subjects in the Diabetes Group ranged in age from 31 to 95 years, while those in the Healthy Group were 47 to 94 years. (Table 1).

The Diabetes Group had a significantly higher BMI, blood glucose, triglyceride and total cholesterol than the Healthy Group.However,there was no significant difference in systolic blood pressure and diastolic blood pressure between the two groups. The tear film function and corneal sensitivity parameters were significantly different between the diabetic and healthy subjects. The corneal sensitivity in the Diabetes Group was much lower than that in the Healthy Group. Both the BUT and Schirmer-Itest scores were significantly lower in the Diabetes group. The diabetic patients had much more unstable tear film than the healthy subjects (Table 2).

A total of 238(17.5%) out of 1360 type 2 diabetic subjects were definitively diagnosed with DED. In the Healthy group, DED was detected in 62 participants (5.9%). There was a significant difference in the prevalence of DED between the two groups (χ^2 = 72.25,p < 0.001). A total of 551 subjects were not in conformity with the DED or non-DED diagnostic criteria, not included in the statistical analysis.

In the Pearson Correlation analysis, age was negatively correlated with BUT and corneal sensitivity (P < 0.05)

Table 1 Demographic characteristics of the diabetes group and healthy group

Characteristic	Sub-group	Diabetes Group	Healthy Group	Statistic Value	P Value
Age(years)		68.91 ± 8.86	68.31 ± 8.09	3.36	0.09
Gender	Female	853	690	2.92	0.09
	Male	507	354		

Prevalence and clinical characteristics of dry eye disease in community-based type 2 diabetic...

33

Table 2 Clinical characteristics of the diabetes group and healthy group

Factor	Diabetes Group	Healthy Group	Statistic Value	P Value
Corneal sensitivity (mm)	54.27 ± 10.64	58.11 ± 4.57	−10.91	0.00
BUT(s)	3.87 ± 2.52	5.65 ± 2.64	−16.81	0.00
Schirmer I test (mm)	8.95 ± 6.24	9.49 ± 6.62	−2.05	0.00
FL	0.60 ± 1.04	0.30 ± 0.97	8.91	0.00
BMI (kg/m^2)	25.53 ± 3.89	24.16 ± 3.71	2.73	0.00
Glucose (mmol/L)	7.92 ± 2.51	6.66 ± 2.74	11.72	0.00
Triglyceride (mmol/L)	1.81 ± 1.32	1.32 ± 1.86	7.55	0.00
Total cholesterol (mmol/L)	5.10 ± 1.17	4.84 ± 0.84	6.08	0.00
SBP (mmHg)	138.27 ± 21.88	134.83 ± 24.48	1.52	0.13
DBP (mmHg)	75.44 ± 18.15	74.19 ± 14.94	1.80	0.07

BUT tear-film break up time, *FL* fluorescein and lissamine green staining, *BMI* Body Mass Index, *SBP* systolic blood *pressure*, *DBP* diastolic blood *pressure*

and positively correlated with FL ($P < 0.05$). The diabetic duration was not correlated with any of the tear film parameters. The HbA1C was negatively correlated with BUT ($P < 0.05$) and positively correlated with FL ($P < 0.05$). The female subjects had shorter BUT, lower SchirmerItest scores and better corneal sensitivity than the males (Tables 3 and 4).

The single factor analysis in diabetic DED patients detected significant variables, including age, gender, corneal sensitivity, blood glucose, HbA1C, diabetes duration, and total cholesterol, as shown in Table 5. No correlation was found between diabetic retinopathy or diabetic nephropathy classification and the prevalence of DED. A dry eye diagnosis was considered to be the dependent variable. The independent variables included age, gender, corneal sensitivity, blood glucose, HbA1C, diabetes duration, and total cholesterol. In the binary logistic regression analysis, the prevalence of DED was significantly associated with a higher glucose ($P < 0.001$, OR1.240) and higher HbA1C ($P < 0.001$, OR1.108). The corneal sensitivity was inversely correlated with the prevalence of DED ($P = 0.02$, OR0.973), indicating that the higher the corneal sensitivity, the lower the prevalence of DED.

Discussion

To the best of our knowledge, this is the first community-based study of DED in type 2 diabetics. In

this study, the prevalence of definitive DED in type2 diabetics was 17.5%, which is much greater than that in the healthy group, but lower than in previously published hospital-based epidemiology studies. First, different diagnostic criteria might affect the prevalence of DED reported in the present and previous studies. For example, Manaviat et al. performed Schirmer and BUT tests and utilized the criterion of one positive test to establish the diagnosis in type 2 hospital-based diabetic patients [5]. Najafi et al. used tear osmolarity values (with a cutoff value of 308 mOsm/L) to diagnose DED in their study [6]. Fuerst et al.showed that 52% of their hospital-based diabetic patients had at least mild DED based on OSDI scores(ranging from 13 to 22) [14]. Second, but more importantly, the poor metabolic status of the hospital-based diabetic patients might also contribute to this difference. For example, HbA1C(%) in one hospital-based study was 8.2 ± 2.2, which was higher than that in the present study [14]. Another significant difference between a hospital-based study and community-based study is the duration of diabetes, which is a well-known correlate of DED. In the study by Manaviat et al., the mean duration of diabetes was 11.48 ± 7.4 years in 108 patients with DED and 9 ± 6.5 years in subjects without DED [5]. However, in our community-based study, the diabetes duration was 9.45 ± 6.24 years in DED patients and 8.01 ± 6.69 years in non-DED patients. Both were

Table 3 Pearson correlation analysis of tear film function and contributing factors in the Diabetic Group

Factor		BUT	SchirmerItest	FL	Corneal Sensitivity
Age	Pearson Correlation	−.104*	.080	.157**	−.246**
	Sig. (2-tailed)	.015	.062	.000	.000
Diabetic duration	Pearson Correlation	.004	−.003	−.072	−.004
	Sig. (2-tailed)	.935	.955	.111	.933
HbA1C	Pearson Correlation	−.111**	.006	.155**	−.051
	Sig. (2-tailed)	.009	.880	.000	.231

BUT tear-film break up time, *FL* fluorescein and lissamine green staining, *HbA1C* glycosylated hemoglobin, * P<0.05, ** P<0.01

Table 4 The tear film function of different gender in the Diabetic Group

Factor	Sub-groups	n	BUT(s)	Schirmer I test	FL	Corneal Sensitivity
Gender	Female	896	3.63 ± 2.10	8.67 ± 5.89	0.59 ± 0.98	55.51 ± 10.21
	Male	464	4.33 ± 2.70	9.59 ± 6.42	0.62 ± 1.16	53.64 ± 10.80
Statistic Value			−5.27	−2.67	− 0.49	3.14
P value			0.00	0.01	0.62	0.00

BUT tear-film break up time, FL fluorescein and lissamine green staining

much shorter than that in the hospital-based study. Therefore, the results of this study provided novel information.

In comparison to the Healthy Group, the Diabetic Group had decreased BUT, Schirmer's test values, and corneal sensitivity and increased FL, in accordance with previous studies [14–17]. In diabetes, damage to the microvasculature feeding the lacrimal gland together with autonomic neuropathy of the lacrimal gland, both of which occur early in the course of diabetes, may contribute to impaired function of the gland [3, 18]. Additionally, sorbitol accumulation within cells can lead to cellular edema and dysfunction, which causes lacrimal gland damage and dysfunction and decreased tear

Table 5 Demographic and clinical characteristics of DED and non-DED subjects among the 1360 community diabetic subjects

Factors	Groups	DED	Non-DED	Statistic Value	P Value
Total Number		238	571		
Age(years)		68.48 ± 8.55	71.30 ± 8.45	4.31	0.00
Gender	Female	157	417		
	Male	81	154	4.07	0.04
Education	Illiterate	18	56		
Level	Primary school	29	87		
	Junior high school	66	142		
	Senior high school	68	189		
	Junior College	32	63		
	Bachelor's degree or higher	25	34	9.24	0.10
Duration of diabetes(years)		9.45 ± 6.24	8.01 ± 6.69	−2.84	0.00
Corneal sensitivity(mm)		52.05 ± 12.52	54.76 ± 10.11	3.23	0.00
BUT(s)		2.70 ± 0.88	5.12 ± 2.99	12.26	0.00
Schirmer I test (mm)		8.62 ± 6.07	9.61 ± 6.28	2.13	0.03
FL		3.74 ± 1.24	0.03 ± 0.20	−69.42	0.00
BMI (kg/m²)		25.50 ± 4.45	25.47 ± 3.97	−0.09	0.92
Glucose (mmol/L)		8.58 ± 2.55	7.33 ± 2.20	−6.61	0.00
HbA1C (%)		7.64 ± 1.55	7.05 ± 1.37	−5.10	0.00
Triglyceride (mmol/L)		1.65 ± 1.22	1.81 ± 1.98	1.16	0.25
Total cholesterol (mmol/L)		5.02 ± 1.05	5.14 ± 1.20	1.34	0.02
DR	Normal	245	407		
	Mild NPDR	5	43		
	Moderate NPDR	19	101		
	Severe NPDR	3	15		
	PDR	3	5	35.67	0.00
Diabetic nephropathy	Normal	391	168		
	microalbuminuria	138	47		
	macroalbuminuria	42	23	2.66	0.26

BUT tear-film break up time, FL fluorescein and lissamine green staining, BMI Body Mass Index, HbA1C glycosylated hemoglobin, DR:diabetic retinopathy, NPDR nonproliferative diabetic retinopathy, PDR proliferative diabetic retinopathy

secretion [19]. Decreased corneal sensitivity is a clinical manifestation of diabetic keratoplasty. A possible mechanism might be that diabetic keratoplasty causes lesions in the corneal epithelial membrane and alters tear protein expression, then tear film function changed and that can lead to DED [20]. Furthermore, reduced corneal sensation can also lead to a reduced blink rate and increased tear evaporation [21]. These potential mechanisms induced DED in the diabetic patients.

The BUT value was found to decrease gradually with increasing age, and the BUT of women was shorter than that of men in the Diabetic Group. However, in contrast to previous studies, age and gender were not found to be relative risk factors for DED in the diabetic group. Possible explanations are that the subjects enrolled in this study were too old (68.91 ± 8.86 years) and that the proportion of male participants in this study was too low. Similarly, Li et al. reported no difference in prevalence of DED between men and women over the age of 60 [10]. The probable cause is reduced tear secretion with aging, or age-related DED, which can affect all exocrine glands in the elderly.

HbA1C is a marker of the average blood glucose level over the 2–3 months prior to measurement. In this study, blood glucose and HbA1C were positively related to the DED prevalence. This result was in accordance with other reports [5, 6, 22]. There are several potential mechanisms for this correlation. Firstly, diabetic patients have an increased level of glucose in their tears, which can increase the expression of advanced glycation end-product(AGE)-modified proteins [23]. The combination of AGEs and receptor for advanced glycation end(RAGE)-products induces a large number of reactive oxygen species (ROS) in corneal epithelial cells, activating downstream signal transduction pathways. The oxidative damage of corneal epithelial cells may result in decreased corneal sensitivity and a delay in wound healing [24]. Secondly, hyperglycemia leads to hyperosmolarity of the tear film and the ocular surface epithelial cells, activating a series of inflammatory responses. Inflammatory cytokines, such as tumor necrosis factor-alpha (TNF-alpha) and matrix metalloproteinase-9 (MMP-9) have been demonstrated to be involved in the pathogenesis of DED [25]. Thirdly, hyperglycemia has also been confirmed to lead to histological alterations in the lacrimal gland. Therefore, diabetes-induced oxidative stress plays an important role in DED [26].

Previous studies have examined the relationship between DED and DR [6, 13]. For example, in a study by Ozdemir et al., the BUT score was lower in participants who had retinal laser treatment than in those who did not have this treatment. This study also showed that subjects with PDR had a lower BUT score compared to subjects with NPDR [13]. However, in our study there was no relationship between the DED prevalence and the DR classification after binary logistic regression analysis. In accordance with Najafi et al. 's study, there was no relationship between the diabetic nephropathy stratification and the prevalence of DED [6]. There may be an indirect correlation between DED and DR, and also between DED and diabietic nephropathy, because all those conditions were more likely to occur in diabetic patients with poor metabolic control.

Our study has some limitations. Firstly, tear osmolarity measurement was not included in dry eye diagnosis. It is important for the diagnosis of Dry Eye, however, it is not widely used in China. Further more, it's difficult to carry out tear osmoloarity measurement which takes a long time and costs high in such a community-based epidemiological investigation. Secondly, the subjects in this study were of old age. The aging of the population is a growing and inevitable social problem. According to census data, 30.2% of the Shanghai population was over the age of 60 at the end of 2015 (the city population was 14.4297 million people). Women were more likely to participate in our study than men, and the gender ratio was suboptimal. Thirdly, meibomian gland function was not included in our study. Since dry eye is associated with meibomian gland dysfunction, future studies should take this aspect into consideration.

Conclusions

In conclusion, DED prevalence was significantly higher in diabetic than healthy subjects, and the overall prevalence of DED was lower in our community-based study than in previous hospital-based studies. Moreover, diabetic patients with poor blood glucose control were more likely to suffer from DED. Therefore, DED testing should be added to the routine screening of diabetes.

Abbreviations
AGE: Advanced glycation end-product; BMI: Body Mass Index; BUT: Tear-film break up time; DBP: Diastolicblood pressure; DED: Dry eye disease; DR: Diabetic retinopathy; FL: Fluorescein and lissamine green stain; HbA1C: Glycosylated hemoglobin; NPDR: Nonproliferative diabetic retinopathy; PDR: Proliferative diabetic retinopathy; RAGE: Receptor for advanced glycation end-products; ROS: Reactive oxygen species; SBP: Systolic blood pressure

Acknowledgements
The authors would like to thank all the staff and participants in the Beixinjing eye study for their valuable skill and support.

Funding
Chinese National Nature Science Foundation (Project number 81670898).
Shanghai Pujiang Program (Project number PJ(2012) 0001652).
Chronic Diseases Prevention and Treatment Project of Shanghai Shen Kang Hospital Development Centre (Grant No. SHDC12015315).
Shanghai Three Year Public Health Action Program (Project No.GWIV-3.3)
Shanghai High-level Oversea Training Team Program on Eye Public Health(Project No.GWTD2015S08).
Shanghai Outstanding Academic Leader Program (Project No.16XD1402300).

Authors' contributions

XZ conducted and analyzed data in this study, wrote and edited the manuscript. LL contributed to concept and design of this epidemiological study. YX, JZ, JH, and BZ participated in data collection and data analysis. HZ participated in the design of this epidemiological study, contributed to the interpretation of the results and discussion, and gave approval to publish this final version. All authors have read and approved the final manuscript.

Competing interests

The authors declare that they have no competing interests.

Author details

[1]Shanghai General Hospital, Nanjing Medical University, No. 100, Haining Road, Hongkou District, Shanghai 200080, China. [2]Department of Preventative Ophthalmology, Shanghai Eye Disease Prevention and Treatment Center, No. 380, Kangding Road, Jingan, Shanghai 200040, China. [3]Department of Ophthalmology, Shanghai General Hospital, Shanghai Jiao Tong University, Shanghai, China. [4]Shanghai Key Laboratory of Fundus Disease, Shanghai, China. [5]Department of Ophthalmology, Fengcheng Hospital, No.9983, Chuannanfeng Road, Fengxian District, Shanghai 201411, China.

References

1. Chen L, Magliano DJ, Zimmet PZ. The worldwide epidemiology of type 2 diabetes mellitus–present and future perspectives. Nat Rev Endocrinol. 2012; 8:228–36.
2. Lemp MA, Foulks GN. The definition and classification of dry eye disease: Report of the definition and classification subcommittee of the international dry eye workshop (2007). Ocul Surf. 2007;5:75–92.
3. Dogru M, Katakami C, Inoue M. Tear function and ocular surface changes in noninsulin-dependent diabetes mellitus. Ophthalmology. 2001;108:586–92.
4. Jin J, Chen LH, Liu XL, Jin GS, Lou SX, Fang FN. Tear film function in non-insulin dependent diabetics [in Chinese]. Zhong Hua Yan Ke Za Zhi. 2003;39:10–3.
5. Manaviat MR, Rashidi M, Afkhami-Ardekani M, Shoja MR. Prevalence of dry eye syndrome and diabetic retinopathy in type 2 diabetic patients. BMC Ophthalmol. 2008;8:10.
6. Najafi L, Malek M, Valojerdi AE, Aghili R, Khamseh ME, Fallah AE, et al. Dry eye and its correlation to diabetes microvascular complications in people with type 2 diabetes mellitus. J Diabetes Complicat. 2013;27:459–62.
7. Shanghai Bureau of Statistics (2016) Statistics bulletin for the national economy and social development in Shanghai [in Chinese]. Available at http://www.stats-sh.gov.cn/html/sjfb/201701/1000339.html. Accessed 4 May 2017.
8. Ayaki M, Kawashima M, Negishi K, Kishimoto T, Mimura M, Tsubota K. Sleep and mood disorders in women with dry eye disease. Sci Rep. 2016;6:35276.
9. Wilkinson CP, Ferris FL 3rd, Klein RE, Lee PP, Agardh CD, Davis M, et al. Proposed international clinical diabetic retinopathy and diabetic macular edema disease severity scales. Ophthalmology. 2003;110:1677–82.
10. Li J, Zheng K, Deng Z, Zheng J, Ma H, Sun L, et al. Prevalence and risk factors of dry eye disease among a hospital-based population in Southeast China. Eye Contact Lens. 2015;41:44–50.
11. Jie Y, Xu L, Wu YY, Jonas JB. Prevalence of dry eye among adult Chinese in the Beijing eye study. Eye. 2009;23:688–93.
12. Liu NN, Liu L, Li J, Sun YZ. Prevalence of and risk factors for dry eye symptom in mainland china: a systematic review and meta-analysis. J Ophthalmol. 2014;2014:748654.
13. Ozdemir M, Buyukbese MA, Cetinkaya A, Ozdemir G. Risk factors for ocular surface disorders in patients with diabetes mellitus. Diabetes Res Clin Pract. 2003;59:195–9.
14. Fuerst N, Langelier N, Massaro-Giordano M, Pistilli M, Stasi K, Burns C, et al. Tear osmolarity and dry eye symptoms in diabetics. Clin Ophthalmol. 2014; 8:507–15.
15. Le Q, Zhou X, Ge L, Wu L, Hong J, Xu J. Impact of dry eye syndrome on vision-related quality of life in a non-clinic-based general population. BMC Ophthalmol. 2012;12:22.
16. Cousen P, Cackett P, Bennett H, Swa K, Dhillon B. Tear production and corneal sensitivity in diabetes. J Diab Complications. 2007;21:371–3.
17. Figueroa-Ortiz LC, Jime´ nezRodrı´guez E, Garcı´a-Ben A,García-Campos J. Study of tear function and the conjunctival surface in diabetic patients. Arch Soc EspOftalmol 2011;86:107–112.
18. Song XJ, Li DQ, Farley W, Luo LH, Heuckeroth RO, Milbrandt J, et al. Neurturin-deficient mice develop dry eye and keratoconjunctivitis sicca. Invest Ophthalmol Vis Sci. 2003;44:4223–9.
19. Ramos-Remus C, Suarez-Almazor M, Russell AS. Low tear production in patients with diabetes mellitus is not due to Sjogren's syndrome. Clin Exp Rheumatol. 1994;12:375–80.
20. Gipson IK, Argueso P. Role of mucins in the function of the corneal and conjunctival epithelia. Int Rev Cytol. 2003;231:1–49.
21. Inoue K, Okugawa K, Amano S, Oshika T, Takamura E, Egami F, et al. Blinking and superficial punctuate keratopathy in patients with diabetes mellitus. Eye (Lond). 2005;19:418–21.
22. Kaiserman I, Kaiserman N, Nakar S, Vinker S. Dry eye in diabetic patients. Am J Ophthalmol. 2005;139:498–503.
23. Liu H, Sheng M, Liu Y, Wang P, Chen Y, Chen L, et al. Expression of SIRT1 and oxidative stress in diabetic dry eye. Int J Clin Exp Pathol. 2015;8:7644–53.
24. Shi L, Yu X, Yang H, Wu X. Advanced glycation end products induce human corneal epithelial cells apoptosis through generation of reactive oxygen species and activation of JNK and p38 MAPK pathways. PLoS One. 2013;8:e66781.
25. Messmer EM, von Lindenfels V, Garbe A, Kampik A. Matrix metalloproteinase 9 testing in dry eye disease using a commercially available point-of-care immunoassay. Ophthalmology. 2016;123:2300–8.
26. Módulo CM, Jorge AG, Dias AC, Braz AM, Bertazolli-Filho R, Jordão AA Jr, et al. Influence of insulin treatment on the lacrimal gland and ocular surface of diabeticrats. Endocrine. 2009;36:161–8.

6

P66Shc expression in diabetic rat retina

Ming-Hui Zhao[1,2], Jianyan Hu[2], Shufeng Li[2], Qiang Wu[2] and Peirong Lu[1]*

Abstract

Background: P66Shc is partially localised within the mitochondrial fraction. It is primarily related to the generation of mitochondrial reactive oxygen species and apoptosis. Based on previous studies, we hypothesize that in the retina, p66Shc may exist and affect the development of diabetic retinopathy. The purpose of this study was to investigate p66Shc expression in retinal in streptozotocin-induced diabetic (SD) rats, which may provide a pathway to study the pathogenesis of diabetic retinopathy.

Methods: Reverse transcription-polymerase chain reaction (RT-PCR) and western blot were used to detect retinal p66Shc mRNA and protein expression in SD rats, respectively. Immunohistochemical staining was applied to detect the location of rat retinal p66Shc expression. TUNEL assay was applied to detect the number of apoptotic cells.

Results: P66Shc expression was found in the retina of normal and diabetic rats, and the level of mRNA and protein expression increased with the progression of diabetes mellitus (DM). P66Shc expression was mainly located in the retinal ganglion cell layer and inner nuclear layer. Compared with the normal group, retinal cell tissue apoptosis rate in the D12w group was significantly increased.

Conclusion: Rat retinal p66Shc expression was mainly in the ganglion cell layer and inner nuclear layer. As the degree of DM progressed, p66Shc expression gradually increased, and the number of apoptotic cells also increased.

Keywords: Diabetic retinopathy, p66Shc, reactive oxygen species, Oxidative stress, Apoptosis

Background

Diabetic retinopathy (DR) is one of the most common complications in both type 1 and type 2 diabetes mellitus (DM). Through a series of mechanisms, such as protein kinase-C activation [1, 2], polyol pathway hyperfunction [3], and the hexosamine pathway [3], reactive oxygen species (ROS) and the advanced glycation end products are generated by hyperglycaemic conditions, which will affect the retinal microvascular structure [4, 5]. Among the spectrum of biochemical changes induced by high-glucose conditions, ROS generation seems to be one of the main pathophysiological mechanisms [6]. Because the eyes constantly exposure to sunlight, atmospheric oxygen, and environmental chemicals, ocular tissues are prone to ROS damage. In addition, free radical-catalysed peroxidation of long-chain polyunsaturated fatty acids (LCPUFAs) will generate LCPUFA metabolites, including isoprostanes and neuroprostanes, which may further exert toxicological and pharmacological actions in ocular tissues [7]. The precise

location and the exact mechanism of physiologically relevant ROS generation within the respiratory chain have not yet been determined, however, it is generally believed that the major site of superoxide production is the respiratory chain in mitochondria. The increase of ROS will activate oxidative stress, and lead to apoptosis. Studies of rats exposed to streptozotocin (STZ) revealed that the apoptosis-specific changes in retinal ganglion cells were observed as early as after 1 month of diabetesspecific metabolic disorders [8, 9]. Noticeably, these changes were not associated with diabetic retinopathy-specific vascular injury [8, 10], which means that the apoptosis is an early pathological feature of DR. Biochemical pathways of apoptosis activation can be extra- or intracellular, and caspase-dependent or caspase-independent [11]. So reducing the extracellular apoptosis inducing signal or interfere with the intracellular apoptosis related signal pathway is important for the prevention and treatment of DR [12, 13].

Adaptor protein p66Shc is a newly recognised mediator of mitochondrial dysfunction. It is expressed in most mammalian tissues. Three isoforms are derived by alternative splicing from the *Shc* locus: p46Shc, p52Shc, and p66Shc [14]. These proteins have 3 same functional

* Correspondence: lupeirongsz@126.com
[1]Department of Ophthalmology, The First Affiliated Hospital of Soochow University, Suzhou 215006, China
Full list of author information is available at the end of the article

domains in structure: a collagen-homology region, Src-homology 2 domain, and a phosphotyrosine-binding domain [14]. Compared with the other two kinds of protein, P66Shc has an additional N-terminal region, which is required for its redox activity [14]. This protein is mainly localised within the mitochondrial fraction, and is primarily associated with mitochondrial ROS generation and apoptosis [15]. Via the oxidation of cytochrome C, p66Shc utilises the mitochondrial electron transfer chain during the generation of hydrogen peroxide (H_2O_2) [16]. P66Shc is entered into the mitochondrial intermembrane space by the form of Ser36 phosphorylation (p-p66Shc) [17]. Former studies showed that p66Shc$^{-/-}$ cells can decrease alterations of mitochondrial DNA, reduce intracellular ROS levels, and resistant apoptosis which was induced by a variety of stimuli, such as ultraviolet radiation, H_2O_2, hypoxia/reoxygenation, and human immunodeficiency virus-1 [17, 18]. Similarly, in p66Shc$^{-/-}$ mice also found increased resistance to oxidative stress and a prolonged life span [18]. They are also prevented the development of diabetic glomerulopathy, possibly by blocking the production of hyperglycaemia-induced ROS [19]. In Graiani et al.'s study, they found that in the ischaemia-reperfusion injury model, mitochondrial dysfunction in renal proximal tubule cells was mediated by p66Shc, which induced apoptosis in myocardial cells [20].

Diabetic nephropathy and DR are the two most common forms of diabetic microvascular complications, and both diseases share a common pathogenesis. Based on these considerations, we postulated that p66Shc could also play a role in the development of DR. The aim of this study was to determine the expression of p66Shc in diabetic retinas.

Methods
Experimental animals
In this study, we used the 3-week-old fasted male Sprague Dawley (SD) rats, which were obtained from Shanghai Sippr-BK laboratory animal Co. Ltd. (Shanghai, China). The mean weight of the SD rats was approximately 150 g. Treatment of animals was compled with the rules of "Instruction and Administration of Experimental Animals", and was approved by the Shanghai Jiaotong University affiliated No.6 hospital. Animals received an intraperitoneal streptozotocin injection (60 mg/kg dissolved in the citric acid solution, pH 4.5) on three successive days. 48 h after STZ injection, the rats with glucose levels > 250 mg/dl were defined as having DM. Non-diabetic age-matched control animals were injected with 0.01 M sodium citrate buffer. According to the DM course, all of the rats were assigned to 3 groups: 15 rats of D4w (4 weeks after diabetes onset) and 15 rats

of D12w (12 weeks after diabetes onset) and 15 rats of not-diabetic control.

Real-time PCR
We used the Trizol method to extract RNA. the primer of *p66Shc* was designed by The PRIMER PREMIER 5.0 software, and was synthesised by Invitrogen Biotechnology Co., LTD (Shanghai, China). Table 1 gives the PCR primer sequences. 1 ml Trizol (Invitrogen Life Technologies, Shanghai, China) was mixed with Retinal tissue, and completely homogenised. Then we put the mixture on ice for about 5 min, in order to allow full denaturation. Then it mixed with 0.25 ml chloroform, oscillated for 15 s and stood for 3 min. At 4 °C, the mixture was centrifuged at 13000 g for 8 min; then supernatant was obtained. After 0.5 ml isopropanol was added and mixed, the mixture stood again for about 10 min at room temperature. At 4 °C, the mixture was centrifuged at 13000 g for 10 min again, and the supernatant was removed. After washed and precipitated the pellet, we added 1.5 ml 75% ethanol, and centrifuged at 13000 g for 5 min at 4 °C. Then we removed supernatant, absorbed the most of the ethanol, precipitated the RNA, and air dried for 5–10 min. Using the RevertAid First Strand cDNA Synthesis Kit (Thermo, Shanghai, China) according to the manufacturer's protocols, total RNA (2 μg) was reverse transcribed. The internal reference gene was *GAPDH*. 95 °C for 10 min, followed by 40 cycles of 95 °C for 15 s and 60 °C for 60 s, the 20 μl reaction mixtures were amplified. The data were analysed using the $2^{-\Delta\Delta Ct}$ method.

Western blot
Retinas were dissected, harvested in radio-immunoprecipitation assay (RIPA) lysis buffer (Beyotime Biotechnology, China), homogenised, and centrifuged at 12000 g for 20 min at 4 °C. The protein sample extracted from the retina was buffered in the liquid, mixed well, and heated in hot water for 10 min, cooled in ice water immediately. We used sodium dodecyl sulphate (SDS)-polyacrylamide gel electrophoresis to conduct gel electrophoresis. Proteins (10–20 μg) were loaded onto an SDS 12% polyacrylamide gel. The proteins were transferred onto polyvinylidene fluoride membranes after electrophoresis. 5% skimmed milk in Tween/Tris-buffered saline (TBST) was used to block nonspecific binding. Membranes were incubated with

Table 1 The PCR primers

Primer	F/R	Sequence (5'-3')
GAPDH	F	TTCCTACCCCCAATGTATCCG
	R	CATGAGGTCCACCACCCTGTT
P66Shc	F	TGTCAATAAGCCCACACGAGG
	R	CTTCACACACCAAACTGATAGCCT

primary antibodies against Shc (1:1000; Santa Cruz, Shanghai, China), and with β-actin (1:2000; KangChen Bio-tech, Shanghai, China) prepared in 5% skimmed milk in TBST overnight at 4 °C. The membrane was washed three times using phosphate buffer solution Tween (PBST) buffer for 15 min in a shaker. The membrane was immersed into the secondary antibody with horseradish peroxidase for 1 h at room temperature. Following three further 15-min washes of the membrane in a shaker using the PBST buffer, by using an enhanced chemiluminescence reaction kit according to the manufacturer's instructions (Goodbio Biological Technology Co., LTD, Wuhan, China), protein bands were visualised and photographed with a Tanon 5500 Imager (Tanon, Shanghai, China). The bands were analysed with AlphaEaseFC (Alpha Innotech, USA). Each band was normalised against the corresponding β-actin band. Changes in expression of protein were expressed as the ratio of diabetic rats versus non-diabetic rats' levels.

Immunohistochemistry (IHC)
Using an abdominal injection of a 2% pentobarbital solution (30 mg/kg) (Goodbio Biological Technology Co., LTD, Wuhan, China), the rats were euthanized. Eyeballs were removed. Then the eyes soaked in 4% paraformaldehyde (phosphate buffer saline (PBS) buffered) for 24 h. In order to eliminate enzymatic activity, retinas were incubated in 3% H_2O_2 for 10 min and washed twice for 5 min using PBS. The samples were blocked using 5% goat serum (diluted in PBS) and incubated at room temperature for 10 min. The blocking serum was removed,primary antibody was added (anti-Shc antibody, 1:125 dilution, Santa Cruz, Shanghai, China), and then be incubated at 4 °C overnight. Retinas were washed twice with PBST, followed by reacting with the secondary immunoglobulin (Dako, Beijing, China) at 37 °C for 30 min. Immunoreactivity was visualised using a Horseradish Peroxidase Colour Development Kit (diaminobenzidine, Goodbio Biological Technology Co., LTD, Wuhan, China), followed by fully washing using running water, and covered with a cover slip. The samples without primary antibody added were as negative controls.

TUNEL assay
In brief, Terminal Deoxynucleotidyl Transferase dUTP Nick End Labeling (TUNEL) assay kit (Roche Applied Science, Sweden) was used to detect tissues apoptosis. Paraffin sections from histological assessment were routinely de-paraffinized, rehydrated, and then rinsed by PBS. TUNEL reaction solution and Converter-POD were added after blocking endogenous peroxidise activity by H_2O_2 in methanol, permeability liquid (1 g/L Triton X-100 was dissolved in 0.1% sodium citrate). 3, 3- diaminobenzidine

(DAB) stained each slice, and then cell apoptosis was observed under a microscope. Cells with brown granules in the nucleus were considered as apoptosis positive cells. Under high magnification field (200×), we randomly selected five fields in each slice. Apoptosis rate means the percentage of apoptosis positive cells relative to the total cell.

Statistical analysis
Statistical analysis was performed using the Statistical Package for Social Sciences (version 11.0, SPSS Inc., Chicago, IL, USA). Data were expressed as the mean standard deviation (SD). The Student's t-test was applied to analyse the difference between the diabetic and control groups. A value of $P < 0.05$ was considered to be statistically significant.

Results
RT-PCR
Rat retinal p66Shc expression was detected by RT-PCR, and was found in the normal, D4w and D12w groups. With the progress of DM, p66Shc expression increased ($P < 0.05$ in D4w, and $P < 0.01$ in D12w, compared to normal group) (Fig. 1).

Western blot
As for mRNA, protein expression was found in the normal, D4w and D12w groups. The expression level increased with the progress of DM (P < 0.05 in D4w, and $P < 0.01$ in D12w, compared to normal group) (Fig. 2).

Immunohistochemistry (IHC)
P66Shc was mainly expressed in the ganglion cell layer (GCL) and inner nuclear layer (INL) of the retina in normal rats. With the progression of DM, the expression was

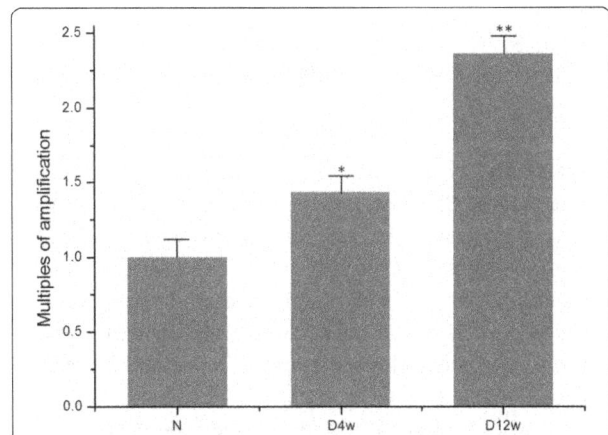

Fig. 1 RT-PCR showed that the level of rat retinal p66Shc mRNA expression significantly increased over 12 weeks of diabetes mellitus (N: control group, D4w: 4 weeks after diabetes onset, D12w: 12 weeks after diabetes onset, *P < 0.05, **P < 0.01, compared to control)

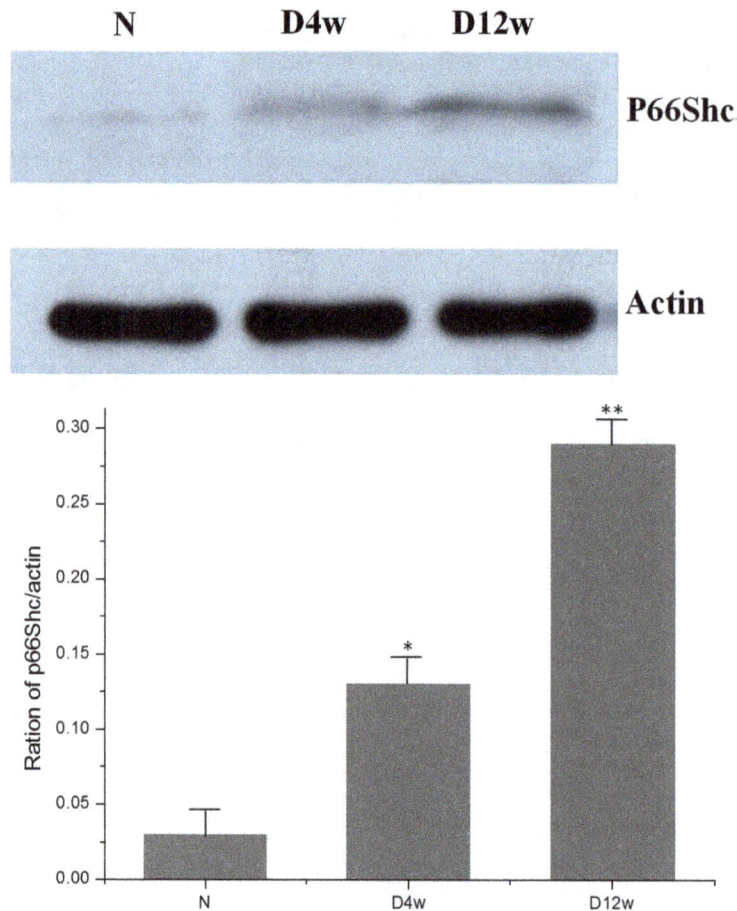

Fig. 2 P66Shc protein expression significantly increased with the progression of diabetes mellitus (N: control group, D4w: 4 weeks after diabetes onset, D12w: 12 weeks after diabetes onset, *$P < 0.05$, ** $P < 0.01$, compared to control)

increased. In the D12w group, p66Shc was expressed in all retinal layers, and was more concentrated in the GCL and INL (Fig. 3).

Apoptosis analysis

Compared with the normal group, retinal cell tissue apoptosis rate in the D12w group was significantly increased ($P < 0.01$) (Fig. 4).

Discussion

DM is one of the most common oxidative-stress related diseases. It seems that oxidative stress from the mitochondrial electron-transport chain and the excessive production of superoxide anion mediate hyperglycaemic damage [21]. Jain and colleagues found that in diabetic patients, peroxidation of membrane lipids was increased, and malonyldialdehyde in erythrocytes was accumulated. The possible reasons for these may be that during periods of poor metabolic control,the blood levels of ketone bodies increased [22], as well as the effect of increased levels of circulating cytokines, including tumour necrosis factor-α and interleukin-6 [23].

Our study followed the course of DM for 12 weeks in the SD rats to investigate whether p66Shc is expressed in the retina and what changes occur in DM. The results showed that p66Shc was expressed in the retina of normal and DM groups both at the mRNA and protein levels. Compared to the normal group, p66Shc expression in the DM groups was statistically increased, which suggested that there was some degree of relationship between the course of the disease and the expression of p66Shc. This was similar to previous studies of p66Shc expression in other diseases. Earlier studies suggested that p66Shc is a vital adaptor protein that regulates oxidative stress and life span in mammalian cells. Genetic deletion of p66Shc attenuated hyperglycaemia-induced endothelial dysfunction and oxidative damage [24, 25]. In ventricular pacing-induced cardiomyopathy dog models, a progressive p66Shc overexpression was induced by increased ROS production and mitochondrial dysfunction, which was correlated with cytochrome c release, parameters of ventricular dysfunction, and activation of procaspases [26]. P66Shc expression and activity are significantly increased in the kidneys of SD

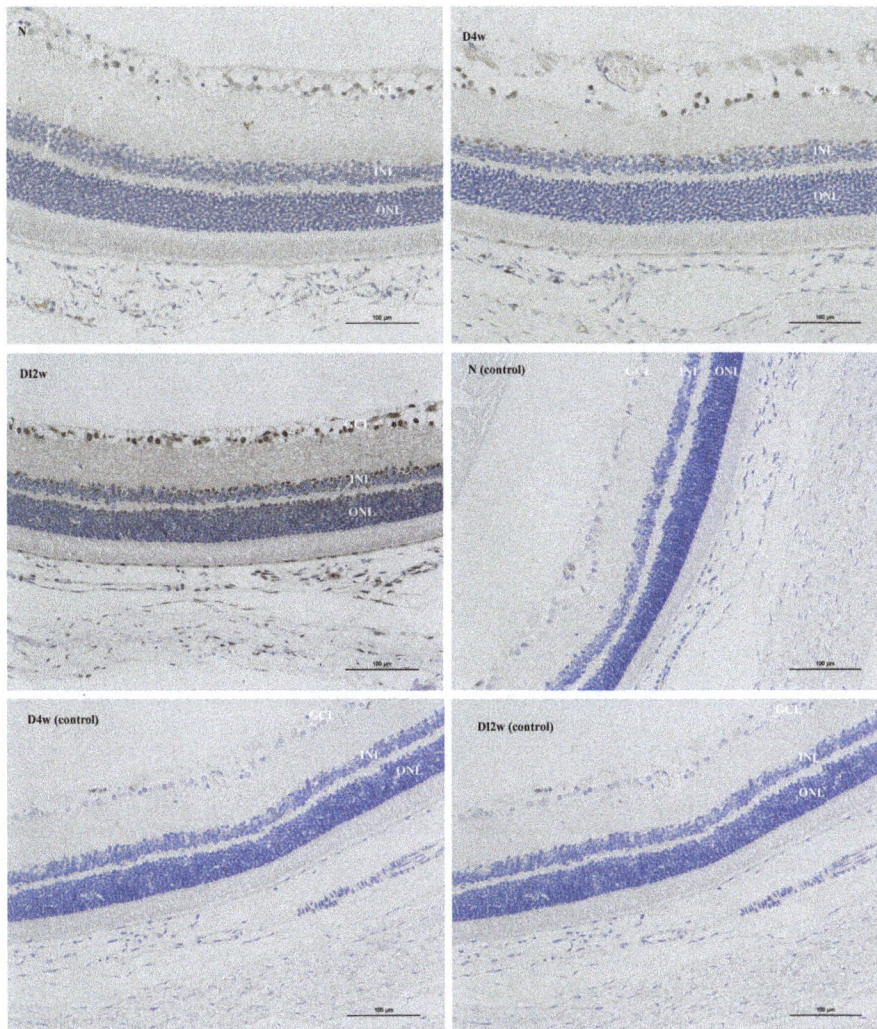

Fig. 3 Immunohistochemical staining of frozen sections. P66Shc was expressed in the retina of normal rats and of rats with diabetes mellitus (DM). Greater p66Shc expression was found in the DM group compared to the control group. The expression increased with the progress of DM. (N: control group, D4w: 4 weeks after diabetes onset, D12w: 12 weeks after diabetes onset, control: the samples without primary antibody added)

rats and db/db mice (a type 2 diabetic mouse model) [27]. In contrast, P66-null Akita mice display marked attenuation of oxidative stress and glomerular/tubular injury and a distinct reduction in urine albumin excretion [27]. The deletion of p66Shc also reduced tissue damage [28] and vascular cell apoptosis [29], as well as protect against ROS-mediated, age-dependent endothelial dysfunction [30]. All these studies suggested that p66Shc is associated with increased oxidative damage [31]. Intracellular ROS availability was increased by P66Shc induction, which in turn affects the rate of oxidative damage.

The p66Shc expression site in the rat retina was detected by frozen-section immunohistochemical staining. It was observed that in normal rat retinas, p66Shc was expressed, mainly in the GCL and INL. As the progression of disease, the expression increased, and in the D12w group, p66Shc was observed in all retinal layers,

mainly in the GCL and INL. TUNEL assay suggested that with the progression of DM, the number of apoptotic cells increased. Barber et al. [32] analyzed paraffin-embedded retinal specimens from STZ-exposed rats, obtained after 30 weeks of experimentally induced diabetes, and found that a 10% reduction in the total number of retinal ganglion cells, along with a 22% decrease in the thickness of the inner ganglion layer of the retina, and a 14% decrease in the thickness of the inner nuclear layer. Interestingly, no changes in the thickness of the outer ganglion cell layer, which suggested that the processes of apoptosis are more intense within the inner layers of the retina [32]. Oxidative stress activates stress-related signalling to trigger apoptosis [33]. Diabetic glomerulopathy in wild-type mice without direct intervention (e.g. STZ injection) was associated with cell-death rate and enhanced extracellular matrix protein

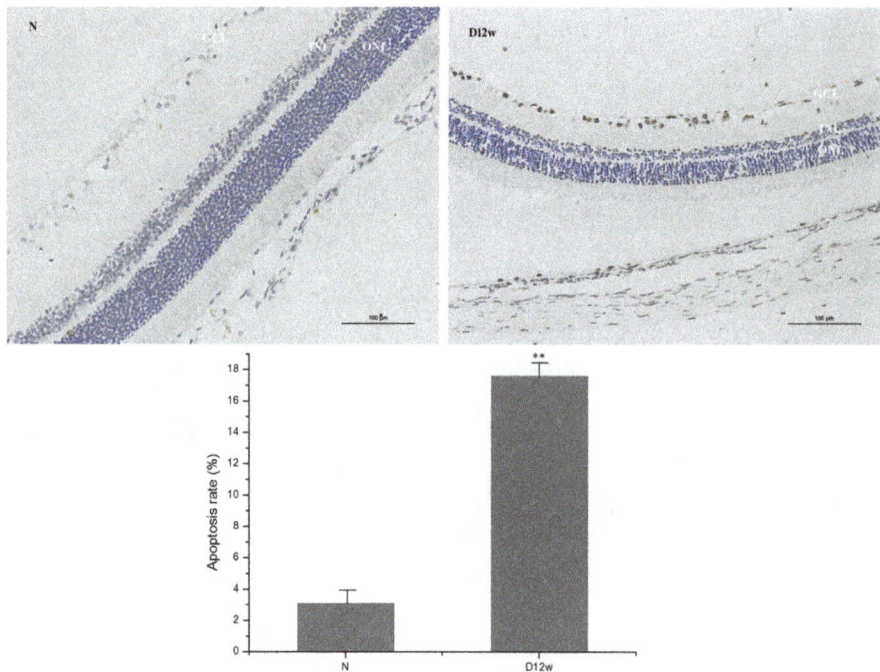

Fig. 4 The detection of apoptotic cells by TUNEL assay for DNA Strand break labeling. TUNEL positive (brown nuclei) and negative cells were further counted for apoptosis rate. (N: control group; D12w: 12 weeks after diabetes onset, **$P < 0.01$, compared with control group)

expression. Renal p66Shc mRNA and protein levels also increased in diabetic wild-type mice [34, 35]. On the contrary, no increase in the glomerular cell-death rate was found in diabetic p66Shc knockout (KO) mice, meanwhile, compared to wild-type diabetic mice, less marked matrix deposition was found in KO mice. ROS levels, glucose-induced apoptosis, and upregulation of extracellular matrix were no or significantly attenuated in mesangial cells from KO mice, which supporting the concept that p66Shc protein deficiency was associated with reduced susceptibility to diabetes-induced oxidative stress, attenuated changes in cell turnover and matrix, and reduced apoptosis [19].

P66Shc expression is regulated by multiple factors. For example, its phosphorylation is regulated by adaptor protein Eps8 together with E3b1; meanwhile Rac1 can reduce ubiquitylation and increase the stability of p66Shc protein [36]. Sos1 and Eps8/E3b1 form a complex, which can activate Rac1 [36]. P66Shc can detach Sos1 from the growth factor receptor-bound protein 2 (Grb2)/Sos1 pool and transfer it with the Eps8/E3b1 pool, which activate Rac1 and result increased generation of oxidants [37]. During severe oxidative stress, the combination of p66Shc with activated epidermal growth factor receptor (EGFR) and Grb2 increased. This binding results in the separation of the Sos1 adaptor protein from the EGFR-recruited signalling complex. Ras/MEK/ERK (extracellular-signal regulated kinase) activation was terminated [38]. Conversely, p66Shc is

tyrosine phosphorylated by receptor tyrosine kinases which were stimulated by growth factors. It is unable to activate the Ras-MAPK-Fos pathways after the tyrosine-phosphorylated P66Shc binds Grb2 [18]. The Ras signalling pathway is also inhibited when p66Shc is over-expressed by the stimulation of cytokines or growth factors [37]. By insulin growth factor, p66Shc inhibit stimulation of the MEK (MAPK-ERK Kinase)/ ERK pathway as well.

In general, p66Shc is implicated in receptor tyrosine kinase signal transduction, and is classically known as a signalling protein. By Ser36 phosphorylation of the protein, p66Shc plays a role in accumulation of intracellular ROS. It has been regarded as a longevity protein and a sensor of oxidative stress-induced apoptosis in mammals. P66Shc expression and/or function changes may play an important role in the pathogenesis of type 2 diabetes, so it may be an effective target for the treatment of DR.

This study has shown that there was p66Shc expression in rat retinal tissues, and the expression was increased along with the progression of DM. These results may offer some explanation about the relationship between p66Sch and DR, and help to understand the mechanism of DR, which may potentially allow its treatment at an earlier stage. Further studies are still required in the p66Shc-specific functional mechanism in DR.

Conclusion

Rat retinal p66Shc expression was mainly in the ganglion cell layer and inner nuclear layer. As the degree of DM progressed, p66Shc expression gradually increased, and the number of apoptotic cells also increased.

Abbreviations

DM: Diabetes mellitus; DR: Diabetic retinopathy; IHC: Immunohistochemistry; LCPUFAs: Long-chain polyunsaturated fatty acids; PBS: Phosphate buffer saline; PBST: Phosphate buffer solution Tween; RIPA: Radio-immunoprecipitation assay; ROS: Reactive oxygen species; RT-PCR: Reverse transcription-polymerase chain reaction; SD: Streptozotocin-induced diabetic; STZ: Streptozotocin; TBST: Tween/Tris-buffered saline; TUNEL: Terminal Deoxynucleotidyl Transferase dUTP Nick End Labeling

Acknowledgements
The authors thank Edanz English editing company for modifying this manuscript.

Funding
No funding was obtained for this study.

Authors' contributions
PR Lu conceived of the study, and participated in its design. MH Zhao participated in the design of the study, feed and handled the animals. JY Hu participated in histochemistry and immunoassay. SF Li performed the statistical analysis. Q Wu participated in immunoassay. All authors read and approved the final manuscript.

Competing interests
The authors declare that they have no competing interests.

Author details
[1]Department of Ophthalmology, The First Affiliated Hospital of Soochow University, Suzhou 215006, China. [2]Department of Ophthalmology, Shanghai Jiaotong University Affiliated Sixth People's Hospital, Shanghai 200233, China.

References
1. Xu X, Zhu Q, Xia X, Zhang S, Gu Q, Luo D. Blood retinal barrier breakdown induced by activation of protein kinase C via vascular endothelial growth factor in streptozotocin induced diabetic rats. Curr Eye Res. 2004;28:251–6.
2. Sheetz MJ, King GL. Molecular understanding of hyperglycemia's adverse effects for diabetic complications. JAMA. 2002;288:2579–88.
3. Naruse K, Nakamura J, Hamada Y, Nakayama M, Chaya S, Komori T, et al. Aldose reductase inhibition prevents glucose induced apoptosis in cultured bovine retinal microvascular pericytes. Exp Eye Res. 2000;71:309–15.
4. Yao D, Taguchi T, Matsumura T, Pestell R, Giardino L, Suske G, et al. High glucose increases angiopoietin 2 transcription in microvascular endothelial cells through methylglyoxal modification of mSin3A. J Biol Chem. 2007;282:31038–45.
5. Pfister F, Feng Y, vom Hagen F, Hoffmann S, Molema G, Hillebrands JL, et al. Pericyte migration: a novel mechanism of pericyte loss in experimental diabetic retinopathy. Diabetes. 2008;57:2495–502.
6. Di Mario U, Pugliese G. 15th Golgi lecture: from hyperglycaemia to the dysregulation of vascular remodelling in diabetes. Diabetologia. 2001;44:674–92.
7. Njie-Mbye YF, Kulkarni-Chitnis M, Opere CA, Barrett A, Ohia SE. Lipid peroxidation: pathophysiological and pharmacological implications in the eye. Front Physiol. 2013;4:366.
8. Fan TJ, Han LH, Cong RS, Liang J. Caspase family proteases and apoptosis. Acta Biochim Biophys Sin. 2005;37:719–27.
9. Yang JH, Kwak HW, Kim TG, Han J, Moon SW, Yu SY. Retinal neurodegeneration in type II diabetic otsuka long-evans Tokushima fatty rats. IOVS. 2013;54:3844–51.
10. Bringmann A, Wiedemann P. Muller glial cells in retinal disease. Ophthalmologica. 2012;227:1–19.
11. Barber AJ, Gardner TW, Abcouwer SF. The significance of vascular and neural apoptosis to the pathology of diabetic retinopathy. IOVS. 2011; 52:1156–63.
12. Rungger-Brandle E, Dosso AA, Leuenberger PM. Glial reactivity, an early feature of diabetic retinopathy. IOVS. 2000;41:1971–80.
13. Du X, Matsumura T, Edelstein D, Rossetti L, Zsengellér Z, Szabó C, Brownlee M. Inhibition of GAPDH activity by ploy (ADP-ribose) polymerase activates three major pathways of hyperglycemic damage in endothelial cells. J Clin Invest. 2003;112:1049–57.
14. Ray PD, Huang BW, Tsuji Y. Reactive oxygen species (ROS) homeostasis and redox regulation in cellular signaling. Cell Signal. 2012;24:981–90.
15. Trinei M, Berniakovich I, Beltrami E, Migliaccio E, Fassina A, Pelicci P, et al. P66Shc signals to age. Aging. 2009;1:503–10.
16. Giorgio M, Migliaccio E, Orsini F, Paolucci D, Moroni M, Contursi C, et al. Electron transfer between cytochrome c and p66Shc generates reactive oxygen species that trigger mitochondrial apoptosis. Cell. 2005;122:221–33.
17. Pinton P, Rimessi A, Marchi S, Orsini F, Migliaccio E, Giorgio M, et al. Protein kinase C beta and prolyl isomerase 1 regulate mitochondrial effects of the life-span determinant p66Shc. Science. 2007;315:659–63.
18. Migliaccio E, Giorgio M, Mele S, Pelicci G, Reboldi P, Pandolfi PP, et al. The p66Shc adaptor protein controls oxidative stress response and life span in mammals. Nature. 1999;402:309–13.
19. Menini S, Amadio L, Oddi G, Ricci C, Pesce C, Pugliese F, et al. Deletion of p66Shc longevity gene protects against experimental diabetic glomerulopathy by preventing diabetes-induced oxidative stress. Diabetes. 2006;55:1642–50.
20. Graiani G, Lagrasta C, Migliaccio E, Spillmann F, Meloni M, Madeddu P, et al. Genetic deletion of the p66Shc adaptor protein protects from angiotensin II-induced myocardial damage. Hypertension. 2005;46:433–40.
21. Brownlee M. Biochemistry and molecular cell biology of diabetic complications. Nature. 2001;414:813–20.
22. Jain SK, Kannan K, Lim G, McVie R, Bocchini JA Jr. Hyperketonemia increases tumor necrosis factor-α secretion in cultured U937 monocytes and type 1 diabetic patients and is apparently mediated by oxidative stress and cAMP deficiency. Diabetes. 2002;51:2287–93.
23. Jain SK, Kannan K, Lim G, Matthews-Greer J, McVie R, Bocchini JA Jr. Elevated blood interleukin-6 levels in hyperketonemic type 1 diabetic patients and secretion by acetoacetate-treated cultured U937 monocytes. Diabetes Care. 2003;26:2139–43.
24. Camici GG, Schiavoni M, Francia P, Bachschmid M, Martin-padura I, Hersberger M, et al. Genetic deletion of p66Shc adaptor protein prevents hyperglycemia-induced endothelial dysfunction and oxidative stress. Proc Natl Acad Sci. 2007;104:5217–22.
25. Tomilov AA, Bicocca V, Schoenfeld RA, Giorgio M, Migliaccio E, Ramsey JJ, et al. Decreased superoxide production in macrophages of long-lived p66Shc knock-out mice. J Biol Chem. 2010;285:1153–65.
26. Cesselli D, Jakoniuk I, Barlucchi L, Beltrami AP, Hintze TH, Nadal-Ginard B, et al. Oxidative stress-mediated cardiac cell death is a major determinant of ventricular dysfunction and failure in dog dilated cardiomyopathy. Circ Res. 2001;89:279–86.
27. Vashistha H, Meggs L. Diabetic nephropathy: lessons from the mouse. Ochsner J. 2013;13:140–6.
28. Zaccagnini G, Martelli F, Fasanaro P, Magenta A, Gaetano C, Di Carlo A, et al. P66Shc a modulates tissue response to hindlimb ischemia. Circulation. 2004; 109:2917–23.

29. Napoli C, Martin-Padura I, de Nigris F, Giorgio M, Mansueto G, Somma P, et al. Deletion of the p66Shc longevity gene reduces systemic and tissue oxidative stress, vascular cell apoptosis, and early atherogenesis in mice fed a high-fat diet. Proc Natl Acad Sci U S A. 2003;100:2112–6.

30. Francia P, delli Gatti C, Bachschmid M, Martin-Padura I, Savoia C, Migliaccio E, et al. Deletion of p66Shc gene protects against age-related endothelial dysfunction. Circulation. 2004;110:2889–95.

31. Sun L, Xiao L, Nie J, Liu FY, Ling GH, Zhu XJ, et al. P66Shc mediates high-glucose and angiotensin II-induced oxidative stress renal tubular injury via mitochondrial-dependent apoptotic pathway. Am J Physiology-Renal Physiol. 2010;299:F1014–25.

32. Barber AJ, Antonetti DA, Kern TS, Reiter CE, Soans RS, Krady JK, et al. The Ins2Akita mouse as a model of early retinal complications in diabetes. IOVS. 2005;46:2210–8.

33. Rozakis-Adcock M, McGlade J, Mbamalu G, Pelicci G, Daly R, Li W, et al. Association of the Shc and Grb2/Sem5 SH2-containing proteins is implicated in activation of the Ras pathway by tyrosine kinases. Nature. 1992;360:689–92.

34. Mishra R, Emancipator SN, Kern T, Simonson MS. High glucose evokes an intrinsic proapoptotic pathway in mesangial cells. Kidney Int. 2005;57:82–93.

35. Lee FT, Cao Z, Long DM, Panagiotopoulos S, Jerums G, Cooper ME, et al. Interactions between angiotensin II and NF-kappaB-dependent pathways in modulating macrophage infiltration in experimental diabetic nephropathy. J Am Soc Nephrol. 2004;15:2139–51.

36. Innocenti M, Tenca P, Frittoli E, Faretta M, Tocchetti A, Di Fiore PP, et al. Mechanisms through which Sos-1 coordinates the activation of Ras and Rac. J Cell Biol. 2002;156:125–36.

37. Pacini S, Pellegrini M, Migliaccio E, Patrussi L, Ulivieri C, Ventura A, et al. P66SHC promotes apoptosis and antagonizes mitogenic signaling in T cells. Mol Cell Biol. 2004;24:1747–57.

38. Arany I, Faisal A, Nagamine Y, Safirstein RL. P66Shc inhibits pro-survival epidermal growth factor receptor/ERK signaling during severe oxidative stress in mouse renal proximal tubule cells. J Biol Chem. 2008;283:6110–7.

7

Evaluation of day care versus inpatient cataract surgery performed at a Jiangsu public Tertiary A hospital

Min Zhuang[1,2], Juan Cao[1], Minglan Cui[1], Songtao Yuan[1], Qinghuai Liu[1] and Wen Fan[1*]

Abstract

Background: High cataract incidence and low cataract surgical rate are serious public health problems in China, despite the fact that efficient day care cataract surgery has been implemented in some public Tertiary A hospitals in China. In this study, we compared not only clinical outcomes, hospitalization time and total costs but also payment manners between day care and inpatient procedures for cataract surgery in a Jiangsu public Tertiary A hospital to put forward several instructional suggestions for the improvement of government medical policies.

Methods: In total, 4151 day care cases and 2509 inpatient cases underwent the same cataract surgery in the day care ward and ordinary ward respectively, and were defined as two groups. General information, complications, postoperative best corrected visual acuity (BCVA), hospitalization time, total costs and especially payment method were analyzed to compare day care versus inpatient.

Results: The general data display no significant differences ($P > 0.05$), and no significant difference between complications and postoperative BCVA were observed between the two groups ($P > 0.05$). The period of stay in hospital was significantly different ($P < 0.001$). The total costs were lower for day care than for inpatients ($P < 0.001$). To avoid sampling error, we analyzed the data of payment manner for each patient among this period. Day care patients tended to pay for the procedure using the Urban Employees Basic Medical Insurance (UEBMI) method, while inpatients tended to use the Out-of-Pocket Medical Treatment (OMT) payment method ($P < 0.001$).

Conclusion: Day surgery of cataract is more cost-effective and efficient than inpatient surgery with equivalent clinical outcomes. As an efficient therapeutic regimen, day care surgery should be further promoted and supported by the government policies.

Keywords: Day care, Inpatient, Cataract

Background

A cataract is an opacity of the lens in the eyes, which can lead to blurry vision or blindness. Cataracts may be classified into three categories: age-related cataracts, metabolic cataracts, and cataracts secondary to other causes. Age-related cataracts are the most common type in adults [1]. With a rapidly growing and aging population, the incidence of cataracts is subsequently increasing. WHO estimated that there were 95 million people visually impaired due to cataracts in 2014. According to the former

therapeutic regimen, patients prefer being hospitalized for several days for cataract surgery, while the concept of day care cataract surgery is currently increasingly introduced [2]. In the U.S. and Europe and America over 60% cases of cataract surgeries are carried out as day care surgeries. Day surgery, a fast and safe therapeutic regimen [3], is a surgical procedure wherein hospitalization, surgery and discharge occur within 24 h after a short post-operative recovery. Ophthalmologic operations are short and quick, making them suitable for day surgery, which allows for a more effective use of medical resources and reduction of average hospitalization days. It has been shown that inpatient care for age-related cataract surgery may not only be cheaper,

* Correspondence: fanwen1029@163.com
[1]Department of Ophthalmology, The First Affiliated Hospital with Nanjing Medical University, Nanjing, China
Full list of author information is available at the end of the article

but also as effective as inpatient treatment after the same surgery [4].

Cataracts are the leading cause of blindness and the second-leading cause of vision loss in China [5]. With the promotion of "Vision 2020-the Right to Sight" propaganda, the rate of cataract surgury has increased in China in recent years [6]. In the past ten years, it has made great progress in blindness prevention and treatment. In 2005, the number of cataract extractions was only 572,000, at the rate of 440 cases per one million people, per year. By 2014, the number of cataract extractions reached 1.9 million cases, a rate of 1400 cases per one million people, per year [7]. Despite this, some patients continue to avoid or refuse cataract surgery due to the costs and fear of surgery [8]. Until now, the high incidence of cataracts and low surgical rate is still a serious public health problem. It is essential to develop day surgery cataract treatment programs due to the fact that they use fewer hospital resources, are cheaper, and more efficient than those procedures which result in ordinary hospitalization.

In 2011, the International Association for Ambulatory Surgery (IAAS) defined day surgery in the UK and Ireland as: the patient must be admitted and discharged on the same day, with day surgery as the intended management [9]. The rate of day care cataract surgery is almost 100% in Denmark and nearly 0% in Austria [10]. In China, day surgery has been implemented only in recent years, later than other countries, but has been implemented in Hong Kong since the 1990s [11]. China joined the IAAS officially in May 2013, as the 22nd member. By October 2014, 28 municipal hospitals performed day surgeries, and from January to October 2014, the daily proportion of day surgeries of the top 10 hospitals accounted for 76.9% of the municipal hospitals in Shanghai [12]. Today, day surgery of cataracts is more widely accepted morethan previously in China [13, 14]. The day care cataract surgery has been implemented by the Ophthalmology of the First Affiliated Hospital of Nanjing Medical University since August 1, 2014, which was the first hospital implementing day surgery in Jiangsu Province.

China launched a government-run mandatory insurance program, the Urban Employee Basic Medical Insurance (UEBMI) at the end of 1998. Current and former employees of urban enterprises and institutions are insured with UEBMI. Rural populations are mainly insured by New Rural Cooperative Medical Care. While the other medical insurances include Urban Residents Basic Medical Insurance (URBMI), Poverty Salvation Free Medical Care, Free medical care. Meanwhile, some citizens pay for their medical care out-of-pocket or are covered by other medical insurances.

In this study, we compared the differences between day care and inpatient cataract surgery, the results of which will guide the further application of day care or inpatient care following cataract surgery.

Methods

Data of patients who underwent cataract operations was pulled from the cataract operation HIS database of the First Affiliated Hospital of Nanjing Medical University from August 1, 2014 to December 31, 2016. There are no absolute contraindications for day surgery patients. Patients with stable chronic medical conditions are considered to be suitable for day surgery [15]. At the First Affiliated Hospital of Nanjing Medical University, patients chose day care or inpatient cataract surgery on a voluntary basis. During this period, all fee standards remained the same, and there was no day care patient transferred to the ordinary ward due to severe surgical complications. In this retrospective cohort study, inclusion and exclusion criteria included: 1) Patients were at least age thirty with a stable state of health and were diagnosed with cataracts in one or both eyes; 2) Patients with other ocular comorbidities that could affect the postoperative prognosis was ruled out by fundus assessment; 3) Each patient underwent surgery for only one eye; 4) All the patients were operated upon under topical anesthesia and were performed cataract surgery by phacoemulsification combined with posterior chamber intraocular lens implantation.These two groups were respectively termed as day care group and inpatient group. The surgeons in the two groups were the same, all of whom were senior doctors with rich clinical experience, performing over 5000 cases of phacoemulsification.The surgical processesfollowed standard procedures [1]. The length from the patient's registration to check-out was called hospitalization time, and less than a day was counted as one day. The costs consisted of the operation treatment fee, cost of the intraocular lens, anesthesia fee, preoperative inspection fee,cost of drugs, and expense of nursing care and hospital bed. All the patients had ophthalmic examinations including BCVA testing, slit-lamp examination, and intraocular pressure at one day, one week, one month, and three months after surgery. BCVA was examined on the basis of standard logarithmic visual acuity chart (GB11533–2011).

Based on these two groups, we analyzed differences of gender, age, and preoperative Best Corrected Visual Acuity (BCVA) between the two groups. Intraoperative posterior capsule rupture was also analyzed. Postoperative complications including cornea edema and intraocular hypertension the first day after surgery, and postoperative BCVA one month after surgery were analyzed. Meanwhile the differences of the hospitalization time, total costs and payment manners between the two groups were also analyzed. All statistical analyses were assessed using a t-test and χ2 test by IBM SPSS Statistics 24, and $P < 0.05$ was considered to be statistically significant.

Results

General information

A total of 2809 males (1724 in the day care group and 1085 in the inpatient group) and 3851 females (2427 in the day care group and 1424 in the inpatient group) patients were included in the current study. The average age was 70.54 ± 11.5 in the day care group and 70.01 ± 12.59 in the inpatient group. The average preoperative BCVA was 3.82 ± 0.48 in the day care group and 3.80 ± 0.50 in the inpatient group. Generally, there were no significant differences in gender ($P = 0.170$), age ($P = 0.150$), or preoperative visual acuity ($P = 0.062$) between day care patients and inpatients (Table 1).

Complications and outcomes

Posterior capsule rupture (PCR) as a intraoperative complication ($P = 0.715$) was noted in 291 cases in the day care group and in 170 cases in the inpatient group (Table 2). The main postoperative complications such as cornea edema ($P = 0.973$) and intraocular hypertension ($P = 0.569$) occurring the first day after surgery were noted in both groups (Table 2). The average postoperative BCVA was 4.84 ± 0.18 in the day care group and 4.86 ± 0.84 in the inpatient group, with no significant difference ($P = 0.290$) between the two groups (Table 3). As aforementioned, there were no significant differences in intraoperative complications, postoperative complications, and postoperative BCVA between the two groups.

Hospitalization time and costs

The average hospitalization time was 1 ± 0 days for the day care group and 4.40 ± 1.69 days for the inpatient group. Those patients who chose the day care option for cataract surgery were hospitalized for a much shorter time ($P < 0.001$) than those who chose the inpatient procedure (Table 3). The average costs paid by patients in the day care group were ¥6893.68 $\pm$ 1362.89. While the average costs paid by inpatients were ¥7849.70 $\pm$ 1432.70, the total costs paid by patients in the day care group were less ($P < 0.001$) than those in inpatient group (Table 3). In

Table 2 Intraoperative and postoperative complications

Complications		Number of participants (%)		P
		Day care (total $n = 4151$)	Inpatient (total $n = 2509$)	
	+	291 (7.0%)	170 (6.8%)	
Posterior capsule rupture				0.715
	–	3860 (93.0%)	2339 (93.2%)	
	+	466(11.2%)	281 (11.2%)	
Cornea edema				0.973
	–	3685 (88.8%)	2228 (88.8%)	
	+	323 (7.8%)	205 (8.2%)	
Intraocular hypertension				0.569
	–	3828 (92.2%)	2304 (91.2%)	

n number of participants; + numbers of participants having complications; – numbers of participants not having complications; $P > 0.05$ shows no significant difference

conclusion, day surgery of cataracts is more efficient and cost-effective than inpatient surgery.

Medical insurances

To minimize sampling error, the data of payment method for each patient who underwentcataract surgery within two years was analyzed. There were over six methods with which to pay for total costs of the medical care. Two main methods were Urban Employees Basic Medical Insurance (UEBMI) and Out-of-pocket Medical Care (OMC) (details in Table 4). There was a significant difference in these main payment methods between these two groups ($P < 0.05$).

Discussion

In our study, the clinical outcomes exhibited by the patients of the day care group were nearly equivalent to those of the inpatient group, underscoring the safety and effectivity of cataract day surgery. The results also demonstrated that day care surgery shortened the patient's hospitalization time, which according to the patients' satisfaction investigations, resulted in a reduction of nervousness, anxiety, and mental stress caused by the long-term hospital stay subsequently reducing the operation burden and improving patient satisfaction. Before the cataract surgery, patients were typically required to undergo general examinations

Table 1 General information before the surgery

Information		Day care (total $n = 4151$)	Inpatient (total $n = 2509$)
Gender	Male	1724	1085
	Female	2427	1424
Age		70.54 ± 11.51	70.01 ± 12.59
Preoperative BCVA		3.82 ± 0.48	3.80 ± 0.50

The data of gender were presented as number of participants (%); the data of age and preoperative BCVA were presented as average ± SD

Table 3 General information after the surgery

Information	Average ± SD		P
	Day care (total $n = 4151$)	Inpatient (total $n = 2509$)	
Postoperative BCVA	4.84 ± 0.18	4.86 ± 0.84	0.290
Hospitalization time (days)	1 ± 0	4.40 ± 1.69	< 0.001
Costs (¥)	6893.68 ± 1362.89	7849.70 ± 1432.70	< 0.001

Total $n = 1000$; $P > 0.05$ shows no significant difference

Table 4 Different payment manners for surgery expenses

Payment manners	Number of participants (%)		P
	Day care (total $n = 4151$)	Inpatient (total $n = 2509$)	
Urban employees basis medical insurance	2029 (48.9%)	765 (30.5%)	< 0.001
Urban residents basic medical insurance	73 (1.8%)	70 (2.8%)	0.006
New rural cooperative medical care	3 (0.1%)	3 (0.1%)	0.533
Poverty salvation	0 (0%)	2 (0.1%)	0.069
Free medical care	197 (4.7%)	102 (4.1%)	0.214
Out-of-pocket medical care	1768 (42.6%)	1529 (60.9%)	< 0.001
Others	81 (2.0%)	38 (1.5%)	0.200

n number of participants; $P > 0.05$ shows no significant difference

and tests, the expenses of which were included in the total costs paid by inpatients and not included in the total costs paid by day surgery patients. As these expenses were a small part of the total cost, they were not the leading cause of the the difference in cost between day care and intpatient procedures. At the same time, hospitalization costs including ward bed expenses, nursing expenses, and treatment expenses were significantly reduced due to the shortened hospitalization time. Day surgery patients were discharged from hospital within 24 h, which had the dual benefit of greatly reducing the total hospitalization costs and accelerating the turnover of hospital beds, leaving more hospital beds available for severe cases and subsequently greatly increasing the efficiency of bed utilization.

UEBMI was the first basic medical insurance established during medical security system reform in China. With the principle of "wide coverage and low level", it provides basic medical insurance for urban workers by combining government subsidies and medical insurance premiums payed by individuals and enterprises together (called "social pooling combined with personal accounts"). [16]. The government has also launched a project called Poverty Salvation For The Poor. Free medical service refers to a social security system implemented by China to cover state staff and offers free medical treatment and preventive service provided by the medical and health departments according to the regulations. Currently, one of the biggest bottlenecks in the development of day surgery in China is the inability to manage the reimbursement. Some studies showed that the reimbursement level of medical insurance was an important factor influencing patients' choice of day surgery [17]. In many areas of China, day care procedures are not reimbursed by the hospital, or only the expenses for the operation can be reimbursed, excluding the preoperative inspection expenses. Although some terms have already been piloted, there is still no national standard for payment, limiting the development of day surgeries in China. Patients in this study mostly chose two methods

(UEBMI and OMC) to pay the expenses, and patients who chose UEBMI in the day care group were more than those in inpatient group, mainly because local residents with UEBMI preferred day care due to the aforementioned advantages. Patients who chose OMC in the inpatient group were more than those in the day care group. For example, most non-Nanjing natives who had other medical insurances at their registered permanent residence, chose inpatient for cataract surgery because they had to pay the medical costs through OMC and apply for reimbursement back to the origin residence. Day care medical expenses not being reimbursed may be the reason why more OMC patients chose regular hospitalization and not day care procedures.

In order to improve day surgery, the Guidelines on Comprehensive Reform Pilot of Urban Public Hospitals announced by General Office of the State Council in May 2015 (No.38 [2015] of the General Office of the State Council) clarified that diagnosis and therapy technologies including day surgery should be gradually brought into the scope of medical insurance payments on the basis of normalizing day surgeries. In 2015, 20 day surgeries including age-related cataract were brought into single diseases in Jiangsu province. Twenty-three day surgeries have been paid according to medical insurance since 2016, with the highest reimbursement rate reaching 85% in Jiangxi province [18]. The Guidelines on Comprehensive Reform Pilot of Urban Public Hospitals announced by General Office of the State Council on June 28, 2017 (No.55 [2017] of the General Office of the State Council) clarifies the importance of medical insurance payments for day surgeries again. In this study, we didn't distinguish the costs of differingartificial lenses, which made the results less rigorous. In further studies, this could be improved by a larger sample size.

In conclusion, our results confirm that cataract day surgery is high-quality and low-cost. Medical insurance payments for day surgery is need urgent improvement. Further optimization and reorganization of the medical service process is essential for day care wards of hospitals to form a high efficiency management and operation system, making it convenient for patients to seek medical treatment and reducing the economic burden patients experience. Along with the rapid economic development in our country, the organization and effective use of medical resources is an urgent and immediate concern.

Conclusions

In this study, we compared the differences between day care and inpatient cataract surgery, the results of which confirm that day care cataract surgery is high-quality and low-cost. Given these results, it is recommendable that the practice of day care cataract surgery be expanded in China.

Abbreviations
BCVA: Best Corrected Visual Acuity; IAAS: International Association for Ambulatory Surgery; OMT: Out-of-Pocket Medical Treatment; PCR: Posterior capsule rupture; UEBMI: Urban Employees Basic Medical Insurance; URBMI: Urban residents basic medical insurance

Funding
No funding was received by any of the authors for the writing of this manuscript.

Authors' contributions
MZ, STY and WF designed the research. MZ, JC and MLC performed all experiments and analyzed the data. MZ, JC and MLC prepared the manuscript. QHL and WF interpreted and edited the manuscript. All authors discussed the results and commented on the manuscript. All authors read and approved the final manuscript.

Competing interests
The authors declare that they have no competing interests.

Author details
[1]Department of Ophthalmology, The First Affiliated Hospital with Nanjing Medical University, Nanjing, China. [2]Department of Ophthalmology, The Fourth Affiliated Hospital of Nantong University, Yancheng, China.

References
1. Liu YC, Wilkins M, Kim T, Malyugin B, Mehta JS. Cataracts. Lancet. 2017; 390(10094):600–12.
2. Ingram RM, Banerjee D, Traynar MJ, Thompson RK. Day-case cataract surgery. Br J Ophthalmol. 1983;67(5):278–81.
3. Nicoll JH. The surgery of infancy—I. Pediatr Anesth. 1998;8(3):248.
4. Hamed W, Fedorowicz Z. Day care versus in-patient surgery for age-related cataract. Cochrane Database Syst Rev. 2011;1:CD004242.
5. Wong TY, Zheng Y, Jonas JB, Flaxman SR, Keeffe JE, Leasher JL, Naidoo K, Pesudovs K, Price H, White RA. Prevalence and causes of vision loss in East Asia: 1990–2010. Br J Ophthalmol. 2014;98(5):599–604.
6. Zhao JL. Chinese ophthalmologists should firmly promote vision 2020 action. Practical Journal of Clinical Medicine. 2010;6:1-3.
7. Zhao J. Change to "prevention of the avoidable blindness and visual impairment" from "prevention of blindness". Zhonghua Yan Ke Za Zhi. 2015;51(7):481–3.
8. Wu M, Yip JLY, Kuper H. Rapid assessment of avoidable blindness in Kunming, China. Ophthalmology. 2008;115(6):969–74.
9. Britainireland AOAOG. Day case and short stay surgery: 2. Anaesthesia. 2011;66(5):417–34.
10. Mojonazzi SM, Mojon DS. The rate of outpatient cataract surgery in ten European countries: an analysis using data from the SHARE survey. Graefes Arch Clin Exp Ophthalmol. 2007;245(7):1041.
11. Hospital CCL. The development of day surgery in Hong Kong. Chinese Hospital Management. 1997(7):31–31.
12. Zhao R, Yang L, Zhang WW, Liu GH, Du N, Liu J, Jia TY, Zhang W. Assessment of the development of ambulatory surgery in shanghai municipal hospitals. Chinese Hospitals. 2015;4:7-10.
13. Wei Y, Liang Y, Wu Y, Chen M. Application of clinical pathway with day-care unit mode among patients with cataract. Chinese Health Quality Management. 2016;23(4):55–7.
14. Lin J, Fang X, Wu S. the management pattern carried out in a cataract surgery day ward. Eye Sci. 2013;28(2):79–83.
15. Ng L, Mercerjones M. Day case surgery guidelines. Surgery (oxford). 2014;32(2):73–8.
16. Lin W, Liu GG, Chen G. The urban resident basic medical insurance: a landmark reform towards universal coverage in China. Health Econ. 2009;(18):83–96.
17. Fang L, Cao J, Wang M, Du N, Yang L, Zhao R, Li G. Comparison research on day surgery in different countries implementing different medical insurance system. Chinese Hospitals. 2014;18(10):78–80.
18. Yu L. Development and Prospect of day surgery in China. Chinese Hospital Management. 2016;36(6):16–8.

8

Characterization, treatment and prognosis of retinoblastoma with central nervous system metastasis

Huimin Hu[1†], Weiling Zhang[1†], Yizhuo Wang[1], Dongsheng Huang[1*] (iD), Jitong Shi[2], Bin Li[2], Yi Zhang[1] and Yan Zhou[1]

Abstract

Background: Retinoblastoma is the most common primary intraocular tumor and more and more attention has been paid to the developing countries. This study was aimed to evaluate the clinical features, treatment, and prognosis of retinoblastoma patients with central nervous system (CNS) metastasis in Beijing Tongren Hospital, one of the largest tertiary eye centers in China.

Methods: Clinical data of 31 consecutive retinoblastoma patients with CNS metastases, who were diagnosed at the Department of Pediatrics in Beijing Tongren Hospital between September 2005 and December 2015, were retrospective analyzed.

Results: The median age at presentation was 29 months (range from 5 to 108 months). Magnetic resonance imaging (MRI) results indicated that 16 patients (56.6%, 16/31) presented with meningeal involvement, 12 (38.7%, 12/31) presented with intracranial mass, 11 (35.5%, 11/31) presented with thickened optic nerve, and 5 (16.1%, 5/31) presented with concurrent meningeal and spinal cord membrane involvement. Retinoblastoma cells were detected in the cerebrospinal fluid (CSF) of 12 patients (44.4%, 12/27). Laboratory examinations on the blood and CSF were performed for 11 patients who had received six cycles of systemic chemotherapy, indicated that the serum level of neurone-specific enolase (NSE) after chemotherapy was significantly lower than that before chemotherapy ($P < 0.05$). At the end of the follow-up, 25 patients were dead with a median survival time of 6 months (1 d – 21 months), and 6 cases were alive and continued to receive treatment.

Conclusion: Our results were basically consistent with previous reports in the developing countries, and it could be guidance for clinical treatment, prognosis and prevention of CNS metastases in retinoblastoma.

Keywords: Retinoblastoma, Central nervous system metastasis, Pediatric

Background

Retinoblastoma is the most common intraocular malignancy in infancy and childhood, with an reported incidence of 1 per 15,000–20,000 live births [1], whereas accounts for 3% of all pediatric cancers [2]. The overall survival rate of retinoblastoma was reported to exceed 95% when children were early diagnosed with localized intraocular phase [3, 4]; however, delayed diagnosis and treatment, which is common situation in the developing countries, may lead to extraocular metastasis, visual loss and death. Meanwhile, secondary to the advanced retinoblastoma cases with central nervous system (CNS) metastasis is associated with exceedingly poor prognosis [5, 6]. Therefore, treatment of retinoblastoma patients with CNS metastases should be tailored to the individual according to the clinical conditions and nature of the tumors. Conventional therapies generally include systematic chemotherapy, enucleation, radiotherapy, even autologous peripheral blood stem cell transplantation (APBSCT), etc. [5].

Management of metastatic retinoblastoma is gaining more and more attention in China, which is a developing

* Correspondence: dongshuang_dr@sina.com
†Equal contributors
[1]Department of Pediatrics, Beijing Tongren Hospital, West South road 2, Yizhuang Economic and Technological Development Zone, Daxing District, Beijing 100176, China
Full list of author information is available at the end of the article

Characterization, treatment and prognosis of retinoblastoma with central nervous system...

51

country with the largest population. The objective of current study was to evaluate and summarize the clinical features, treatment, and prognosis of retinoblastoma patients with CNS metastases, who were treated at the Department of Pediatrics in Beijing Tongren Hospital, one of the largest and best-known tertiary eye centers in China.

Methods

A total of 1404 retinoblastoma patients were received at the Department of Pediatrics in Beijing Tongren Hospital, Beijing, China, between September 2005 and December 2015. Then 31 consecutive retinoblastoma patients who diagnosed with CNS metastasis were eligible for this study and clinical data were analyzed retrospectively. The study protocol was approved by the Medical Ethics Committee of the Beijing Tongren Hospital, and all participants gave their written informed consent. Orbital computed tomography (CT) scan, cranial CT scan and/or cranial magnetic resonance imaging (MRI) examination were performed in all patients. Trilateral retinoblastoma was excluded from the study. American Joint Committee on Cancer TNM clinical classification system [7] was used for the assessment of the whole patient by extent of extraocular disease (Additional file 1: Table S1). Orbital enhanced MRI, cranial MRI, contrast enhanced CT scan of the lungs, bone marrow cytology, hepatobiliary lymph node ultrasonography, superficial lymph nodes ultrasound and cerebrospinal fluid cytology examination were performed for extraocular patients in order to definite specific TNM stages.

Multi-drug combination chemotherapy was adopted in our treatment, including vincristine (1.5 mg/m^2, day 1), etoposide/teniposide (100 mg/m^2, day 2–3), carboplatin (560 mg/m^2, day 1), and cyclophosphamide (65 mg/kg, day 2). In each cycle of the chemotherapy, lumbar puncture and intrathecal injection were performed for every patient with methotrexate (MTX), cytosine arabinoside (Ara-c), and dexamethasone (Dex) according to the following regimen: age < 12 months: MTX (5.0 mg), Ara-c (12.0 mg), Dex (2.0 mg); age 12–24 months: MTX (7.5 mg), Ara-c (15.0 mg), Dex (2.0 mg); age 25–35 months: MTX (10.0 mg), Ara-c (25.0 mg), Dex (5.0 mg); age ≥ 36 months: MTX (12.5 mg), Ara-c (35.0 mg), Dex (5.0 mg). Routine biochemistry of Cerebrospinal fluid (CSF) and cytology examinations were performed; moreover, neuron specific enolase (NSE) in serum and CSF of patients were analyzed using the electrochemiluminescence with the NSE Kit (Roche, US).

Cranial and orbital contrast-enhanced MRI examinations were routinely performed every two chemotherapy cycles. Children patients with CNS metastases were received radiation therapy at the dose of 40 Gy after chemotherapy. Tumor spreads through the cerebrospinal fluid was generally required craniospinal irradiation, and the

dose of radiotherapy is not more than 40 Gy. Adverse reactions to radiotherapy and chemotherapy were evaluated according to CTCAE standard [8]. APBSCT treatment (APBSCT regimen: CBP 425 mg/ (m^2.d); from − 6 to − 3 days + VP-16: 338 mg/ (m^2.d); From − 6 to − 3 days + CTX: 1.5 g / (m^2.d) was performed for 2 patients after achieving a stable disease condition.

Table 1 Clinical characteristics of retinoblastoma patients with CNS metastasis

Characteristics	Data
Gender (male), n (%)	14 (45.2)
Age at presentation (months), median (range)	29 (5 to 108)
Laterality	
Bilateral, n (%)	8 (25.8)
Unilateral, n (%)	23 (74.2)
Right eyes, n (%)	14 (60.9)
Family history, n (%)	1 (3.2)
Lag period between first symptom and initiation of treatment (months), median (range)	3 (0.03–21)
T stages at first diagnosis	1 (1–24)
M stage at first diagnosis	6 (0.5–12)
TNM stages at first diagnosis, n (%)	
T1	3 (9.7)
T2	0
T3	10 (32.3), (T3a:6; T3b:4)
T4	4 (12.9), (T4a:3; T4b:1)
M	14 (45.2)
MRI features, n (%)	
Meningeal involvement	16 (56.6)
Meningeal and spinal cord membrane involvement	5 (16.1)
Intracranial mass	12 (38.7)
Thickened optic nerve	11 (35.5)
Involvement of other systematic organs, n (%)	
CNS with intraorbital involvement	12 (38.7)
CNS with bone	10 (32.3)
CNS with bone marrow	1 (3.2)
CNS with lung	2 (6.5)
CNS with pleura	1 (3.2)
CNS with mass of the lateral wall of pelvis	1 (3.2)
Surgery	
Enucleation	24 (77.4)
Exenteration	5 (16.1)
CSF cytology positive	12 (44.4, 12/27)

CNS: central nervous system; MRI: magnetic resonance imaging; CSF: cerebrospinal fluid

Statistical analysis was performed using SPSS software (version 20.0, IBM, USA). For continuous variables, data were presented as mean ± standard deviation or median (Q25, Q75), and were compared using Student's paired t-tests or Wilcoxon matched-pairs signed-rank test. A value of $P < 0.05$ was considered statistically significant. Kaplan-Meier survival curve was plotted to analyze the survival time after the diagnosis of CNS metastasis, the median survival time was also calculated.

Results

Of the enrolled 31subjects, 14 retinoblastoma cases were diagnosed CNS metastasis at the time of first RB diagnosis. 17 retinoblastoma cases were detected CNS metastases at some later point, the median time/range from RB diagnosis to CNS metastasis was 9 months (3-23 months). 23 (74. 2%) were unilateral, and 8 (25.8%) were bilateral advanced retinoblsatoma. The median age at the time of patient visit was 29 months (range from 5 to 108 months). The median lag period of 31 patients between first symptom and initiation of treatment was 3 months. The median lag period of subjects at T stage (17/31) between first symptom and initiation of treatment was 1 month, whereas the median lag period was 6 months for patients at M stage (14/31). Detailed clinical characteristics are shown in Table 1. MRI results showed that the proportion of subjects with meningeal involvement accounts for 56.6% (16/31), followed by presented with, 12 intracranial mass (38.7%, 12/31) and thickened optic nerve (35.5%, 11/31).Representative MRI results of retinoblastoma patients with CNS metastases are also shown in Fig. 1. In addition, a positive rate of retinoblastoma cells in CSF cytology was 44.4% (12/27). Two patients' parents were unable to accept eye enucleation, although all images of retinoblastoma showed an indication of enucleation. Images of CSF cytology and histopathology examinations are shown in Fig. 2. Autopsy was

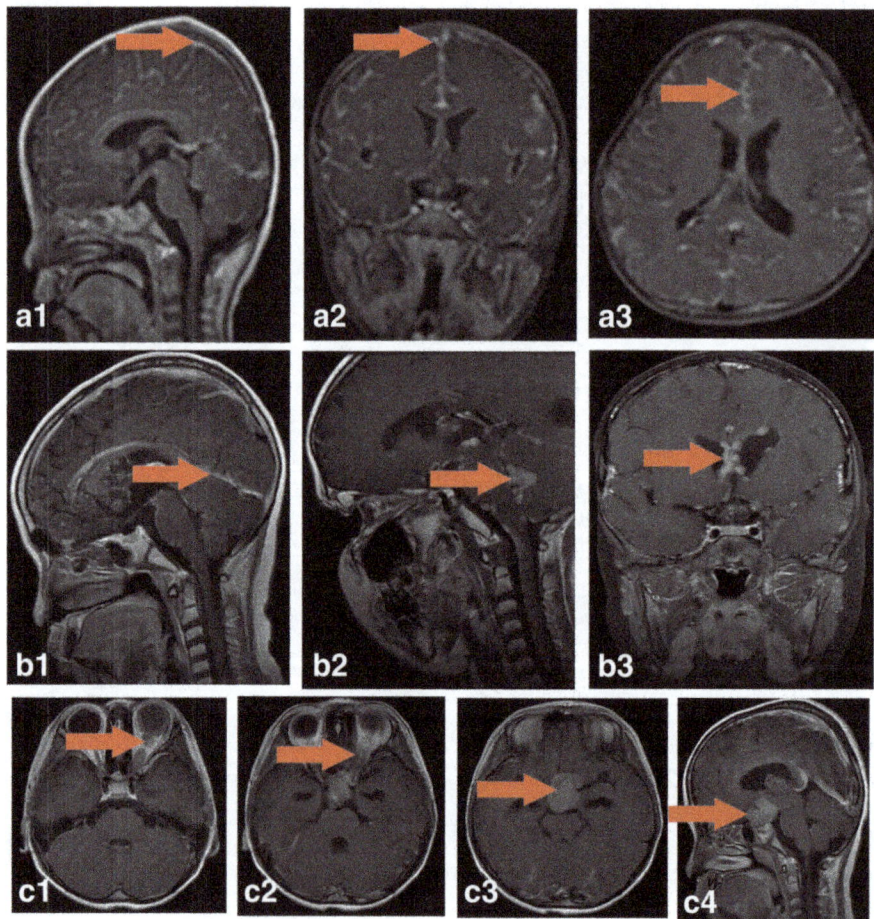

Fig. 1 Representative MRI results of retinoblastoma patients with CNS metastasis. (**a**1–3) Head contrast-enhanced MRI: visible diffuse enhancement of the intracranial pial from sagittal, axial, and coronal imaging, respectively, cervical spinal cord membrane also show enhancement. (**b**1–3) Head and orbital contrast-enhanced MRI: sagittal image shows thickened meninges of the anterior, middle and posterior cranial fossa, brain stem surface, and the cerebellum (**b**1); and orbital MRI images show enhanced signaling of nodules, possibly spreading via the cerebrospinal fluid (**b**2–3). (**c**1–4) Head MRI: signs of optical nerve, optic chiasma, and supra sella cistern involvement, respectively (**c**1–3); visible mass formed in the supra sella cistern, and enhanced signal of the cerebral falx (**c**4). MRI: magnetic resonance imaging; CNS: central nervous system

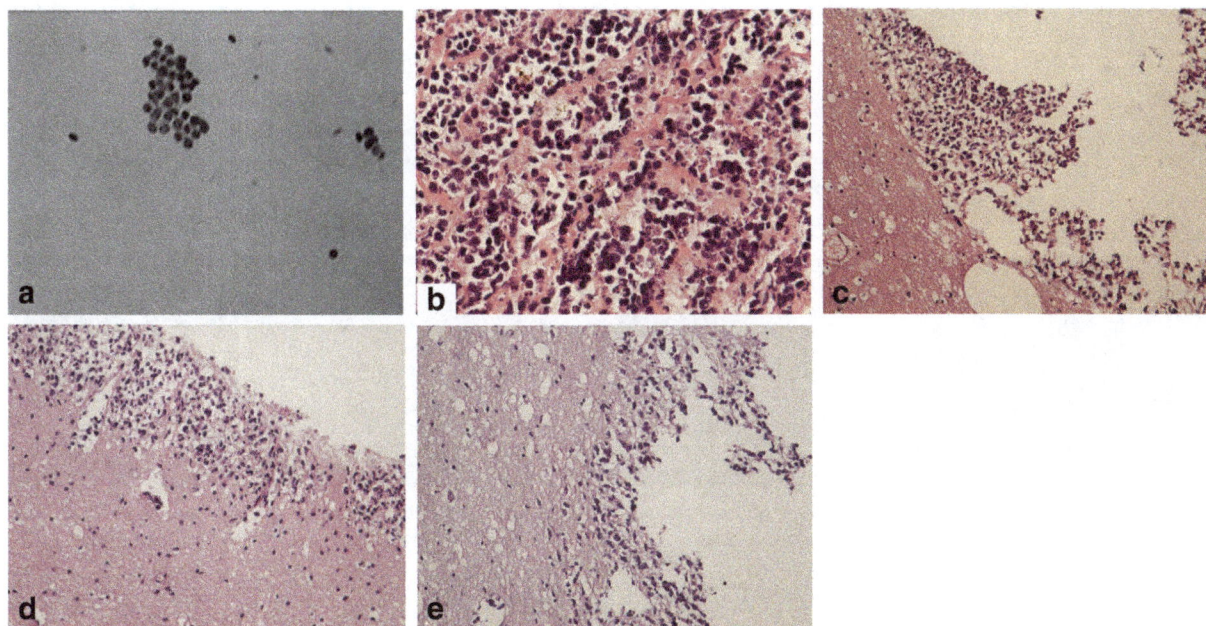

Fig. 2 Representative images of CSF cytology and histopathology in retinoblastoma patients with CNS metastasis. Retinoblastoma cells as shown in the CSF smear (**a**, × 200), and tumor cells spreading in the optic nerve (**b**, × 200), left temporal lobe (**c**, × 100), mesencephalon (**d**,× 100), and cerebellomedullary (**e**,× 100) as stained by haematoxylin and eosin. CSF: cerebrospinal fluid; CNS: central nervous system

suggested and performed in one patient, who was the first retinoblastoma patient with orbital exente ation diagnosed in our department, but no metastasis was found by cranial MRI. Then the patient was dead after six months of chemotherapy. The autopsy results indicated that the optic nerve, left temporal lobe, antennal lobe, mesencephalon, and cerebellomedullary were all affected. Complications of chemo-radiotherapy were evaluated, and mainly including headache, vomit, fever, and myelo suppression, and all attenuated after the treatment. Neither hemorrhagic cystitis nor peripheral nervous system damage was found.

Laboratory examinations were performed for the serum and CSF samples after six cycles of systemic chemotherapy (11 cases). As shown in Table 2, the level of neurone-specific enolase (NSE) in serum was found to be significantly decreased after chemotherapy (31.70 (26.50, 45.60) µg/L versus 91.20 (45.50, 6.20) µg/L, $P < 0.05$), and white blood cell count in CSF was also reduced after chemotherapy (4.27 ± 1.60 × 10^6/L versus 80.36 ±

18.69 × 10^6/L, $P < 0.05$). Contrast-enhanced MRI results showed tumor size and meningeal enhancement were attenuated after treatment (Fig. 3).

All patients were followed up until March 31, 2016, and at the end point death. Among the 31 cases, 25 patients were dead with a median survival time of 6 months (1 day – 21 months), and 6 patients with disease were alive with a median follow-up time of 6 months (2–36 months) and were continually under therapy. Kaplan-Meier survival curve is plotted as shown in Fig. 4.

Discussion

In the present study, among the 31 cases of retinoblastoma patients with CNS metastasis, 12 cases were found to have intraorbital involvement; consistently, it was reported that retinoblastoma patients with intraorbital involvement tend to have systemic metastasis and a high mortality rate, and the CNS metastasis is the most common [6]. As previously reported, retinoblastoma with invasion of the

Table 2 Laboratory examination results of the blood and CSF samples from 11 patients after six cycles of systemic chemotherapy

Parameters	Normal range	Pre-chemotherapy	Post-chemotherapy
Serum NSE, µg/L	0–16.3	91.20 (45.50, 6.20)	31.70 (26.50, 45.60)*
CSF NSE, µg/L	0–16.3	54.60 (31.50, 196.40)	24.00 (9.60, 51.20)
CSF protein, g/L	0.15–0.45	0.34 (0.08, 0.83)	0.30 (0.07, 0.45)
CSF white blood cell, ×10^6/L	0–10	80.36 ± 18.69	4.27 ± 1.60*

Data are presented as median (Q25, Q75), or mean ± standard deviation. *$P < 0.05$ versus pre-chemotherapy. *CNS*: central nervous system; *NSE*: neurone-specific enolase; *CSF*: cerebrospinal fluid

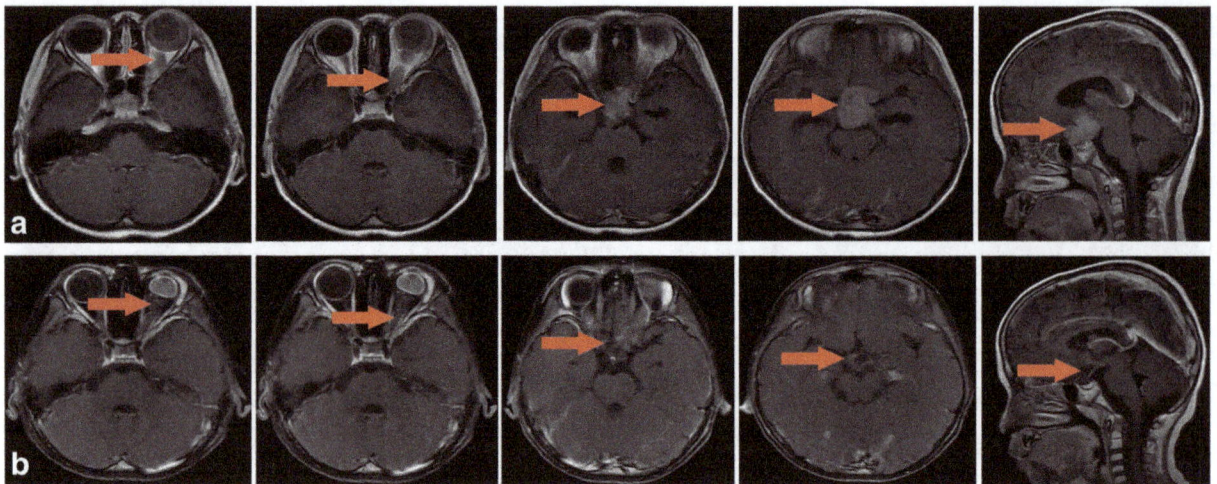

Fig. 3 Contrast-enhanced MRI images of tumor regression and attenuated meningeal enhancement after chemotherapy. Coronal, and sagittal images show the mass in the supra sella cistern and enhanced signal of cerebral falx before chemotherapy (**a**), which were improved after chemotherapy (**b**). MRI: magnetic resonance imaging

postlaminar optic nerve is at high risk of metastasis and death [9]. We also found that the percentage of optic nerve involvement was as high as 35.5% (11/31). The median lag period between first symptom and initiation of treatment for patients with M stage is 6 months, whereas 1 month for T stage patients. There has been demonstrated that the longer lag period was associated with higher risk of CNS metastasis [10]. Thus, shortening the lag period has been considered as an important target of treatment.

It is well known that retinoblastoma is the most common intraocular malignancy in childhood in developed

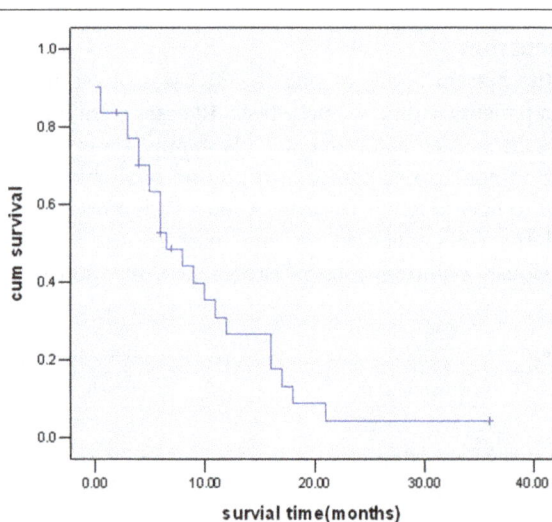

Fig. 4 Kaplan-Meier survival curve of retinoblastoma patients with CNS metastasis. CNS: central nervous system

countries. Secondary to late presentation, advanced retinoblastoma with metastatic disease is more common in developing countries and is associated with delayed diagnosis and extremely poor prognosis. Secondary to the poor overall prognosis of retinoblastoma cases with CNS metastases can be classified metastatic retinoblastoma patients into those presenting with or without CNS disease. MRI can serve as a useful adjunct method for diagnosis in retinoblastoma with CNS metastasis [11]. Our results show that, meningeal and/or spinal cord membrane involvement, and intracranial mass were most common image features in retinoblastoma patients with CNS metastasis, which is consistent with a previous report [7]. The metastasis occurrence was mainly due to direct invasion of the optic chiasma, intracranial optical nerve, supra sella cistern, meninges, even locally brain parenchyma. Meningeal involvement combined with spinal cord membrane involvement might be due to the meninges invasion and/or the spreading of CSF. Meanwhile, other metastasis pathways such as hematogenous metastasis might be also involved cases with bone and bone marrow metastasis, and pulmonary and pleural metastasis. Thus systemic contrast-enhanced MRI is necessary for the diagnosing and monitoring.

CSF examination was regarded as a gold standard for diagnosing CNS metastasis in retinoblastoma patients, and repeated could increase the sensitivity [12, 13]. In the present study, a positive rate of CSF cytology (44.4%) was consistent with reported previously. One of the reasons for negative results (15 cases) in our study was not received repeated CSF examinations. Therefore, we suggest that repeated CSF cytology examination can elevate the detection rate of CNS metastasis during the process of treatment.

NSE, a 78-kDa dimeric γ-isoenzyme of the glycolytic enzyme enolase, is localized predominately in the cytoplasm of neurons and neuroendocrine cells. The elevated NSE levels have been shown in retinoblastoma patients. Thus, NSE levels of CSF and the serum are the standard at our institution. The CSF was taken from the patients with optic nerve invasion and CNS metastasis before intrathecal injection to perform CSF and biochemical routine examinations, also included NSE and pathological examinations [14, 15]. In the present study, NSE levels were found to be elevated in both serum and CSF samples of retinoblastoma patients with CNS metastasis. It might be more NSE was released into the serum and CSF due to tumor invasion. Meanwhile, retinoblastoma cells might also contribute to the NSE secretion. In addition, NSE levels were decreased after systematic chemotherapy, indicating that NSE might have a potential role in the diagnosis and therapeutic effect.

Regarding the fact that extraocular retinoblastoma is very common in the developing countries. Palliative-care protocols such as chemo- and radiotherapy are urgently needed, also it is necessary to optimize. Based on previous reports [16–19], chemotherapy provides a good palliation of extraocular retinoblastoma, even multi-drug combination chemotherapy was adopted in our department, including vincristine, etoposide/teniposide, carboplatin, and cyclophosphamide, combined with intrathecal injection treatment in each cycle of the chemotherapy. Our results also showed that NSE level in the serum and white blood cell count were significantly reduced after chemo and radiotherapy [20]. Furthermore, findings of the present study are consistent with Palma et al. who reported a significantly improved in treatment with APBSCT [21], suggesting it play a potential role in the treatment of retinoblastoma.

Although varied in different studies, the prognosis of retinoblastoma with CNS metastasis is fairly poor, especially in the developing countries [6, 22, 23]. Consistently, in our study, the median survival time was as short as 6 months; this might be due to missed diagnosis or mismanagement before the referral, and denial of management by parents, etc.

Conclusion

In the present study, we reported the characteristics, treatment, and prognosis of retinoblastoma with CNS metastasis at the Department of Pediatrics in Beijing Tongren Hospital,.one of the largest and best-known tertiary eye centers in China. The outcomes of our study were similar to those expected in the developing countries. Since the early diagnosis and timely treatment are vital for a good prognosis, thus, much more efforts are needed to increase the public awareness, implement appropriated education programs for pediatricians and ophthalmologists, and improve the health care accessibility.

Abbreviations
APBSCT: Autologous Peripheral Blood Stem Cell Transplantation; CNS: Central Nervous System; CSF: Cerebrospinal Fluid; CT: Computed Tomography; MRI: Magnetic Resonance Imaging; MTX: Methotrexate; NSE: Neuron Specific Enolase; NSE: Neurone-specific Enolase

Funding
The funding was Beijing Key Laboratory of Intraocular Tumor Diagnosis and Treatment (No. 2016YNZL04).

Authors' contributions
DSH, HMH and WLZ conceived the design. HMH and YZW wrote the manuscript. JTS and BL analyzed the data. YZ, YZ and YZ W collected the data. All authors have read and approved the manuscript.

Competing interests
The authors declare that they have no competing interests.

Author details
[1]Department of Pediatrics, Beijing Tongren Hospital, West South road 2, Yizhuang Economic and Technological Development Zone, Daxing District, Beijing 100176, China. [2]Department of Ophthalmology, Beijing Tongren Hospital, Capital Medical University, Beijing 100176, China.

References
1. Kivelä T. The epidemiological challenge of the most frequent eye cancer: retinoblastoma, an issue of birth and death. Br J Ophthalmol. 2009;93:1129–31.
2. Abramson DH, Schefler AC. Update on retinoblastoma. Retina. 2004;24:828–48.
3. Temming P, Lohmann D, Bornfeld N, Sauerwein W, Goericke SL, Eggert A. Current concepts for diagnosis and treatment of retinoblastoma in Germany: aiming for safe tumor control and vision preservation. Klin Padiatr. 2012;224: 339–47.
4. Huang D, Zhang Y, Zhang W, Wang Y, Zhang P, Hong L, Zhou Y, Han T, Zhi T. Study on clinical therapeutic effect including symptoms, eye preservation rate, and follow-up of 684 children with retinoblastoma. Eur J Ophthalmol. 2013;23:532–8.
5. Dimaras H, Kimani K, Dimba EA, Gronsdahl P, White A, Chan HS, Gallie BL. Retinoblastoma. Lancet. 2012;379:1436–46.
6. Gündüz K, Müftüoglu O, Günalp I, Unal E, Taçyildiz N. Metastatic retinoblastoma clinical features, treatment, and prognosis. Ophthalmology. 2006;113:1558–66.
7. Chantada GL, Sampor C, Bosaleh A, Solernou V, Fandiño A, de Dávila MT. Comparison of staging systems for extraocular retinoblastoma: analysis of 533 patients. JAMA Ophthalmol. 2013;131:1127–34.
8. Trotti A, Colevas AD, Setser A, Rusch V, Jaques D, Budach V, Langer C, Murphy B, Cumberlin R, Coleman CN, Rubin P. CTCAE v3.0: development of a comprehensive grading system for the adverse effects of cancer treatment. Semin Radiat Oncol. 2003;13:176–81.
9. Kaliki S, Shields CL, Shah SU, Eagle RC, Shields JA, Leahey A. Postenucleation adjuvant chemotherapy with vincristine, etoposide, and carboplatin for the treatment of high-risk retinoblastoma. Arch Ophthalmol. 2011;129:1422–7.
10. Lim FP, Soh SY, Iyer JV, Tan AM, Swati H, Quah BL. Clinical profile, management, and outcome of retinoblastoma in Singapore. J Pediatr Ophthalmol Strabismus. 2013;50:106–12.
11. Schueler AO, Hosten N, Bechrakis NE, Lemke AJ, Foerster P, Felix R, Foerster MH, Bornfeld N. High resolution magnetic resonance imaging of retinoblastoma. Br J Ophthalmol. 2003;87:330–5.
12. Baiges-Octavio JJ, Huerta-Villanueva M. Meningeal carcinomatosis. Rev Neurol. 2000;31:1237–41.

13. Ota KV, Dimaras H, Héon E, Babyn PS, Yau YC, Read S, Budning A, Gallie BL, Chan HS. Toxocariasis mimicking liver, lung, and spinal cord metastases from retinoblastoma. Pediatr Infect Dis J. 2009;28:252–4.

14. Shine BS, Hungerford J, Vaghela B, Sheraidah GA. Electrophoretic assessment of aqueous and serum neurone-specific enolase in retinoblastoma and ocular malignant melanoma. Br J Ophthalmol. 1990;74:427–30.

15. Nakajima T, Kato K, Kaneko A, Tsumuraya M, Morinaga S, Shimosato Y. High concentrations of enolase, alpha- and gamma-subunits, in the aqueous humor in cases of retinoblastoma. Am J Ophthalmol. 1986;101:102–6.

16. Chantada G, Fandiño A, Dávila MT, Manzitti J, Raslawski E, Casak S, Schvartzman E. Results of a prospective study for the treatment of retinoblastoma. Cancer. 2004;100:834–42.

17. Dunkel IJ, Khakoo Y, Kernan NA, Gershon T, Gilheeney S, Lyden DC, Wolden SL, Orjuela M, Gardner SL, Abramson DH. Intensive multimodality therapy for patients with stage 4a metastatic retinoblastoma. Pediatr Blood Cancer. 2010;55:55–9.

18. Kwong YL, Yeung DY, Chan JC. Intrathecal chemotherapy for hematologic malignancies: drugs and toxicities. Ann Hematol. 2009;88:193–201.

19. Doz F, Neuenschwander S, Plantaz D, Courbon B, Gentet JC, Bouffet E, Mosseri V, Vannier JP, Mechinaud F, Desjardins L. Etoposide and carboplatin in extraocular retinoblastoma: a study by the Société Française d'Oncologie Pédiatrique. J Clin Oncol. 1995;13:902–9.

20. Bhasker S, Bajpai V, Turaka A. Palliative radiotherapy in paediatric malignancies. Singap Med J. 2008;49:998–1001.

21. Palma J, Sasso DF, Dufort G, Koop K, Sampor C, Diez B, Richard L, Castillo L, Chantada GL. Successful treatment of metastatic retinoblastoma with high-dose chemotherapy and autologous stem cell rescue in South America. Bone Marrow Transplant. 2012;47:522–7.

22. Cozza R, De Ioris MA, Ilari I, Devito R, Fidani P, De Sio L, Demelas F, Romanzo A, Donfrancesco A. Metastatic retinoblastoma: single institution experience over two decades. Br J Ophthalmol. 2009;93:1163–6.

23. Bekibele CO, Ayede AI, Asaolu OO, Brown BJ. Retinoblastoma: the challenges of management in Ibadan, Nigeria. J Pediatr Hematol Oncol. 2009;31:552–5.

9

Ocular surface health in Shanghai University students: a cross-sectional study

Shanshan Li[1,2], Jiangnan He[1], Qiuying Chen[1], Jianfeng Zhu[1,2*], Haidong Zou[1] and Xun Xu[1]

Abstract

Background: Our study aimed to investigate the ocular surface health of Shanghai University students.

Methods: This is a cross-sectional study carried out among freshmen and sophomores on the main campus of Shanghai University. Questionnaires including the widely-used ocular surface disease index (OSDI) and the Zung Self-rating Anxiety Scale (SAS) were completed first, and then ocular examinations were conducted regarding height & weight, blood pressure and heart rate, optometry, intraocular pressure exam, vision and subjective refraction, Aladdin, Macular pigment density measurement, tear test, anterior segment examination, fundus photography, ophthalmologist check, TOPCON OCT check, and Collin's fundus blood test.

Results: Totally 901 students were involved in our five-day study. The prevalence of myopia was 92% (the spherical equivalent refraction (SER) < − 0.50 D), and that of high myopia was 23% (SER < − 6.0D). The prevalence of dry eye disease (DED) was 10%. The corneal epithelial loss rate (corneal fluorescein staining > 1) was 10%, and corneal sensation decline rate (≤ 30 mm) was 12%. 4.5% of subjects ($n = 40$) had moderate or severe anxiety, 78% were mild and a small portion (17.5%) didn't have anxiety at all. No statistical significant association was found between anxiety with DED, fluorescein staining or with corneal sensation (all $p > 0.05$). However, subjects with DED had more symptoms of anxiety. Results also showed that students who kept eye strain for a long time were more inclined to have DED (12.5%: 6.9%, $p = 0.0407$, 95% CI); those who watched mobile phones and/or computers for over eight hours daily were more vulnerable to DED and fluorescein staining than others (14.1%: 8.6%, $p = 0.0129$; 13.0%: 8.3%, $p = 0.0233$, 95% CI).

Conclusions: Keeping eye strain or near work for a long time is associated with DED, while students with DED tend to encounter anxiety symptoms. The prevalence of myopia in Chinese university students is still high. We consider it necessary to provide education to university students about the good eye-using habits, and to diagnose anxiety for student patients with DED.

Keywords: Ocular surface health, Eye health, Dry eye disease, Anxiety, Students

Background

Eye health, including ocular surface health, is an integral part of the human physical health. Statistics from the World Health Organization (WHO) alarms us against the severity of eye health. A total of nearly 50 million persons are blind and another 150 million are victims of severe visual disability, and this number will probably double in the year 2020 [1].

China, with its 1.5 billion population, has a huge number of students. As reported in the 2016 National Statistical Communiqué on Development of Education published by the Ministry of Education, there were about 160 million students from grade 1 to 12, and over 41 million college/university students (including nearly 2 million post-graduate students) at school at the survey time [2]. College students form a distinctive group with their own obvious characteristics. They are young in relatively good physical conditions (having passed the physical examination for entering the colleges); have finished 12-year basic education with good academic scores; have more opportunities (compared with elementary and middle school students) and spare time to use video display terminals (VDT) at a short distance for a long time; often

* Correspondence: jfzhu1974@hotmail.com
[1]Shanghai Eye Disease Prevention and Treatment Center, Shanghai, China
[2]Shanghai General Hospital, Shanghai, China

stay up late; and many of them bear the pressure of studying. As revealed by the General Administration of Sport in the Communiqué on National Physical Health Monitoring conducted in 2014, physical fitness of college students in China is worse than the year 2010, while the prevalence of myopia was higher with a tendency to younger ages at the time of incidence [3].

According to the 2004 National Students Physical Health Monitoring Report, the poor sight detection rate was 32.5% among pupils aged 7 to 12. The rate was 59.4% among junior middle school students and 77.3% among senior middle school students. A larger proportion (80.0%) of university students were detected with poor sight and some of them even had high myopia [4]. High myopia often causes pathological changes of eyes with symptoms like decline of eye sight, fast worsening of myopia, proptosis, bad dark adaptation, dark shadows, etc. Complications may include macular degeneration, retinal detachment and other diseases that may cause blindness [5, 6].

With the popularity of computers and smart phones/ video display terminals (VDT), more and more Chinese students suffer from refractive errors and have to wear glasses if the error is not detected and corrected in a timely manner [7]. While wearing glasses is an obvious sign of damaged eye health, some ocular surface diseases (OSD) are more concealed, as well as fundus oculi diseases.

Dry eye is a multifactorial disease characterized by unstable tear film causing a variety of symptoms and/or visual impairment, potentially accompanied by ocular surface damage. In 2016, the Asia Cornea Society (ADES) and the Dry Eye Society Japan implemented new diagnostic criteria for DED that enabled diagnosis with two positive items, namely subjective symptoms and decreased TBUT (≤ 5 s) [8].

To date, teenagers-based studies in China have been focusing on myopia/high myopia, good examples of which may be the Shunyi Study [9, 10], the Guangzhou Study [11], and the Yangxi Study [12]. On the other hand, college/ university-based studies are rare, though Jing Sun et al. had carried out a survey on diopter and myopia in Shanghai Donghua University in 2012 [13]. Our study aimed to investigate the ocular surface health of Shanghai University students.

The obvious strength of the updated study is that it is the first to pay attention to ocular surface health condition of Chinese university students, as well as to explore the association of their anxiety status with their eye health.

Methods

This is an observational cross-sectional study, comprising a questionnaire survey and ophthalmologic examinations. It was carried out on Baoshan Campus of Shanghai University in September 2016. Located in Shanghai with three campuses, Shanghai University is one of the national key universities with over 54,000 students from various areas across the country to study in the university by February 27, 2017 [14]. Baoshan Campus is the main and largest campus containing almost all the colleges/departments where all their freshmen and sophomores receive undergraduate education. Our study is designed to include only freshmen and sophomores rather than senior students, because we had a 3-year visit plan for students with eye diseases. Students of higher grades would graduate and leave the school pretty soon, making the 3-year visit plan difficult to carry out. The school, the students' union and the Youth League Committee were responsible for informing the students, who visited our booths on the campus at their own willingness. Subjects first read and signed the informed consent, then completed a questionnaire on iPad designed and provided by the investigators. Incomplete questionnaires could not be submitted. After completing the questionnaires (see Additional file 1) including but not limited to the widely-used ocular surface disease index (OSDI) and the Zung Self-rating Anxiety Scale (SAS) [15], subjects went through examinations, i.e. height & weight, optometry, intraocular pressure exam, vision and subjective refraction (< 0.8, one eye), Aladdin (Topcon, made in Japan), Macular pigment density measurement, tear test, anterior segment examination, fundus photography, ophthalmologist check, TOPCON (made in Japan, TOPCON CORPOERATION) OCT check, Collin's fundus blood test, blood pressure and heart rate. Around ten medical staff worked together with five doctors to implement the study on site. Examination data were logged into computer by a data entry operator. The survey lasted for five days from September 9 through September 13, 2016.

Statistical analysis was performed with SAS® software, version 9.2 (SAS Institute, NC, USA). Spherical equivalent refraction (SER) was calculated as the spherical value of the refractive error plus half of the cylindrical value. Myopia was defined as a SER ≤ 0.5 diopters (D) and high myopia was defined as a SER ≤ 6.0 D. The OSD was determined based on the OSDI scores and the ophthalmologic examination results. Corneal epithelial loss was identified when the corneal fluorescein staining > 1. Corneal sensation ≤ 30 mm was considered as decline. Statistical analysis focused on OSDs, specifically the dry eye disease (DED), cornea fluorescein staining and corneal sensation. All P values were two-sided and were considered statistically significant when the P values were < 0.05. Person Chi-Square test was used to analyze associations with genders and ages, different eye-using habits and anxiety status. Cochran-Armitage Trend Test was performed to identify the trend of association between anxiety and DED.

Results

Our study involved 901 students in total in Shanghai University. The subjects, at an equal sex ratio, responded with questionnaires and ophthalmologic examinations. Most of the subjects were freshmen and sophomores whose ages ranged from 18 to 22 (Table 1), and no one was under the age of 17, as per the automatic calculation of the system after dates of birth were entered.

The prevalence of myopia was 92% (the spherical equivalent refraction (SER) < – 0.50 D), and that of high myopia was 23% (SER < – 6.0D). The prevalence of DED was 10%. The corneal epithelial loss rate (corneal fluorescein staining > 1) was 10%, and corneal sensation decline rate (≤ 30 mm) was 12%.

Statistical analysis indicated that 4.5% of subjects (*n* = 40, see Table 3) had moderate or severe anxiety, 78% were mild and a small portion (17.5%) didn't have anxiety at all. No statistical significant association was found between anxiety with DED, fluorescein staining or corneal sensation (all *p* > 0.05). However, subjects with DED had more symptoms of anxiety (see Table 3), such as feeling afraid for no reason at all (*p* = 0.0023), getting upset easily or feeling panicky (*p* = 0.0004), and being bothered by headaches neck and back pain (*p* = 0.0101), feeling weak and getting tired easily (*p* = 0.0004), being bothered by dizzy spells (p = 0.0004), having fainting spells or feeling like it (*p* = 0.0175), being bothered by a stomach aches or indigestion (*p* = 0.0001), face getting hot and blushes (*p* = 0.0039). Cochran-Armitage Trend Test identified a trend of anxiety among DED subjects (see Table 4). Adjusted *p*-values also showed worse anxiety status of subjects with DED, mainly with symptoms of getting upset easily or feeling panicky (*p* = 0.0216), feeling weak and getting tired easily (*p* = 0.0340), being bothered by dizzy spells (*p* = 0.0120), and being bothered by a stomach aches or indigestion (*p* = 0. 0190).

Results also showed that students who kept eye strain for a long time were more inclined to have DED (12.5%: 6.9%, *p* = 0.0407, 95% CI); those who watched mobile phones and/or computers for over eight hours daily were more vulnerable to DED and fluorescein staining than others (14.1%: 8.6%, *p* = 0.0129; 13.0%: 8.3%, *p* = 0.0233, 95% CI). No significant differences were found among other variables such as age, gender, near work and improper reading gestures; no significant differences/associations for corneal sensation (see Table 2). However, none of the comparison results in Table 2 was significant (*p* < 0.05) after adjustment.

Discussion

We carried out a cross-sectional study using both questionnaires and ophthalmologic examinations for 901 students in Shanghai University for the purpose of getting real data of ocular surface health of university students in China. The obvious strength of the updated study is that it is the first to pay attention to ocular surface health condition of Chinese university students, as well

as to explore the association of their anxiety status with their eye health.

The study results showed that the prevalence of myopia was 92% (SER < – 0.50 D), that of high myopia was 23% (SER < – 6.0D), and dry eye disease 10%. The corneal epithelial loss rate (corneal fluorescein staining > 1) was 10%, and the corneal sensation decline rate (≤ 30 mm) was 12%.

There are quite a few published studies on myopia and ocular surface health of Chinese university students. The study implemented by Jing Sun et al. in Shanghai Donghua University found that 95.5% of the subjects were myopic (SER < – 0.50 D), 19.5% were highly myopic (SER < – 6.0 D) [13]. This is similar to our study results. There are no published study results on OSD conditions of Chinese university/college students yet. However, studies in other countries may provide references. A cross-sectional survey conducted in students from the University of Monterrey using Ocular Surface Disease Index (OSDI) questionnaire in 2016 have found that University students have a prevalence of 70.4% of ocular surface disease, and OSD was associated with gender (women have a higher prevalence), smoking and the use of eye drops [16]. Another study by Kofi Asiedu et al. concluded that the prevalence of symptomatic dry eye among undergraduate students in Ghana is high (44.3% (95% confidence interval [CI], 40.6–48.2%) and it is associated with self-medication with over-the-counter eye drops, allergies, use of oral contraceptive, windy conditions, very low humid areas, air-conditioned rooms, and sex [17]. Compared to those two studies, prevalence of OSDs in our study was not high. It may be because we took into consideration the ophthalmologic examination results to determine the OSD, instead of using OSDI scores only. We had investigated the contact lens wearing of these students, and analysis was reported in Table 2. However, no significant relations were found between contact lens wearing and DED, cornea fluorescein staining or corneal perception (*P* > 0.05), which may be due to the shorter and less frequent use of contact lenses by these freshmen.

Mental disorder, specifically anxiety, was explored in our study. As currently known, these factors are related to anxiety: Biological factors, such as genetic and physiological diseases, social factors, tension, and high work pressure, psychological factors, hormone levels, and so on. Published results of studies have already found correlation of eye diseases, especially the DED, with mental disorders. A study by Li M et al. in 2011 showed that the prevalence of anxiety or depression symptoms in dry eye syndrome subjects was significantly higher than in the control group (*p* = 0.003; *p* < 0.001, respectively) [18]. A meta-analysis concluded that depression and anxiety are more prevalent in DED patients than in controls,

Table 1 Demographics and eye examination results by disease types and in total

	Total (N = 901)	Dry eye disease			Cornea fluorescein staining			Corneal sensation		
		Absent (N = 733)	Present (N = 94)	P-value	≤1 (N = 796)	>1 (N = 89)	P-value	>30 mm (N = 780)	≤30 mm (N = 105)	P-value
Age, years	19.7 (2.7)	19.7 (2.7)	19.9 (2.5)	0.4721[a]	19.7 (2.7)	19.8 (2.5)	0.5520[a]	19.7 (2.7)	19.7 (2.5)	0.8036[a]
Age, years [n (%)]				0.6914[b]			0.0860[b]			0.8003[b]
< 18	102 (11.3%)	85 (11.6%)	6 (6.4%)		88 (11.1%)	14 (15.7%)		91 (11.7%)	11 (10.5%)	
18 ≤ age < 19	322 (35.7%)	264 (36.0%)	34 (36.2%)		294 (36.9%)	21 (23.6%)		275 (35.3%)	40 (38.1%)	
19 ≤ age < 20	124 (13.8%)	101 (13.8%)	13 (13.8%)		107 (13.4%)	14 (15.7%)		109 (14.0%)	12 (11.4%)	
20 ≤ age < 21	94 (10.4%)	77 (10.5%)	11 (11.7%)		85 (10.7%)	8 (9.0%)		85 (10.9%)	8 (7.6%)	
21 ≤ age < 22	89 (9.9%)	70 (9.5%)	12 (12.8%)		73 (9.2%)	14 (15.7%)		76 (9.7%)	11 (10.5%)	
≥22	170 (18.9%)	136 (18.6%)	18 (19.1%)		149 (18.7%)	18 (20.2%)		144 (18.5%)	23 (21.9%)	
Gender [n (%)]				0.4143[b]			0.6014[b]			0.7361[b]
Male	397 (44.1%)	321 (43.8%)	37 (39.4%)		354 (44.5%)	37 (41.6%)		343 (44.0%)	48 (45.7%)	
Female	504 (55.9%)	412 (56.2%)	57 (60.6%)		442 (55.5%)	52 (58.4%)		437 (56.0%)	57 (54.3%)	
Height(cm)	158.3 (37.9)	159.0 (36.9)	157.2 (38.1)	0.6505[a]	158.4 (37.7)	157.7 (39.3)	0.8593[a]	159.3 (35.8)	151.7 (50.0)	0.0560[a]
Weight(Kg)	54.9 (16.6)	55.2 (16.6)	53.9 (15.3)	0.4793[a]	55.0 (16.3)	55.0 (19.0)	0.9694[a]	55.4 (16.1)	52.2 (19.8)	0.0649[a]
BMI(Kg/m^2)	19.7 (5.2)	19.7 (5.2)	19.6 (4.9)	0.8058[a]	19.7 (5.1)	19.6 (5.9)	0.9738[a]	19.8 (5.0)	18.6 (6.4)	0.0216[a]
Axial length R, mm	25.0 (2.6)	25.0 (2.7)	25.0 (2.8)	0.9968[a]	25.0 (2.6)	24.9 (2.9)	0.7163[a]	25.1 (2.3)	24.6 (4.4)	0.1407[a]
Axial length L, mm	24.8 (3.0)	24.8 (3.0)	24.9 (2.8)	0.8640[a]	24.8 (2.9)	24.6 (3.9)	0.5279[a]	24.8 (2.8)	24.5 (4.4)	0.3616[a]
Intraocular pressure R, mmHg	13.9 (3.4)	13.9 (3.4)	13.7 (3.4)	0.5859[a]	13.9 (3.4)	14.0 (3.2)	0.7750[a]	13.9 (3.3)	13.7 (3.8)	0.5143[a]
Intraocular pressure L, mmHg	14.0 (3.5)	14.1 (3.4)	13.5 (3.4)	0.1393[a]	14.0 (3.5)	13.8 (3.3)	0.6580[a]	14.0 (3.5)	13.8 (3.4)	0.6178[a]
Diopter R, D	398.7 (259.5)	400.3 (256.3)	408.2 (257.9)	0.7782[a]	400.4 (264.8)	377.4 (205.1)	0.4278[a]	397.7 (259.4)	400.7 (260.9)	0.9119[a]
Diopter L, D	368.4 (264.7)	365.8 (265.1)	404.0 (237.4)	0.1835[a]	368.4 (269.8)	361.7 (215.6)	0.8189[a]	366.4 (261.8)	377.7 (286.8)	0.6810[a]

BMI body mass index, L left eye, R right eye, SD standard deviation
[a] ANOVA
[b] Pearson Chi-Square test

Table 2 Prevalence of eye diseases by demographics, eye care habits and in total

	Dry eye disease %(95% CI)[a] (N = 94)	P-value	Cornea fluorescein staining >1%(95% CI)[a] (N = 89)	P-value	Corneal perception test ≤ 30 mm %(95% CI)[a] (N = 105)	P-value
Age, years [n(%)]		0.6914[b]		0.0860[b]		0.8003[b]
< 18	6.6%(2.5,13.8)		13.7%(7.7,22.0)		10.8%(5.5,18.5)	
18 ≤ age < 19	11.4%(8.0,15.6)		6.8%(4.3,10.2)		12.7%(9.3,16.9)	
19 ≤ age < 20	11.4%(6.2,18.7)		11.3%(6.3,18.2)		9.7%(5.1,16.3)	
20 ≤ age < 21	12.5%(6.4,21.3)		8.5%(3.7,16.1)		8.5%(3.7,16.1)	
21 ≤ age < 22	14.6%(7.8,24.2)		15.7%(8.9,25.0)		13.5%(7.2,22.4)	
≥ 22	11.7%(7.1,17.8)		10.6%(6.4,16.2)		13.5%(8.8,19.6)	
Gender [n (%)]		0.4143[b]		0.6014[b]		0.7361[b]
Male	10.3%(7.4,14.0)		9.6%(6.9,12.9)		12.6%(9.5,16.3)	
Female	12.2%(9.3,15.5)		10.3%(7.8,13.3)		11.3%(8.7,14.4)	
Near work [n (%)]		0.1296[b]		0.8785[b]		0.9049[b]
No	10.0%(6.9,13.8)		10.6%(7.5,14.4)		11.2%(8.1,15.1)	
Yes	13.6%(10.5,17.2)		10.3%(7.7,13.4)		10.9%(8.2,14.2)	
View for long time [n (%)]		0.0683[b]		0.4039[b]		0.0169[b]
No	8.1%(4.5,13.2)		12.1%(7.7,17.7)		15.9%(10.9,22.1)	
Yes	13.2%(10.6,16.3)		9.9%(7.7,12.6)		9.6%(7.4,12.2)	
Incorrect reading gesture [n (%)]		0.0624[b]		0.5986[b]		0.2197[b]
No	9.5%(6.5,13.2)		9.8%(6.8,13.4)		9.5%(6.6,13.1)	
Yes	14.0%(10.8,17.6)		10.9%(8.2,14.1)		12.2%(9.4,15.6)	
Play computers or video games for a long time [n (%)]		0.7056[b]		0.5224[b]		0.6531[b]
No	11.6%(8.7,15.2)		11.1%(8.3,14.4)		10.6%(7.9,13.9)	
Yes	12.5%(9.2,16.5)		9.7%(6.8,13.2)		11.6%(8.5,15.4)	
Study for over 8 h every day [n (%)]		0.0303[b]		0.7818[b]		0.3854[b]
No	9.1%(6.5,12.2)		10.3%(7.7,13.5)		11.0%(8.3,14.2)	
Yes	13.9%(10.6,17.6)		9.8%(7.1,13.0)		12.9%(9.8,16.4)	
Use mobile phone/computer for over 8 h every day [n (%)]		0.0099[b]		0.0233[b]		0.6436[b]
No	9.1%(6.8,12.0)		8.3%(6.1,10.9)		12.3%(9.6,15.3)	
Yes	15.0%(11.2,19.5)		13.0%(9.6,17.1)		11.2%(8.0,15.1)	
Often stay up late [n (%)]		0.2960[b]		0.6277[b]		0.0517[b]
No	9.0%(5.0,14.6)		9.0%(5.1,14.5)		16.3%(11.0,22.8)	
Yes	11.9%(9.6,14.6)		10.3%(8.2,12.7)		10.8%(8.7,13.4)	
Often wear eye makeup [n (%)]		0.0541[b]		0.2297[b]		0.4444[b]
No	10.9%(8.8,13.3)		9.8%(7.9,12.0)		11.7%(9.6,14.0)	
Yes	21.1%(9.6,37.3)		15.8%(6.0,31.3)		15.8%(6.0,31.3)	
Do outdoor exercises, eye exercises or overlooking with eyes [n (%)]		0.3515[b]		0.7346[b]		0.6941[b]
No	12.9%(8.9,17.8)		10.5%(7.1,15.0)		12.5%(8.7,17.2)	
Yes	10.7%(8.3,13.4)		9.8%(7.6,12.4)		11.6%(9.2,14.3)	
Do you wear contact lenses? [n (%)]		0.3279[b]		0.0766[b]		0.7296[b]
No	11.5%(8.9,14.5)		9.2%(6.9,11.9)		11.5%(9.0,14.5)	
Yes	14.1%(9.6,19.8)		13.6%(9.2,19.2)		10.6%(6.7,15.8)	

BMI body mass index, *L* left eye. *R* right eye, *SD* standard deviation
[a]The Exact Unconditional Confidence Interval
[b]Pearson Chi-Square test

Table 3 Various mental statuses by disease types and in total

	Total (N = 901)	Dry eye disease			Cornea fluorescein staining			Corneal sensation		
		Absent (N = 733)	Present (N = 94)	P-value	≤1 (N = 796)	>1 (N = 89)	P-value	>30 mm (N = 780)	≤30 mm (N = 105)	P-value
I feel more nervous and anxious than usual.				0.1332[a]			0.9415[a]			0.4303[a]
A little or some of the time	491 (56.1%)	414 (57.1%)	46 (48.9%)		442 (56.1%)	49 (55.7%)		437 (56.5%)	54 (52.4%)	
Good part or most of the time	385 (43.9%)	311 (42.9%)	48 (51.1%)		346 (43.9%)	39 (44.3%)		336 (43.5%)	49 (47.6%)	
I feel afraid for no reason at all.				0.0023[a]			0.6147[a]			0.6648[a]
A little or some of the time	684 (78.4%)	576 (79.8%)	62 (66.0%)		614 (78.1%)	70 (80.5%)		605 (78.6%)	79 (76.7%)	
Good part or most of the time	189 (21.6%)	146 (20.2%)	32 (34.0%)		172 (21.9%)	17 (19.5%)		165 (21.4%)	24 (23.3%)	
I get upset easily or feel panicky.				0.0004[a]			0.7419[a]			0.5343[a]
A little or some of the time	551 (63.0%)	472 (65.0%)	43 (46.2%)		497 (63.2%)	54 (61.4%)		489 (63.3%)	62 (60.2%)	
Good part or most of the time	324 (37.0%)	254 (35.0%)	50 (53.8%)		290 (36.8%)	34 (38.6%)		283 (36.7%)	41 (39.8%)	
I feel like I'm falling apart and going to pieces.				0.1458[a]			0.5045[a]			0.7820[a]
A little or some of the time	757 (86.3%)	634 (87.3%)	77 (81.9%)		679 (86.1%)	78 (88.6%)		669 (86.4%)	88 (85.4%)	
Good part or most of the time	120 (13.7%)	92 (12.7%)	17 (18.1%)		110 (13.9%)	10 (11.4%)		105 (13.6%)	15 (14.6%)	
I feel that everything is all right and nothing bad will happen.				0.3091[a]			0.1519[a]			0.4895[a]
A little or some of the time	142 (16.2%)	122 (16.9%)	12 (12.8%)		123 (15.6%)	19 (21.6%)		128 (16.6%)	14 (13.9%)	
Good part or most of the time	732 (83.8%)	600 (83.1%)	82 (87.2%)		663 (84.4%)	69 (78.4%)		645 (83.4%)	87 (86.1%)	
My arms and legs shake and tremble.				0.3031[a]			0.3375[a]			0.5465[a]
A little or some of the time	761 (87.2%)	633 (87.8%)	79 (84.0%)		688 (87.5%)	73 (83.9%)		674 (87.4%)	87 (85.3%)	
Good part or most of the time	112 (12.8%)	88 (12.2%)	15 (16.0%)		98 (12.5%)	14 (16.1%)		97 (12.6%)	15 (14.7%)	
I am bothered by headaches neck and back pain.				0.0101[a]			0.2039[a]			0.6391[a]
A little or some of the time	503 (57.5%)	432 (59.7%)	43 (45.7%)		458 (58.2%)	45 (51.1%)		446 (57.8%)	57 (55.3%)	
Good part or most of the time	372 (42.5%)	292 (40.3%)	51 (54.3%)		329 (41.8%)	43 (48.9%)		326 (42.2%)	46 (44.7%)	
I feel weak and get tired easily.				0.0004[a]			0.6428[a]			0.1817[a]
A little or some of the time	322 (36.8%)	281 (38.8%)	19 (20.2%)		292 (37.0%)	30 (34.5%)		278 (36.0%)	44 (42.7%)	
Good part or most of the time	554 (63.2%)	444 (61.2%)	75 (79.8%)		497 (63.0%)	57 (65.5%)		495 (64.0%)	59 (57.3%)	
I feel calm and can sit still easily.				0.3764[a]			0.2911[a]			0.7117[a]
A little or some of the time	274 (31.4%)	232 (32.0%)	25 (27.5%)		251 (32.0%)	23 (26.4%)		240 (31.2%)	34 (33.0%)	
Good part or most of the time	598 (68.6%)	492 (68.0%)	66 (72.5%)		534 (68.0%)	64 (73.6%)		529 (68.8%)	69 (67.0%)	

Table 3 Various mental statuses by disease types and in total (Continued)

	Total (N = 901)	Dzry eye disease			Cornea fluorescein staining			Corneal sensation		
		Absent (N = 733)	Present (N = 94)	P-value	≤1 (N = 796)	>1 (N = 89)	P-value	>30 mm (N = 780)	≤30 mm (N = 105)	P-value
I can feel my heart beating fast.				0.0550[a]			0.9174[a]			0.6683[a]
A little or some of the time	653 (74.5%)	545 (75.2%)	62 (66.0%)		587 (74.5%)	66 (75.0%)		578 (74.8%)	75 (72.8%)	
Good part or most of the time	223 (25.5%)	180 (24.8%)	32 (34.0%)		201 (25.5%)	22 (25.0%)		195 (25.2%)	28 (27.2%)	
I am bothered by dizzy spells.				0.0004[a]			0.8430[a]			0.5927[a]
A little or some of the time	692 (78.7%)	587 (80.7%)	61 (64.9%)		622 (78.6%)	70 (79.5%)		613 (79.0%)	79 (76.7%)	
Good part or most of the time	187 (21.3%)	140 (19.3%)	33 (35.1%)		169 (21.4%)	18 (20.5%)		163 (21.0%)	24 (23.3%)	
I have fainting spells or feel like it.				0.0175[a]			0.8478[a]			0.2952[a]
A little or some of the time	772 (88.1%)	646 (89.1%)	75 (80.6%)		695 (88.2%)	77 (87.5%)		678 (87.7%)	94 (91.3%)	
Good part or most of the time	104 (11.9%)	79 (10.9%)	18 (19.4%)		93 (11.8%)	11 (12.5%)		95 (12.3%)	9 (8.7%)	
I can breathe in and out easily.				0.8312[a]			0.4371[a]			0.9660[a]
A little or some of the time	424 (48.3%)	352 (48.5%)	44 (47.3%)		378 (47.9%)	46 (52.3%)		374 (48.3%)	50 (48.5%)	
Good part or most of the time	453 (51.7%)	374 (51.5%)	49 (52.7%)		411 (52.1%)	42 (47.7%)		400 (51.7%)	53 (51.5%)	
I get numbness and tingling in my fingers and toes.				0.9498[a]			0.8044[a]			0.5168[a]
A little or some of the time	763 (87.2%)	634 (87.3%)	81 (87.1%)		687 (87.3%)	76 (86.4%)		672 (86.9%)	91 (89.2%)	
Good part or most of the time	112 (12.8%)	92 (12.7%)	12 (12.9%)		100 (12.7%)	12 (13.6%)		101 (13.1%)	11 (10.8%)	
I am bothered by stomach aches or indigestion.				0.0001[a]			0.1914[a]			0.0392[a]
A little or some of the time	574 (65.4%)	494 (68.0%)	45 (47.9%)		522 (66.1%)	52 (59.1%)		498 (64.2%)	76 (74.5%)	
Good part or most of the time	304 (34.6%)	232 (32.0%)	49 (52.1%)		268 (33.9%)	36 (40.9%)		278 (35.8%)	26 (25.5%)	
I have to empty my bladder often.				0.3573[a]			0.0958[a]			0.8032[a]
A little or some of the time	609 (69.5%)	511 (70.6%)	62 (66.0%)		541 (68.7%)	68 (77.3%)		537 (69.4%)	72 (70.6%)	
Good part or most of the time	267 (30.5%)	213 (29.4%)	32 (34.0%)		247 (31.3%)	20 (22.7%)		237 (30.6%)	30 (29.4%)	
My hands are usually dry and warm.				0.6917[a]			0.2221[a]			0.4782[a]
A little or some of the time	288 (32.8%)	240 (33.1%)	33 (35.1%)		254 (32.2%)	34 (38.6%)		251 (32.4%)	37 (35.9%)	
Good part or most of the time	589 (67.2%)	486 (66.9%)	61 (64.9%)		535 (67.8%)	54 (61.4%)		523 (67.6%)	66 (64.1%)	
My face gets hot and blushes.				0.0039[a]			0.0704[a]			0.0303[a]
A little or some of the time	625 (71.3%)	528 (72.8%)	55 (58.5%)		555 (70.3%)	70 (79.5%)		543 (70.1%)	82 (80.4%)	
Good part or most of the time	252 (28.7%)	197 (27.2%)	39 (41.5%)		234 (29.7%)	18 (20.5%)		232 (29.9%)	20 (19.6%)	

Table 3 Various mental statuses by disease types and in total (Continued)

	Total (N = 901)	Dry eye disease			Cornea fluorescein staining			Corneal sensation		
		Absent (N = 733)	Present (N = 94)	P-value	≤1 (N = 796)	>1 (N = 89)	P-value	>30 mm (N = 780)	≤30 mm (N = 105)	P-value
I fall asleep easily and get a good night's rest.				0.9241[a]			0.3199[a]			0.8477[a]
A little or some of the time	291 (33.1%)	243 (33.5%)	31 (33.0%)		266 (33.7%)	25 (28.4%)		256 (33.0%)	35 (34.0%)	
Good part or most of the time	587 (66.9%)	483 (66.5%)	63 (67.0%)		524 (66.3%)	63 (71.6%)		519 (67.0%)	68 (66.0%)	
I have nightmares.				0.3115[a]			0.2875[a]			0.2757[a]
A little or some of the time	637 (72.5%)	531 (73.0%)	64 (68.1%)		569 (71.9%)	68 (77.3%)		567 (73.1%)	70 (68.0%)	
Good part or most of the time	242 (27.5%)	196 (27.0%)	30 (31.9%)		222 (28.1%)	20 (22.7%)		209 (26.9%)	33 (32.0%)	

[a]Pearson Chi-Square test

Table 4 Summary of Zung self-rating anxiety scale

	Dry eye disease			Cornea fluorescein staining			Corneal sensation		
	Absent (N = 733)	Present (N = 94)	P-value	≤1 (N = 796)	>1 (N = 89)	P-value	>30 mm (N = 780)	≤30 mm (N = 105)	P-value
Severity of anxiety			0.0136[a]			0.1364[a]			0.8399[a]
None (<35)	85 (12.2%)	5 (5.6%)		85 (11.2%)	12 (14.3%)		88 (11.8%)	9 (9.3%)	
Mild (≥35,<55)	582 (83.4%)	76 (85.4%)		632 (83.6%)	71 (84.5%)		618 (83.2%)	85 (87.6%)	
Moderate (≥55,<65)	28 (4.0%)	6 (6.7%)		35 (4.6%)	0		33 (4.4%)	2 (2.1%)	
Severe (≥65)	3 (0.4%)	2 (2.2%)		4 (0.5%)	1 (1.2%)		4 (0.5%)	1 (1.0%)	
Missing	35	5		40	5		37	8	
Sum of scores			<0.0001[b]			0.9229[b]			0.7769[b]
Number	698	89		756	84		743	97	
Mean (SD)	42.5 (7.2)	45.8 (7.5)		42.8 (7.3)	42.8 (7.0)		42.9 (7.4)	42.6 (6.6)	
Median	42.5	45.0		42.5	43.8		43.8	42.5	
Min: Max	25: 79	29: 66		25: 79	26: 65		25: 79	25: 65	

[a]CMH SCORES = RANK
[b]ANOVA

irrespective of the underlying etiologies of DED and ethnic differences of the patients [19]. Investigators of our study have also noticed, from their clinical practice, that many patients with ocular surface diseases had mental disorders to some extent. However, no significant association was found with DED, fluorescein staining or corneal sensation (all $p > 0.05$). A reasonable explanation may be that the subjects included in our study were young people (mean age 19.7 ± 2.7) with relatively good physical and mental health (they passed the university entrance examination and relevant physical checks). Results of a study by van der Vaart et al. also found associations between DED and anxiety differed across age groups with the elders having stronger associations [20].

Nonetheless, subjects with DED in our study were found to have more symptoms of anxiety, e.g. feeling afraid for no reason at all, getting upset easily or feeling panicky, feeling weak and getting tired easily, etc. (see Table 3). A statistically significant trend was found between anxiety and DED (see Table 4). This is in agreement with clinical experience. Patients with DED usually have more complaints and discomforts than those who only have refractive error. In addition to artificial tears and other medication, it is necessary for doctors to explain reasons and console them. For student patients, eye irritation symptoms such as foreign body sensation and dryness are common as a result of over-regulation of the eyes and/or reduction of blinks [21] during/after excessive reading or computer/mobile phone use. Some students may grow anxious as these symptoms occur from time to time.

Therefore, school doctors, acting as the primary care taker for university students, are suggested to pay attention to mental statuses of students with DED symptoms rather than just cure DED alone. Consolation or soothing, or even psychological counseling can be performed whenever necessary. Medical-psychological health intervention mode may be adopted to provide science education, eye health survey, counseling and other interventions. To our knowledge, ours is the first study to call on school doctors to address anxiety status for university students with DED symptoms.

Regarding habits, statistical significance was found in two habits out of ten (see Table 2): (1) keeping eye strain for a long time, associated with the DED ($p = 0.0407$); and (2) watching mobile phones and/or computers for over 8 h every day, associated with the DED and corneal fluorescein staining ($p = 0.0129$, $p = 0.0233$). Near work, though considered as one of the reasons for refraction error [22–25], was found uncorrelated with DED, fluorescein staining or corneal sensation ($p > 0.05$). One possible explanation may be that the variable of near work is a vague expression without a specific standard for subjects to make better or precise judgments. Another

reason may be near work itself doesn't do much harm to ocular surface disease, but it will do if combined with a long time and/or continuous use of VDT, a good example of which is the variable "watching mobile phones and/or computers for over 8 hours every day". Our study identified the importance of period of time, either for eye strain or watching VDTs. This is consistent with findings of previous studies [22, 25]. The blinking action prevents the lipid layer from contacting the mucus layer, maintains the thickness of the tear layer in the tear film, and keeps the tear film stable [26]. The number of blinks is reduced when eyes focus on close things. This is typical in VDT users. They tend to blink less when focus on computers and such terminals as a smart phone for a long time at a very short distance. This will cause an abnormal distribution of tears and tear secretion, which in turn leads to an increase in eye discomfort. Hence, it's suggested to pay more attention to the duration of one continuous near work (watching or reading). Keeping time of the continuous near work as short as possible may be beneficial to students' eye health. However, further studies may be needed to explore the exact length of time proper for one continuous near work.

Our study has obvious limitations. Firstly, the subjects were a specific group, and results may not be proper for a general population-based generalization. Besides, the sample size was not very big, which might cause statistical bias. Thirdly, only one university participated in the study. Future studies may involve more universities to cover as many majors as possible.

Conclusions

Our study has revealed the fact the prevalence of myopia in Chinese university students is still high, that keeping eye strain or near work for a long time is associated with DED, and that students with dry eye disease/syndrome tend to encounter anxiety symptoms of one kind or another. This conclusion might be used by school doctors to educate university students about the good eye-using habits, and to diagnose anxiety for patients with DED. Further studies are warranted to cover more universities.

Abbreviations

CI: Confidence interval; DED: Dry eye disease; OSD: Ocular surface diseases; OSDI: Ocular surface disease index; SAS: The Zung Self-rating anxiety scale; SER: Spherical equivalent refraction; VDT: Video display terminals; WHO: The World Health Organization

Acknowledgments

We'd like to express our appreciations to Sam Zhong (SZ) and Cui-Ling Yin (CLY) for their generous support with this study.

Funding

This article is funded by the following projects: "Epidemiological survey of ophthalmopathy" (The project of Shanghai Municipal Health and Family Planning Commission: Key subjects of eye hygiene No.15GWZK0601) and "Epidemiological investigation of pathological myopia of college students in Shanghai". (The project of Shanghai Municipal Health and Family Planning Commission No.20134215).

Authors' contributions

All the authors have contributed to the study and manuscript, and approved this submission. XX, JZ, HZ and SL were responsible for concept and design of the study. SL, and JZ were responsible for administration, ethical review and publication of the study. SL drafted the manuscript.
JZ reviewed. SL, JH and QC were responsible for the On-site research implementation. Statistical analysis was implemented by SL and JH. All authors have read and approved the manuscript, and ensure that this is the case.

Competing interests

The authors declare that they have no competing interests.

References

1. WHO: VISION 2020: The Right to Sight. 2005. https://www.v2020.org. Accessed 28 Aug 2017.
2. National Statistical Communiqué on Development of Education. 2016. http://www.moe.gov.cn/jyb_sjzl/sjzl_fztjgb/201707/t20170710_309042.html. Accessed 28 Aug 2017.
3. Communiqué on National Physical Health Monitoring. China Sports. 2014. November 27, 2015, V004.
4. National Students Physical Health Monitoring Report. Sports, health and art Department of the Ministry of Education. Higher Education Press. 2004. Version 1, December 1, 2006. ISBN: 9787040208696, 7040208695.
5. Curtin BJ, Iwamoto T, Renaldo DP. Normal and Staphylomatous sclera of high myopia: an electron microscopic study. Arch Ophthalmol. 1979;97(5):912–5.
6. Liu KR, Chen MS, Ko LS. Electron microscopic studies of the scleral collagen Fiber in excessively high myopia. J Formos Med Assoc. 1986;85(11):1032–8.
7. Impact of Gazing at Video Display Terminals on Eye Health of Teenagers. Guangxi Med J 2006, 28 (4):522–523.
8. Tsubota K, Yokoi N, Shimazaki J, Watanabe H, et al. New perspectives on dry eye definition and diagnosis: a consensus report by the Asia dry eye society. Asia Dry Eye Society Ocul Surf. 2017;15(1):65–76. https://doi.org/10.1016/j.jtos.2016.09.003.
9. Zhao J, Pan X, Sui R, Munoz SR, Sperduto RD, Ellwein LB. Refractive error study in children: results from Shunyi District, China. Am J Ophthalmol. 2000;129:427–35.
10. Zhao J, Mao J, Luo R, Li F, Munoz SR, Ellwein LB. The progression of refractive error in school-age children: Shunyi district. China Am J Ophthalmol. 2002;134:735–43.
11. He M, Zeng J, Liu Y, Xu J, Pokharel GP, Ellwein LB. Refractive error and visual impairment in urban children in southern China. Invest Ophthalmol Vis Sci. 2004;45:793–9.
12. He M, Huang W, Zheng Y, Huang L, Ellwein LB. Refractive error and visual impairment in school children in rural southern China. Ophthalmology. 2007;114:374–82.
13. Sun J, Zhou J, Zhao P, Lian J, Zhu H, Zhou Y, Sun Y, Wang Y, Zhao L, Wei Y, Wang L, Cun B, Ge S, Fan X. High prevalence of myopia and high myopia in 5060 Chinese university students in shanghai. Invest Ophthalmol Vis Sci. 2012;53(12):7504. 2012:53 (12) :7504–7505.
14. http://www.shu.edu.cn/Default.aspx?tabid=10591. Last accessed: 7 Sept 2017.
15. Zung WW. A rating instrument for anxiety disorders. Psychosomatics. 1971;12:371–9.
16. Garza-León M, Valencia-Garza M, Martínez-Leal B, Villarreal-Peña P, Marcos-Abdala HG, Cortéz-Guajardo AL, Jasso-Banda A. Prevalence of ocular surface disease symptoms and risk factors in group of university students in Monterrey, Mexico. J Ophthalmic Inflamm Infect 2016;6(1):44. Epub 2016 Nov 18.
17. Asiedu K, Kyei S, Boampong F, Ocansey S. Symptomatic Dry Eye and Its Associated Factors: A Study of University Undergraduate Students in Ghana. Eye contact Lens. Jul. 2017;43(4):262–6.
18. Li MI, Gong L, Sun X, Chapin WJ. Anxiety and depression in patients with dry eye syndrome. Curr Eye Res. 2011;36(1):1–7.
19. Wan1 KH, Chen1 LJ, Young1 AL. Depression and anxiety in dry eye disease: a systematic review and meta-analysis. Eye. 30(12):1558–67.
20. van der Vaart R, Weaver MA, Lefebvre C, Davis RM. The association between dry eye disease and depression and anxiety in a large population-based study. Am J Ophthalmol. 2015;159(3):470–4.
21. Alex A, Edwards A, Daniel Hays J, Kerkstra M, Shih A, de Paiva CS, Pflugfelder SC. Factors predicting the ocular surface response to desiccating environmental stress. Invest Ophthalmol Vis Sci. 2013;54(5):3325–32.
22. Huang HM, Chang DS, Wu PC. The Association between Near Work Activities and Myopia in Children-A Systematic Review and Meta-Analysis. PLoS One. 2015;10(10):e0140419.
23. Sivaraman V, Rizwana JH, Ramani K, Price H, Calver R, Pardhan S, Vasudevan B, Allen PM. Near work-induced transient myopia in Indian subjects. Clin Exp Optom. 2015;98(6):541–6.
24. Muhamedagic L, Muhamedagic B, Halilovic EA, Halimic JA, Stankovic A, Muracevic B. Relation between near work and myopia progression in student population. Mater Sociomed. 2014;26(2):100–3.
25. Ip JM, Saw SM, Rose KA, Morgan IG, Kifley A, Wang JJ, Mitchell P. Role of near work in myopia: findings in a sample of Australian school children. Invest Ophthalmol Vis Sci. 2008;49(7):2903–10.
26. Braun RJ, King-Smith PE, Begley CG, Li L, Gewecke NR. Dynamics and function of the tear film in relation to the blink cycle. Prog Retin Eye Res. 2015;0:132–64. https://doi.org/10.1016/j.preteyeres.2014.11.001.

10

Species-specific characteristics of the biofilm generated in silicone tube: an in vitro study

Dong Ju Kim, Joo-Hee Park and Minwook Chang[*]

Abstract

Background: To investigate characteristics of biofilm which is usually found in silicone tube for nasolacrimal duct surgery and can be the root of chronic bacterial infections eventually resulted in surgical failure.

Methods: To form a biofilm, sterile silicone tube was placed in culture media of *Staphylococcus aureus*, *Corynebacterium matruchotii*, *Pseudomonas aeruginosa*, or *Streptococcus pneumonia*. Biofilms formed on these silicone tubes were fixed with 95% ethanol and stained with 0.1% crystal violet. After staining, the optical densities of biofilms were measured using spectrophotometer on a weekly basis for 12 weeks.

Results: *Staphylococcus aureus* group and *Pseudomonas aeruginosa* group formed significantly more amounts of biofilms compared to the control group. The maximum optical densities of the two groups were found on week 3–4 followed by a tendency of decrease afterwards. However, the amounts of biofilms formed in other groups of silicone tubes were not statistically significant from that of the control group.

Conclusions: Bacterial species that could form biofilm on silicone tube included *Staphylococcus aureus* (week 3) and *Pseudomonas aeruginosa* (Week 4). It is important to first consider that the cause of infection around 1 month after silicone tube intubation can be *Staphylococcus aureus* and *Pseudomonas aeruginosa*.

Keywords: Dacryocystorhinostomy, Biofilms, Silicone tube, Nasolacrimal duct obstruction, Pseudomonas, Staphylococcus

Background

Nasolacrimal duct obstruction (NLDO) mainly occurs in inflammation and fibrosis of lacrimal system. Either external or endoscopic dacryocystorhinostomy (DCR) is commonly used for NLDO [1–3]. DCR with silicone tube intubation has been commonly used to treat NLDO [4–8]. Although the beneficial effects of silicone tube intubation remain controversial [4, 9], silicone tube intubation is usually performed in order to maintain ostium patency and reinstate lacrimal drainage function, especially in case of distal or common canalicular obstruction [10, 11]. However, silicone tube intubation is associated with complications such as granulation formation, fibrosis and inflammation of nasolacrimal system, patient discomfort, infection of silicone tube, and cost related to intubation [12, 13]. Infection of silicone tube can result in

* Correspondence: mdjacob@naver.com
Department of Ophthalmology, Dongguk University, Ilsan Hospital, 814, Siksadong, Ilsan-dong-gu, Goyang, Gyeonggido 410-773, South Korea

postoperative failure [14, 15]. Bacteria can form biofilms, a complex of microbial communities enclosed in an exopolysaccharide matrix adherent to surface of prosthetics or living organism [16]. Biofilms enable bacteria to survive by reducing their metabolic needs and increasing their inherent resistance to antimicrobial agents. Biofilms formed on silicone tube could be the root of persistent and chronic bacterial infections. They can lead to chronic inflammatory response [17, 18]. Thus, it is important to find out the pathogen that formed biofilm on silicone tube.

In previous studies, both Gram-positive and Gram-negative bacteria have been isolated from extubated silicone tubes. Lee et al. [19] have reported culture positivity of 60% from extruded polyurethane nasolacrimal stents, with *Pseudomonas aeruginosa* being isolated from 40% of these stents. Ali et al. [20] have reported a positive culture of 94%, with *Pseudomonas aeruginosa* being isolated in 24% of cases. Kim et al. [14] have reported a positive culture of 94.9% from extubated silicone tubes, with 73% of the isolated bacteria being Gram-positive. They have also reported that *Pseudomonas aeruginosa* is associated with complications such as prolonged intubation, revision surgeries, and surgery failure [14].

The objective of this study was to investigate the characteristics of biofilms formed by four bacteria species (*Staphylococcus aureus, Corynebacterium matruchotii, Pseudomonas aeruginosa,* and *Streptococcus pneumonia*) usually found in silicone tubes used for nasolacrimal duct surgery [14, 19, 20]. The results of this study will improve our understanding on the characteristics of biofilms depending on bacteria, such as the amount of biofilms formed and the peak time of biofilm formation. These information will help us decide the treatment plan such as prophylactic use of antibiotics, the timing of stent removal and may aid in development of future strategies in treating silicone tube infection.

Methods

Bacteria culture

Staphylococcus aureus (KTCT#1621, ATCC#25923), *Corynebacterium matruchotii* (KTCT#19325,) *Pseudomonas aeruginosa* (KTCT#2513, ATCC#9027), and *Streptococcus pneumonia* (KTCT#5765, ATCC#BAA-960) were used in this study. *Staphylococcus aureus, Corynebacterium matruchotii,* and *Streptococcus pneumonia* are Gram-positive bacteria while *Pseudomonas aeruginosa* is Gram-negative bacterium. All bacteria were obtained from the Korean Collection for Type cultures (KCTC). Bacteria were maintained in Nutrient broth media (234,000; BD), BBL Trypticase soy broth media (211,768; BD), or Bacto Tryptic soy broth (211,825; BD), and cultured in an incubator at 37 °C except *Streptococcus pneumonia. Streptococcus pneumonia* was cultured in an incubator at 37 °C in an atmosphere of 5% CO_2.

Biofilm formation on silicon tube

Silicon tube (60–411-40; HelixMark) was cut into 2 cm in length and autoclaved. One silicone tube was cut into 6 pieces. Each group had 6 samples. To maintain the culture condition, we change the media as follows. *Staphylococcus aureus* culture media (Nutrient Broth media, 37 °C) was changed every 2 days. *Corynebacterium matruchotii* culture media (Trypticase soy broth, 37 °C) was changed every 4 days. *Pseudomonas aeruginosa* culture media (Trypticase soy broth, 37 °C) was changed every 2 days. *Streptococcus pneumonia* culture media (Bacto Tryptic soy broth, in 5% carbon dioxide at 37 °C) was changed every 4 days. The control group was not in contact with the bacteria in culture media (Nutrient Broth media).

Biofilm formation measurement on silicon tube

Silicon tubes incubated in cultured media were moved to new well and washed three times with distilled water. Biofilms formed on these silicon tubes were fixed with 95% ethanol. Tubes were washed twice with distilled water and stained with 0.1% crystal violet (V5265; SIGMA) for 30 min. After staining, silicon tubes were washed three times with distilled water. The crystal violet remained inside the silicon tube was removed using 22G syringe. These silicone tubes were dried on paper towel. The stained silicone tube was cut into 5 mm in thickness. These 5 mm tubes were placed in 96-well plate and filled with 95% ethanol (100 μl). The 96-well plate was sealed and incubated at 4 °C for 24 h. The optical density of the solubilized crystal violet in each well was then measured at wavelength of 570 nm using a spectrophotometer (SpectraMax plus 384 microplate reader, Molecular Devices, Sunnyvale, CA, USA). Each sample (Fig. 1) was measured for 12 weeks.

Statistical analysis

The normality of data was checked by using Sapiro-Wilk test. All data showed normal distribution. The sphericity of the data was checked using Mauchly's test. Repeated measure analysis of variance (RM-ANOVA) was used to compare time and optical density between control and bacteria. Post hoc test was conducted using the Bonferroni procedure. Statistical analyses were carried out using IBM SPSS ver. 21.0(IBM Corp., Armonk, NY, USA). *P*-value less than 0.05 was considered as statistically significant.

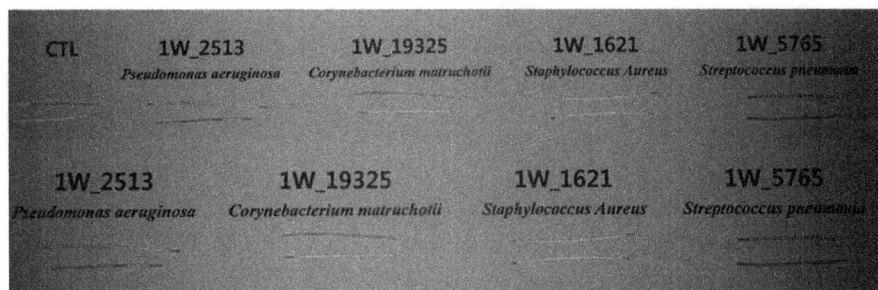

Fig. 1 Sample of biofilm formed on silicone tube stained by crystal violet before measuring optical density by spectrophotometer

Results

Six tubes from each group were evaluated for 12 weeks. *Staphylococcus aureus* group ($P = 0.000$, RM-ANOVA) and *Pseudomonas aeruginosa* ($P = 0.004$, RM-ANOVA) group formed significantly higher optical density of biofilms compared to control groups. Specifically, significantly higher optical densities were observed at week 3, 4, 5, 8 in *Pseudomonas aeruginosa* group and at week 3, 4, 6 in *Staphylococcus aureus* group (Table 1, Fig. 2).

The maximum optical density of *Pseudomonas aeruginosa* was found in week 4. It was then decreased afterwards but increased temporarily in week 8. Similarly, the maximum optical density of *Staphylococcus aureus* was found in week 3 with a tendency to decrease afterwards. A second peak occurred in week 6. The amounts of biofilms formed by *Corynebacterium matruchotii* and *Streptococcus pneumonia* were not significantly ($P > 0.05$, RM-ANOVA) different from those of the control groups.

Discussion

Biofilm have been associated with ocular prosthetic materials infection [21]. A biofilm is a complex organization of bacteria adherent to a biotic or an abiotic surface by living together in organized structures and communicating with one another in a co-operative manner [22, 23]. The bacteria self-produced polymeric matrix is embedded. This structure provides many advantages to bacteria, such as helping them endure environmental changes, resistant to host defense mechanisms, and resist conventional antibiotics. The presence of biofilm on a biomaterial could eventually lead to chronic inflammation and serve as a reservoir for bacteria. Therefore, bacterial biofilm has been increasingly recognized as playing an important role in surgical failure [24].

DCR and their surgical variants have been known as effective treatment for nasolacrimal duct problem. Among these surgical variants, nasolacrimal tube insertion is one of the most popular methods. However, complications related to postoperative infections associated with biofilms formed on tubes have been recently reported [12–15, 20].

Kim et al. [14] have reported that *Pseudomonas aeruginosa* infection is significantly associated with membranous obstruction of nasal mucosa, prolonged silicone intubation, and surgical failure. Balikoglu-Yilmaz et al. [25] have reported that *Staphylococcus epidermidis* and *Pseudomonas aeruginosa* are commonly culture positive on lacrimal stent. Ali et al. [20] have also reported that the most common bacterial organisms on lacrimal stents are *Pseudomonas aeruginosa* and *Staphylococcus aureus*. However, biofilm may be formed even if the culture was negative for bacterial growth. [26] due to limitation of conventional culture techniques [27]. Therefore, the possibility of chronic infection caused by biofilm could not be ruled out when the culture was negative.

Bacteriology of dacryocystitis has been gradually changed. Imatiaz A. Chaudhry et al. and Hartikainen J et al. have reported that *Staphylococcus* species were usually the most common organisms in Gram-positive bacteria while *Pseudomonas aeruginosa* and *Haemophilus* species were common Gram-negative bacteria found in dacryocystitis. Corynebacterium species were also detected [28–30]. Also, *Pseudomonas aeruginosa* and *Staphylococcus aureus* are well known producers of biofilms in paranasal sinus disease [31]. However, according to studies by David B. Samimi et al., nontuberculosis mycobacteria(NTM) was detected in silicone tube. Particularly, NTM was found in patients with clinically significant

Table 1 Change of optical density according to time

| | Optical density | | | | |
	Control	P.aeruginosa	C.matruchotti	S.aureus	S.pneumoniae
Week 1	0.1394 ± 0.0378	0.2154 ± 0.0740	0.1257 ± 0.0401	0.1272 ± 0.0406	0.2474 ± 0.1002
Week 2	0.1003 ± 0.0007	0.2299 ± 0.1030	0.0913 ± 0.0151	0.2583 ± 0.1249	0.1058 ± 0.0029
Week 3	0.1209 ± 0.0447	0.3414 ± 0.1359*	0.1301 ± 0.0459	1.5018 ± 0.2985*	0.0944 ± 0.0084
Week 4	0.1008 ± 0.0301	0.9106 ± 1.0651*	0.1388 ± 0.0517	0.4858 ± 0.1167*	0.1438 ± 0.0416
Week 5	0.0963 ± 0.0352	0.2415 ± 0.0691*	0.0967 ± 0.0228	0.2147 ± 0.0679	0.0863 ± 0.0074
Week 6	0.0902 ± 0.0028	0.1326 ± 0.1189	0.0946 ± 0.0034	0.8363 ± 0.2872*	0.1317 ± 0.0389
Week 7	0.1157 ± 0.0319	0.1659 ± 0.0416	0.1322 ± 0.0344	0.2579 ± 0.1053	0.1021 ± 0.0202
Week 8	0.0834 ± 0.0053	0.3392 ± 0.0757*	0.1094 ± 0.0332	0.1672 ± 0.0385	0.0911 ± 0.0222
Week 9	0.2378 ± 0.0257	0.1874 ± 0.0480	0.1616 ± 0.0410	0.4937 ± 0.1167	0.2217 ± 0.0179
Week 10	0.2635 ± 0.0613	0.2711 ± 0.0621	0.2808 ± 0.0388	0.3295 ± 0.0653	0.2539 ± 0.0357
Week 11	0.2412 ± 0.0403	0.3468 ± 0.0742	0.3209 ± 0.0746	0.3978 ± 0.0905	0.2320 ± 0.0035
Week 12	0.1701 ± 0.0461	0.1801 ± 0.0629	0.1712 ± 0.0519	0.7783 ± 0.2538	0.1738 ± 0.0210

Values are presented as mean ± standard deviation
*RM-ANOVA with post-hoc by Bonferroni ($P < 0.004$)

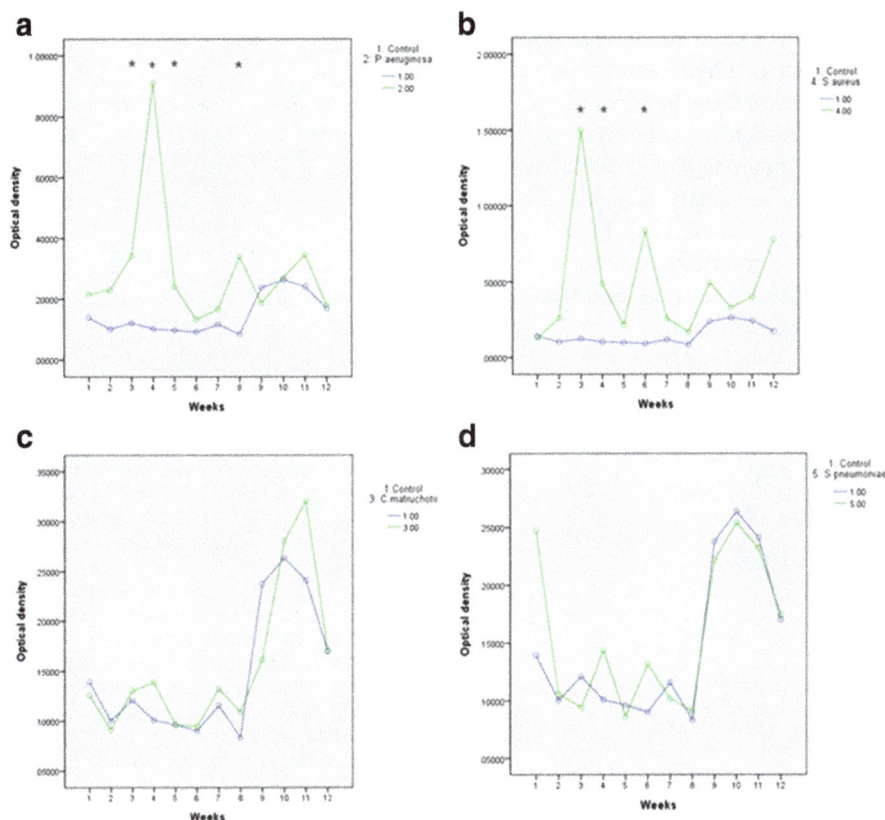

Fig. 2 Overall tendency of optical density of biofilms formed according to time

infection of silicone tube. But this study was a single institutional study in South Florida, so it is difficult to apply it to other region [32, 33]. Considering all above studies, we selected four bacterial species in this study, including *Staphylococcus aureus* and *Pseudomonas aeruginosa*.

The optical densities of the *Staphylococcus aureus* group and the *Pseudomonas aeruginosa* group were found to be higher than those of the control groups. This result suggests that the formation of biofilm depends on bacteria species. In terms of the amount of biofilm formed, the maximum value was achieved in 3 or 4 weeks with a tendency of decrease afterwards. A secondary peak occurred at 3 or 4 weeks after the first peak. This result can be used as a basis to use prophylactic antibiotics for 4 weeks to 8 weeks after silicone tube intubation. Once infection occurs, to treat infection and prevent recurrences, the prosthetic medical devices must be removed and antibiotics must be used at stronger doses or more often. It has been reported that if lacrimal stents are left longer than 1 month, biofilms may influence postoperative healing and the ultimate outcome [34]. Our results also support the use of prophylactic antibiotics after surgery.

This study has some limitations. First, this is an in-vitro study. Therefore, interaction of bacteria and immune system could not be evaluated. The causative relationship between biofilm and surgical failure was difficult to determine. To evaluate this, an in-vivo study is required. Second, many studies have reported that both bacteria and fungus are isolated from silicone stents, with fungus being isolated from 3.8% to 60% of cases [14, 20, 26, 34]. Symbiotic biofilms are more resistant to antibiotics with more complicated complex compared to non-symbiotic biofilms [35, 36]. However, we only investigated bacteria in this study.

Third, there are many methods for quantifying and detecting biofilms such as scanning electron microscopy morphology as a predictor [32, 37], biomass using confocal scanning laser microscope [34]. However, there is no standard method. We selected optical density using spectrophotometer at wavelength of 570 nm. This method had limited ability in assessing the depth of biofilm, thickness, or maturity. However, it can be quantified for comparison purpose and one study reported that crystal violet detect biofilm matrix for monitoring overall biofilm architecture [38, 39]. Antibiotic sensitivity or resistance associated with optical density could provide better information on treatment decision.

Conclusions

In conclusion, this study found that, of four bacterial species tested, *Staphylococcus aureus* and *Pseudomonas aeruginosa* could significantly form biofilms on silicone tube. The maximum optical density of biofilms occurred at around 1 month after incubating silicone tubes with bacterial culture media. A secondary peak occurred at around 2 months after incubation. On this basis, we first consider that the cause of infection around 1 month after silicone tube intubation can be *Staphylococcus aureus* and *Pseudomonas aeruginosa*.

Abbreviations

DCR: dacryocystorhinostomy; NLDO: nasolacrimal duct obstruction; NTM: nontuberculosis mycobacteria; OD: optical density

Acknowledgements

This work was supported by the Dongguk University Research Fund (grant No. S-2014-G0001-00024). The funding organization had no role in the design or conduct of this research.

Authors' contributions

DJK and MC were responsible for the conception and design of the study. DJK and JHP carried out culture, making biofilm, measurment of biofilm. DJK and JHP acquired the data. DJK, MC analyzed and interpreted the data. DJK wrote the draft. MC revised the manuscript critically. All authors have read and approved the final manuscript.

Competing interests

The authors declare that they have no competing interests.

References

1. Huang J, Malek J, Chin D, Snidvongs K, Wilcsek G, Tumuluri K, Sacks R, Harvey RJ. Systematic review and meta-analysis on outcomes for endoscopic versus external dacryocystorhinostomy. Orbit. 2014;33(2):81–90.
2. Ben Simon GJ, Joseph J, Lee S, Schwarcz RM, McCann JD, Goldberg RA. External versus endoscopic dacryocystorhinostomy for acquired nasolacrimal duct obstruction in a tertiary referral center. Ophthalmology. 2005;112(8):1463–8.
3. Jawaheer L, MacEwen CJ, Anijeet D. Endonasal versus external dacryocystorhinostomy for nasolacrimal duct obstruction. Cochrane Database Syst Rev. 2017;2:CD007097.
4. Chong KK, Lai FH, Ho M, Luk A, Wong BW, Young A. Randomized trial on silicone intubation in endoscopic mechanical dacryocystorhinostomy (SEND) for primary nasolacrimal duct obstruction. Ophthalmology. 2013; 120(10):2139–45.
5. Gu Z, Cao Z. Silicone intubation and endoscopic dacryocystorhinostomy: a meta-analysis. J Otolaryngol Head Neck Surg. 2010;39(6):710–3.
6. Marcet MM, Kuk AK, Phelps PO. Evidence-based review of surgical practices in endoscopic endonasal dacryocystorhinostomy for primary acquired nasolacrimal duct obstruction and other new indications. Curr Opin Ophthalmol. 2014;25(5):443–8.
7. Xie C, Zhang L, Liu Y, Ma H, Li S. Comparing the success rate of Dacryocystorhinostomy with and without silicone intubation: a trial sequential analysis of randomized control trials. Sci Rep. 2017;7(1):1936.
8. Feng YF, Cai JQ, Zhang JY, Han XH. A meta-analysis of primary dacryocystorhinostomy with and without silicone intubation. Can J Ophthalmol. 2011;46(6):521–7.
9. Syed MI, Head EJ, Madurska M, Hendry J, Erikitola OC, Cain AJ. Endoscopic primary dacryocystorhinostomy: are silicone tubes needed? Our experience in sixty three patients. Clin Otolaryngol. 2013;38(5):406–10.
10. Paik JS, Cho WK, Yang SW. Bicanalicular double silicone stenting in endoscopic dacryocystorhinostomy with lacrimal trephination in distal or common canalicular obstruction. Eur Arch Otorhinolaryngol. 2012; 269(6):1605–11.
11. Buttanri IB, Serin D, Karslioglu S, Akbaba M, Fazil K, Acar B, Sevim MS. The outcome of silicone intubation and tube removal in external dacryocystorhinostomy patients with distal canalicular obstruction. Eur J Ophthalmol. 2012;22(6):878–81.
12. Smirnov G, Tuomilehto H, Terasvirta M, Nuutinen J, Seppa J. Silicone tubing is not necessary after primary endoscopic dacryocystorhinostomy: a prospective randomized study. Am J Rhinol. 2008;22(2):214–7.
13. Smirnov G, Tuomilehto H, Terasvirta M, Nuutinen J, Seppa J. Silicone tubing after endoscopic dacryocystorhinostomy: is it necessary? Am J Rhinol. 2006; 20(6):600–2.
14. Kim SE, Lee SJ, Lee SY, Yoon JS. Clinical significance of microbial growth on the surfaces of silicone tubes removed from dacryocystorhinostomy patients. Am J Ophthalmol. 2012;153(2):253–7. e251
15. Ibanez A, Trinidad A, Garcia-Berrocal JR, Gomez D, San Roman J, Ramirez-Camacho R. Biofilm colonisation in nasolacrimal stents. B-ENT. 2011;7(1):7–10.
16. Bispo PJ, Haas W, Gilmore MS. Biofilms in infections of the eye. Pathogens. 2015;4(1):111–36.
17. Costerton JW. Introduction to biofilm. Int J Antimicrob Agents. 1999;11(3–4): 217–21. discussion 237-219
18. Davies D. Understanding biofilm resistance to antibacterial agents. Nat Rev Drug Discov. 2003;2(2):114–22.
19. Lee JH, Kang MS, Yang JW. Clinicopathologic findings after nasolacrimal polyurethane stent implantations. Korean J Ophthalmol. 2005;19(4):252–7.
20. Ali MJ, Manderwad G, Naik MN. The microbiological spectrum and antibiotic sensitivity profile of extubated silicone stents following dacryocystorhinostomy. Orbit. 2013;32(5):298–303.
21. Zegans ME, Becker HI, Budzik J, O'Toole G. The role of bacterial biofilms in ocular infections. DNA Cell Biol. 2002;21(5–6):415–20.
22. Mirani ZA, Aziz M, Khan MN, Lal I, Hassan NU, Khan SI. Biofilm formation and dispersal of Staphylococcus aureus under the influence of oxacillin. Microb Pathog. 2013;61-62:66–72.
23. Veerachamy S, Yarlagadda T, Manivasagam G, Yarlagadda PK. Bacterial adherence and biofilm formation on medical implants: a review. Proc Inst Mech Eng H. 2014;228(10):1083–99.
24. Costerton JW, Stewart PS, Greenberg EP. Bacterial biofilms: a common cause of persistent infections. Science. 1999;284(5418):1318–22.
25. Balikoglu-Yilmaz M, Yilmaz T, Cetinel S, Taskin U, Banu Esen A, Taskapili M, Kose T. Comparison of scanning electron microscopy findings regarding biofilm colonization with microbiological results in nasolacrimal stents for external, endoscopic and transcanalicular dacryocystorhinostomy. Int J Ophthalmol. 2014;7(3):534–40.
26. Parsa K, Schaudinn C, Gorur A, Sedghizadeh PP, Johnson T, Tse DT, Costerton JW. Demonstration of bacterial biofilms in culture-negative silicone stent and jones tube. Ophthal Plast Reconstr Surg. 2010;26(6):426–30.
27. Fux CA, Costerton JW, Stewart PS, Stoodley P. Survival strategies of infectious biofilms. Trends Microbiol. 2005;13(1):34–40.
28. Hartikainen J, Lehtonen OP, Saari KM. Bacteriology of lacrimal duct obstruction in adults. Br J Ophthalmol. 1997;81(1):37–40.
29. Sainju R, Franzco AA, Shrestha MK, Ruit S. Microbiology of dacryocystitis among adults population in southern Australia. Nepal Med Coll J. 2005; 7(1):18–20.
30. Chaudhry IA, Shamsi FA, Al-Rashed W. Bacteriology of chronic dacryocystitis in a tertiary eye care center. Ophthal Plast Reconstr Surg. 2005;21(3):207–10.
31. Bendouah Z, Barbeau J, Hamad WA, Desrosiers M. Biofilm formation by Staphylococcus aureus and Pseudomonas aeruginosa is associated with an unfavorable evolution after surgery for chronic sinusitis and nasal polyposis. Otolaryngol Head Neck Surg. 2006;134(6):991–6.

32. Samimi DB, Ediriwickrema LS, Bielory BP, Miller D, Lee W, Johnson TE. Microbiology and biofilm trends of silicone lacrimal implants: comparing infected versus routinely removed stents. Ophthal Plast Reconstr Surg. 2016; 32(6):452–7.

33. Samimi DB, Bielory BP, Miller D, Johnson TE. Microbiologic trends and biofilm growth on explanted periorbital biomaterials: a 30-year review. Ophthal Plast Reconstr Surg. 2013;29(5):376–81.

34. Murphy J, Ali MJ, Psaltis AJ. Biofilm quantification on nasolacrimal Silastic stents after Dacryocystorhinostomy. Ophthal Plast Reconstr Surg. 2015;31(5): 396–400.

35. Peleg AY, Hogan DA, Mylonakis E. Medically important bacterial-fungal interactions. Nat Rev Microbiol. 2010;8(5):340–9.

36. Wargo MJ, Hogan DA. Fungal–bacterial interactions: a mixed bag of mingling microbes. Curr Opin Microbiol. 2006;9(4):359–64.

37. Wilson A, Gray D, Karakiozis J, Thomas J. Advanced endotracheal tube biofilm stage, not duration of intubation, is related to pneumonia. J Trauma Acute Care Surg. 2012;72(4):916–23.

38. Bakke R, Kommedal R, Kalvenes S. Quantification of biofilm accumulation by an optical approach. J Microbiol Methods. 2001;44(1):13–26.

39. Elkhatib WF, Khairalla AS, Ashour HM. Evaluation of different microtiter plate-based methods for the quantitative assessment of Staphylococcus aureus biofilms. Future Microbiol. 2014;9(6):725–35.

11

Acquired distance esotropia associated with myopia in the young adult

Ke Zheng, Tian Han, Yinan Han and Xiaomei Qu[*]

Abstract

Background: To describe the clinical features of acquired progressive esotropia, with a larger angle at distance than near, associated with myopia in young adults.

Methods: Eleven adults (ages ranging from 18 to 37 years) with constant or intermittent horizontal diplopia at distance were recruited. Subjective refraction, ocular alignment, fusional amplitudes and horizontal eye movements were measured at distance and near.

Results: Distance esotropia varied from 20 to 60 prism diopters (PD). At near, the esotropic deviation ranged from 10 to 30 PD. Spherical equivalents (SE) of the right eye ranged from − 3.50 to − 8.25 diopters (D) while SE of the left eye ranged from − 0.375 to − 7.25 D. Ten of the eleven patients presented with constant diplopia at distance. Horizontal ductions and versions were full in all patients. The pathological report of seven patients who underwent lateral rectus resection showed that there were no muscle fibres, but rather, collagenous fibres.

Conclusions: This unusual sub-type of strabismus is a benign entity with slow progression that can occur in young adults with myopia. The cause of this condition is still unknown, and may be related to long periods of near work.

Keywords: Distance esotropia, Diplopia, Myopia

Background

Comitant esotropia is generally divided into three main categories: infantile-onset esotropia, accommodative esotropia, and non-accommodative acquired esotropia. In a previous report, age-related distance esotropia was proposed as a new subcategory. David Mittelman [1] reported this kind of non-accommodative acquired esotropia occurring in older patients with a median age of 77 years. Daisy Godts [2] reported this form of esotropia as being observed in patients over the age of 60, and this form was not associated with any neurological abnormalities or lateral rectus underaction. Divergence insufficiency (DI) presented comitant esotropia that is greater at distance than at near due to the progressive loss of fusional divergence amplitudes [3]. The patients usually were without neurological abnormalities and presented with the insidious onset of horizontal diplopia at distance.

In our clinical practice, the young adults who have acquired distance esotropia have some similarities with the signs of acquired progressive esotropia, typically a larger angle at distance than near and they tend to present with an insidious onset of horizontal diplopia at distance. This is usually associated with prolonged near work and myopia. By describing the clinical characteristics of these patients, hopefully it can be understood whether these patients belong to a special type of esotropia, and the possible pathogenesis can be explored.

Subjects

Eleven adult patients with myopia and distance esotropia were recruited and assessed between January 2015 and February 2015. The inclusion criteria included normal ductions, onset of symptoms before the age of 40, comitancy of esotropia in lateral gazes, symptoms of diplopia at distance and an esotropia greater at distance than near by five prism diopters (PD) or more. The patients who had a history of orbital trauma, childhood strabismus, previous strabismus surgery, accommodative disorders, coexisting vertical strabismus, myasthenia gravis,

* Correspondence: quxiaomei2002@126.com
Department of Ophthalmology, Eye and ENT Hospital of Fudan University and Myopia Key Laboratory of Ministry of Health, Shanghai, China

thyroid eye disease, cranial nerve palsies or supranuclear palsies would be excluded.

All patients had corrected visual acuities of 20/20 or better. All were evaluated using the duochrome test to ensure that they were not overcorrected. Vergence fusional amplitudes were measured with a phoropter. Binocular alignment was measured using the prism cover test. Ocular motility was evaluated clinically in all directions of gaze with an emphasis on lateral gaze. A portion of the lateral rectus muscle was taken for Haematoxylin-Eosin staining in patients who underwent lateral rectus resection.

This study followed the tenets of the Declaration of Helsinki and was approved by the ethics committee of the Eye and ENT Hospital of Fudan University. Informed consent was obtained from all participants.

Results

Eleven young adults were selected for this study: five females and six males. The patients ranged in age from 18 to 37 years, with a median age of 25 years. Table 1 shows that the spherical equivalents (SE) of the right eye ranged from − 3.50 to − 8.25 diopters (D), and the mean SE was − 5.65 DS; the SE of the left eye ranged from − 0.375 to − 7.25 D, and the mean SE was − 5.09 D. All patients complained of horizontal diplopia on distance fixation. The duration of these symptoms ranged from three months to seven years, with a mean of 32 months. Constant diplopia was the presenting complaint in 10 of the 11 individuals. All the patients had a history of prolonged near work, ranging from 6 h to 13 h per day (a median time of 12 h per day), before the onset of diplopia. Table 2 shows that the distance deviation varied from 20 PD esotropia to 60 PD esotropia, with a median angle of 30 PD esotropia. At near fixation, the measurements ranged from 10 PD esotropia to 30 PD esotropia, with a median deviation of 20 PD esotropia. Ductions and versions were full. There was no

evidence of lateral rectus paresis. The deviation difference was less than 5 PD in various positions of gaze. None of the patients had an obvious underlying neurological disease such as tumour or stroke. Three patients had previously undergone computed axial tomography (CT) or magnetic resonance imaging (MRI) after the onset of diplopia, the results of which were found to be normal for their age. None of the patients displayed a vertical deviation.

Seven patients were successfully treated with lateral rectus resection, and all samples underwent pathological examination, which showed that there were no muscle fibres but rather collagenous fibres from the lateral rectus. Figure 1.

Discussion

A previous population-based study reported that distance esotropia with orthotropia at near may include as many as 10.6% of adults with strabismus [4]. The present study is the first to report the features of distance esotropia in young adults. However, the classification of esotropia at distance has not been entirely clear because many clinical situations may produce an esotropia greater at distance than near. Divergence palsy affects all age groups and is often associated with various neurological disorders, and the sudden onset of distance esotropia is associated with loss of divergence [1]. None of the patients in the presented study had any neurological pathology.

Medial rectus muscle restriction with Graves' disease may cause comitant esotropia at distance [5]; however, none of the patients in the present study showed any ocular or systemic symptoms or signs of Graves' disease. Orbital lipoatrophy can reduce muscle tension in extraocular muscles by a relative decrease in muscle strain. The stronger medial rectus muscle, which is associated with relative relaxation of the lateral rectus muscle, may

Table 1 Patient characteristics

Case No.	SE of OD(D)	SE of OS(D)	Medical History	Head Scan	prolonged near work time(h)	Onset (months)
1	−7	−7.25	–	–	6	84
2	−5.5	−5.25	–	–	8	3
3	−5.5	−5.125	–	CT/MRI:normal	6	84
4	−8.25	−6.875	–	CT:normal	13	60
5	−5	−5.25	–	–	10	24
6	−6.875	−6.75	–	–	12	24
7	−3.875	−0.375	–	–	12	24
8	−3.5	−3.75	–	–	8	12
9	−6.725	−5.5	–	–	12	8
10	−4.75	−5	–	MRI:normal	12	5
11	−5.25	−4.875	–	–	13	24

SE Spherical equivalents, *D* Diopter

Table 2 Deviation and fusional amplitudes at distance and near

Case No.	Distance Deviation(PD)	Near Deviation(PD)	Distance BI(PD)	Distance BO(PD)	Near BI(PD)	Near BO(PD)
1	20	10	5.2/21.8/18.8	5.8/7.4/5	x/3.2/1.6	x/3.4/2.8
2	40	30	diplopia	diplopia	diplopia	diplopia
3	60	10	diplopia	diplopia	3/7.2/6	25/> 40/26
4	30	20	diplopia	diplopia	diplopia	diplopia
5	30	20	diplopia	diplopia	diplopia	diplopia
6	30	25	diplopia	diplopia	5.8/8/0.8	11/> 40/12
7	40	20	diplopia	diplopia	x/3.2/0.4	20/34.8/28.2
8	30	20	diplopia	diplopia	diplopia	diplopia
9	40	30	diplopia	diplopia	diplopia	diplopia
10	20	10	diplopia	diplopia	5.2/5.8/1	28/> 40/30
11	35	30	diplopia	diplopia	diplopia	diplopia

PD Prism diopters, *BI:*Base in, *BO* Base out;

result in a distant esotropia [6]. The finding is often associated with a relative and/or progressive enophthalmos, which was not seen in the present study group, making this aetiology less likely. Recently, Rutar and Demer [7] showed that orbital connective tissue degeneration led to a sudden decline in three elderly patients. However, the patients in the present study are young adults.

The aetiology of this uncommon type of strabismus is unknown by the authors, but there is a tendency to speculate that progressive myopathy affects the lateral rectus. The elderly may appear to have similar limitations. Bothun and Archer [5] reported a series of eight older patients (mean age of 60 years) with progressive distance esotropia; all patients were healthy and didn't have any neurological diseases. Robert E. Wiggins [8], in his series of elderly patients (mean age of 72 years), defined the divergence weakness as comitant esotropia with diplopia at distance and fusion at near. Horizontal ductions and versions should be normal. Christine Berscheid [9] showed that patients with secondary DI have the tendency to present with diplopia at a younger age than those with primary DI. The average age of patients with DI in the study was 51 years, compared with 62 years in patients with primary DI. It is suggested that the distance esotropia was possibly due to vascular factors in elderly patients. In the present study, the mean patient age is 25 years, which is much younger than the ages in previous studies.

Guyton [10] has proposed that tight adduction from near-target convergence leads to a shortening of the medial rectus muscle and reduced ability to maintain orthographic position at distance. In the present study, it was found that all patients spent a prolonged period performing tasks requiring near vision, ranging from six hours to 13 h per day (a median time of 12 h per day), before the onset of double vision. Therefore, it is hypothesized that the esotropia described in this article is due to the weakening of the lateral rectus muscle from prolonged near work, resulting in a slow progressive esodeviation that manifests initially at distance. Seven patients underwent a pathological examination of their lateral rectus muscles, which showed that there were no muscle fibres but rather collagenous fibres. Small esodeviations can be easily corrected because divergent fusion is often prioritized. However, divergent fusional amplitudes are much smaller at distance. Therefore, when the eyes deviate progressively inwards, patients are unable to compensate, resulting in horizontal diplopia at distance. Akiko Tanaka [11] reported that exotropia was more common than esotropia in patients with pathologic myopia. High myopia prescriptions are often undercorrected for high refractive error, which would induce less accommodation and exotropia. However, in the present study, all patients were myopic and had distance esotropia. Clearly, many more patients need to be studied in the future.

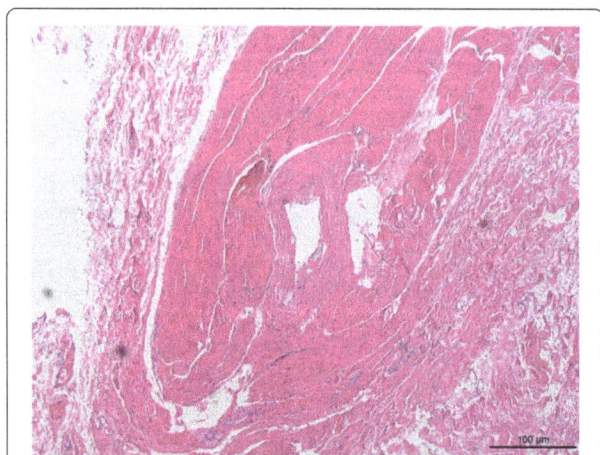

Fig. 1 Lateral rectus histopathology of patient 5

Conclusions

In conclusion, acquired distance esotropia with diplopia was observed in young adults with myopia; however, the aetiology is still unclear. It can be hypothesized that the esotropia described is due to the weakening of the lateral rectus muscle from prolonged near work, resulting in a slow, progressive esodeviation that manifests initially at distance.

Abbreviations
BI: Base in; BO: Base out; CT: Computed axial tomography; D: Diopters; DI: Divergence insufficiency; MRI: Magnetic resonance imaging; PD: Prism diopter; SE: Spherical equivalents

Acknowledgements
Not Applicable.

Funding
Xiaomei Qu provided financial support in the form of Scientific research projects of Shanghai funding (14411969500).

Authors' contributions
Study concept and design (KZ); data collection (KZ); analysis and interpretation of data (TH,YH); drafting of the manuscript (KZ, YH); critical revision of the manuscript (XQ); supervision (XQ). All authors read and approved the final manuscript.

Competing interests
The authors declare that they have no competing interests.

References
1. Mittelman D. Age-related distance esotropia. J AAPOS. 2006;10:212–3.
2. Godts D, Mathysen DG. Distance esotropia in the elderly. Br J Ophthalmol. 2013;97:1415–9.
3. Rambold H, Neumann G, Sander T, Helmchen C. Age-related changes of vergence under natural viewing conditions. Neurobiol Aging. 2006;27:163–72.
4. Martinez-Thompson JM, Diehl NN, Holmes JM, Mohney BG. Incidence, types, and lifetime risk of adult-onset strabismus. Ophthalmology. 2014;121:877–82.
5. Bothun ED, Archer SM. Bilateral medial rectus muscle recession for divergence insufficiency pattern esotropia. J AAPOS. 2005;9:3–6.
6. Reader AR. Age-related distance esotropia. J AAPOS. 2007;11:69–70. author reply 70
7. Rutar T, Demer JL. "heavy eye" syndrome in the absence of high myopia: a connective tissue degeneration in elderly strabismic patients. J AAPOS. 2009;13:36–44.
8. Wiggins RJ, Baumgartner S. Diagnosis and management of divergence weakness in adults. Ophthalmology. 1999;106:1353–6.
9. Berscheid C. Divergence insufficiency. Am Orthopt J. 2005;55:106–11.
10. Guyton DL. The 10th Bielschowsky lecture. Changes in strabismus over time: the roles of vergence tonus and muscle length adaptation. Binocul Vis Strabismus Q. 2006;21:81–92.
11. Tanaka A, Ohno-Matsui K, Shimada N, Hayashi K, Shibata Y, Yoshida T, et al. Prevalence of strabismus in patients with pathologic myopia. J Med Dent Sci. 2010;57:75–82.

12

Prevalence of depression and anxiety among participants with glaucoma in a population-based cohort study: The Gutenberg Health Study

J. Rezapour[1]* ⓘD, S. Nickels[1], A. K. Schuster[1], M. Michal[2], T. Münzel[3], P. S. Wild[4,5,6], I. Schmidtmann[7], K. Lackner[8], A. Schulz[5], N. Pfeiffer[1] and M. E. Beutel[2]

Abstract

Background: To investigate the prevalence of depression and anxiety among subjects with self-reported glaucoma and the association between self-reported glaucoma and depression respectively anxiety in a European cohort.

Methods: A study sample of 14,657 participants aged 35 to 74 years was investigated in a population-based cohort study. All participants reported presence or absence of glaucoma. Ophthalmological examinations were carried out in all participants and demographic and disease related information were obtained by interview. Depression was assessed with the Patient Health Questionnaire (PHQ-9), and generalized anxiety with the two screening items (GAD-2) of the short form of the GAD-7 (Generalized Anxiety Disorder-7 Scale). Prevalence of depression and generalized anxiety were investigated for subjects with and without self-reported glaucoma. Logistic regression analyses with depression, respectively anxiety as dependent variable and self-reported glaucoma as independent variable were conducted and adjusted for socio-demographic factors, systemic comorbidities (arterial hypertension, myocardial infarction, stroke, diabetes mellitus, chronic obstructive pulmonary disease, cancer), ocular diseases (cataract, macular degeneration, corneal diseases, diabetic retinopathy), visual acuity, intraocular pressure, antiglaucoma eye drops (sympathomimetics, parasympathomimetics, carbonic anhydrase inhibitors, beta-blockers, prostaglandins) and general health status.

Results: 293 participants (49.5% female) reported having glaucoma. Prevalence of depression among participants with and without self-reported glaucoma was 6.6% (95%-CI 4.1–10.3) respectively 7.7% (95%-CI 7.3–8.2), and for anxiety 5.3% (95%-CI 3.1–8.7) respectively 6.6% (95%-CI 6.2–7.1). Glaucoma was not associated with depression (Odds ratio 1.10, 95%-CI 0.50–2.38, p = 0.80) or anxiety (1.48, 95%-CI 0.63–3.30, p = 0.35) after adjustment for socio-demographic factors, ocular/systemic diseases, ocular parameters, antiglaucoma drugs and general health status. A restriction to self-reported glaucoma cases either taking topical antiglaucoma medications or having a history of glaucoma surgery did not alter the result.

Conclusions: This is the first study analyzing both depression and anxiety among glaucoma patients in a European cohort. Subjects with and without self-reported glaucoma had a similar prevalence of depression and anxiety in our population-based sample. Self-reported glaucoma was not associated with depression or anxiety. A lack of a burden of depressive symptoms may result from recruitment from a population-based sample as compared to previous study groups predominantly recruited from tertiary care hospitals.

Keywords: Glaucoma, Depression, Anxiety, Prevalence, Population-based cohort study, European cohort

* Correspondence: jasmin.rezapour@gmail.com
[1]Department of Ophthalmology, University Medical Center Mainz, Mainz, Germany
Full list of author information is available at the end of the article

Background

Glaucoma is a chronic, progressive eye disease, which is characterized by optic nerve damage and visual field loss [1]. It is the second leading cause of irreversible blindness worldwide [2], with approximately 8 million cases of bilateral blindness in 2010 [3]. The number of people with glaucoma was estimated to be 64 million in 2013 [4], increasing to 80 million by 2020 [3]. Treatment often includes the use of multiple eye drops and surgery, however, optic nerve damage cannot be reversed and many patients present disease progression despite therapy. The fear of potential vision loss may result in a higher prevalence of depression and anxiety among glaucoma patients compared to the general population. Depression is a frequent comorbid condition observed in chronic diseases [5, 6] and consequently it has been debated in the past years, whether depression is increased in glaucoma patients or not. Several studies showed a higher prevalence of depressive symptoms among glaucoma patients [7–11], while Wilson et al. did not confirm this finding [12]. The prevalence of depression in subjects with glaucoma has been estimated to be between 10 and 32% in previous studies [7, 11].

Anxiety frequently co-occurs with depression, and anxiety disorders may rise in subjects with glaucoma due to fear of potential blindness and restrictions in everyday activities [13]. Several community-based studies analyzed the prevalence of depression [8, 14] in glaucoma patients, but so far, to the best of our knowledge, this is the first study analyzing both depression and anxiety in a European cohort.

The Gutenberg Health Study (GHS) is a population-based, prospective cohort study in Germany. It includes physical examinations, interviews and questionnaires, related to physical and mental health conditions. This database can be used to determine the prevalence of depression and anxiety among subjects with self-reported glaucoma, and to identify associated factors modifying possible relationships between self-reported glaucoma and psychological disturbances. The results of this study can be used to improve understanding and awareness of mental diseases in glaucoma patients.

Methods

The Gutenberg Health Study (GHS) is an ongoing population-based, interdisciplinary, prospective, observational single-center cohort study in the Rhein-Main Region in western mid-Germany. It was approved by the ethics committee (Ethics Commission of the State Chamber of Physicians of Rhineland-Palatinate, reference no. 837.020.07, original vote: 22.3.2007, latest update: 20.10.2015). According to the Declaration of Helsinki, written informed consent was obtained from all subjects before entering the study. The population sample was randomly drawn via local residents' registration offices and equally stratified by sex and residence (urban/rural) for each decade of age. Exclusion criteria were physical and mental disability to visit the study center on their own and an insufficient knowledge of the German language. A detailed description of the study design has been published elsewhere [15].

Study sample

The baseline sample of 15,010 participants aged 35 to 74 years of the Gutenberg Health Study (GHS) was analyzed in this study.

Materials and assessment

The baseline-examination was carried out between 2007 and 2012, lasted 5 h and included evaluation of prevalent classical cardiovascular risk factors and clinical variables, laboratory examinations from a venous blood sample, blood pressure and anthropometric measurements, as well as ophthalmological examinations and computer-assisted personal interviews [16].

Ophthalmological examinations

The ophthalmic part was described in detail by Höhn et al. [16]. In brief, the ophthalmic examinations included objective refraction and distance-corrected visual acuity (DCVA) (Humphrey Automated Refractor / Keratometer [HARK] 599; Carl Zeiss Meditec AG, Jena, Germany) and intraocular pressure (IOP) (Nidek NT-2000; Nidek, Co., Gamagori, Japan).

Self-reported eye diseases and history of any form of glaucoma surgery were assessed by questions during the eye examination. Participants were asked if they suffer from glaucoma, cataract, macular degeneration, corneal diseases or diabetic retinopathy. Additionally, participants were asked if they used any eye drops. Antiglaucoma eye drops were classified using the Anatomic Therapeutic Chemical (ATC) code, including following substance groups: Sympathomimetics (S01EA), Parasympathomimetics (S01 EB), Carbonic anhydrase inhibitors (S01EC), Beta-blockers (S01ED), Prostaglandins (S01EE).

Questionnaires

Depression was assessed with the Patient Health Questionnaire (PHQ-9), which evaluates how often subjects have been bothered by any of the nine diagnostic criteria of Major depression over the last two weeks. The total points for each of the items were summed up to create a score between 0 and 27 points. Depression was defined as a sum score of ≥ 10. A prior study showed a sensitivity of 81% and a specificity of 82% for any depressive disorder [17]. In addition, depressive symptoms were classified as "minimal" (score 5 to 9), "mild" (score 10 to 14), "moderately severe" (score 15 to 19) and "severe"

(score > 20) [18]. Generalized anxiety was measured with
the two screening items of the short form of the GAD-7
(Generalized Anxiety Disorder [GAD]-7 Scale), a screening tool for all anxiety disorders. Participants rated
"Feeling nervous, anxious or on edge" and "Not being
able to stop or control worrying" by 0 = "not at all", 1
= "several days", 2 = "over half the days", and 3 = "nearly
every day". Generalized anxiety (GAD-2) was defined as
a sum score of ≥3, corresponding to a sensitivity of 86%
and a specificity of 83% [19].

Computer-assisted personal interview
During the computer-assisted personal interview subjects were asked if they had the history of any depressive
or anxiety disorder. According to Lampert and Kroll, the
socioeconomic status (SES) was defined by education,
income and job position, with a range from 3 to 21,
while 3 indicated the lowest SES and 21 the highest SES
[20]. For statistical analyses, three groups were defined
including low SES (3–8 points), medium SES (9–14
points) and high SES (15–21 points) [21].Furthermore,
subjects were asked to classify their general health condition into four categories (Excellent = 1, good = 2, fair =
3 and poor = 4), and the following self-reported general
diseases were collected from the personal interview:
arterial hypertension, myocardial infarction, stroke, diabetes mellitus, chronic obstructive pulmonary disease
(COPD) and cancer.

Statistical analysis
Descriptive analyses were performed as absolute and
relative proportions for categorical data, mean and
standard deviation for continuous variables with approximately normal distribution and median with inter-
quartile range if not fulfilling this criterion.
Prevalence rates of depression and depressive symptoms,
resp. generalized anxiety were given for subjects with and
without self-reported glaucoma in our study sample.
To validate self-reported glaucoma data, we conducted
a sensitivity analysis and included only those self-reported
glaucoma subjects, who reported the use of antiglaucoma
drugs or having history of glaucoma surgery. Furthermore,
a subgroup analysis was performed, to evaluate only
glaucoma-subjects with advanced disease. Prevalence of
depression and anxiety was computed for subjects with
and without self-reported glaucoma and a visual acuity
>0.5 logMar in the worse eye. Comparisons between
groups were done with chi-squared-test for categorical
variables and with Mann-Whitney U-test and t-test for
continuous variables.
To determine a relationship between self-reported glaucoma and depression (caseness: PHQ-9 sum score < 10 vs.
PHQ-9 sum score ≥ 10), resp. generalized anxiety (caseness: GAD-2 sum score < 3 vs. GAD-2 sum score ≥ 3) we

performed logistic regression analysis with depression
(PHQ-9 sum score) resp. anxiety (GAD-2 sum score)
as the dependent variable. In model 1, self-reported
glaucoma was included as independent variable, adjusted for age, sex and socio-economic status. In the
following models, we additionally adjusted stepwise
for systemic comorbidities (arterial hypertension,
myocardial infarction, stroke, diabetes mellitus,
chronic obstructive pulmonary disease, cancer), ocular diseases (cataract, macular degeneration, corneal
diseases, diabetic retinopathy), visual acuity of the
worse eye, IOP, antiglaucoma eye drops (Sympathomimetics, Parasympathomimetics, Carbonic anhydrase inhibitors, Beta-blockers, Prostaglandins) and
general health status. The last model included all the
above mentioned independent variables.
All p-values should be regarded as a continuous
parameter that reflect the level of statistical evidence
and are therefore reported exactly. Statistical analysis
was carried out using R version 3.3.1 [22].

Results
14,657 (98% of 15,010) subjects were analyzed and 293
(2.0%) reported having glaucoma. Characteristics of the
total study sample and participants with and without
self-reported glaucoma are described in Table 1.
The mean age of subjects with glaucoma was 11 years
older compared to the non-glaucoma group. Subjects
with glaucoma presented more often with a low SES
compared to the non-glaucoma group. General comorbidities such as diabetes mellitus, arterial hypertension,
stroke, COPD, bronchial asthma and cancer were more
often seen in the glaucoma-group. For ocular comorbidities, the distributions were similar in both groups except
for cataract. Mean visual acuity in the worse eye was
relatively good for both groups (0.1 vs. 0 logMar).
Ophthalmological data are presented in Table 2.
There was no difference in the prevalence of depression between subjects with and without self-reported
glaucoma. The prevalence of depression was 6.6% (95%
CI 4.1–10.3) for participants with self-reported glaucoma
compared to 7.7% (95% CI 7.3–8.2) for participants
without self-reported glaucoma (p = 0.58).
For both groups, the prevalence of severe depression
was very low compared to minimal depressive symptoms
and the distribution of depression severity was comparable
(Table 3). Of the participants with self-reported glaucoma
69.1% presented no depressive symptoms (vs. 64.8%; p =
0.14), 24.3% minimal (vs. 27.5%; p = 0.26), 4.9% mild (vs.
5.8%; p = 0.61), 1.7% moderately severe (vs. 1.5%; p = 0.62)
and 0.0% severe (vs. 0.4%; p = 0.63) depressive symptoms.
With respect to anxiety, prevalence did not differ between the glaucoma and non-glaucoma group. Prevalence for anxiety was 5.3% (95% CI 3.1–8.7) in the

Table 1 Characteristics and general health condition of participants with and without self-reported glaucoma in the Gutenberg Health Study (GHS), 2007–2012

	All (N = 14,657)	No self-reported glaucoma (N = 14,364) mean or %	Self-reported glaucoma (N = 293) mean or %	P value
Demographics				
Age, years	55	55	66	<0.0001
Sex (women) (%)	49.5	49.5	51.2	0.6
SES	12.0	12.0	11.0	0.0001
High (3–8) (%)	18.3	18.1	25.0	0.004
Medium (9–14) (%)	46.2	46.2	48.6	0.4
Low (15–21) (%)	5.5	35.7	26.4	0.001
Comorbidities and general health status				
Diabetes mellitus (%)	9.3	9.2	17.1	<0.0001
Arterial hypertension (%)	49.6	49.1	71.7	<0.0001
Myocardial infarction (%)	2.9	2.9	3.8	0.38
Stroke (%)	1.9	1.9	2.4	0.51
COPD (%)	5.0	4.9	8.5	0.01
Bronchial asthma (%)	2.9	2.8	5.5	0.01
Cancer (%)	9.9	8.9	13.7	0.01
General health status	2.11 ± 0.64	2.10 ± 0.64	2.18 ± 0.61	0.03
Excellent (%)	12.7	12.8	7.5	0.01
Good (%)	66.9	66.8	70.2	0.23
Fair (%)	17.4	17.4	18.5	0.64
Poor (%)	12.7	12.8	7.5	0.01

SES socioeconomic status, *COPD* chronic obstructive pulmonary disease

glaucoma group vs. 6.6% (95% CI 6.2–7.1) in the non-glaucoma group ($p = 0.47$) (Table 3).

To validate self-reported glaucoma data, we analyzed glaucoma defined as self-reported glaucoma and the use of antiglaucoma eye medications or history of glaucoma surgery. According to this definition, 333 subjects had glaucoma. Comparable prevalence of anxiety (5.3% in the glaucoma group vs. 6.6% in the non-glaucoma group, $p = 0.37$) and of depression (7.0% vs. 7.7% in the non-glaucoma group, $p = 0.75$) was found (Table 4).

Table 2 Ocular characteristics of participants with and without self-reported glaucoma in the Gutenberg Health Study (GHS), 2007–2012

	All (N = 14,657)	No self-reported glaucoma (N = 14,364) mean or %	Self-reported glaucoma (N = 293) mean or %	P value
logMar DCVA	0.05	0	0.1	<0.0001
IOP (mmHg)	14	14	15.75	0.0001
Ocular diseases				
AMD (%)	0.5	0.5	1.4	0.05
Corneal diseases (%)	2.0	2.0	3.8	0.05
Cataract (%)	30.7	30.3	49.5	<0.0001
Diabetic retinopathy (%)	0.5	0.5	0.7	0.66
Antiglaucoma drugs				
Sympathomimetics (%)	0.3	0.0	11.6	<0.0001
Parasympathomimetics (%)	0.0	0.0	1.4	<0.0001
Carbonic anhydrase inhibitors (%)	0.3	0.1	12.6	<0.0001
Beta-blockers (%)	1.4	0.2	61.1	<0.0001
Prostaglandins (%)	0.7	0.0	30.4	<0.0001

IOP intraocular pressure, *DCVA* distantce-corrected visual acuity

Table 3 Prevalence of anxiety and depression and severity of depressive symptoms in participants with and without self-reported glaucoma in the Gutenberg Health Study (GHS), 2007–2012

	All (N = 14,657)	No self-reported glaucoma (N = 14,364) mean or %	Self-reported glaucoma (N = 293) mean or %	P-value
Depression				
PHQ-9 ≥ 10 (%)	7.7	7.7	6.6	0.58
History of depression (%)	12.0	12.1	9.6	0.24
None (%)	64.9	64.8	69.1	0.14
Minimal (%)	27.4	27.5	24.3	0.26
Mild (%)	5.8	5.8	4.9	0.61
Moderately (%)	1.5	1.5	1.7	0.62
Severe (%)	0.4	0.4	0.0	0.63
Anxiety				
GAD-2 ≥ 3 (%)	6.6	6.6	5.3	0.47
History of Anxiety (%)	7.3	7.3	6.5	0.65

PHQ-9 Patient Health Questionnaire, *GAD-2* Generalized Anxiety Disorder-2 Scale

To identify subjects with an advanced disease, we performed a subsample analysis between those having a visual acuity >0.5 logMar in the worse eye. Only 4.1% (597) of the sample had a visual acuity >0.5 logMar. In the glaucoma group 8.9% had a visual acuity >0.5% compared with 4.0% in the non-glaucoma group. Both prevalence of depression and anxiety were higher for the non-glaucoma group in this subsample analysis (Table 5). Prevalence for depression in glaucoma and non-glaucoma subjects with VA logMar >0.5 were 0 and 8.7% ($p = 0.25$). Prevalence for anxiety in glaucoma and non-glaucoma subjects with VA logMar >0.5 were 4.2 and 5.4% ($p = 1.0$).

To investigate associations between self-reported glaucoma and depression, resp. anxiety we performed logistic regression analyses. After adjusting for age, sex and SES we found no association between self-reported glaucoma and depression (OR 1.08, 95% CI 0.69–1.62), resp.

anxiety (OR 1.15, 95% CI 0.7–1.78). After additional adjustment for general comorbidities (namely arterial hypertension, diabetes mellitus, myocardial infarction, stroke, COPD, cancer), visual acuity (worse eye), IOP, ocular diseases (namely cataract, AMD, corneal diseases, diabetic retinopathy), antiglaucoma drugs (namely eye drops categorized into sympathomimetics, carbonic anhydrase inhibitors, beta-blockers, prostaglandins) and general health status we also found no association (Table 6).

Discussion

This is the first population-based study in a large European cohort analyzing the association between a) self-reported glaucoma and depression and b) self-reported glaucoma and anxiety.

Table 4 Sensitivity Analysis of participants with new glaucoma definition: Self-reported glaucoma + antiglaucoma drugs and/or history of glaucoma surgery

	All (N = 14,657)	No glaucoma (N = 14,324) mean or %	Glaucoma (N = 333) mean or %	P-value
Depression				
PHQ-9 ≥ 10 (%)	7.7	7.7	7.0	0.75
History of depression (%)	12.0	12.0	10.6	0.49
None (%)	64.9	64.8	69.1	0.11
Minimal (%)	27.4	27.5	23.9	0.15
Mild (%)	5.8	5.8	5.2	0.72
Moderately (%)	1.5	1.5	1.8	0.48
Severe (%)	0.4	0.4	0.0	0.64
Anxiety				
GAD-2 ≥ 3 (%)	6.6	6.6	5.3	0.37
History of Anxiety (%)	7.3	7.3	5.7	0.34

PHQ-9 Patient Health Questionnaire, *GAD-2* Generalized Anxiety Disorder Scale

Table 5 Subsample Analysis of participants with logMar BCVA>0.5 in the worse eye

	All (N = 597)	Self-reported no glaucoma (N = 571) mean or %	Self-reported glaucoma (N = 26) mean or %	P-value
Depression				
PHQ-9 ≥ 10 (%)	8.3	8.7	0.0	0.25
History of depression (%)	13.6	14.3	0.0	0.04
None (%)	59.5	59.2	66.7	0.53
Minimal (%)	32.1	32.1	33.3	1.00
Mild (%)	6.7	7.1	0.0	0.40
Moderately (%)	1.4	1.5	0.0	1.00
Severe (%)	0.2	0.2	0.0	1.00
Anxiety				
GAD-2 ≥ 3 (%)	5.4	5.4	4.2	1.00
History of Anxiety (%)	9.1	9.5	0.0	0.16

PHQ-9 Patient Health Questionnaire, *GAD-2* Generalized Anxiety Disorder Scale

The present study did not show a higher prevalence of depression or anxiety in self-reported glaucoma subjects compared to control subjects and there was no statistically significant association between glaucoma and depression or anxiety.

In our study sample the prevalence for depression was 6.6% in the glaucoma group and 7.7% in the non-glaucoma group. The prevalence for anxiety was 5.3% in the glaucoma group and 6.6% in the non-glaucoma group.

Prior studies showed a great inconsistency in depression prevalences among subjects with glaucoma. Depression prevalences varied between 4.3 and 32.1% [7, 8, 10–12, 14, 23–25]. Anxiety prevalences among glaucoma patients were reported to be as high as 13.0% in Japan [7], 22.9% in China [25] and 64% in Singapore [10]. However, it should be noted that these studies differed in study design, sample size and study population. For example, Lim et al. [10] showed depression and anxiety prevalence of 30 and 64%, which is much higher than in our study and compared to other studies. This study was conducted as a case-control study with the study population recruited from tertiary care hospitals. Those studies with subjects recruited from a tertiary care hospital seem to have higher prevalence rates in general which may be an overestimation due to increased severity of cases.

Glaucoma patients treated in hospitals present more often disease progression and complex medical records and consequently may have a higher risk for depression or generalized anxiety. Most of the participants of the GHS probably did not require medical treatment in a tertiary care hospital due to their glaucoma disease. Population-based studies have a more heterogeneous study sample, representative of the general population. Prevalence for depression in two other population based studies were 4.3% [14] and 10.9% [8]. It should be considered that an underestimation in a population based study is possible, since severe depression may prevent subjects from attending such studies. Regarding the distribution of depression classes in the current study, there is a low prevalence of moderately severe and severe depression in both groups. In the glaucoma and non-glaucoma group moderately severe depression was seen in 1.7 and 1.5% (p = 0.62) and severe depression in only 0.4% of the non-glaucoma group (p = 0.63). A recent cross-sectional study evaluating 1520 patients for glaucoma status, dry eye, mood and sleep disorders showed similar depression and anxiety rates in the glaucoma group receiving prostaglandin monotherapy and the non-glaucoma group. These findings are consistent with our results. The authors assume that social awareness of glaucoma and advanced diagnostics

Table 6 Associations of self-reported glaucoma with depression and anxiety in the Gutenberg Health Study (GHS), 2007–2012

	Model 1				Model 2			
	OR	CI	P-Value	n	OR	CI	P-Value	n
Depression (PHQ-9 ≥ 10)	1.08	0.69–1.62	0.72	14,359	1.10	0.50–2.38	0.80	14,061
Anxiety (GAD-2 ≥ 3)	1.15	0.70–1.78	0.55	14,288	1.48	0.63–3.30	0.35	13,991

PHQ-9 Patient Health Questionnaire, *GAD-2* Generalized Anxiety Disorder Scale, *OR* Odds ratio, *CI* 95% confidence Interval
Model 1: logistic regression analysis adjusted for age, sex, socio-economic status; Model 2 additionally adjusted for systemic comorbidities (arterial hypertension, myocardial infarction, stroke, diabetes mellitus, chronic obstructive pulmonary disease, cancer), ocular diseases (cataract, macular degeneration, corneal diseases, diabetic retinopathy), visual acuity of the worse eye, IOP, antiglaucoma eye medications (Sympathomimetics, Parasympathomimetics, Carbonic anhydrase inhibitors, Beta-blockers, Prostaglandins) and general health status

tools have led to an improvement in disease management and may contribute to the prevention of psychiatric disorders in glaucoma patients [26].

Our study provides a wide range of socio-demographic factors and comorbidities to assess a possible independent association between glaucoma and depression or anxiety.

In both groups the prevalence of self-reported cataract is high, with 49.5% in the glaucoma group and 30.3% in the non-glaucoma group and might be a confounding factor. Population-based studies showed that depressive symptoms and anxiety were associated with self-reported cataract [14, 27]. However adjusting for ophthalmological diseases including cataract did not alter our findings.

We conducted multiple regression analyses to evaluate a potential relationship. In none of the models could we find an association between glaucoma and depression or anxiety. This is consistent with the results of Wang et al., who also did not observe a significant association after including self-reported general health condition in the regression model. Glaucoma was also self-reported in this population based study [8]. Wilson et al. enrolled a prospective case-control study and stated that self-reported glaucoma patients are not more depressed than patients without glaucoma [12]. The survey instrument used for identifying depression was different from ours, in contrast to the study of Wang et al., where also the PHQ-9 was applied. Both are established survey instruments with a high reliability and validity and useful screening tests for identifying symptoms of depression [17, 28]. The results of Wang et al. might suggest that the perception of having poor general health, induced by an eye disease may be the causal link between eye disease and depression. Consistent with their findings, objective measures of glaucoma such as visual acuity and visual field defects were not associated with depression, in contrast to self-reported measures of visual disability. Self-reported measures were determined from a validated instrument for self-reporting visual disability (the National Eye Institute Visual Function Questionnaire). Su et al. also demonstrated a high impact of systemic comorbidities on depression rates among glaucoma patients in a case-control study. They compared glaucoma patients with a diagnosis of depression to age- and sex-matched glaucoma control subjects without depression. A significantly higher percentage of subjects with a high comorbidity index score was found in the depression group ($p < 0.0001$) [24]. Other previous studies showed that self-reported measures like General Health Status, rather than objective parameters were predictors of depression in glaucoma [8, 11].

The percentage of ß-blockers use is relatively high (61.1%) in our study. The use of systemic ß-blockers was proposed to have neuropsychiatric side effects and to be a possible risk factor for depression [29]. Therefore, some clinicians presume that glaucoma patients may have a higher risk of depression due to the side effects of topically applied ß-blockers [30]. Prior studies could not find the use of topical β-blockers to be associated with depression or anxiety in the multivariate logistic regression model [8, 10, 12, 24]. Presumably the systemic concentration of topically applied ß-blockers is not sufficient to contribute to psychiatric side effects.

The strength of this present study is the population-based design, with a large sample size, standardized examinations and a broad variety of potential confounders. Furthermore, we used established survey instruments with high reliability and validity to identify depression and general anxiety. However, our study also has some limitations. Due to the population-based study design the sample size of the glaucoma group is small, compared to the control group. Glaucoma diagnosis was self-reported, which may lead to recall-error. In our study design optical coherence tomography (OCT) was not included. OCT is an imaging technology that can be used for visualizing and analysing retinal tissue quickly and noninvasively [31]. It enables the detection of structural loss in the retinal nerve fiber layer (RNFL) before perimetric visible visual field defects and has become standard of care for detection of glaucoma and monitoring its progression and for detecting macular and retinal diseases [32]. However, we diminished the recall error of self-reported glaucoma diagnosis by analyzing a subsample, which included only self-reported glaucoma subjects with an additional use of antiglaucoma medications or having a history of glaucoma surgery. This subsample analysis revealed similar results. Additional examination of glaucoma subjects with a visual acuity >0.5 (logMar) in the worse eye again led to the same results. Generally, the number of subjects with reduced visual acuity in our study was low. Only 4.1% (597) of the total sample had a visual acuity >0.5 in the worse eye. Subjects with severe visual impairment might not participate in such a study. This study also comprised only a small number of participants with severe depressive symptoms. A reason could be that severe depression prevents subjects from participating in studies. Finally, the study did not include quantitative visual field measurements to categorize glaucoma severity. A categorization by glaucoma severity might reveal different depression and anxiety prevalence in different glaucoma stages. However, a previous study indicated that the worse eye's visual acuity was a stronger predictor of depression than the mean deviation, implying that central visual impairment may be more likely to contribute to depression than peripheral visual loss [11].

Conclusions

We did not find participants with self-reported glaucoma to be more depressed or anxious than participants without self-reported glaucoma. Adjustment for potential confounders did not alter our findings substantially. Future studies are needed to analyze the risk of mental disorders in glaucoma of different severities.

Abbreviations
AMD: Age-related macular degeneration; ATC: Anatomic therapeutic chemical code; COPD: Chronic obstructive pulmonary disease; DCVA: Distance-corrected visual acuity; GAD: Generalized anxiety disorder scale; GHS: The Gutenberg Health Study; IOP: Intraocular pressure; PHQ: Patient health questionnaire; SES: Socioeconomic status

Acknowledgements
GHS thanks all participants who took part in this study, and the whole GHS team, which includes study assistants, interviewers, computer and laboratory technicians, research scientists, managers and statisticians.

Funding
The Gutenberg Health Study is funded through the government of Rheinland-Pfalz ("Stiftung Rheinland-Pfalz für Innovation", contract AZ 961–386261/733), the research programs "Wissen schafft Zukunft" and "Center for Translational Vascular Biology (CTVB)" of the Johannes Gutenberg University of Mainz, and its contract with Boehringer Ingelheim, PHILIPS Medical Systems and Novartis Pharma, including an unrestricted grant for the Gutenberg Health Study. PSW is funded by the Federal Ministry of Education and Research (BMBF 1EO1003) Funders were involved in the development of the study design as scientific consultants. The funders had no role in study design, data collection and analysis, decision to publish, or preparation of the manuscript.

Authors' contributions
JR analyzed and interpreted the data and was a major contributor in writing the manuscript. AKS, SN, NP and MB made substantive intellectual contributions to conception and design and were involved in drafting and revising the manuscript. AS and IS made substantial contributions to statistical analysis of data. MM made substantial contributions to aquisition of psychiatric data and KL to aquistion of labarotory data. PSW and TM were involved in study design. All authors read and approved the final manuscript.

Competing interests
The authors declare that they have no competing interests. Boehringer Ingelheim, PHILIPS Medical Systems and Novartis Pharma provided funding towards this study. There are no patents, products in development or marketed products to declare. This does not alter the authors' adherence to all the BMC Ophthalmology policies on sharing data and materials. The funders had no role in study design, data collection and analysis, decision to publish, or preparation of the manuscript.

Author details
[1]Department of Ophthalmology, University Medical Center Mainz, Mainz, Germany. [2]Department of Psychosomatic Medicine and Psychotherapy, University Medical Center Mainz, Mainz, Germany. [3]Center for Cardiology I, University Medical Center Mainz, Mainz, Germany. [4]Preventive Cardiology and Preventive Medicine / Center for Cardiology, University Medical Center Mainz, Mainz, Germany. [5]Center for Thrombosis and Hemostasis (CTH), University Medical Center Mainz, Mainz, Germany. [6]German Center for Cardiovascular Research (DZHK), partner site Rhine-Main, Mainz, Germany. [7]Institute for Medical Biostatistics, Epidemiology and Informatics, University Medical Center Mainz, Mainz, Germany. [8]Institute for Clinical Chemistry and Laboratory Medicine, University Medical Center Mainz, Mainz, Germany.

References
1. Jonas JB, Aung T, Bourne RR, Bron AM, Ritch R, Panda-Jonas S. Glaucoma. Lancet. 2017;390(10108):2183–193. https://doi.org/10.1016/S0140-6736(17)31469-1. Epub 2017 May 31.
2. Resnikoff S, Pascolini D, Etya'ale D, Kocur I, Pararajasegaram R, Pokharel GP, Mariotti SP. Global data on visual impairment in the year 2002. Bull World Health Organ. 2004;82:844–51.
3. Quigley HA, Broman AT. The number of people with glaucoma worldwide in 2010 and 2020. Br J Ophthalmol. 2006;90:262–7.
4. Tham YC, Li X, Wong TY, Quigley HA, Aung T, Cheng CY. Global prevalence of glaucoma and projections of glaucoma burden through 2040: a systematic review and meta-analysis. Ophthalmology. 2014;121:2081–90.
5. Kimmel PL, Thamer M, Richard CM, Ray NF. Psychiatric illness in patients with end-stage renal disease. Am J Med. 1998;105:214–21.
6. Amato L, Paolisso G, Cacciatore F, Ferrara N, Canonico S, Rengo F, Varricchio M. Non-insulin-dependent diabetes mellitus is associated with a greater prevalence of depression in the elderly. The Osservatorio Geriatrico di Campania Region Group. Diabetes Metab. 1996;22:314–8.
7. Mabuchi F, Yoshimura K, Kashiwagi K, Shioe K, Yamagata Z, Kanba S, Iijima H, Tsukahara S. High prevalence of anxiety and depression in patients with primary open-angle glaucoma. J Glaucoma. 2008;17:552–7.
8. Wang SY, Singh K, Lin SC. Prevalence and predictors of depression among participants with glaucoma in a nationally representative population sample. Am J Ophthalmol. 2012;154:436–44. e432
9. Cumurcu T, Cumurcu BE, Celikel FC, Etikan I. Depression and anxiety in patients with pseudoexfoliative glaucoma. Gen Hosp Psychiatry. 2006;28:509–15.
10. Lim NC, Fan CH, Yong MK, Wong EP, Yip LW. Assessment of depression, anxiety, and quality of life in Singaporean patients with glaucoma. J Glaucoma. 2016;25:605–12.
11. Skalicky S, Goldberg I. Depression and quality of life in patients with glaucoma: a cross-sectional analysis using the geriatric depression Scale-15, assessment of function related to vision, and the glaucoma quality of Life-15. J Glaucoma. 2008;17:546–51.
12. Wilson MR, Coleman AL, Yu F, Fong Sasaki I, Bing EG, Kim MH. Depression in patients with glaucoma as measured by self-report surveys. Ophthalmology. 2002;109:1018–22.
13. Geldel MGD, Mayou R. Oxford Textbook of Psychiatry. 2nd ed. London: Oxford University Press; 1984.
14. Eramudugolla R, Wood J, Anstey KJ. Co-morbidity of depression and anxiety in common age-related eye diseases: a population-based study of 662 adults. Front Aging Neurosci. 2013;5:56.
15. Wild PS, Zeller T, Beutel M, Blettner M, Dugi KA, Lackner KJ, Pfeiffer N, Munzel T, Blankenberg S. The Gutenberg Health Study. Bundesgesundheitsblatt Gesundheitsforschung Gesundheitsschutz. 2012;55:824–9.
16. Hohn R, Kottler U, Peto T, Blettner M, Munzel T, Blankenberg S, Lackner KJ, Beutel M, Wild PS, Pfeiffer N. The ophthalmic branch of the Gutenberg Health Study: study design, cohort profile and self-reported diseases. PLoS One. 2015;10:e0120476.
17. Lowe B, Grafe K, Zipfel S, Witte S, Loerch B, Herzog W. Diagnosing ICD-10 depressive episodes: superior criterion validity of the Patient Health Questionnaire. Psychother Psychosom. 2004;73:386–90.
18. Wiltink J, Michal M, Wild PS, Schneider J, Konig J, Blettner M, Munzel T, Schulz A, Weber M, Fottner C, et al. Associations between depression and diabetes in the community: do symptom dimensions matter? Results from the Gutenberg Health Study. PLoS One. 2014;9:e105499.
19. Kroenke K, Spitzer RL, Williams JB, Monahan PO, Lowe B. Anxiety disorders in primary care: prevalence, impairment, comorbidity, and detection. Ann Intern Med. 2007;146:317–25.
20. Lampert T, Kroll LE, Muters S, Stolzenberg H. Measurement of the socioeconomic status within the German Health Update 2009 (GEDA). Bundesgesundheitsblatt Gesundheitsforschung Gesundheitsschutz. 2013;56:131–43.
21. Lampert T, Kroll LE, Muters S, Stolzenberg H. [Measurement of the socioeconomic status within the German Health Update 2009 (GEDA)]. Bundesgesundheitsblatt, Gesundheitsforschung, Gesundheitsschutz. 2013;56(1):131–43.
22. Team RC. R: A language and environment for statistical computing. Vienna: R Foundation for Statistical Computing; 2016.
23. Yochim BP, Mueller AE, Kane KD, Kahook MY. Prevalence of cognitive impairment, depression, and anxiety symptoms among older adults with glaucoma. J Glaucoma. 2012;21:250–4.

24. Su CC, Chen JY, Wang TH, Huang JY, Yang CM, Wang IJ. Risk factors for depressive symptoms in glaucoma patients: a nationwide case-control study. Graefes Arch Clin Exp Ophthalmol. 2015;253:1319–25.

25. Zhou C, Qian S, Wu P, Qiu C. Anxiety and depression in Chinese patients with glaucoma: sociodemographic, clinical, and self-reported correlates. J Psychosom Res. 2013;75:75–82.

26. Ra S, Ayaki M, Yuki K, Tsubota K, Negishi K. Dry eye, sleep quality, and mood status in glaucoma patients receiving prostaglandin monotherapy were comparable with those in non-glaucoma subjects. PLoS One. 2017;12:e0188534.

27. Freeman EE, Gresset J, Djafari F, Aubin MJ, Couture S, Bruen R, Laporte A, Boisjoly H. Cataract-related vision loss and depression in a cohort of patients awaiting cataract surgery. Can J Ophthalmol. 2009;44:171–6.

28. Mcdowell I. Measuring Health: A Guide to Rating Scales and Questionnaires. New York: In Oxford University Press, vol. 2nd ed., 2nd edition; 1996.

29. Keller S, Frishman WH. Neuropsychiatric effects of cardiovascular drug therapy. Cardiol Rev. 2003;11:73–93.

30. Shore JH, Fraunfelder FT, Meyer SM. Psychiatric side effects from topical ocular timolol, a beta-adrenergic blocker. J Clin Psychopharmacol. 1987;7:264–7.

31. Schuman JS. Optical Coherence Tomography in High Myopia. JAMA Ophthalmol. 2016;134:1040.

32. Harwerth RS, Carter-Dawson L, Smith EL 3rd, Barnes G, Holt WF, Crawford ML. Neural losses correlated with visual losses in clinical perimetry. Invest Ophthalmol Vis Sci. 2004;45:3152–60.

13

General analysis of factors influencing cataract surgery practice in Shanghai residents

Yi Xu[1], Jiangnan He[1], Senlin Lin[1], Bo Zhang[1], Jianfeng Zhu[1], Serge Resnikoff[2], Lina Lu[1*] and Haidong Zou[1]

Abstract

Background: It was reported that lack of knowledge, less confidence of medical services, commute difficulties, and poor economic conditions would be the main barriers for cataract surgery practice. The influencing factors could have changed in cities with high developing speed. Shanghai is one of the biggest cities in China and the world. The purpose of the study was to explore the factors influencing cataract surgery practice in Shanghai.

Methods: This was a population-based, cross-sectional study. A total of 2342 cataract patients older than 50 years old with cataract-induced visual impairment or who had undergone cataract surgery were recruited from rural and urban areas of Shanghai. Participants accepted a face-to-face structured questionnaire. Data were collected on patient demographics, education, work, income, health insurance, awareness about cataracts disease, treatment and related medical resources and deration policy, transportation and degree of satisfaction with hospitals.

Results: There were 417 patients who had received cataract surgery, 404 of them supplied complete information in the questionnaire. More female subjects (64.6%) than male subjects (35.4%) accepted cataract surgery among the 404 patients. Of the patients with cataract history, 36.4% of surgery patients were equal or older than 80. More people with urban medical insurance received surgery ($p = 0.036$). Patients who received surgery were more satisfied with local medical service ($p = 0.032$). In urban area, Lower income and difficulties with commutes were related to a higher rate of surgery.

Conclusions: Cataract patients with the following features were more inclined to receive surgery: female, old age, better awareness. In urban areas low income and difficult commutes did not represent barriers for cataract surgery, probably because of appropriate cataract surgery promotion policies recent years in Shanghai. In rural areas, better healthcare reimbursement policies would likely lead to a higher uptake of cataract surgery. Further cohort studies with more controls could supply stronger evidence for our viewpoint.

Keywords: Cataract surgery, Influencing factor, Economy, Policy, Questionnaire

Background

According to the World Health Organization (WHO) report, cataracts were responsible for blindness in 10.8 million people around the world, or 33.4% of all blindness [1]. As such, it is a leading cause of avoidable blindness [2–4]. By 2020, the estimated cost required to treat the burden of avoidable blindness and visual impairment over 10 years will be US$23.1 billion [5]. In China, age-related cataracts are still the leading cause of treatable blindness [6, 7]. However, China has one of the lowest cataract surgery rates (CSR) in Asia [8–10], with clear disparities across different areas [11]. In 2014, the CSR was 1125 per 1,000,000 per year [12]. China's CSR was much lower than that of developed countries and some developing areas such as Latin America [13]. In areas with low CSR, cataract surgeries are often postponed until the disease progresses to a worse condition, by which time there are more surgery risks and complications [14]. There is no standardized medical referral

---

* Correspondence: linaluoph@163.com
[1]Shanghai Eye Disease Prevention & Treatment Center / Shanghai Eye Hospital; Shanghai Key Laboratory of Ocular Fundus Diseases; Shanghai General Hospital; Shanghai Engineering Center for Visual Science and Photomedicine, 380 Kangding Road, Shanghai 200040, China
Full list of author information is available at the end of the article

system in China; nearly all of the hospitals are walk-in, and a severe imbalance exists in the distribution of ophthalmologic medical resources. Cataract patients who want to receive surgery have to travel a long way if there are no cataract hospitals near their home. It was reported that [15] the following four problems could be primary barriers to basic cataract surgery: lack of knowledge about cataracts, low confidence in the quality of local medical services, transportation difficulties, and poor economic conditions. However, the major factors influencing cataract surgery may differ across various areas [16].

In recent years, rapid development has occurred in many areas of China, and an imbalance exists across various geographical districts and people with regard to medical resources, infrastructure, financial conditions, education level, health awareness status, and so on [17, 18]. Shanghai, which is undergoing dramatic urbanization, has one of the most rapid rates of development in China and in the world. The availability and affordability of medical services in Shanghai is relatively optimal compared to most developing districts of China [19, 20]. Over the past 15 years, the Shanghai government has been putting policies into practice to promote cataract surgeries. Shanghai's cataract surgery rate has been rapidly increasing during the last 10 years. However, the administration of cataract surgery practice is still met with big problems in some populations. To analyse the major factors influencing cataract surgery, we enrolled 2342 Shanghai residents who had undergone cataract surgery or with cataract-induced visual impairment whose presenting visual acuity (PVA) was less than 20/40, and collected various information on population features, social economics, medical resources and patients' health awareness status. The aim was to investigate the possible reasons for unoperated cataracts, which cause vision impairment, in a population-based study.

Methods

Study setting and population

This study was approved by the Ethics Committee of the Shanghai Eye Disease Prevention & Treatment Center. It was carried out in accordance with the Declaration of Helsinki. It was executed from June to November 2014 [21]. The Baoshan and Xuhui districts were randomly selected as representative rural and urban areas in the present study, respectively. Cluster sampling was used based on community unit, the sample of individuals were randomly selected. The study sampling frame for each community was constructed using geographically defined clusters based on register census data. Each cluster contained a population of approximately 1000 individuals (all ages). Basing on the percentage of population of older than 50 years old, we randomly selected 24 and

19 clusters (with equal probability) from the sampling frame of Baoshan and Xuhui districts. Finally, 11,644 residents ≥50 years old were enrolled [21, 22]. Ophthalmologic examinations were performed on each subject. Those patients who had undergone cataract surgery or who presented with cataracts and presented visual acuity (PVA) in the better eye worse than 20/40 (mild visual impairment) were chosen for the questionnaire survey. The diagnostic criteria for cataract was that patients' lens opacity was commensurate with visual impairment and no other abnormality could account for the decrease in visual acuity. The definition of cataract-induced visual impairment was: Besides cataract, there were no other abnormality could account for the decrease in visual acuity, and PVA in the better eye worse than 20/40 [22]. Participation in the study was encouraged by the mayors of the communities. A total of 2542 patients were eligible for the study, and 2342 patients accepted the questionnaire survey, 2234 of them supplied complete information required by the questionnaire. The response rate was 92%.

District information

The Baoshan district is in the northern part of Shanghai, and the Xuhui district is located in the southwest. The land areas of Baoshan and Xuhui cover 270.99 km^2 and 54.76 km^2, respectively. According to the report from the "Shanghai Statistical Yearbook 2015", the year-end populations in 2014 were 2.024 million (Baoshan) and 1. 110 million (Xuhui). According to the 2014 report from the Shanghai eye diseases prevention and treatment information management system, the district CSRs were 2951 (Baoshan) and 4548 (Xuhui), and the CSR for the entire city was 3807. The details are shown in Table 1.

Medical resources

There are 5 hospitals in Baoshan district in which 16 cataract surgeons perform surgery regularly. Compared to Baoshan district, Xuhui district has many more hospitals and cataract doctors (8 hospitals and 120 cataract surgeons) (Table 1).

Patients

Door-to-door recruitment was conducted and written informed consent was acquired from each participant. Ophthalmic examination and questionnaire surveys were conducted at local community healthcare centers. All of the participants were 50 years old or older. Patients underwent ophthalmic examinations performed by professional optometrists and an ophthalmologist, including distance-presenting visual acuity (PVA) tested by a retro illuminated tumbling E LogMAR chart; intraocular pressure (IOP); fundus photography; and slit-lamp examination of eyelid, ocular globe, pupillary reflex, lens grade

Table 1 District information and cataract medical resources in Baoshan & Xuhui districts

	Land area (km^2)	Population (million)	CSR in 2014	Number of hospitals for cataract treatment	Number of doctors being able to do cataract surgery
Baoshan	270.99	2.024	2951	5	16
Xuhui	54.76	1.110	4548	8	120
Total	325.75	3.134	3750	13	136

and fundus. Cataract was assigned when lens opacity was observed, if a previous cataract surgery was reported, or if signs of cataract or previous cataract surgery were observed in slit-lamp examination. For patients who had received cataract surgery, we recorded the surgery type, IOL (intraocular lens) position, posterior capsule status and other complications. A total of 2542 cataract patients (1312 rural, 1230 urban) with PVA in the better eye worse than 20/40 were selected for the following questionnaire survey.

Questionnaires

There were 2342 cataract patients who accepted the interview. Face-to-face visits were conducted by four primary healthcare professionals. The four professionals were well-trained before they conducted the work, and consistency checks were performed. The following information was collected during the survey:

1. Basic information: age, gender, education, work, medical insurance, family disposable income per month.
2. Patients' awareness: awareness about cataracts (4 questions); awareness about cataract surgery, including treatment and proper surgery access, long-term complications from untreated cataracts, whether it is painful and how long it takes to recover after the surgery (7 questions); awareness about cataract medical resources and deration policy, including whether they know which hospitals in the district perform cataract surgery, knowledge about cataract surgery cost and the reimbursement policy (6 questions). Each question in this part was scored "1", "2", "3" or "4" when the answer was "nothing", "a little knowledge", "basic knowledge" or "good knowledge", respectively. Scores from 17 questions about awareness were summed for each patient.
3. Transportation: How long does it take to travel from your home to the nearest cataract surgery hospital? How many transfer times of the transportation would you need? The reason that we identified transfer times as a potential risk factor is that most older people in China do not know how to drive or do not drive; instead, they usually take public transportation. Transfer times could therefore limit accessibility to cataract hospitals.
4. Satisfaction with local hospitals: Are you satisfied with the facilities and medical service of the hospitals nearby?

The study abided by the tenets of the Declaration of Helsinki. It was approved by the Shanghai Eye Disease Preventive & Treatment Center Committee of Ethics.

Statistical analyses

All statistical analyses were performed using STATISTICAL ANALYSIS SYSTEM (SAS 9.2, SAS Institute, Inc., Cary, NC. USA). Statistical significance was determined at $p < 0.05$. Absolute frequency (n) and relative frequency (%) were calculated, and Pearson chi-square (χ^2) tests were used for the qualitative variables. Means and SDs (mean ± SD) were calculated, and logistic analysis and univariate ANOVA were applied to the quantitative variables. Multivariate logistic regression models were constructed to assess the association with surgery status, including gender, age, income, education, social insurance, hospital accessibility, satisfaction about hospital facilities, satisfaction about medical service, awareness score and district as the independent variables. The subgroup analysis within rural area or urban area about the association with surgery status were also shown. Odds ratios (ORs), 95% confidence intervals (CIs), and p value are also presented in Table 4.

Results

Clinical information derived from questionnaire interview

All of the selected patients underwent ophthalmologic examination. PVA, IOP and lens status are shown in Table 2. Most of the patients in rural and urban areas had PVA between 20/63 to < 20/40. Of patients in rural and urban areas, 13.2% and 15.4%, respectively, had PVA worse than 20/400. The average IOPs were 16.9 ± 3.9 mmHg in rural patients and 15.8 ± 4.0 mmHg in urban patients ($p = 0.12$). Among the 2342 interviewees, there were 417 patients who had received cataract surgery and 1925 patients had not.

Table 2 Ophthalmologic examination of subjects accepted questionnaire interview in rural and urban

	Rural n = 1312	Urban n = 1230	P value
PVA			0.16
< 20/40–20/63	803(61.2%)	758(61.5%)	
20/63–20/200	312(23.8%)	259(21.1%)	
20/200–20/400	24(1.8%)	24(2.0%)	
< 20/400	173(13.2%)	189(15.4%)	
IOP (mmHg)	16.9 ± 3.9	15.8 ± 4.0	0.12
Lens status			0.004
cataract	1084(82.6%)	937(83.6%)	
IOL	129(10.5%)	176(15.7%)	
aphakic	3(0.2%)	3(0.3%)	
others	5(0.4%)	5(0.4%)	

Information about gender, age, family income, education, medical insurance type, commute, satisfaction, awareness and district of patients who had received or not received cataract surgery

Two thousand two hundred thirty-four patients supplied complete information required in the questionnaire. It showed that more female subjects (64.6%) than male subjects (35.4%) accepted cataract surgery among the 404 patients who had surgery history. Of the 404 patients, 36.4% of surgery patients were equal or older than 80. However, the most common age range in no surgery population were 60 to 70 years old (34.9%) and 70 to 80 years old (33.6%). The constituent ratio of age in surgery group and no surgery group were significantly different ($p < 0.0001$). There were no significant differences between patients who had received surgery and those who had not with regard to family income level. For patients who received surgery, 92.1% had urban medical insurance; for patients who did not receive surgery, 87.0% had urban medical insurance ($p = 0.036$). Commute times were longer among those who had received surgery ($p = 0.0115$). Patients in the surgery group were more satisfied with local medical service than people in the "no surgery" group ($p = 0.0048$). Most of the patients in the surgery group were from urban area (55.2%), whereas patients from rural area composed a larger portion (54.5%) of the "no surgery" group ($p = 0.0004$). Details are shown in Table 3.

In order to investigate different personal reasons for unacceptance of cataract surgery, we designed a question in the questionnaire: Why haven't you accepted cataract surgery previously before the survey? There were 287 patients supplied their answers. Several kinds of answers were collected. The most frequent answers were that "I don't think that cataract has much influence on my life. My present visual acuity still makes do" and "I did not

know that my visual acuity was impaired by cataract". Details were shown in Table 4.

Correlations between gender, age, family income, education, medical insurance type, commute, satisfaction, awareness, district and surgery status among cataract patients with vision impairment

To investigate the correlations between possible factors influencing cataract surgery among interviewees, we performed multivariable linear regression analysis. The results indicated that gender, age, awareness, district type, family income and commute time were significantly correlated with cataract surgery. Patients with the following features were more likely to receive cataract surgery: female (OR(95%CI) for male = 0.649 (0.506, 0.833), $p = 0.0007$), over 80 years old (OR(95%CI) = 2.521(1.535, 4.140), $p = 0.0003$), better awareness (OR(95%CI) = 1.034 (1.028, 1.040), $p < 0.0001$), lower family income (OR(95%CI) for income ≥5000 = 0.579 (0.400, 0.837), $p = 0.0036$) and longer commute time (OR(95%CI) for one transfer = 1.344 (1.033, 1.749), $p = 0.0278$). The latter two features represent a significant departure from several previous reports. To clarify the reasons that patients with lower income and inconvenient commutes were more prone to receive cataract surgery than people with higher income and more convenient transportation conditions, we further analysed patients from rural and urban areas separately. We found that these phenomena existed in urban but not rural residents. Details are shown in Table 5.

Discussion

Surgery remains the major option for cataract treatment. However, many patients in developing countries only seek cataract surgery in later stages of cataract progression. Severe complications, such as phacolytic and phacomorphic glaucoma, could occur at these later stages. In this study, patients who had visual impairment caused by cataracts completed a questionnaire survey. The survey was executed in the form of a face-to-face interview. Compared to some other studies [23–25] that were conducted by telephone, this form of survey was more appropriate for collecting broader information.

To ensure the necessity of cataract surgery in those patients, we performed ophthalmologic examination of all interviewees. Subjects suffering from other visual impairments, such as high myopia, corneal opacity, age-related macular degeneration, diabetic retinopathy and glaucoma, were excluded, as these comorbidities could confound our results. With regard to lens status, there were more "IOLs" implanted in Xuhui than in Baoshan (15.7% vs 10.5%, respectively, $p = 0.004$). This result was in accordance with the fact that the surgery rate was lower in Baoshan district.

Table 3 Gender, age, family income, education, medical insurance type, commute, satisfaction, awareness, district of patients accepted and unaccepted cataract surgery

	Cataract surgery history		P value
	Yes	No	
	n = 404	n = 1830	
Gender [n(%)]			0.0127
Male	143 (15.6%)	771 (84.4%)	
Female	261 (19.8%)	1059 (80.2%)	
Total	404 (17.8%)	1830 (82.2%)	
Age [n(%)]			< 0.0001
50- < 60	30 (14.6%)	176 (85.4%)	
60- < 70	94 (12.8%)	638 (87.2%)	
70- < 80	133 (17.8%)	614 (82.2%)	
≥ 80	147(26.8%)	402 (73.2%)	
Total	404 (17.8%)	1830 (82.2%)	
Disposable family Income per month [n(%)]			0.5624
< 1000 RMB	8 (11.6%)	61 (88.4%)	
1000–2999 RMB	207 (18.4%)	918 (81.6%)	
3000–4999 RMB	124 (18.2%)	556 (81.8%)	
≥ 5000 RMB	65 (18.1%)	295 (81.9%)	
Total	404 (17.8%)	1830 (82.2%)	
Education [n(%)]			0.0323
illiteracy	70 (16.9%)	344 (83.1%)	
Primary school	103 (19.5%)	424 (80.5%)	
middle school	179 (16.6%)	902 (83.4%)	
College and above	52 (24.5%)	160 (75.5%)	
Total	404 (17.7%)	1830 (82.3%)	
Medical Insurance [n(%)]			0.0363
No insurance	1 (5.6%)	17 (94.4%)	
Urban medical insurance	372 (18.9%)	1593 (81.1%)	
Rural medical insurance	21 (11.9%)	156 (88.1%)	
Non-local medical insurance	10 (13.5%)	64 (86.5%)	
Total	404 (17.8%)	1830 (82.2%)	
Transfer times [n(%)]			0.0115
0	181 (15.7%)	970 (84.3%)	
1	164 (20.7%)	630 (79.3%)	
≥ 2	59 (20.4%)	230 (79.6%)	
Total	404 (17.8%)	1830 (82.2%)	
Satisfaction about facilities of hospitals nearby [n(%)]			0.0319
Very satisfied	118 (21.1%)	441 (78.9%)	
Other	286 (17.1%)	1389 (82.9%)	
Total	404 (17.8%)	1830 (82.2%)	
Satisfaction about service of hospitals nearby [n(%)]			0.0048

Table 3 Gender, age, family income, education, medical insurance type, commute, satisfaction, awareness, district of patients accepted and unaccepted cataract surgery *(Continued)*

	Cataract surgery history		P value
	Yes	No	
	n = 404	n = 1830	
Very satisfied	127 (22.0%)	451 (78.0%)	
Other	277 (16.7%)	1379 (83.3%)	
Total	404 (17.8%)	1830 (82.2%)	
District [n(%)]			0.0004
Rural	181 (15.4%)	998 (84.6%)	
Urban	223 (21.1%)	832 (78.9%)	
Total	404 (17.8%)	1830 (82.2%)	
[a]Awareness evaluation score			< 0.0001
Mean (standard deviation)	55.0 (23.4)	38.8 (24.2)	
	404	1830	

Pearson Chi-square (χ^2) test and [a]type III ANOVA test were used for qualitative and quantitative variables separately

Table 4 The reason for that patients did not accept cataract surgery treatment before the survey

	District		P value
	Rural (n = 160)	Urban (n = 180)	
Why haven't you accepted cataract surgery previously before the survey?			< 0.0001
I did not know that my visual acuity was impaired by cataract.	4 (3.3%)	29 (17.5%)	
I don't think that cataract has much influence on my life. My present visual acuity still makes do.	79 (65.3%)	74 (44.6%)	
I did not know that cataract could be treated by surgery.	1(0.8%)	5 (3.0%)	
I am worried about the effect of cataract surgery, especially the possibility of resurgence.	5 (4.1%)	21 (12.7%)	
I am worried about that I could not be able to work after surgery.	0 (0.0%)	11 (6.6%)	
I am worried about that nobody would take care of me during perioperative period.	0 (0.0%)	4 (2.4%)	
It was inconvenient for me to go to hospital and ask for help.	2 (1.7%)	3 (1.8%)	
I don't trust on the surgery treatment.	0 (0.0%)	2 (1.2%)	
I could not afford the surgery cost.	6 (5.0%)	3 (1.8%)	
Religion reasons	0 (0.0%)	0 (0.0%)	
Others	24 (19.8%)	14 (8.4%)	
Total	121	166	

Pearson Chi-square (χ2) test

Table 5 Logistic regression of the correlation between gender, age, family income, education, medical insurance type, commute, satisfaction, awareness, district and surgery status

Factors		Rural & urban			Rural			Urban		
		OR	95% CI	P value	OR	95% CI	P value	OR	95% CI	P value
Gender	Female	reference			reference			reference		
	Male	0.649	0.506 0.833	0.0007	0.635	0.439 0.918	0.0158	0.660	0.467 0.931	0.0178
Age	50- < 60	reference			reference			reference		
	60–69	0.801	0.494 1.298	0.3675	0.627	0.340 1.155	0.1343	1.259	0.548 2.893	0.5876
	70–79	1.182	0.733 1.908	0.4931	0.875	0.469 1.632	0.6739	1.872	0.829 4.229	0.1313
	> 79	2.521	1.535 4.140	0.0003	1.841	0.947 3.582	0.0721	4.132	1.808 9.444	0.0008
Income	≤2999	reference			reference			reference		
	3000–4999	0.720	0.545 0.950	0.0203	0.731	0.477 1.120	0.1501	0.709	0.486 1.032	0.0728
	≥ 5000	0.579	0.400 0.837	0.0036	0.904	0.484 1.688	0.7506	0.501	0.313 0.804	0.0042
Education	illiteracy	reference			reference			reference		
	primary school	1.282	0.880 1.867	0.1963	1.154	0.693 1.921	0.5814	1.485	0.831 2.652	0.1816
	middle school	1.104	0.751 1.622	0.6159	0.923	0.536 1.589	0.7735	1.325	0.744 2.360	0.3391
	college and above	1.375	0.831 2.275	0.2151	0.867	0.402 1.869	0.7151	2.141	1.043 4.392	0.0379
Social insurance	without insurance & non-local insurance	0.762	0.382 1.522	0.4419	0.747	0.330 1.693	0.4855	0.718	0.188 2.744	0.6284
	urban health insurance	reference			reference			reference		
	rural health insurance	0.904	0.526 1.555	0.7158	0.812	0.446 1.479	0.4956	2.875	0.500 16.515	0.2366
Hospital accessibility	through bus	reference			reference			reference		
	one transfer	1.344	1.033 1.749	0.0278	1.143	0.762 1.716	0.5185	1.466	1.030 2.0872	0.0336
	≥ twice transfer	1.419	0.988 2.039	0.0581	1.120	0.650 1.931	0.6826	1.760	1.068 2.901	0.0266
Satisfaction about hospital facilities	others	reference			reference			reference		
	satisfied	0.667	0.369 1.203	0.1780	0.654	0.284 1.506	0.3184	0.676	0.285 1.605	0.3747
Satisfaction about medical service	others	reference			reference			reference		
	satisfied	1.632	0.918 2.903	0.0952	1.363	0.617 3.012	0.4435	1.786	0.756 4.219	0.1858
Awareness score	–	1.034	1.028 1.040	< 0.0001	1.039	1.030 1.047	< 0.0001	1.031	1.023 1.039	< 0.0001
District	Baoshan	reference			–			–		
	Xuhui	1.524	1.181 1.967	0.0012						

The Logistic analysis (full model)

There are many factors influencing cataract surgery in rural and urban populations. After referring to the reported studies and the local features of Shanghai city, we chose these factors described in the study to do the questionnaire survey. According to our results, 17.8% of subjects (417 out of 2342) had received cataract surgery. The surgery rate in patients with the following features was higher: female, over 80 years old, low family income, longer commute time, better health awareness, and urban residents. Patients with disposable family income greater than 3000 Chinese Yuan (about 470 US Dollars) per month were less willing to commit to surgery. Some of our results were similar to previous reports. However, a unique observation was that patients in urban areas with lower family income and longer commutes were even more prone to receive surgery. This is distinct from other studies which reported that economic and commute difficulties could pose a barrier to cataract surgery among patients with visual impairment. A possible reason for this may be that partial reimbursement of surgery costs by the Social Security Administration is profitable for hospitals providing medical service. Thus, this may be an important income source for many public hospitals. Before 2015, the reimbursement ratio of urban health insurance was much higher than that of rural health insurance (70% versus 50%) in Shanghai, which means that hospitals could benefit more from patients having urban health insurance. In recent years, cataract surgery promotion policies for patients from poor economic backgrounds have been widely promoted by the Shanghai government. Hospitals were encouraged to screen proper cataract patients with poor economy background to perform cataract surgeries, and there were shuttle buses from hospitals to pick up patients in inconvenient areas to surgery performing hospitals and send them back to home after surgeries. In such situations, more patients with low income and inconvenient commutes accepted cataract surgeries on the contrary. Due to the reimbursement profit gap between urban health insurance and rural health insurance, hospitals were much more willing to perform such screenings among populations in urban areas. The reasons listed above could cause more patients in urban area to receive cataract surgery even though their family income is low and their commute is inconvenient. This study indicates the important influence of government policy on cataract surgery promotion even though economic and commute difficulties still exist. Better policy support is needed for patients with rural health insurance. Visual impairment in different distance and cataract surgery practice was another important research topic. It was possible that patients with distant visual impairment may not have surgery because that they could still handle with daily life with near vision. It is worthy to do further study to investigate this topic.

According to the survey, the most frequent answers to why the patients did not accept cataract surgery were that "I don't think that cataract has much influence on my life. My present visual acuity still makes do" and "I did not know that my visual acuity was impaired by cataract". It could be explained by the reasons as follows:most of the patients were old people and work did not play an important role in their life, most of the patients did not ask for much for their quality of life, and their awareness about cataract needed improving. Health education could be effective for improving the awareness and cataract surgery practice in those patients.

During the investigation, we did general ophthalmologic evaluation for the patients. However, in the present study, we mainly used the clinical data to screen out those subjects with visual impairment caused by cataract and did questionnaire survey to the patients, so the basic clinical data related to cataract were shown, including visual acuity, intraocular pressure and lens status. In further study derived from the investigation, we will focus on the clinical examination and more clinical data would be analysed.

Patients' health awareness is an important factor influencing surgery in general. Our results show that the surgery rate was higher among patients with better health awareness level, which in turn demonstrates the importance of health awareness in promoting cataract surgery. Since 1998, a large number of public health system building projects have been executed and promoted by the Shanghai Municipal government, the Center for Disease Control and the Shanghai Eye Disease Prevention & Treatment Center. Patient education has been widely promoted at each community health care centre. This work has improved health awareness in both rural

and urban areas and has promoted cataract surgery in general.

The patients included in the study have different awareness status about the cataract disease. The awareness status was influenced by various reasons, such as patients' education level, the health literacy, the health service access, and the health service quality [26]. All those factors could have influence on the patients' awareness and the surgery practice, and it is very important to clarify the influence of the health service access on the awareness. We will do further study to discuss the influence of various factors on awareness on surgery practice.

Conclusions
Shanghai is the city with the largest population in China, and it is one of the biggest cities worldwide. As a municipality, its administrative level is equal to that of a province in China. The scale and importance of this city indicates the degree to which our study may be representative of many metropolitan cities and their adjacent rural areas in China. In order to prove the effectiveness of government policies, further cohort studies with more controls will be needed, which could supply stronger evidence to support our viewpoint. This study provides information for policymakers to consider how to increase cataract surgery rates and reduce vision impairment caused by cataracts across the entire country of China.

Abbreviations
CSR: Cataract surgery rate; PVA: Presented visual acuity

Acknowledgements
We thank all patients and their families for kindly participating in the study.

Funding
This study was financially supported by the Shanghai Municipal Commission of Health and Family Planning Grant (No. 201440529).

Authors' contributions
YX Design and execution of the study, data collection and manuscript preparation; JH Design and execution of the study, data collection and analysis; SL Execution of the study, data collection and analysis; BZ Execution of the study; JZ Design of the study; SR manuscript preparation and review; LL Design and execution of the study, manuscript preparation; HZ Design of the study, manuscript preparation. All authors read and approved the final manuscript.

Competing interests
The authors declare that they have no competing interests.

Author details
[1]Shanghai Eye Disease Prevention & Treatment Center / Shanghai Eye Hospital; Shanghai Key Laboratory of Ocular Fundus Diseases; Shanghai General Hospital; Shanghai Engineering Center for Visual Science and Photomedicine, 380 Kangding Road, Shanghai 200040, China. [2]Brien Holden Vision Institute and SOVS, University of New South Wales, Sydney, NSW, Australia.

References

1. Khairallah M, Kahloun R, Bourne R, Limburg H, Flaxman SR, Jonas JB, et al. Number of people blind or visually impaired by cataract worldwide and in world regions, 1990 to 2010. Invest Ophthalmol Vis Sci. 2015;56:6762–9.
2. Gonzalez-Salinas R, Guarnieri A, Guirao Navarro MC, Saenz-de-Viteri M. Patient considerations in cataract surgery - the role of combined therapy using phenylephrine and ketorolac. Patient Prefer Adherence. 2016;10:1795–801.
3. Blindness in the elderly [editorial]. Lancet. 2008;372(9646):1273.
4. Brian G, Taylor H. Cataract blindness—challenges for the 21st century. Bull World Health Organ. 2001;79:249–56.
5. PwC (PricewaterhouseCoopers). The price of sight: the global cost of eliminating avoidable blindness. Final report for the Fred hollows foundation. Melbourne: PricewaterhouseCoopers; 2012.
6. Liang Yb1, Friedman DS, Wong TY, Zhan SY, Sun LP, Wang JJ, et al. Prevalence and causes of low vision and blindness in a rural Chinese adult population: the Handan eye study. Ophthalmol. 2008;115:1965–72.
7. Tang Y, Wang X, Wang J, Huang W, Gao Y, Luo Y, et al. Prevalence of age-related cataract and cataract surgery in a Chinese adult population: the Taizhou eye study. Invest Ophthalmol Vis Sci. 2016;57:1193–200.
8. China Disabled Person's Federation (CDPF). Statistics yearbook on the undertakings of people with disabilities in China. Beijing: CDPF Information Center; 2005. p. 3–99.
9. Zhao JL. To promote "vision 2020" initiative under the new situation in China. Zhonghua Yan Ke Za Zhi. 2011;47:769–72.
10. Chen T, Jin L, Zhou Z, Huang Y, Yan X, Liu T, et al. Factors influencing the output of rural cataract surgical facilities in China: the SHARP study. Invest Ophthalmol Vis Sci. 2015;56:1283–91.
11. Zhao J, Ellwein LB, Cui H, Ge J, Guan H, Lv J, et al. Prevalence and outcomes of cataract surgery in rural China the China nine-province survey. Ophthalmol. 2010;117:2120–8.
12. Information about national cataract surgery operations in 2014. National health and family planning commission of the people's republic of China. 2015. http://www.moh.gov.cn/yzygj/s7653/201503/9aa3cc022c744b28845c121209166491.shtml. Accessed 31 Mar.
13. Showcase - VISION 2020 Latin America. Graph. Regional CSR, 2005-2013. 2013. https://www.iapb.org/iapb-membership/council-of-members-meetings/council-meetings-archive/paris-2014/showcase-vision-2020-latin-america/.
14. Chu CJ, Johnston RL, Buscombe C, Sallam AB, Mohamed Q, Yang YC, et al. Risk factors and incidence of macular edema after cataract surgery: a database study of 81984 eyes. Ophthalmol. 2016;123:316–23.
15. Yin Q, Hu A, Liang Y, Zhang J, He M, Lam DS, et al. A two-site, population-based study of barriers to cataract surgery in rural China. Invest Ophthalmol Vis Sci. 2009;50:1069–75.
16. Xu L, Cui T, Zhang S, Sun B, Zheng Y, Hu A, et al. Prevalence and risk factors of lens opacities in urban and rural Chinese in Beijing. Ophthalmol. 2006;113:747–55.
17. Lin H, Lin D, Long E, Jiang H, Qu B, Tang J, et al. Patient participation in free cataract surgery: a cross-sectional study of the low-income elderly in urban China. BMJ Open. 2016;6:e011061.
18. Wang Y, Wang J, Maitland E, Zhao Y, Nicholas S, Lu M. Growing old before growing rich: inequality in health service utilization among the mid-aged and elderly in Gansu and Zhejiang provinces, China. BMC Health Serv Res. 2012;12:302.
19. Jin Y, Zhang Q, Shan L, Li SP. Characteristics of venture capital network and its correlation with regional economy: evidence from China. PLoS One. 2015;10:e0137172.
20. Sun J, Guo Y, Wang X, Zeng Q. mHealth for aging China: opportunities and challenges. Aging Dis. 2016;7:53–67.
21. He J, Lu L, He X, Xu X, Du X, Zhang B, et al. The relationship between crystalline lens power and refractive error in older Chinese aldults: the shanghai eye study. PLoS One. 2017;12:e0170030.
22. Zhao J, Xu X, Ellwein LB, Cai N, Guan H, He M, et al. Prevalence of Vision Impairment in Older Adults in Rural China in 2014 and Comparisons With the 2006 China Nine-Province Survey. Am J Ophthalmol. 2018;185:81–93.
23. Plonczak AM, McArthur GJ, Goldsmith N, Horwitz M. Hand Therapist Led Follow-up for Paediatric Hand Trauma – a Retrospective Study of 139 Closed Hand Injuries. Ortop Traumatol Rehabil. 2017;19:531–6.
24. Zhu Z, Wang L, Young CA, Huang S, Chang BH, He M. Cataract-related visual impairment corrected by cataract surgery and 10-year mortality: the Liwan eye study. Invest Ophthalmol Vis Sci. 2016;57:2290–5.
25. Zhang XJ, Jhanji V, Leung CK, Li EY, Liu Y, Zheng C, et al. Barriers for poor cataract surgery uptake among patients with operable cataract in a program of outreach screening and low-cost surgery in rural China. Ophthalmic Epidemiol. 2014;21:153–60.
26. Shrestha MK, Guo CW, Maharjan N, Gurung R, Ruit S. Health literacy of common ocular diseases in Nepal. BMC Ophthalmol. 2014;14:2.

Prospective study of bilateral mix-and-match implantation of diffractive multifocal intraocular lenses in Koreans

Chan Min Yang[1†], Dong Hui Lim[1,2†], Sungsoon Hwang[1], Joo Hyun[3] and Tae-Young Chung[1*]

Abstract

Background: To evaluate monocular and binocular visual outcomes for near, intermediate, and far distance in patients implanted with diffractive multifocal intraocular lenses (IOLs) with different add power contralaterally.

Methods: This is a prospective contralateral study. Two diffractive multifocal IOLs with different added power were implanted bilaterally in twenty patients. TECNIS® ZKB00 (+ 2.75 D) was implanted in a dominant eye, and TECNIS® ZLB00 (+ 3.25 D) was implanted in a non-dominant eye. Uncorrected distance visual acuity (UDVA), uncorrected intermediate visual acuity (UIVA), uncorrected near visual acuity (UNVA), and manifest refraction (MR) values were measured at 1 month and 3 months postoperatively. At the 3-month follow-up, defocus curve, contrast sensitivity, and reading performance were evaluated. Quality of vision, overall satisfaction, and spectacle independence were evaluated by questionnaire.

Results: Postoperative binocular UDVA, visual acuity at 80 cm, 60 cm, 50 cm, 43 cm, 33 cm were − 0.08 ± 0.10, 0.12 ± 0.14, 0.09 ± 0.09, 0.07 ± 0.11, 0.14 ± 0.09, 0.25 ± 0.11 logMAR. The binocular defocus curve showed an extended range of good visual acuity with sharp vision being observed from 0 D to − 2.50 D defocus (logMAR≤0.1). Reading performance was significantly improved compared to baseline. All patients were spectacle-free at distance, and 94.74% of the patients did not require glasses for near and intermediate vision.

Conclusions: Mix-and-match implantation of diffractive multifocal IOLs with different add power provides an excellent wide range of vision, as well as high levels of visual quality and patient satisfaction.

Background

A monofocal intraocular lens (IOL) implanted after cataract extraction to replace the focusing power of the crystalline lens has a fixed focal length. Although patients can achieve a good uncorrected-distance visual acuity after monofocal IOL implantation, most patients need glasses for reading or other activities at close distance.

However, in recent years, the increasing use of smartphones and tablets and new leisure activities require a fast alternation of far and near distance tasks, also in

elderly people. So spectacle dependence after cataract surgery can be inconvenient in the daily life of patients. In order to solve both cataract and presbyopia simultaneously, a variety of intraocular lenses have been developed. Diffractive bifocal IOLs with various levels of additional power have been widely used for correcting presbyopia after cataract surgery. The additional power of diffractive bifocal IOLs was selected according to patients' lifestyle. Although diffractive bifocal IOL implantation is an effective way to satisfy patients who want to stop using their glasses after cataract surgery, it often results in visual symptoms, including diminished contrast sensitivity and dysphotopsia due to the IOLs' diffractive surface [1, 2]. Other disadvantages of the implantation of bifocal IOLs is

* Correspondence: tychung@skku.edu
†Equal contributors
[1]Department of Ophthalmology, Samsung Medical Center, Sungkyunkwan University School of Medicine, #81 Irwon-ro, Gangnam-gu, Seoul 06351, South Korea
Full list of author information is available at the end of the article

a suboptimal intermediate visual acuity compared to near and distance visual acuities [3, 4].

Diffractive trifocal IOLs aim to provide a wider range of spectacle independence especially at an intermediate distance compared to bifocal IOLs. Trifocal IOLs provide three foci to enhance intermediate visual acuity. However, the distribution of light energy for a third focus could negatively affect near and distance visual acuity [5]. Decreased contrast sensitivity and unwanted visual symptoms may also occur after trifocal IOLs implantation [6, 7].

Recently, several methods of combining different types IOLs have been introduced to meet the diverse needs of the patients [8, 9]. And bilateral mix-and-match implantation of diffractive multifocal IOLs with different add power may be another option for enhancing intermediate visual acuity. However, previous studies of contralateral implantation of diffractive multifocal IOLs with different add power have used AcrySof IQ ReSTOR [10, 11].

The purpose of this study was to evaluate the clinical outcomes following bilateral mix-and-match implantation of the recently developed Tecnis diffractive bifocal IOLs with + 2.75 and + 3.25 add power.

Methods

This prospective, contralateral study comprised 20 patients affected by bilateral senile cataract. The study was approved by the Institutional Review Board of the Samsung Medical Center, and adhered to the tenets of the Declaration of Helsinki. Written informed consent was obtained from all patients.

The inclusion criteria were patients with bilateral senile cataract and the desire to be spectacle-free for all distances. Exclusion criteria were ages younger than 21 years, corneal astigmatism greater than 1.00 D, previous ocular surgery or trauma and ocular disease other than cataract. Hole-in-the card test was conducted in all patients for detection of dominant eye preoperatively.

The implanted IOLs were TECNIS ZKB00 (add power + 2.75 diopter [D], theoretical working distance 50 cm; Abbott Medical Optics, Santa Ana, California, USA) and TECNIS ZLB00 (add power + 3.25D, theoretical working distance 42 cm). The + 2.75D IOL was implanted in the dominant eye and that + 3.25D IOL in the non-dominant eye. Emmetropic intraocular lens power was selected from SRK/T, SRKII, Haigis, or Hoffer Q formulas according to corneal curvature, axial length and anterior chamber depth measured by IOLMaster version 5.4 (Carl Zeiss Meditec, Jena, Germany).

Surgical technique

One experienced surgeon (T.Y.C) performed all surgical procedures under topical anesthesia using a standardized sutureless phacoemulsification with a 2.75 mm clear corneal incision. Steep axis corneal incision was created in eyes with corneal astigmatism of more than 0.5D, and temporal corneal incision was made in eyes with corneal astigmatism less than 0.5D. The non-dominant eye was operated first. After that contralateral surgery was performed at an interval of one week. Postoperative gatifloxacin and fluometholone 0.1% eye drops were used 4 times a day for 1 month.

Patient evaluation

Preoperatively, all patients underwent a complete ophthalmologic examination including corrected and uncorrected visual acuity, manifest refraction, slit-lamp bio-microscopy, and fundus examination.

Patients were evaluated postoperatively at 1 day, 1 week, and 1 and 3 months. At 1 and 3 months after surgery, corrected and uncorrected visual acuity, manifest refraction, defocus curve, contrast sensitivity, reading performance, and subjective satisfaction were examined.

All patients underwent measurement of corrected and uncorrected distance visual acuity at 5 m (CDVA and UDVA). Uncorrected intermediate visual acuities (UIVA) were measured at 60 cm and 80 cm and uncorrected near visual acuities (UNVA) at 33 cm, 43 cm, and 50 cm using the ETDRS chart. All visual acuity were measured monocularly and binocularly.

Defocus curves were plotted by measuring the visual acuity under photopic condition at 5 m, adding lenses in 0.5D increments from − 4.0 to + 2.0D.

Contrast sensitivity at 3, 6, 12, and 18 cycles per degree was measured using a CSV-1000 chart (Vector Vision, Greenville, OH) under photopic (85 cd[cd]/m^2) and mesopic (~ 3 cd/m^2) conditions at 3 months after surgery. Results were converted in log units for statistical analysis using a specific table for the CSV-1000 [12].

At baseline and 3 months postoperatively, reading performance was measured using an iPad application at 50 cm [13]. The print size of the reading chart ranges from 1.0 to 0 logarithm of the minimal angle of resolution (logMAR). Average reading speed in words per minute (wpm) was calculated with the iPad application. Critical print size was defined as the last acuity measured before the reading speed was reduced below the 95% confidence interval of that individual's average reading speed [14]. Threshold print size was determined as the smallest print size that could be read and expressed in logarithm of the reading acuity determination (logRAD).

One and three months after surgery, all patients were asked to complete the questionnaire regarding overall satisfaction, presence of visual artifacts, and dependency on spectacles for near, intermediate and far vision. Overall satisfaction was evaluated using 5 levels (very satisfied, satisfied, neither satisfied nor dissatisfied, unsatisfied, very unsatisfied). Severity of visual artifacts, divided into 4 levels (none, minimal, moderate and severe), were assessed using a Quality of Vision questionnaire [15]. Furthermore, patients were asked if they would choose the same IOL again.

Statistical analysis

All data are presented as mean ± standard deviation. The statistical analysis was performed using SPSS software version 18.0 (SPSS, Inc., Chicago, IL). Measured decimal visual acuities were converted to logMAR for data analysis. Because the variables did not follow a normal distribution, non-parametric statistical analysis was used. The Wilcoxon signed-rank test was applied to assess the difference between preoperative and postoperative data. The Mann-Whitney U test was used to compare the dominant and non-dominant eyes. A sample size of 17 patients would allow the detection of a minimum clinical relevant difference in depth of focus with a standard deviation of 5.8. The sample sizes took into account a significance level of 5% and a power of 80% for a 2-sided test. Assuming an proportion of withdrawal of 10%, 20 patients were included.

Results

A total of 20 patients were enrolled, of which 19 completed the study. Patient recruitment was from August 2015 to January 2016. The study was finished after 3 months postoperative follow-up visit was completed for all patients in April 2016. All patients received regular follow-up examinations for at least 3 months. The mean age was 60.1 ± 6.61 years (range: 45 to 70 years), 63.1% (12 of 19) of the patients were female. Preoperative mean axial length was 24.74 ± 1.43 mm (range: 22.19 mm to 27.87 mm), mean keratometric value was 43.18 ± 1.25 D (range: 40.91 D to 45.18 D). Preoperative mean anterior chamber depth was 3.15 ± 0.49 mm (range: 2.42 mm to 4.53 mm). The mean IOL power implanted was 18.5 ± 4.4 D (range: 7.5 D to 25.5 D). Table 1 shows preoperative and postoperative monocular refractive results and visual acuities. At 3 months, there were statistically significant improvements in CDVA, UDVA, UIVA, and UNVA ($p < 0.001$). However, UNVA at 33 cm of eye with ZKB00 was not significantly different compared to the preoperative value ($p = 0.178$). No significant differences between eyes implanted with ZKB00 and eyes implanted with ZLB00 were found in uncorrected and corrected visual acuity at all distances ($p > 0.05$).

Table 2 shows preoperative and postoperative binocular visual acuities. Postoperative binocular visual acuities were significantly better than preoperative values, except for binocular UNVA at 33 cm. Cumulative binocular UNVA, UIVA, and UDVA at 1 and 3 months after surgery are shown in Figs. 1, 2 and 3.

Monocular and binocular defocus curves are shown in Fig. 4. Eyes implanted with ZKB00 and ZLB00 had two peaks at 0 and – 2 D. When comparing both eyes,

ZKB00 eyes had a slightly better visual acuity from – 1.0 to – 2.0 D. However, these differences were not statistically significant ($p = 0.84$, $p = 0.103$ and $p = 0.908$, respectively). Eyes with ZLB00 showed significantly better visual acuity at – 2.5, – 3.0, and – 3.5D compared to eyes implanted with ZKB00 ($p = 0.003$, $p = 0.022$ and p = 0.022, respectively). The binocular defocus curve also showed two peaks and overlapping curves with monocular defocus curves, as well as a wider range of good visual acuity from 0 to – 3.0 D (log MAR < 0.2 [range; – 0 ~ – 3.0 D], logMAR < 0.1 [range: 0–2.5 D]) Eyes with ZKB00 had a slightly better visual acuity from – 1.0 to – 2.0 diopters (D) compared to eyes with ZLB00. Eyes with ZLB00 showed significantly better visual acuity at – 2.5, – 3.0, and – 3.5 D (Mann-Whitney U test, p values < 0.05). Binocular defocus curve showed good visual acuity better than 0.1 logMAR from 0 to – 2.5 D.

Postoperative contrast sensitivity at 3 months was statistically significantly better at some spatial frequencies than that measured preoperatively (Fig. 5).

The mean reading speed increased from 76.93 ± 17.47 wpm (range: 44.33 to 106.17 wpm) at baseline to 86.83 ± 17.45 wpm (range: 64.99 to 123.53 wpm) at 3 months after surgery. The mean critical print size decreased from 0.65 ± 0.22 logRAD (range: 0.1 to 0.8 logRAD) at baseline to 0.24 ± 0.13 logRAD (range: 0 to 0.5 logRAD) at 3 months after surgery. The threshold print size also decreased from 0.35 ± 0.22 logRAD (range: 0 to 0.8 logRAD) at baseline to 0.14 ± 0.13 logRAD (range: 0 to 0.4 logRAD) at 3 months after surgery. There were statistically significant differences in mean reading speed, critical print size, and threshold print size between baseline and 3 months after surgery ($p = 0.07$, $p = 0.01$ and $p = 0.03$, respectively).

Overall satisfaction, visual symptoms and spectacle dependence are summarized in Table 3. Postoperative overall satisfaction with distance vision was statistically significant regarding the improvement achieved compared to preoperative ($p < 0.05$). Although halo and starburst were increased at 1 and 3 months after surgery, there were no significant differences compared to baseline (halo: $p = 0.108$ and $p = 0.301$, respectively; starburst: $p = 0.890$ and $p = 0.209$, respectively). All patients reported complete spectacle independence for distance after surgery. One patient required spectacles for near vision and another one patient sometimes for intermediate vision after surgery. A total of 94.7% of the patients (18 of 19) answered that they would choose the same IOLs again and 89.4% (17 of 19) did not feel dizzy and recognized the difference between both eyes.

Discussion

In this prospective study, the clinical outcomes of mix-and-match implantations of ZKB00 and ZLB00

Table 1 Monocular refractive results and visual acuities in patients implanted with ZKB00 and ZLB00 multifocal IOLs at preoperative, 1 month and 3 months after surgery

Measurement	Preoperative		1 month				3 months			
	Dominant eye	non-dominant eye	Dominant eye	P value[a]	non-dominant eye	P value[b]	Dominant eye	P value[c]	non-dominant eye	P value[d]
Spherical equivalent (D)	−1.61 ± 3.71	−1.69 ± 3.92	−0.01 ± 0.32		0.00 ± 0.30		−0.03 ± 0.22		0.06 ± 0.27	
CDVA at 5 m	0.09 ± 0.13	0.21 ± 0.24	−0.04 ± 0.08	0.005	−0.04 ± 0.07	<0.001	−0.06 ± 0.07	<0.001	−0.06 ± 0.07	<0.001
UDVA at 5 m	0.53 ± 0.45	0.62 ± 0.45	−0.03 ± 0.09	<0.001	−0.02 ± 0.10	<0.001	−0.02 ± 0.10	<0.001	−0.01 ± 0.10	<0.001
UIVA at 80 cm	0.61 ± 0.27	0.67 ± 0.32	0.26 ± 0.17	0.002	0.27 ± 0.16	0.001	0.19 ± 0.14	<0.001	0.19 ± 0.12	<0.001
UIVA at 60 cm	0.66 ± 0.15	0.66 ± 0.27	0.12 ± 0.12	0.003	0.18 ± 0.14	0.005	0.16 ± 0.12	0.003	0.25 ± 0.13	<0.001
UNVA at 50 cm	0.62 ± 0.23	0.65 ± 0.26	0.13 ± 0.12	<0.001	0.14 ± 0.12	<0.001	0.14 ± 0.13	<0.001	0.16 ± 0.12	<0.001
UNVA at 43 cm	0.58 ± 0.21	0.69 ± 0.18	0.24 ± 0.15	<0.001	0.22 ± 0.13	<0.001	0.21 ± 0.11	<0.001	0.16 ± 0.10	<0.001
UNVA at 33 cm	0.46 ± 0.29	0.53 ± 0.31	0.41 ± 0.21	0.441	0.30 ± 0.20	0.005	0.36 ± 0.18	0.178	0.30 ± 0.13	0.008

CDVA Corrected distance visual acuity, UDVA Uncorrected distance visual acuity, UIVA Uncorrected intermediate visual acuity, UNVA Uncorrected near visual acuity

[a]Dominant eye: Preoperative to 1 month after surgery

[b]Nondominant eye: Preoperative to 1 month after surgery

[c]Dominant eye: Preoperative to 3 months after surgery

[d]Nondominant eye: Preoperative to 3 months after surgery

Table 2 Binocular visual acuities in patients implanted with ZKB00 and ZLB00 multifocal IOLs at preoperative, 1 month and 3 months after surgery

Measurements	Preoperative	1 month	p value[a]	3 months	p value[b]
CDVA at 5 m	0.03 ± 0.12	− 0.11 ± 0.08	0.001	−0.12 ± 0.08	0.001
UDVA at 5 m	0.36 ± 0.27	−0.10 ± 0.10	< 0.001	−0.08 ± 0.10	< 0.001
UIVA at 80 cm	0.50 ± 0.27	0.21 ± 0.23	0.013	0.12 ± 0.14	< 0.001
UIVA at 60 cm	0.51 ± 0.18	0.10 ± 0.14	0.003	0.09 ± 0.09	0.003
UNVA at 50 cm	0.43 ± 0.19	0.10 ± 0.10	< 0.001	0.07 ± 0.11	< 0.001
UNVA at 43 cm	0.45 ± 0.17	0.16 ± 0.15	< 0.001	0.14 ± 0.09	< 0.001
UNVA at 33 cm	0.31 ± 0.30	0.27 ± 0.23	0.491	0.25 ± 0.11	0.348

CDVA Corrected distance visual acuity, UDVA Uncorrected distance visual acuity, UIVA Uncorrected intermediate visual acuity, UNVA Uncorrected near visual acuity
[a]Preoperative to 1 month
[b]Preoperative to 3 months

were showed good UCVA and UNVA as well as UIVA and high satisfaction without visual disturbance such as glare and halo. Although there was previous study comparing ZMB00, ZKB00 and ZLB00, we could confirm that depth of focus was increased through contralateral mix-and-match implantation of ZKB00 and ZLB00. Compared with previous studies using the trifocal diffractive IOLs, our results revealed that contrast sensitivity was not reduced and visual disturbance was less. The previous version, ZMB00 Tecnis multifocal IOLs with + 4.0 D add power has the same design as the studied IOLs; however, the study IOLs have a relatively lower add power of + 2.75 D and + 3.25 D. All IOLs of this platform have a refractive zone on the anterior surface to provide distance vision and a full diffractive posterior surface for near vision. The fewer diffractive rings of ZKB00 and ZLB00 compared to ZMB00 are considered to reduce unwanted visual symptoms [16].

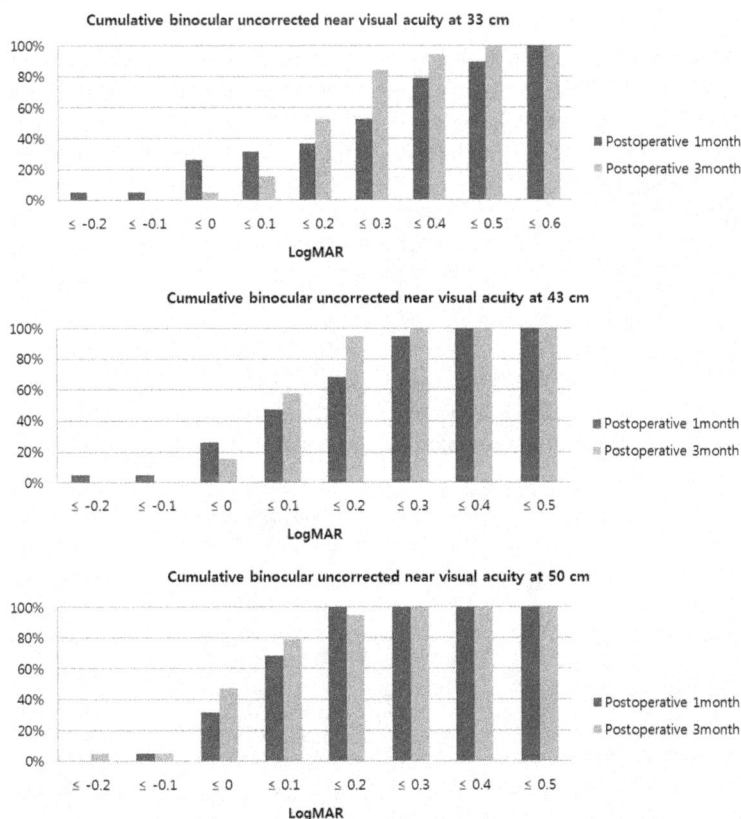

Fig. 1 Postoperative cumulative binocular uncorrected near visual acuity (UNVA) in patients implanted with ZKB00 and ZLB00 multifocal intraocular lens at 33 cm, 43 cm, and 50 cm in logarithm of the minimal angle of resolution (logMAR)

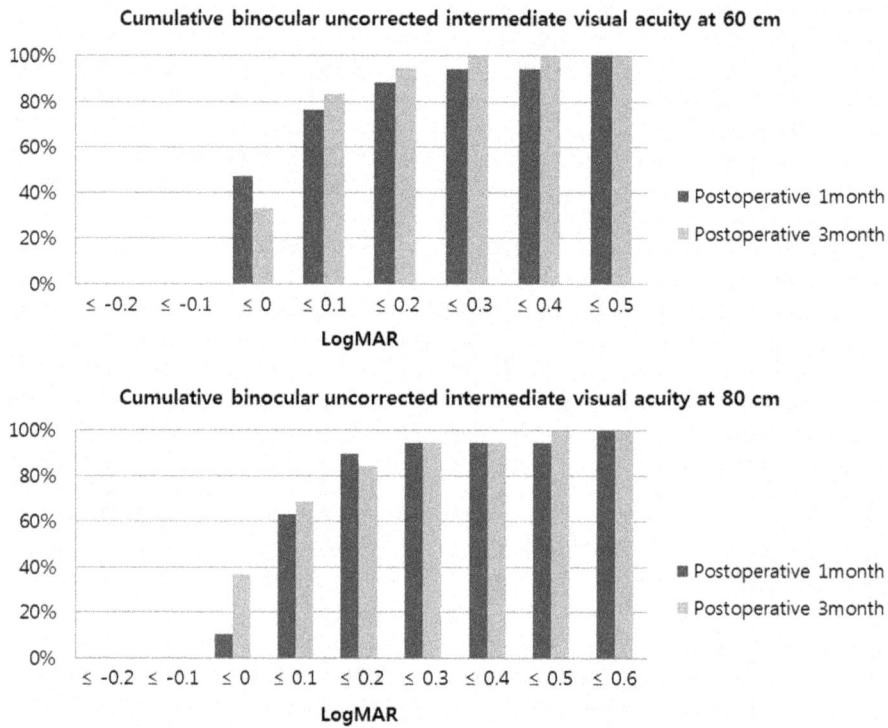

Fig. 2 Postoperative cumulative binocular uncorrected intermediate visual acuity (UIVA) in patients implanted with ZKB00 and ZLB00 multifocal intraocular lens at 60 cm and 80 cm in logarithm of the minimal angle of resolution (logMAR)

Regardless of pupil size, the light is evenly distributed between distance and near foci. Other optical principles of multifocal IOLs are dependent on pupil size [17].

Other studies with ZKB00 and ZLB00 IOL implantation report that subjects implanted with low add power bifocal IOLs had good intermediate and distance visual acuity with a high level of satisfaction [16, 18, 19]. Kretz et al. [19] reported 63.3% of the patients implanted with ZKB00 in both eyes achieved a binocular UIVA at 80 cm of 0.1 logMAR or better. In this study, the percentage of patients with binocular logMAR UIVA better than 0.1 logMAR at 80 cm was 68.5%. Kretz et al. [18] reported that bilaterally implantation of the ZLB00 IOL revealed a

binocular UIVA of 0.06 ± 0.09 logMAR at 60 cm. In our study, we found comparable results with 0.09 ± 0.09 logMAR. However, previous studies did not include the defocus curve which makes it difficult to compare the achieved visual acuity at various distances directly. Previous studies of bilateral mix-and-match implantation of diffractive bifocal IOLs reported a better visual acuity over a wider range compared to bilateral implantation of IOLs with the same add power [11]. Our study with mix-and-match implantations of Tecnis ZKB00 and ZLB00 found a 0.1 logMAR or better visual acuity in the 0 to – 2.5 D range of the defocus curve. We could speculate that outcomes of mix-and-match implantation

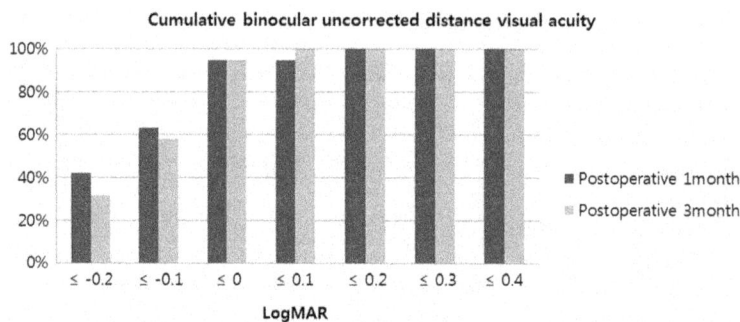

Fig. 3 Postoperative cumulative binocular uncorrected distance visual acuity (UDVA) in patients implanted with ZKB00 and ZLB00 multifocal intraocular lens in logarithm of the minimal angle of resolution (logMAR)

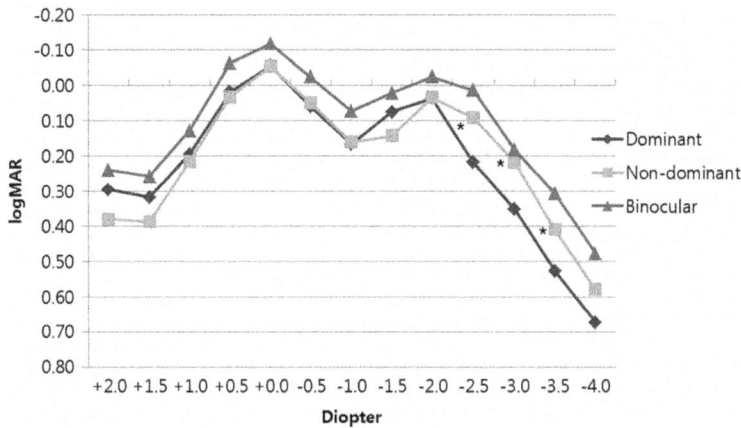

Fig. 4 Monocular and binocular defocus curve plotted in logarithm of the minimal angle of resolution (logMAR) in patients implanted with ZKB00 and ZLB00 multifocal intraocular lens at 3 months postoperatively. (*: $p < 0.05$, between dominant and non-dominant eye)

of Tecnis ZKB00 and ZLB00 might be better visual acuity at a broader range than bilateral implantation of IOLs with the same add power (ZKB00 or ZLB00).

This study is the first prospective study applying the bilateral mix-and-match implantation of Tecnis ZKB00 and ZLB00. All previous studies on mix-and-match implantations of diffractive bifocal IOLs used the AcrySof ReSTOR IOL [10, 11]. Nakamura et al. [10] reported that contralateral implantation of ReSTOR IOLs with + 3.0 and + 4.0 D addition was an effective way to get a broad range of good uncorrected visual acuity in the defocus curve. Mastropasqua R et al. [11] also reported that patients, implanted with ReSTOR IOLs with contralateral + 2.5 and + 3.0 D additions, had good uncorrected visual acuity over a wide range, and contrast sensitivity and visual quality did not decrease compared to bilateral implantation of diffractive multifocal IOLs with the same additional power. Compared with the

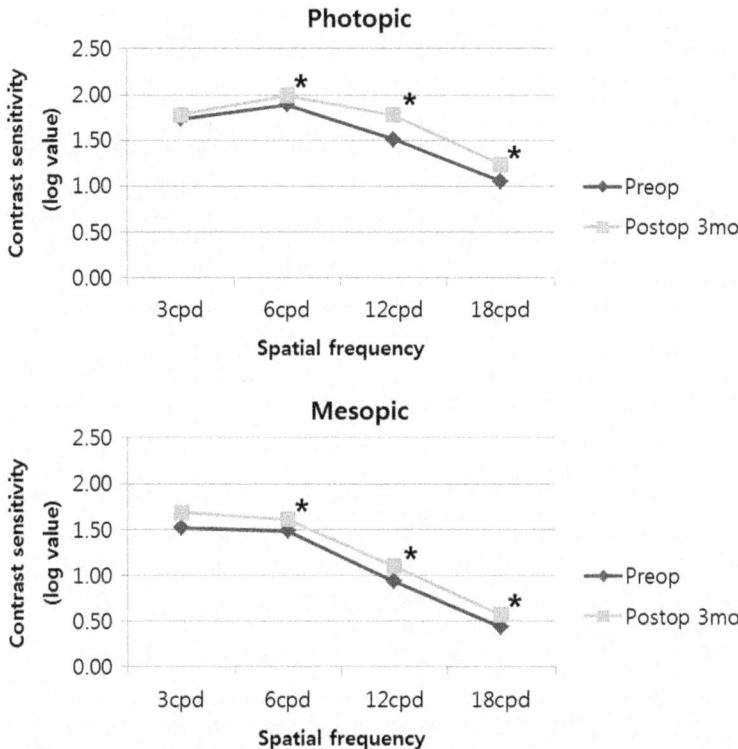

Fig. 5 Mean binocular photopic (Top) and mesopic (Bottom) contrast sensitivity in patients implanted with ZKB00 and ZLB00 multifocal intraocular lens

Table 3 Overall satisfaction, visual artifact questionnaire response and spectacle dependence in patients implanted with ZKB00 and ZLB00 multifocal IOLs at preoperative, 1 month and 3 months after surgery

	Preoperative	1 month	p value[a]	3 months	p value[b]
Overall satisfaction					
Far	2.68 ± 0.89	4.37 ± 0.50	< 0.001	4.42 ± 0.51	0.001
Intermediate	2.68 ± 0.89	3.95 ± 1.13	0.003	4.11 ± 0.81	0.001
Near	2.84 ± 1.01	3.84 ± 0.90	0.013	3.89 ± 0.88	0.008
Visual artifact					
Glare	0.47 ± 1.02	0.58 ± 1.07	0.777	0.21 ± 0.71	0.334
Halo	0.47 ± 1.02	1.11 ± 1.33	0.108	0.84 ± 1.12	0.164
Starburst	0.37 ± 0.96	0.32 ± 0.75	0.890	0.79 ± 1.13	0.179
Spectacle use					
Far	73.68%	0.00%	< 0.001	0.00%	< 0.001
Intermediate	78.94%	5.26%	< 0.001	5.26%	< 0.001
Near	63.16%	5.26%	< 0.001	5.26%	< 0.001

Overall satisfaction: 1 = very dissatisfied; 2 = dissatisfied; 3 = neither satisfied nor dissatisfied; 4 = satisfied; 5 = very satisfied
Visual artifacts: 0 = none; 1 = minimal; 2 = moderate; 3 = severe
Visual artifact was assessed using the Quality of Vision questionnaire
[a]Preoperative to 1 month
[b]Preoperative to 3 months

defocus curve of Mastropasqua et al., our study revealed 0.1 logMAR or better vision from 0 to – 2.5 D, whereas Mastropasqua et al. report 0.1 logMAR or better in the range from 0D and – 1.5 ~ – 2.5D. In the range of intermediated distance from – 0.5D to – 1.5D, the results of ours study appear better than those of Mastropasqua et al. Although the add power differs slightly between studies, it seems that the IOL design is responsible for the better intermediate vision. And it may be due to differences in clinical characteristics of patients, such as axial length that can affect effective lens position.

Recently, trifocal diffractive IOLs were developed to provide better intermediate visual acuity. So far, no direct comparative study between bilateral implantation of diffractive trifocal IOLs and contralateral implantation of diffractive bifocal IOLs has been published. Ours study shows 0.1 logMAR or better visual acuity in the range from 0 to – 2.5D in the defocus curve and it was comparable to or slightly better than that reported in previous studies on trifocal diffractive IOLs [20].

Multifocal IOLs had a drawback in decreasing contrast sensitivity However, for Tecnis multifocal IOLs it was known as the prolate anterior surface could improve the mesopic contrast sensitivity [17, 21]. Gierek-Ciaciura et al. [22] reported that eyes with ZM900 Tecnis multifocal IOLs had better contrast sensitivity than eyes with other diffractive multifocal IOLs or refractive multifocal IOLs. Kim et al. [16] found that contrast sensitivity was higher in subjects with ZKB00 or ZLB00 than subjects with ZM900. This study, using ZKB00 and ZLB00, also showed improvement of contrast sensitivity compared

with preoperative contrast sensitivity, and statistically significant improvement in some spatial frequency.

Diffractive multifocal IOLs with fewer diffractive rings and lower add power could theoretically improve the quality of vision after cataract surgery. Trifocal IOLs need it split more light energy to form the third focal point compared to bifocal IOLs and more diffractive rings are used for the trifocal IOLs compared to the IOLs used in our study. This might have an effect on the quality of vision for near and distance [5–7]. Montes-Mico R et al. [5] used optical bench testing to confirm the quality of the apodized trifocal IOL (Finevision Micro F, Phys-IOL, Liege, Belgium), and report a worse quality of vision compared bifocal diffractive IOLs. Kohnen T et al. [7] reported that halo and glare appeared in 60% and 28% of patients, respectively, after the implantation of AT LISA tri839MP, another trifocal IOL (Carl Zeiss Meditec, Jena, Germany). Our study showed halo and glare in 31.5% and 5.3% of patients, respectively, less visual artifacts compared to the results of Kohnen et al. Jonker et al. [6] also reported that mesopic contrast sensitivity was slightly decreased in eyes with diffractive trifocal IOLs compared to diffractive bifocal IOLs. Future studies should compare the quality of vision between groups with bilaterally implanted with diffractive trifocal IOLs and contralaterally implanted diffractive bifocal IOLs.

Reading performance, such as reading speed, critical print size, and threshold print size, were significantly improved postoperatively compared to baseline. Alfonso et al. [14] reported critical print size and threshold size after bilateral implantation of AcrySof + 3.0 toric multifocal IOLs were

0.28 ± 0.12 logRAD and 0.08 ± 0.08 logRAD, respectively. Schmickler et al. [23] reported that critical print size was 0.27 ± 0.12 logRAD in patients after bilateral implantation of Tecnis ZMB00 + 4.0 diffractive multifocal IOLs. Our results of critical print size and threshold print size were 0.24 ± 0.13 logRAD and 0.14 ± 0.13 logRAD, respectively, and comparable to previous studies [14, 23]. In our study, postoperative reading speed was 86.83 ± 17.45 wpm. Alfonso et al. [14] reported a reading speed of 132.68 ± 23.69 wpm after the implantation of diffractive multifocal IOLs. Reading speed in our study is slightly lower compared to results from Western regions [14, 24]. One study using the same application as in our study to test reading speed in Koreans reported a reading speed of 129.7 ± 25.9 wpm for adults in their 20s and 30s [13]. Considering that the reading speed of young adults without presbyopia is faster than that of the older adults with presbyopia, it is possible that the difference in the testing method and characteristics of the languages are the reason for the variance between the results [6, 14, 24].

When the overall satisfaction was evaluated on a five-point scale, satisfaction with distance, intermediate and near vision was 4.42 ± 0.51, 4.11 ± 0.81, and 3.89 ± 0.88, respectively. The results showed that most patients were satisfied. When patients were asked if they would choose the same IOLs again and if they would recommend the IOLs to others, 68.4% of the patients (13 of 19) would choose the same IOLs and recommend it to others.

In this study, ocular dominance was tested prior to cataract surgery, and ZKB00 (add power + 2.75D) was implanted in the dominant eyes and ZLB00 (add power + 3.25D) was implanted in the non-dominant eyes. We assumed that the 'relatively far' near focus (ZKB00) in the dominant eye and 'relatively near' near focus (ZLB00) in the non-dominant eye would benefit according to the classic monovision trial. However, due to conflicting results with cross monovision results, it may be necessary to conduct additional research to compare the results with cross monovision [25]. Although both eyes of each patient were implanted with different add power, visual acuities of the dominant and non-dominant eyes at each distances were not statistically different. This may be due to the fact that difference in add power between the two IOLs was only 0.5 D. When patients were asked whether they could feel differences between eyes, 17 out of 19 patients did not perceive any difference between both eyes and they did not feel uncomfortable with it. It would be interesting to apply the mix-and-match technique using IOLs with an add power of + 2.75 D and + 4.00 D.

The strength of this prospective contralateral study is the first study applying bilateral mix-and-match implantation of Tecnis multifocal IOLs. Second strength is visual acuities were measured at 6 different distances and that an objective measure of the expected vision at different distances was performed with a defocus curve. Previous studies measured intermediate and near visual acuity only at a single distance. And we comprehensively evaluate clinical outcomes including reading performance, contrast sensitivity and questionnaire. The limitation of this study is the missing direct comparison with bilaterally implanted IOLs with the same add power. However, the results of defocus curve of this study were good and not inferior to those of previous studies.

Conclusions
In conclusion, the mix-and-match technique using Tecnis multifocal IOLs with low add power is an effective way to achieve good visual acuity over a wide range without affecting quality of vision. The mix-and-match technique is an interesting option for patients who want to be spectacle-free after cataract surgery.

Abbreviations
CDVA: Corrected distance visual acuity; IOL: Intraocular lens; logMAR: Logarithm of the minimal angle of resolution; logRAD: Logarithm of the reading acuity determination; MR: Manifest refraction; UDVA: Uncorrected distance visual acuity; UIVA: Uncorrected intermediate visual acuity; UNVA: Uncorrected near visual acuity; WPM: Words per minute

Acknowledgements
None.

Funding
This research received no specific grant from any funding agency.

Authors' contributions
Involved in conception and design (DHL, T-YC) and conduct of the study (CMY, DHL, T-YC); collection, management and interpretation of data (CMY, DHL, SH, JH); data analysis (CMY, DHL); writing the article (CMY, DHL); and preparation, review, and approval of the manuscript (CMY, DHL, T-YC). CMY and DHL contributed equally to the manuscript as the first authors. T-YC contributed to the manuscript as the corresponding authors.

Competing interests
No conflicts of interest and have no proprietary interest in any of the materials mentioned in this article.

Author details
[1]Department of Ophthalmology, Samsung Medical Center, Sungkyunkwan University School of Medicine, #81 Irwon-ro, Gangnam-gu, Seoul 06351, South Korea. [2]Department of Preventive Medicine, Catholic University School

of Medicine, Seoul, South Korea. [3]Department of Ophthalmology, Saevit Eye Hospital, Goyang, South Korea.

References

1. Packer M, Chu YR, Waltz KL, et al. Evaluation of the aspheric tecnis multifocal intraocular lens: one-year results from the first cohort of the food and drug administration clinical trial. Am J Ophthalmol. 2010;149:577–84e1.
2. Ang R, Martinez G, Cruz E, et al. Prospective evaluation of visual outcomes with three presbyopia-correcting intraocular lenses following cataract surgery. Clin Ophthalmol. 2013;7:1811–23.
3. Maxwell WA, Cionni RJ, Lehmann RP, et al. Functional outcomes after bilateral implantation of apodized diffractive aspheric acrylic intraocular lenses with a +3.0 or +4.0 diopter addition power Randomized multicenter clinical study. J Cataract Refract Surg. 2009;35:2054–61.
4. de Vries NE, Webers CA, Montes-Mico R, et al. Visual outcomes after cataract surgery with implantation of a +3.00 D or +4.00 D aspheric diffractive multifocal intraocular lens: comparative study. J Cataract Refract Surg. 2010;36:1316–22.
5. Montes-Mico R, Madrid-Costa D, Ruiz-Alcocer J, et al. In vitro optical quality differences between multifocal apodized diffractive intraocular lenses. J Cataract Refract Surg. 2013;39:928–36.
6. Jonker SM, Bauer NJ, Makhotkina NY, et al. Comparison of a trifocal intraocular lens with a +3.0 D bifocal IOL: results of a prospective randomized clinical trial. J Cataract Refract Surg. 2015;41:1631–40.
7. Kohnen T, Titke C, Bohm M. Trifocal intraocular lens implantation to treat visual demands in various distances following lens removal. Am J Ophthalmol. 2016;161:71–7 e1.
8. Yoon SY, Song IS, Kim JY, et al. Bilateral mix-and-match versus unilateral multifocal intraocular lens implantation: long-term comparison. J Cataract Refract Surg. 2013;39:1682–90.
9. Pepose JS, Qazi MA, Davies J, et al. Visual performance of patients with bilateral vs combination Crystalens, ReZoom, and ReSTOR intraocular lens implants. Am J Ophthalmol. 2007;144:347–57.
10. Nakamura K, Bissen-Miyajima H, Yoshino M, et al. Visual performance after contralateral implantation of multifocal intraocular lenses with +3.0 and +4.0 diopter additions. Asia Pac J Ophthalmol (Phila). 2015;4:329–33.
11. Mastropasqua R, Pedrotti E, Passilongo M, et al. Long-term visual function and patient satisfaction after bilateral implantation and combination of two similar multifocal IOLs. J Refract Surg. 2015;31:308–14.
12. Schmitz S, Dick HB, Krummenauer F, et al. Contrast sensitivity and glare disability by halogen light after monofocal and multifocal lens implantation. Br J Ophthalmol. 2000;84:1109–12.
13. Song J, Kim JH, Hyung S. Validity of Korean version reading speed application and measurement of reading speed: pilot study. J Korean Ophthalmol Soc DE - 2016-04-28. 2016;57:642–9.
14. Alfonso JF, Knorz M, Fernandez-Vega L, et al. Clinical outcomes after bilateral implantation of an apodized +3.0 D toric diffractive multifocal intraocular lens. J Cataract Refract Surg. 2014;40:51–9.
15. McAlinden C, Pesudovs K, Moore JE. The development of an instrument to measure quality of vision: the quality of vision (QoV) questionnaire. Invest Ophthalmol Vis Sci. 2010;51:5537–45.
16. Kim JS, Jung JW, Lee JM, et al. Clinical outcomes following implantation of diffractive multifocal intraocular lenses with varying add powers. Am J Ophthalmol. 2015;160:702–9 e1.
17. Gil MA, Varon C, Rosello N, et al. Visual acuity, contrast sensitivity, subjective quality of vision, and quality of life with 4 different multifocal IOLs. Eur J Ophthalmol. 2012;22:175–87.
18. Kretz FT, Koss MJ, Auffarth GU. Intermediate and near visual acuity of an aspheric, bifocal, diffractive multifocal intraocular lens with +3.25 D near addition. J Refract Surg. 2015;31:295–9.
19. Kretz FT, Gerl M, Gerl R, et al. Clinical evaluation of a new pupil independent diffractive multifocal intraocular lens with a +2.75 D near addition: a European multicentre study. Br J Ophthalmol. 2015;99:1655–9.
20. Sheppard AL, Shah S, Bhatt U, et al. Visual outcomes and subjective experience after bilateral implantation of a new diffractive trifocal intraocular lens. J Cataract Refract Surg. 2013;39:343–9.
21. Cillino G, Casuccio A, Pasti M, et al. Working-age cataract patients: visual results, reading performance, and quality of life with three diffractive multifocal intraocular lenses. Ophthalmology. 2014;121:34–44.
22. Gierek-Ciaciura S, Cwalina L, Bednarski L, et al. A comparative clinical study of the visual results between three types of multifocal lenses. Graefes Arch Clin Exp Ophthalmol. 2010;248:133–40.
23. Schmickler S, Bautista CP, Goes F, et al. Clinical evaluation of a multifocal aspheric diffractive intraocular lens. Br J Ophthalmol. 2013;97:1560–4.
24. Alio JL, Plaza-Puche AB, Pinero DP, et al. Optical analysis, reading performance, and quality-of-life evaluation after implantation of a diffractive multifocal intraocular lens. J Cataract Refract Surg. 2011;37:27–37.
25. Jain S, Ou R, azar DT. Monovision outcomes in presbyopic individuals after refractive surgery. Ophthalmology. 2001;108:1430–3.

15

Surgical peripheral iridectomy via a clear-cornea phacoemulsification incision for pupillary block following cataract surgery in acute angle closure

Aiwu Fang, Peijuan Wang, Rui He and Jia Qu* (ID)

Abstract

Background: To describe a technique of surgical peripheral iridectomy via a clear-cornea tunnel incision to prevent or treat pupillary block following phacoemulsification.

Methods: Description of technique and retrospective description results in 20 eyes of 20 patients with acute angle closure with coexisting visually significant cataract undergoing phacoemulsification considered at risk of postoperative papillary block as well as two pseudo-phakic eyes with acute postoperative pupillary-block. Following phacoemulsification and insertion of an intraocular lens, a needle with a bent tip was inserted behind the iris through the corneal tunnel incision. A blunt iris repositor was introduced through the paracentesis and placed above the iris to exert posterior pressure and create a puncture. The size of the puncture was enlarged using scissors. For postoperative pupillary block the same technique was carried out through the existing incisions created for phacoemulsification.

Results: Peripheral iridectomy was successfully created in all 22 eyes. At a mean follow-up of 18.77 ± 9.72 months, none of the iridectomies closed or required enlargement. Two eyes had mild intraoperative bleeding and one eye a small Descemet's detachment that did not require intervention. No clinically significant complications were observed. Visual acuity and IOP improved or was maintained in all patients. The incidence of pupillary block in our hospital was 0.09% overall, 0.6% in diabetics and 3.5% in those with diabetic retinopathy.

Conclusions: This technique of peripheral iridectomy via the cornea tunnel incision can be safely used during phacoemulsification in eyes at high risk of pupillary block or in the treatment of acute postoperative pupillary-block after cataract surgery. The technique is likely to be especially useful in brown iris, or if a laser is not available.

Keywords: Surgical peripheral iridectomy, Phacoemulsification, Pupillary block, Acute angle closure

Background

Pupillary block is a rare complication in cataract surgery wit IOL in lens bag [1]. Accordingly peripheral iridectomy (PI) is not performed during routine phacoemulsification but may be indicated in special situations such as implantation of an anterior chamber (or iris-fixated) lens and perhaps in patients prone to inflammation and pupillary block [1, 2].

Phacoemulsification is increasingly being used for the primary management of acute angle closure (AAC) [1, 3–7], where, theoretically the shorter axial length and higher risk of post-operative inflammation may increase the risk of postoperative pupillary block, especially if other risk factors like diabetes are present [1, 6, 8]. An elective intra-operative iridectomy is difficult to execute through the length of the corneal tunnel incision. The alternatives are to create an additional limbal incision for this purpose, or perform a laser peripheral iridotomy (LPI) either prior to or after surgery if required. In the setting of inflammatory post-operative pupillary block, LPI is more difficult to perform and is prone to occlusion. In this situation, it is even more difficult to perform LPI on Chinese people due to the brown irises, which are thicker than blue irises. Furthermore, a Neodymium-YAG laser is not universally available,

* Correspondence: wzjiaqu@126.com
Wenzhou Medical University Eye Hospital, Wenzhou 325027, China

especially in poorly resourced countries. We describe a surgical technique and retrospectively describe the results of performing a surgical iridectomy through the cornea tunnel incision used for phacoemulsification.

Methods

This was a retrospective case series. The technique was used on a series of patients with AAC seen between September 2009 and January 2013 at the glaucoma unit of the eye hospital, Wenzhou Medical University. Patients were included if they had concomitant visually significant cataract where the surgeon considered the risk of pupillary block (AAC concomitant diabetic retinopathy, uveitis and short axial length) following phacoemulsification for AAC warranted an intra-operative iridectomy. The institutional review board approved the study and informed consent was obtained from all patients.

The inclusion criteria were: (1) AAC concomitant diabetic retinopathy, uveitis and short axial length (<22 mm); (2) visually significant cataract or pseudophakic eye following phacoemulsification recently; (3) IOP and inflammation was under control prior to surgery. Exclusion criteria were: (1) AAC was not caused by non-pupillary block glaucoma such as neovascular glaucoma, trauma; (2) corneal opacity prevent to perform a surgical iridectomy; (3) AAC with clear opening of laser peripheral iridotomy.

Surgical procedure

Surgery was performed by a single surgeon under topical or peribulbar anesthesia. A standard clear-cornea phacoemulsification was performed with implantation of a foldable post chamber intraocular lens (IOL). The position of the clear-cornea tunnel was located in the nasal superior quadrant. Following insertion of the IOL in the capsular bag, a viscoelastic agent was injected into the anterior chamber and the posterior chamber at the site of the intended surgical iridectomy. A 26G needle with its tip bent to approximately 45 degrees about 1 mm from the tip was inserted into the corneal tunnel and advanced behind the iris, anterior to capsule and IOL to the selected site. The tip was kept horizontal to avoid snagging the iris. A blunt iris repositor was introduced into the eye through the paracentesis and placed above the iris adjacent to the needle. The needle tip was then turned anteriorly towards the iris and posterior pressure exerted with the repository to create a temperal inferior puncture. The size of the puncture was enlarged using fine long bladed microsurgical scissors to excise a small piece of iris tissue and the excised iris tissue removed with microsurgery forceps. The surgical technique can also create a nasal iridectomy through a temporal corneal tunnel. In the first three cases intra-cameral Carbamylcholine Chloride (0.01%) was administered to constrict the pupil following intraocular lens implantation. The surgical steps are illustrated in Fig. 1 and a typical post-operative result is shown in Fig. 2. Viscoelastic material was evacuated as is routine at the end of surgery.

The technique was used in twenty eyes of 20 patients with AAC and coexisting visually significant cataract considered to be at high risk of postoperative pupillary block due to the presence of factors such as poorly controlled diabetes, uveitis and short axial length. Two pseudophakic eyes that developed acute postoperative pupillary-block following phacoemusificatoin for AAC (in whom intraoperative iridectomy was not performed) also underwent this procedure.

Clinical observations

Preoperative examination included decimal visual acuity (VA), applanation tonometry, biomicroscopy, ophthalmoscopy, gonioscopy, specular microscopy, and ultrasound biomicroscopy (UBM, OTI, Inc. CA). Anterior chamber depth was measured with UBM, Keratometry, and axial length were measured with an IOL Master (Carl Zeiss Meditec, Inc. Dublin, CA).

In all patients the acute attack was controlled with medications and/or paracentesis prior to surgery. Phacoemusification was undertaken as soon as the IOP decreased and the inflammation was under control. The time to surgery was 2 to 30 days.

Postoperative care included topical steroids and antibiotics, as is routine following phacoemulsification. Systemic steroids were administered if a fibrin reaction was seen in the anterior chamber. Patients were followed up on day 1 and 2, week 1 and 2, months 1, 2, 3, 6, 9, and 12 and then every 6 months thereafter. VA, intraocular pressure (IOP), disc assessment and postoperative complications were recorded.

Statistical analysis

Statistical analysis was performed using the SPSS 20 software package (SPSS Inc., Munich, Germany). Results are reported as the mean ± standard deviation. A paired t test was used to evaluate changes in IOP and VA before and after surgery. VA was analyzed after conversion to the logarithm of the minimal angle resolution (logMAR) score. Hand-motion VA and counting fingers were assigned decimal equivalents of 0.001(+ 3.0 logMAR) and 0.01 (+ 2.0 logMAR). A p value less than 0.05 was considered statistically significant.

Results

A patent surgical peripheral iridectomy was successfully achieved in the twenty eyes that underwent phacoemulsification for AAC and the two pseudophakic eyes with pupillary block that followed phacoemulsification.

Three patients were male and 19 were females. Mean patient age was 56.86 ± 12.90 years (range: 27 to 75). The table details demographics, eye characteristics and results. There were no complications during phacoemulsification

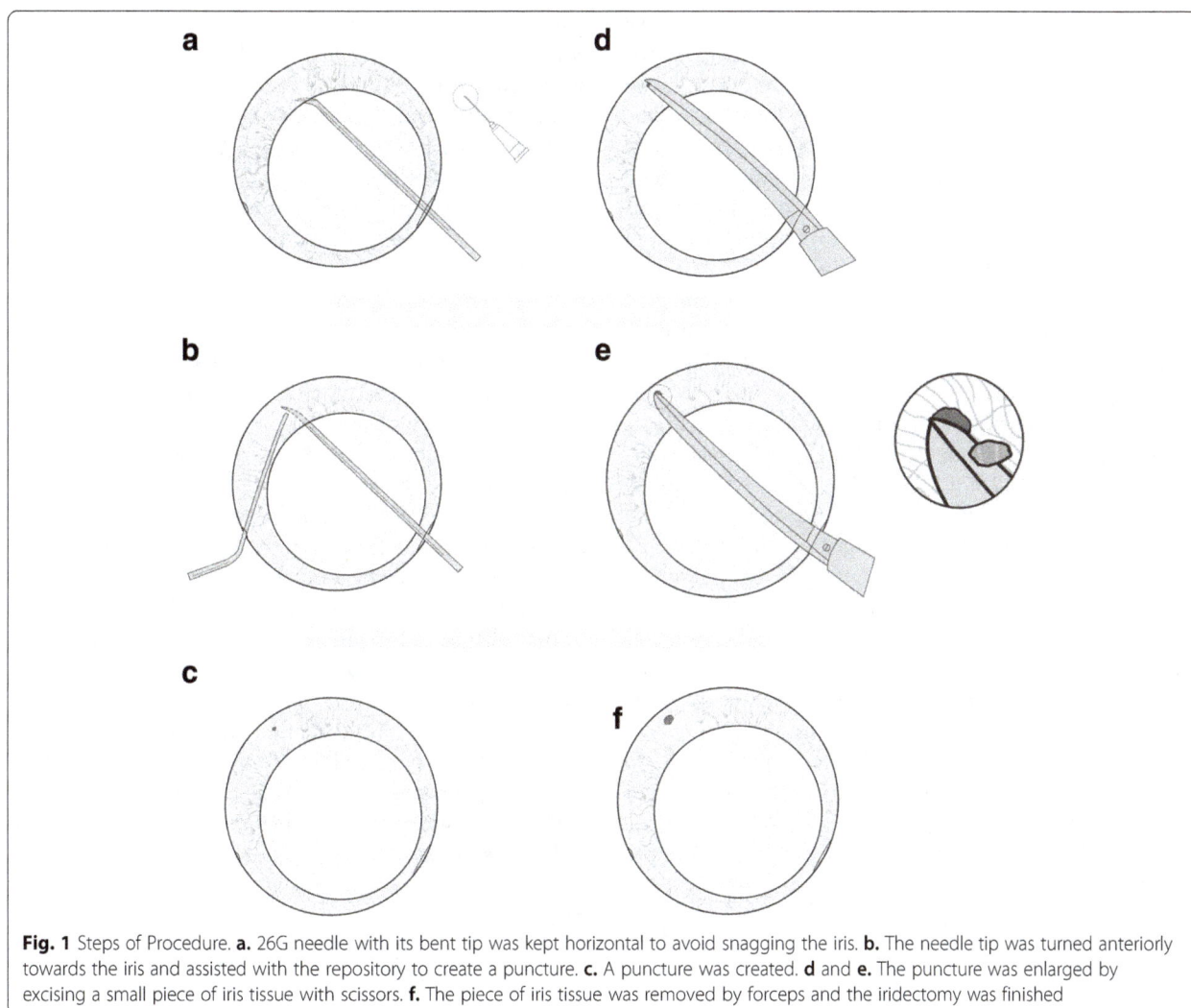

Fig. 1 Steps of Procedure. **a.** 26G needle with its bent tip was kept horizontal to avoid snagging the iris. **b.** The needle tip was turned anteriorly towards the iris and assisted with the repository to create a puncture. **c.** A puncture was created. **d** and **e.** The puncture was enlarged by excising a small piece of iris tissue with scissors. **f.** The piece of iris tissue was removed by forceps and the iridectomy was finished

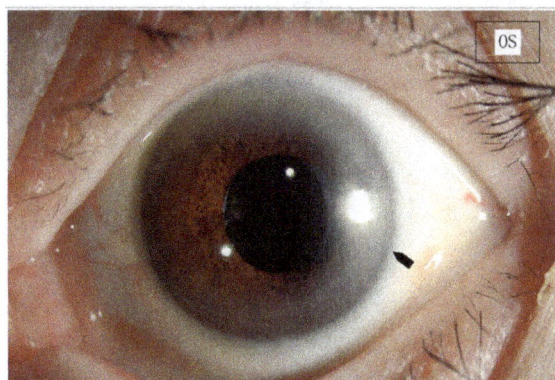

Fig. 2 Patent Surgical Iridectomy. The iridectomy remained patent over a follow up of 12 months

and the IOL was implanted in capsular bag in all 20 eyes. During surgical peripheral iridectomy, two eyes had intraoperative bleeding resulting in a 1–2 mm hypaema that resolved spontaneously within a week. One eye had a small (approximately 1 mm^2) Descemet's detachment caused by the needle tip, but did not require any intervention. Two eyes that underwent phacoemulsification within two weeks of the acute attack developed intraoperative corneal edema that did not preclude completion of iridectomy. Complications such as iridodialysis/cyclodialysis were not observed and none of the patients reported dysphotopsia. All iridectomies remained patent through the mean follow-up of 18.8 ± 9.7 months (range 12–48 months).

Two patients had an IOP elevation on the first postoperative day. The IOP was lowered by pressure on the posterior lip of the paracentesis with a 26G needle at the slit lamp to allow egress of aqueous and any residual viscoelastic. None of the patients required long term anti-glaucoma medications.

Significant postoperative inflammation and corneal edema were the most common complications. Four eyes that developed a fibrin aqueous reaction and/or corneal edema had undergone surgery within 2 weeks of the acute attack. Three of the eyes had received intracameral Carbamylcholine Chloride; two eyes developed the fibrin reaction immediately after injection of this miotic. Four eyes developed significant stromal edema of the cornea, which subsided within 4 weeks.

Postoperative visual acuities improved or remained unchanged (Table 1). Visual acuity improved from 0.96 ± 1.03logMAR preoperatively to 0.18 ± 0.21 logMAR after surgery ($p = 0.01$).

The mean preoperative IOP at presentation was 50.81 ± 6.0 mmHg (range, 41–60 mmHg) (Table 1). At the final examination for IOP was 12.95 ± 3.36 mmHg (range, 8–20 mmHg) without medication (Table 1). The difference in pre and post-operative IOP was statistically significant ($p = 0.000$).

Discussion

Postoperative pupillary block is a rare complication following phacoemulsification [1]. A surgical iridectomy may be indicated in high risk situations such as implantation of an anterior chamber (AC) or iris-fixed intraocular lens, perhaps in patients who are more prone to inflammation such as diabetics and those with current and past inflammation, especially where a YAG laser is not available [1, 2, 8]. In eyes with posterior chamber IOL, papillary block may be related to excessive postoperative inflammation, with the formation of posterior synechiae [9, 10]. This risk is higher in diabetics [1, 8], and in angle closure glaucoma [11].

Phacoemulsification is increasingly being used for the primary management of AAC [1, 3–7]. Two randomized trials have investigated phacoemulsification as a primary treatment for AAC [3, 6]. None of the patients undergoing phacoemulsification in those studies developed pupillary block; as numbers were small the upper end of the confidence interval is actually compatible with a true rate of 10–22% [3, 6].

A short axial length and higher risk of post-operative inflammation may increase the risk of pupillary block [1, 2]. Gaton's series of pupillary block following posterior IOL implantation included two patients (2/6) with known diabetic retinopathy and four (4/6) with glaucoma [1]. Diabetes was also present in 3 of 4 patients who developed acute postoperative pupillary-block following phacoemulsification [12]. Acute postoperative pupillary block occurred in 11 eyes (11 patients) of 12,016 phacoemulsifications (0.09%) performed by one unit in our hospital between 2011 and 2014 (unpublished data). 10 of the 11 patients that developed pupillary block were diabetic while one had uveitis. Pupillary block occurred in 10 of 1704 (0.6%) diabetics undergoing phacoemulsification; all had diabetic retinopathy. The incidence of pupillary block in those with diabetic retinopathy was 3.5% (10 of 290).

Table 1 The demographics, eye characteristics and results of this study

Patient characteristics	Mean ± SD (range)	
Number of patients	22	
Female/male ratio	19/3	
Age	56.86 ± 12.90 (27–75)	
Follow-up range (months)	18.9 ± 9.72 (12–48)	
Diagnosis		
a. AAC with cataract (n = 20)		
PAS (clock hours)	6.95 ± 3.15 (0–12)	
ACD (mm)	1.59 ± 0.20 (1.22–1.90)	
AL (mm)	21.44 ± 0.58 (19.65–21.97)	
b. Postoperative pupillary block after phacoemulsification (n = 2)	Case 1	Case 2
PAS (clock hours)	9	11
ACD (mm)	3.75	3.15
AL (mm)	22.86	23.26
Preoperative data		
IOP at presentation (mmHg)	50.81 ± 6.01 (41–60)	
LogMAR BCVA	0.96 ± 1.03 (0.1–3)	
Postoperative data		
IOP at last follow up (mmHg)	12.95 ± 3.36 (8–20)	
LogMAR BCVA	0.18 ± 0.21 (0–0.8)	

PAS Periphery anterior aynechia, *ACD* Anterior chamber depth, *AL* Axial lenth, *IOP* Intraocular pressure, *BCVA* Best corrected visual acuity, *SD* Standard deviation

A surgical iridectomy may be warranted in cases considered high risk for postoperative pupillary block. Performing LPI postoperatively only if papillary block occurs is certainly an option. However LPI in the situation of postoperative pupillary block, especially in the presence of inflammation that follows an acute attack is more difficult and associated with more complications [13–16]. Moreover it is also more difficult to perform LPI in brown irises in this situation, and in many locations a YAG laser may not be available. If YAG laser is not available, the described technique can also be used for the pupillary block that may follow AC or iris fixated IOL's.

Performing a surgical iridectomy through a tunnel incision can be technically challenging. An elegant technique that creates a small incision in the bed of a 4–5 mm scleral tunnel during the course of manual small incision cataract surgery has been described and can be used if a scleral tunnel is employed for phacoemulsification [17, 18]. This method can also be used with a corneal tunnel, but is easier with a longer incisional length and width. Also, an incision in the bed of a corneal tunnel has the potential to distort the wound and cause leakage; a watertight closure in this situation needs a larger tunnel length which can make phacoemulsification more difficult.

Other alternatives include an additional limbal incision for the iridectomy or the use of a vitrector. An extra limbal incision that requires a suture will be unattractive to most surgeons. We tend to avoid a vitrector primarily because it adds considerable expense to the procedure but also because it is more difficult and traumatic in a dilated pupil [19, 20].

Proper positioning of the iridectomy when performed through the tunnel is difficult in patients with the dilated pupils encountered in AAC. While miochol can be used to constrict the pupil, some pupils are unreactive, and, in our experience, inflammation in eyes that have recently suffered AAC is aggravated by Miochol [3, 6].

Potential complications of this method include complications related to introduction of a sharp needle behind the iris. While damage to the posterior capsule is conceivable, the needle is introduced under viscoelastic with the tip oriented horizontally and the maneuvers are undertaken following intraocular lens implantation. Introducing a scissor into the AC can cause damage to tissues. While an iridotomy alone might suffice, we elected to excise tissue, as the larger opening is less likely to occlude in the presence of inflammation. Bleeding from the iris and damage to Descemets membrane (as occurred in one case) and to the corneal endothelium is also possible. In order to avoid the immediate postoperative pressure spike, residual viscoelastic agent should be removed completely at the end of the surgery.

We acknowledge that an iridectomy adds an extra step to surgery and as there is potential for complications, it is only indicated in cases at higher risk of pupillary block. We also acknowledge that it is difficult to accurately predict post-operative pupillary block and that our own data suggests that some of the iridectomies were probably unnecessary. A risk of 3.5% has a number needed to treat of 29 and may help the decisions in specific situations/locations [21].

To conclude, this surgical technique for iridectomy can be safely and conveniently used for cases with or at high risk of postoperative pupillary block following cataract surgery, especially in settings where a YAG laser is not available.

Abbreviations

AAC: Acute angle closure; AC: Anterior chamber; IOL: Intraocular lens; IOP: Intraocular pressure; logMAR: Logarithm of the minimal angle resolution; LPI: Laser peripheral iridotomy; PI: Peripheral iridectomy; UBM: Ultrasound biomicroscopy; VA: Visual acuity

Acknowledgments

We appreciate the generous help and contributions made by professor Ravi Thomas to this manuscript.

Authors' contributions

AWF performed the surgery, participated in the design of the study, and drafted the manuscript; PJW analyzed the data and revised the manuscript; RH collected and analyzed the data; JQ participated in the design of the study and gave final approval of the version to be published. All authors read and approved the final manuscript.

Competing interests

The authors declare that they have no competing interests.

References

1. Gaton DD, Mimouni K, Lusky M, Ehrlich R, Weinberger D. Pupillary block following posterior chamber intraocular lens implantation in adults. Br J Ophthalmol. 2003;87(9):1109–11.
2. Stamper RL, Lieberman MF, Drake MV. Becker-Shaffer's diagnosis and therapy of the glaucomas. 7th ed. San Diego: Harcourt Publishers Limited; 2001.
3. Husain R, Gazzard G, Aung T, Chen Y, Padmanabhan V, Oen FT, Seah SK, Hoh ST. Initial management of acute primary angle closure: a randomized trial comparing phacoemulsification with laser peripheral iridotomy. Ophthalmology. 2012;119(11):2274–81.
4. Imaizumi M, Takaki Y, Yamashita H. Phacoemulsification and intraocular lens implantation for acute angle closure not treated or previously treated by laser iridotomy. J Cataract Refract Surg. 2006;32(1):85–90.
5. Hwang JU, Yoon YH, Kim DS, Kim JG. Combined phacoemulsification foldable intraocular lens implantation, and 25-gauge transconjunctival sutureless vitrectomy. J Cataract Refract Surg. 2006;32(5):727–31.
6. Lam DS, Leung DY, Tham CC, Li FC, Kwong YY, Chiu TY, Fan DS. Randomized trial of early phacoemulsification versus peripheral iridotomy to

prevent intraocular pressure rise after acute primary angle closure. Ophthalmology. 2008;115(7):1134–40.

7. Teekhasaenee C, Ritch R. Combined phacoemulsification and goniosynechialysis for uncontrolled chronic angle-closure glaucoma after acute angle-closure glaucoma. Ophthalmology. 1999;106(4):669–74. discussion 674-5

8. Naveh N, Wysenbeek Y, Solomon A, Melamed S, Blumenthal M. Anterior capsule adherence to iris leading to pseudophakic pupillary block. Ophthalmic Surg. 1991;22(6):350–2.

9. Ferris FL 3rd, Kassoff A, Bresnick GH, Bailey I. New visual acuity charts for clinical research. Am J Ophthaloml. 1982;94(1):91–6.

10. Vajpayee RB, Angra SK, Titiyal JS, Sharma YR, Chabbra VK. Pseudophakic pupillary-block glaucoma in children. Am J Ophthalmol. 1991;111(6):715–8.

11. Weinreb RN, Wasserstrom JP, Forman JS, Ritch R. Pseudophakic papillary block with angle-closure glaucoma in diabetic patients. Am J Ophthalmol. 1986;102(3):325–8.

12. Khor WB, Perera S, Jap A, Ho CL, Hoh ST. Anterior segment imaging in the management of postoperative fibrin pupillary-block glaucoma. J Cataract Refract Surg. 2009;35(7):1307–12.

13. Sihota R, Lakshmaiah NC, Walia KB, Sharma S, Pailoor J, Agarwal HC. The trabecular meshwork in acute and chronic angle closure glaucoma. Indian J Ophthalmol. 2001;49(4):255–9.

14. Saw SM, Gazzard G, Friedman DS. Interventions for angle-closure glaucoma: an evidence-based update. Ophthalmology. 2003;110(10):1869–78.

15. Sakai H, Ishikawa H, Shinzato M, Nakamura Y, Sakai M, Sawaguchi S. Prevalence of ciliochoroidal effusion after prophylactic laser iridotomy. Am J Ophthalmol. 2003;136(3):537–8.

16. Athanasiadis Y, de Wit DW, Nithyanandrajah GA, Patel A, Sharma A. Neodymium: YAG laser peripheral iridotomy as a possible cause of zonular dehiscence during phacoemulsification cataract surgery. Eye (Lond). 2010; 24(8):1424–5.

17. Blumenthal M, Kahana M. Performing peripheral Iridectomy via a scleral tunnel incision: a new technique. Ophthalmic Surg and Lasers. 1997; 28(2):162–4.

18. Thomas R, Parikh R, Muliyil J. Comparison between phacoemulsification and the Blumenthal technique of manual small-incision cataract surgery combined with trabeculectomy. J Glaucoma. 2003;12(4):333–9.

19. Bitrian E, Caprioli J. Pars plana anterior vitrectomy, hyaloido-zonulectomy, and iridotomy for aqueous humor misdirection. Am J Ophthalmol. 2010; 150(1):82–7.

20. Debrouwere V, Stalmans P, Van Calster J, Spileers W, Zeyen T, Stalmans I. Outcomes of different management options for malignant glaucoma: a retrospective study. Graefes Arch Clin Exp Ophthalmol. 2012;250(1):131–41.

21. Thomas R, Padma P, Braganza A, Muliyil J. Assessment of clinical significance: the number needed to treat. Indian J Ophthalmol. 1996; 44(2):113–5.

16

Predictive multi-imaging biomarkers relevant for visual acuity in idiopathic macular telangiectasis type 1

Jingli Guo, WenYi Tang, Xiaofeng Ye, Haixiang Wu, Gezhi Xu, Wei Liu* and Yongjin Zhang*⬤

Abstract

Background: To evaluate the structural changes associated with visual acuity (VA) in patients with idiopathic macular telangiectasia (MT) type 1 using multimodal imaging modalities.

Methods: A retrospective study of 14 patients with MT type 1 and of 10 eyes from 10 healthy individuals as age-matched controls was conducted. The medical records of patients who had undergone colour fundus photography, spectral domain optical coherence tomography (OCT), fluorescein angiography and OCT angiography were reviewed. Central macular thickness (CMT), the areas of macular oedema and ellipsoid zone (EZ) disruption, EZ length, disorganization of the retinal inner layers (DRIL) and external limiting membrane (ELM) disruption, as measured by spectral domain OCT; and vascular density and the foveal avascular zones (FAZ) of the superficial capillary plexus (SCP) and deep capillary plexus (DCP), as measured by OCT angiography, were assessed in MT type 1 eyes and correlated with VA.

Results: The mean baseline best-corrected VA of MT type 1 eyes was 0.45 ± 0.28. The mean CMT was 385.19 ± 75.21 μm in MT type 1 eyes and 252.43 ± 15.77 μm in contralateral eyes ($Z = -4.113$, $p < 0.001$). The mean vessel density of the DCP was lower in MT type 1 eyes ($47.25 \pm 4.69\%$) than in contralateral eyes ($53.93 \pm 2.94\%$) and normal eyes ($59.37 \pm 2.50\%$) ($Z = -3.492$, -4.099; $p < 0.001$, < 0.001). The baseline logMAR VA was correlated with CMT ($r = 0.682$, $p = 0.007$), SCP density ($r = -0.652$, $p = 0.012$), DCP density ($r = -0.700$, $p = 0.005$), total area of EZ disruption ($r = 0.649$, $p = 0.012$); and total lengths of EZ ($r = 0.681$, $p = 0.007$), ELM ($r = 0.699$, $p = 0.005$) and DRIL ($r = 0.707$, $p = 0.005$) disruption in the 1-mm-diameter foveal region in MT type 1 eyes.

Conclusions: Decreased DCP density and the presence of DRIL may be predictive biomarkers of VA in MT type 1. CMT, SCP density, total area of EZ disruption, and lengths of EZ and ELM disruption within the 1-mm-diameter central region were strongly associated with VA.

Keywords: Macular telangiectasia type 1, Disorganization of the retinal inner layers, Optical coherence tomography angiography, Ellipsoid zone disruption

Background

Idiopathic macular telangiectasia (MT) is characterized by abnormally dilated and tortuous capillaries around the fovea for no known reason. MT was originally termed idiopathic juxtafoveolar retinal telangiectasis, and was classified by Gass and Oyakawa into three categories: exudation, non-exudation and combination

with or without nervous system vasculopathy [1]. Based on recent advances in imaging that have led to better characterization of the disease, Yannuzzi et al. have recently defined two distinct forms of the disease, MT type 1 (aneurysmal telangiectasia) and MT type 2 (perifoveal telangiectasia) [2].

MT type 1 is typically a unilateral disease that is found more often in men and is clinically associated with loss of retinal transparency, salient extensive ectasia, lipid exudates, arteriolar aneurysms, deeply right-angled venules, and intra-retinal cystoid degeneration

* Correspondence: bfgf14@aliyun.com; yongjinzhang@yahoo.com
Department of Ophthalmology, Eye and ENT Hospital of Fudan University, Shanghai Key Laboratory of Visual Impairment and Restoration, Shanghai 200031, China

mainly on the temporal side of the macula [2]. Previous studies of patients with MT type 1 have assessed the correlations of visual acuity (VA) with photoreceptor inner segment–outer segment (IS/OS) disruption and the cystoid space using spectral domain optical coherence tomography (SD-OCT), and that with the microvascular density of the superficial capillary plexus (SCP) and deep capillary plexus (DCP) using OCT angiography (OCTA) [3, 4]. However, few studies have explored the associations of SD-OCT- and OCTA-derived parameters with VA.

Although SD-OCT can be effective for evaluating the thickness of vascularized layers by automatic segmentation [5, 6], OCTA provides more detailed information of the vascular networks. OCTA is a new technology used as an auxiliary examination to provide high-resolution imaging of retinal morphology and sensitive identification of the vascular layers [7], and has become a critical method for evaluating retinal vascular disorders such as diabetic retinopathy [8, 9], retinal vein occlusion [10, 11] and MT types 1 [4, 12, 13] and 2 [14, 15].

The aims of our study were to evaluate the OCTA and SD-OCT features of MT type 1, to compare SCP and DCP microvascular densities between normal and contralateral eyes, and to correlate VA with central macular thickness (CMT), areas of macular oedema and ellipsoid zone (EZ) disruption, lengths of the EZ, disorganization of the retinal inner layers (DRIL) and external limiting membrane (ELM) disruption, as measured by OCT; and with vascular density and the foveal avascular zone (FAZ) areas of the SCP and DCP, as measured by OCTA.

Methods

This was a retrospective study that enrolled consecutive patients with MT type 1 diagnosed from December 2014 to September 2017 at the outpatient clinic of the Eye & ENT Hospital of Fudan University, Shanghai, China. This study was approved by the Institutional Review Board of the Eye and ENT Hospital of Fudan University. All procedures were performed according to the principles of the Declaration of Helsinki. Written informed consent was obtained from all participants or their guardians.

Patients underwent comprehensive ocular examinations in both eyes, including best-corrected VA (BCVA) evaluation, intraocular pressure reading, slit-lamp biomicroscopic ophthalmoscopic exam, dilated fundoscopy, fundus photography (Topcon TRC50LX; Topcon, Tokyo, Japan), OCTA (Optovue RTVue XR 100 Avanti, Fremont, CA, USA), SD-OCT (Heidelberg Engineering, Heidelberg, Germany) and fluorescein angiography (FA, Topcon TRC501X; Topcon). None of the patients in this study had undergone previous ocular treatment. As

the control group, 10 right eyes imaged by SD-OCT and OCTA from 10 healthy individuals without any ocular diseases who were of similar age and sex as the MT type 1 cases were evaluated.

The clinical criteria used for diagnosing MT type 1 were confirmed by FA and included the following: (1) FA detection of unilateral, visible telangiectasis, aneurysms during the early stage and fluorescein leakage during the late stage of MT type 1, (2) OCTA detection of telangiectasis, aneurysms and decreased vascular densities of the SCP and DCP and (3) SD-OCT detection of intra-retinal oedema and hard exudates. Patients with neovascular maculopathies (e.g., age-related macular degeneration, polypoidal choroidal vasculopathy, retinal angiomatous proliferation, angioid streaks and other causes of secondary MT, including Coats' disease, Leber disease, retinal vein occlusion and radiation retinopathy) were excluded. Also excluded were patients with diabetes, hypertension, ischemic heart disease, a history of vitreoretinal surgery, ophthalmic disorders excluding mild refractive errors and mild cataracts, or an oral history of anti-oestrogen tamoxifen for breast cancer.

SD-OCT was performed with 6-mm line scans (vertical and horizontal) across the centre of the fovea. A 19 line scans that covered a $20 \times 15°$ (5.8×4.3 mm) area centred on the fovea was obtained in all eyes, with 20 automated real-time means per scan on high-resolution mode. The CMT in the 1-mm-diameter central region of the macula according to the Early Treatment of Diabetic Retinopathy Study thickness map was measured using Spectralis software. The ELM is formed by the junctions between the inner segments of photoreceptors and Müller cells [16]. The EZ is formed by the reflectivity generated from the high mitochondrial density of the outermost portion of the inner photoreceptor segments [17]. To calculate the area of EZ disruption, the intensity of the EZ band and border of the EZ disruption were measured using the plot profile function in ImageJ software (National Institutes of Health, Bethesda, MD, USA) and the grayscale image obtained by SD-OCT. The border of the disrupted EZ area was defined as a decrease in EZ reflectivity of 2 SD compared with an EZ band in the normal retina [18]. DRIL was defined as the inability to identify and differentiate any of the boundaries of the ganglion cell layer–inner plexiform layer (IPL) complex, inner nuclear layer, and outer plexiform layer (OPL) [19]. All images were obtained by well-trained operators (GJL, TWY). All data were measured within a 1-mm-diameter region encompassing the foveal centre and also on three B-scans performed immediately above and below.

Two independent observers (GJL, TWY) assessed the OCTA data using the best-quality 3×3-mm scan and controlled the corrected segmentation for the 14 patients before reporting the data. Vascular retinal layers were divided into the SCP, DCP, outer retina and choroidal layers by OCTA. The FAZ and density of the macula were assessed using flow density map software Angio-Analytics (Optovue RTVue XR 100 Avanti). The signal strength index of all images was greater than 60. Whole-image data were used to measure the microvascular densities in the SCP and DCP layers.

Statistical analysis

BCVA values were converted into logarithm of the minimum angle of resolution values (logMAR) for statistical evaluation. Quantitative data (mean BCVA, CMT, vascular density, FAZ areas of the SCP and DCP) were compared among MT type 1, contralateral and normal eyes by the Mann–Whitney test and Wilcoxon test using IBM SPSS Statistics v19 (SPSS Inc., Chicago, IL, USA). Significance was defined as $P < 0.05$. Pearson's correlation coefficient analyses were used to identify the factors associated with VA. The correlation was defined as none/very weak at $r < 0.1$, weak at $0.1 < r < 0.3$, moderate at $0.3 < r < 0.6$, strong at $0.6 < r < 0.8$, or very strong at $0.8 < r < 1$ [19].

Results

A total of 14 eyes in 14 patients (8 men and 6 women) were included in the study. The mean $\pm$ SD age was 55.07 ± 12.74 years (range, 34–75 years). The BCVA values (mean $\pm$ SD) in the MT type 1, contralateral and control eyes at baseline (logMAR) were 0.45 ± 0.28 (range, 20/20 to 20/200), 0.07 ± 0.07 (range, 20/20 to 20/32) and 0.02 ± 0.04 (range, 20/20 to 20/25), respectively. The CMT values (mean $\pm$ SD) in the MT type 1, contralateral and normal eyes were 385.19 ± 75.21 (range, 224–487) μm, 252.43 ± 15.77 (range, 225–280) μm and 230.30 ± 7.04 (221–241) μm, respectively (Fig. 1). The fundus photography revealed oedematous maculae in 13 eyes, in which macular oedema appeared as hypo-reflective areas, and hard exudates and a few aneurysms appeared as hyper-reflective areas on SD-OCT at the first visit. In the remaining patient, SD-OCT displayed multiple disorganized hyper-reflective points from the IPL to the OPL (Fig. 2). The CMT values were higher in the 14 MT type 1 eyes than in the contralateral and normal eyes (Z = – 3.296, Z = – 4.101; $p < 0.001$, $p < 0.001$). An interrupted EZ structure was found in 13 patients. On FA, abnormally dilated and tortuous capillaries and aneurysms were observed during the early phase and intense hyperfluorescence and parafoveal leakage during the late

phase, mainly in the temporal hemisphere. The demographic characteristics of the patients are listed in Table 1.

In the OCTA examination, decreased vessel density and telangiectasis in the SCP and DCP were observed in all of the MT type 1 eyes, and these observations were much clearer compared with those on FA or OCT when observing telangiectasis variations in real time. The high resolution of OCTA enabled the clearest view of the vascular structure of the retina. The mean vessel density value of the DCP ($47.25 \pm 4.69\%$) was lower in MT type 1 eyes than in contralateral eyes ($53.93 \pm 2.94\%$) and normal eyes ($59.37 \pm 2.50\%$) (Z = – 3.492, Z = – 4.099; $p < 0.001$, $p < 0.001$). The FAZ areas of the SCP and DCP were larger in MT type 1 eyes (0.45 ± 0.15 mm^2 and 0.78 ± 0.35 mm^2, respectively) than in normal eyes (0.28 ± 0.14 mm^2 and 0.35 ± 0.13 mm^2, respectively) (Z = – 2.372, Z = – 3.455; $p = 0.018$, $p = 0.001$; Fig. 1).

The baseline logMAR VA was correlated with the CMT ($r = 0.682$, $p = 0.007$), densities of the SCP ($r = – 0.652$, $p = 0.012$) and DCP ($r = – 0.700$, $p = 0.005$), total area of EZ disruption ($r = 0.649$, $p = 0.012$); and the lengths of EZ ($r = 0.681$, $p = 0.007$), ELM ($r = 0.699$, $p = 0.005$) and DRIL ($r = 0.707$, $p = 0.005$) disruption in the 1-mm-diameter foveal region in MT type 1 eyes. The associations of baseline SD-OCT and OCTA parameters with baseline logMAR VA are shown in Table 2.

Early-stage MT type 1 was observed in Patient 4 (Fig. 2). In this patient, central macular oedema (CME) was not detected by SD-OCT (Fig. 2g), but the patient had blurred vision and abnormal microvascular variations in the IPL and OPL. Aneurysms were subsequently seen on FA (Fig. 2b) and OCTA. The telangiectasis of SCP and DCP was clearly revealed by OCTA (Fig. 2c). The vascular changes were barely evident in the SCP but prominent in the DCP.

In addition, the DCP density was decreased in MT type 1 eyes compared with contralateral and normal eyes. The FAZ areas in the SCP and DCP were larger in MT type 1 eyes than in contralateral and normal eyes.

Discussion

Few studies have evaluated the correlations between anatomic factors and baseline VA in MT type 1 [3, 4]. Takayama et al. reported strong associations between intra-retinal cystoid spaces and IS/OS alterations and retinal sensitivity [3]. Matet et al. found that logMAR VA was inversely correlated with SCP and DCP densities [4]. The current study demonstrated strong correlations of baseline logMAR VA with DRIL and microvascular DCP density, and associations were also found between baseline logMAR VA and CMT, SCP density, lengths of EZ and ELM disruption within the

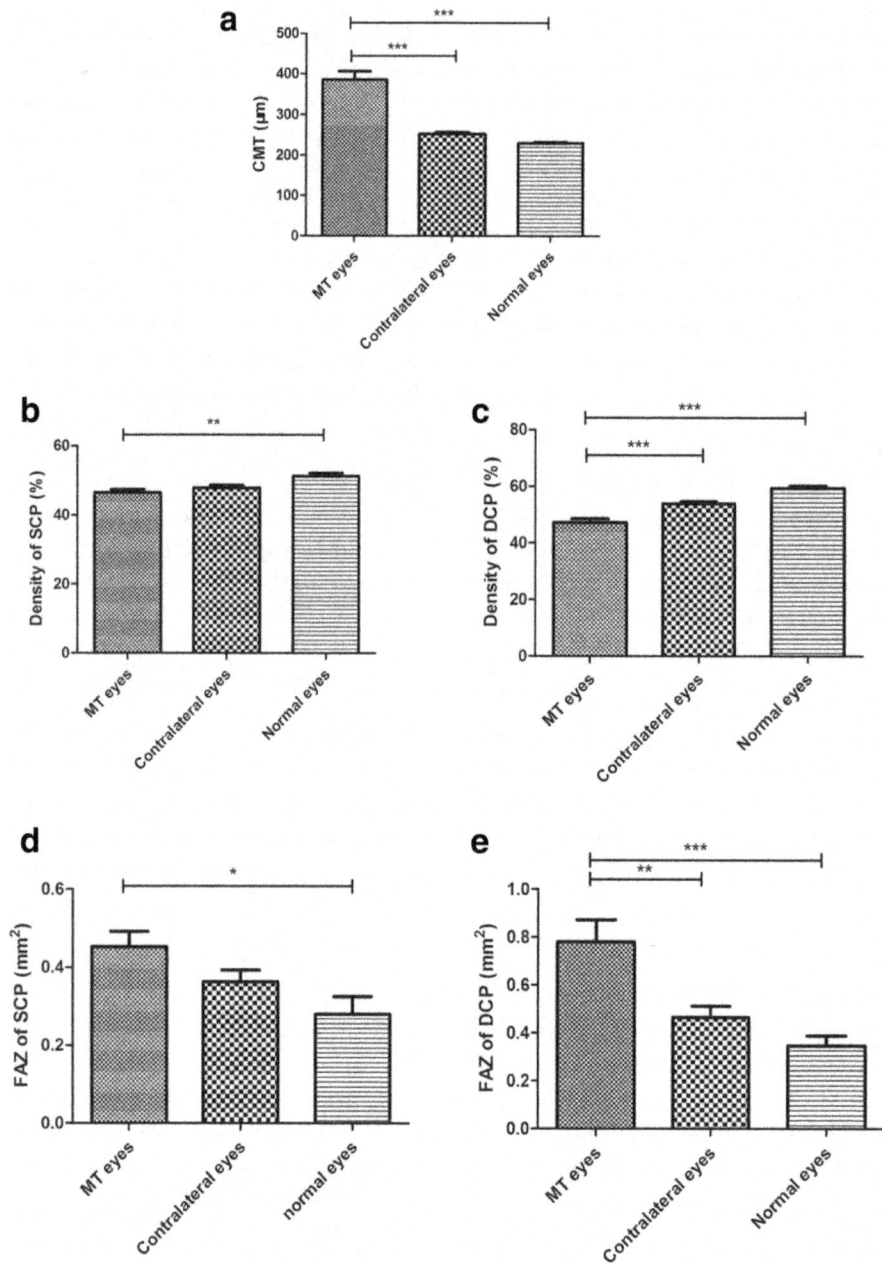

Fig. 1 Comparisons among idiopathic macular telangiectasia (MT) type 1 eyes, contralateral eyes and normal eyes. (**a**) Central macular thickness (CMT). (**b**) Density of the superficial capillary plexus (SCP). (**c**) Density of the deep capillary plexus (DCP). (**d**) Foveal avascular zone (FAZ) area of the SCP. (**e**) FAZ area of the DCP. *$p < 0.05$, ** $p < 0.01$, *** $p < 0.001$

1-mm-diameter central region of the macula, and the total area of EZ disruption. Because these SD-OCT- and OCTA-derived anatomic parameters can provide further information on VA, they could be useful in determining therapeutic regimens and for developing patient counselling strategies.

In the present study, a strong correlation was found between baseline logMAR VA and DRIL. The inner retinal layers play crucial roles in neural transmission from the photoreceptors to the retinal ganglion cells. The inability to distinguish the retinal layer boundaries likely represents partial destruction of the inner retinal cells, thus interrupting transmission between the photoreceptors and the ganglion cells [20]. Sun et al. were the first to report that DRIL is correlated with worse VA in eyes with diabetic macular oedema [21]. All of the MT type 1 eyes in the present study had DRIL, which was positively correlated with baseline logMAR VA. Furthermore, the reduced viable tissue in DRIL may further decrease the demand for a blood supply, resulting in loss of the deep

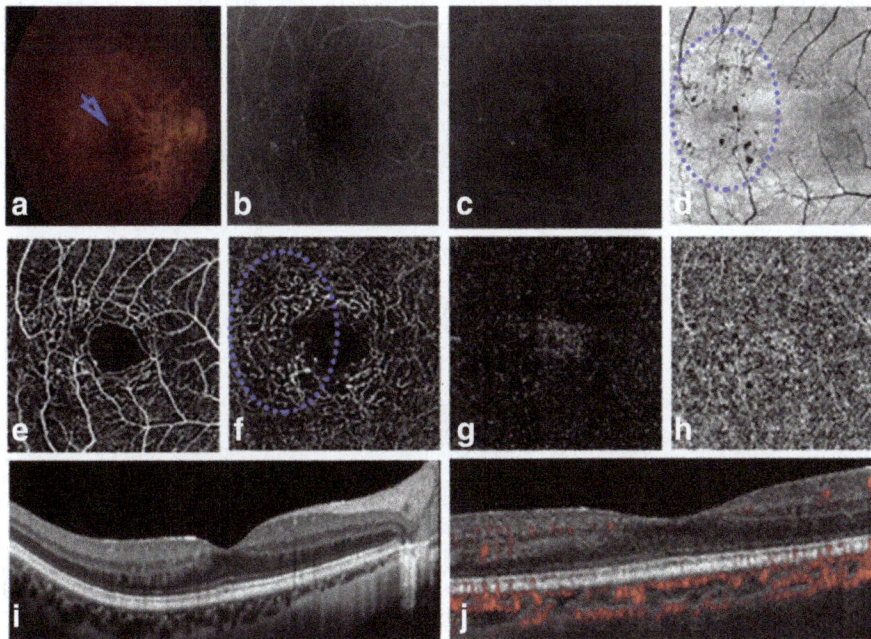

Fig. 2 Imaging of the right eye of Patient 4. Capillary variations are visible from the inner to the outer plexiform layers on the temporal side of the macula. (**a**) Blue arrow shows sparse micro-aneurysms. (**b**) Fluorescein angiography (FA) reveals hyperfluorescence from micro-aneurysms on the temporal side of the macula during the early stage of MT type 1. (**c**) FA showing leakage of fluorescein due to vascular endothelial cell injury during the late stage of MT type 1. (**d**) No lesion is visible in the inner and outer segment junction (IS/OS) and blue-dotted oval shows sparse micro-aneurysms on en-face OCT. (**e**) OCT angiography (OCTA) reveals decreased capillary density in the superficial capillary plexus. (**f**) OCTA image showing the transformational foveal avascular zone (FAZ), aneurysms, and telangiectasia in the deep capillary plexus (DCP) on the temporal side of the macula. (**g** and **h**) OCTA images show no changes in the outer or choroidal layers, respectively. (**i**) SD-OCT shows areas of hyper-reflectance from the inner to the outer plexiform layers on the temporal side. (**j**) OCTA showing blood flow

vascular plexus [22]. This view was confirmed by our findings that the DCP density was decreased in all patients with MT type 1 and was correlated with logMAR VA. The ELM, which exhibits several different junctional complexes between Muller and rod/cone photoreceptor cells, may be an indispensable factor for the survival of photoreceptor cells. The integrity of the ELM and EZ may be regarded as predictors of a better VA prognosis [10]. In our study, the lengths of EZ and ELM disruption within the 1-mm-diameter central region and the total area of EZ disruption were positively correlated with the baseline logMAR VA.

With the rapid development of imaging techniques, OCTA has become a convenient and noninvasive method

Table 1 Characteristics of idiopathic macular telangiectasia type 1 patients and normal patients

	MT eyes	Fellow eyes	Normal eyes
Number of eyes	14	14	10
Age (years)	55.07 ± 12.74 (34-75)	55.07 ± 12.74 (34-75)	48.80 ± 9.32(36-60)
Sex (men/women)	8/6	8/6	6/4
BCVA(LogMAR)	0.45 ± 0.28	0.07 ± 0.07	0.02 ± 0.04
BCVA (Snellen equivalent)	20/44 (20/20-20/200)	20/23 (20/20-20/32)	20/21 (20/20-20/25)
Microvascular density of SCP(%)	46.47 ± 3.42 (38.25-51.90)	47.78 ± 2.89 (42.52-52.33)	51.30 ± 2.81 (46.46-54.50)
Microvascular density of DCP(%)	47.25 ± 4.69 (39.90-54.60)	53.93 ± 2.94 (48.36-57.83)	59.37 ± 2.50 (54.62-61.96)
FAZ of SCP (mm^2)	0.45 ± 0.15 (0.22-0.71)	0.36 ± 0.11 (0.21-0.59)	0.28 ± 0.14 (0.07-0.55)
FAZ of DCP (mm^2)	0.78 ± 0.35 (0.25-1.45)	0.47 ± 0.17 (0.33-0.94)	0.35 ± 0.13 (0.11-0.57)
CMT (μm)	385.19 ± 75.21 (224-487)	252.43 ± 15.77 (225-280)	230.30 ± 7.04(221-241)
Mean areas with photoreceptor damage (mm^2)	3.22 ± 2.02 (0-5.81)		

BCVA best-corrected visual acuity, *SCP* superficial plexus, *DCP* deep plexus, *FAZ* foveal avascular zone, *CMT* centre macular thickness, *MT* idiopathic macular telangiectasia

Table 2 Associations of baseline spectral-domain optical coherence tomography and optical coherence tomography angiography parameters with baseline logMAR visual acuity

Parameters	MT type 1 eyes	r	p value
FAZ of SCP (mm^2)	0.45 ± 0.15	0.451	0.106
FAZ of DCP (mm^2)	0.78 ± 0.35	0.521	0.056
Microvascular density of SCP (%)	46.47 ± 3.42	−0.652	0.012
Microvascular density of DCP (%)	47.25 ± 4.69	− 0.700	0.005
CMT (μm)	385.19 ± 75.21	0.682	0.007
Total area of macular oedema (mm^2)	0.08 ± 0.10	0.443	0.112
Largest area of macular edema (mm^2)	0.08 ± 0.09	0.512	0.061
Length of EZ disruption (μm)	642.26 ± 349.66	0.681	0.007
Area of EZ disruption (mm^2)	0.93 ± 1.22	0.27	0.351
Total area of EZ disruption (mm^2)	3.22 ± 2.02	0.649	0.012
Length of ELM disruption (μm)	372.57 ± 279.16	0.699	0.005
Length of DRIL disruption (μm)	480.79 ± 340.73	0.707	0.005

p-values indicate the relationships between logMAR VA and spectral domain OCT and OCTA parameters

OCT spectral domain optical coherence tomography, OCTA optical coherence tomography angiography, logMAR logarithm of the minimal angle of resolution, VA visual acuity, MT idiopathic macular telangiectasia, FAZ foveal avascular zone, SCP superficial capillary plexus, DCP deep capillary plexus, CMT central macular thickness, EZ ellipsoid zone, ELM external limiting membrane, DRIL disorganization of retinal inner layers, r Pearson's correlation coefficient

for evaluating ocular variations in retinal vascular diseases (particularly variations in the deep capillary) that can be used at every visit to the clinic [23]. SD-OCT and FA enable gross evaluation of changes in the vascular network. Because of the limited visualization of FA due to dye leakage, we were unable to observe the deep vascular plexus in more detail using this method. However, OCTA has the particular advantage of visualizing real-time dynamic changes in various retinal layers, and enables gross quantification of capillary density in several retinal layers simultaneously [23]. Accordingly, we can use OCTA to assess the reductions in capillary density in both the SCP and DCP in comparison with those of the contralateral healthy eye, despite the lack of an accurate measuring technique. Moreover, the alterations in DCP density and FAZ area are specific parameters for analysis at follow-up. Two unique characteristics of MT type 1 eyes were revealed in the present patients by OCTA. First, there was a negative correlation between DCP density in the lesion and logMAR VA in our cases. Second, decreased capillary density variation in the deep layer was a predictor of very-early-stage MT type 1. Birol et al. confirmed in an animal model that the deep capillary bed is conducive to the oxygen requirements of the photoreceptor layer [24]. In their study, the primary oxygen supply to photoreceptor layers was derived from the choroidal circulation, but 10%–15% was derived from the retinal circulation. As oxygenation of the fovea is somewhat different from that of the perifoveal retina, it would be useful to discuss this and any other potentially relevant correlations regarding the foveal and perifoveal areas. We speculate that the vascular variation in the DCP and DRIL may predict hypoxidosis in the

photoreceptor layer. Of the 13 patients in the study of Birol et al., 12 had characteristics of macular oedema rather than retinal atrophy. However, among our cases, patient 4, who had obviously distorted capillaries and aneurysms during the early stage, and leakage during the late stage according to FA, had slightly blurred vision without CME, but the DCP density and FAZ area already showed obvious transformations. One possible explanation for this finding is that the abnormal morphology and structure from the IPL to OPL on the temporal side of the macula are also related to telangiectasia. Gass and Oyakawa [1] suggested that disruption of the deeper capillary plexus predominantly causes variation in the retinal vasculature and that the late diffuse fluorescence is derived from the outer retina. It has been reported that in MT type 1, changes occur earlier in the deep capillary bed than in the superficial capillary bed [25], which was confirmed in the present series.

The limitations of our study included its retrospective design and the small sample size due to the low prevalence of MT type 1. The captured images inevitably have artefacts despite being obtained by two experienced observers (GJL and TWY).

Conclusion

The greater the scale of EZ disruption and/or lengths of DRIL and ELM disruption in the lesion, the worse the vision. Decreased DCP density is potentially an earlier indicator of MT type 1 than are macular oedema and EZ layer disruption. We speculate that variation in structure from the IPL to the OPL on OCT and morphological changes on OCTA are manifestations of very-early-stage MT type 1.

Abbreviations
BCVA: best-corrected visual acuity; CMT: central macular thickness; DCP: deep capillary plexus; DRIL: disorganization of the retinal inner layers; ELM: external limiting membrane; EZ: ellipsoid zone; FA: fluorescein angiography; FAZ: foveal avascular zone; MT type 1: idiopathic macular telangiectasia type 1; OCTA: optical coherence tomography angiography; SCP: superficial capillary plexus; SD-OCT: spectral-domain optical coherence tomography; VA: visual acuity

Acknowledgements
We would like to thank all of the participants and staff for their valuable contributions to this research.

Funding
This study was supported by grant SHDC12016116 from the Science and Technology Commission of Shanghai Municipality.

Authors' contributions
GJL: substantial contributions to the study conception and design and data acquisition, analysis and interpretation; TWY: substantial contributions to data analysis and interpretation; YXF: acquisition of data and research design; WHX: acquisition of data and research design; XGZ: acquisition of data and research design. LW: final approval of the version to be published, research design and manuscript preparation. ZYJ: final approval of the version to be published, research design, data analysis and manuscript preparation. All authors have read and approved the final manuscript.

Competing interests
The authors declare that they have no competing interests.

References
1. Gass JD, Oyakawa RT. Idiopathic juxtafoveolar retinal telangiectasis. Arch Ophthalmol. 1982;100:769–80.
2. Yannuzzi LA, Bardal AM, Freund KB, Chen KJ, Eandi CM, Blodi B. Idiopathic macular telangiectasia. Arch Ophthalmol. 2006;124:450–60.
3. Takayama K, Ooto S, Tamura H, Yamashiro K, Otani A, Tsujikawa A, et al. Retinal structural alterations and macular sensitivity in idiopathic macular telangiectasia type 1. Retina. 2012;32:1973–80.
4. Matet A, Daruich A, Dirani A, Ambresin A, Behar-Cohen F. Macular telangiectasia type 1: capillary density and microvascular abnormalities assessed by optical coherence tomography angiography. Am J Ophthalmol. 2016;167:18–30.
5. Demirkaya N, van Dijk HW, van Schuppen SM, Abramoff MD, Garvin MK, Sonka M, et al. Effect of age on individual retinal layer thickness in normal eyes as measured with spectral-domain optical coherence tomography. Invest Ophthalmol Vis Sci. 2013;54(7):4934–40.
6. Abdolrahimzadeh S, Parisi F, Scavella V, Recupero SM. Optical coherence tomography evidence on the correlation of choroidal thickness and age with vascularized retinal layers in normal eyes. Retina. 2016;36(12):2329–38.
7. Wylegala A, Teper S, Dobrowolski D, Wylegala E. Optical coherence angiography: a review. Medicine (Baltimore). 2016;95(41):e4907.
8. Ishibazawa A, Nagaoka T, Yokota H, Takahashi A, Omae T, Song YS, et al. Characteristics of retinal neovascularization in proliferative diabetic retinopathy imaged by optical coherence tomography angiography. Invest Ophthalmol Vis Sci. 2016;57(14):6247–55.
9. Soares M, Neves C, Marques IP, Pires I, Schwartz C, Costa MA, et al. Comparison of diabetic retinopathy classification using fluorescein angiography and optical coherence tomography angiography. Br J Ophthalmol. 2017;101(1):62–8.
10. Kang JW, Yoo R, Jo YH, Kim HC. Correlation of microvascular structures on optical coherence tomography angiography with visual acuity in retinal vein occlusion. Retina. 2017;37(9):1700–9.
11. Balaratnasingam C, Inoue M, Ahn S, McCann J, Dhrami-Gavazi E, Yannuzzi LA, et al. Visual acuity is correlated with the area of the foveal avascular zone in diabetic retinopathy and retinal vein occlusion. Ophthalmology. 2016;123(11):2352 67.
12. Yannuzzi NA, Gregori NZ, Roisman L, Gupta N, Goldhagen BE, Goldhardt R. Fluorescein angiography versus optical coherence tomography angiography in macular telangiectasia type I treated with bevacizumab therapy. Ophthalmic Surg Lasers Imaging Retina. 2017;48(3):263–6.
13. Pappuru RR, Peguda HK, Dave VP. Optical coherence tomographic angiography in type 1 idiopathic macular telangiectasia. Clin Exp Optom. 2018;101(1):143–4.
14. Mao L, Weng SS, Gong YY, Yu SQ. Optical coherence tomography angiography of macular telangiectasia type 1: comparison with mild diabetic macular edema. Lasers Surg Med. 2017;49(3):225–32.
15. Chidambara L, Gadde SG, Yadav NK, Jayadev C, Bhanushali D, Appaji AM, et al. Characteristics and quantification of vascular changes in macular telangiectasia type 2 on optical coherence tomography angiography. Br J Ophthalmol. 2016;100(11):1482–8.
16. Toto L, Di Antonio L, Mastropasqua R, Mattei PA, Carpineto P, Borrelli E, et al. Multimodal imaging of macular telangiectasia type 2: focus on vascular changes using optical coherence tomography angiography. Invest Ophthalmol Vis Sci. 2016;57(9):T268–76.
17. Drexler W, Sattmann H, Hermann B, Ko TH, Stur M, Unterhuber A, et al. Enhanced visualization of macular pathology with the use of ultrahigh-resolution optical coherence tomography. Arch Ophthalmol. 2003;121(5):695–706.
18. Staurenghi G, Sadda S, Chakravarthy U, Spaide RF. Proposed lexicon for anatomic landmarks in normal posterior segment spectral domain optical coherence tomography. The IN•OCT consensus. Ophthalmology. 2014;121(8):1572–8.
19. Wakazono T, Ooto S, Hangai M, Yoshimura N. Photoreceptor outer segment abnormalities and retinal sensitivity in acute zonal occult outer retinopathy. Retina. 2013;33(3):642–8.
20. Grewal DS, O'Sullivan ML, Kron M, Jaffe GJ. Association of disorganization of retinal inner layers with visual acuity in eyes with uveitic cystoid macular edema. Am J Ophthalmol. 2017;177:116–25.
21. Sun JK, Lin MM, Lammer J, Prager S, Sarangi R, Silva PS, et al. Disorganization of the retinal inner layers as a predictor of visual acuity in eyes with center-involved diabetic macular edema. JAMA Ophthalmol. 2014;132(11):1309–16.
22. Spaide RF. Volume-rendered optical coherence tomography of diabetic retinopathy pilot study. Am J Ophthalmol. 2015;160(6):1200–10.
23. Abreu-Gonzalez R, Diaz-Rodriguez R, Rubio-Rodriguez G, Gil-Hernandez MA, Abreu-Reyes P. Macular vascular flow area and vascular density in healthy population using optical coherence tomography angiography. Invest Ophthalmol Vis Sci. 2016;57(15):6713.
24. Birol G, Wang S, Budzynski E, Wangsa-Wirawan ND, Linsenmeier RA. Oxygen distribution and consumption in the macaque retina. Am J Physiol Heart Circ Physiol. 2007;293(3):H1696–704.
25. Sugiura Y, Okamoto F, Okamoto Y, Hiraoka T, Oshika T. Visual function in patients with idiopathic macular telangiectasia type 1. Acta Ophthalmol. 2016;94(7):e672–3.

17

Analysis of pre-operative factors affecting range of optimal vaulting after implantation of 12.6-mm V4c implantable collamer lens in myopic eyes

Hun Lee[1,2], David Sung Yong Kang[3], Jin Young Choi[3], Byoung Jin Ha[3], Eung Kweon Kim[2,4], Kyoung Yul Seo[2] and Tae-im Kim[2*]

Abstract

Background: To evaluate clinical factors affecting postoperative vaulting in eyes that had achieved optimal vaulting within the range of 250–750 μm following implantation of 12.6-mm V4c implantable collamer lenses (ICL).

Methods: A total of 236 eyes of 236 patients that had achieved optimal vaulting following implantation of a 12.6-mm V4c ICL were retrospectively analyzed. Associations between postoperative vaulting and age, preoperative anterior chamber depth (ACD), preoperative axial length (AL), preoperative white-to-white diameter, preoperative pupil size, preoperative sulcus-to-sulcus diameter, and preoperative manifest refraction spherical equivalent were investigated using simple regression, stepwise multiple regression, and multinomial logistic regression analyses.

Results: Mean central vaulting at the 6-month follow-up was 519.0 ± 112.8 μm. Variables relevant to postoperative vaulting were, in order of influence, preoperative ACD ($\beta = 0.305$, $p < 0.001$), preoperative pupil size ($\beta = 0.218$, $p < 0.001$), and preoperative AL ($\beta = 0.171$, $p = 0.006$). Low preoperative pupil size was associated with low optimal vaulting (250 to 450 μm), relative to that observed in the mid optimal vaulting group (451 to 550 μm) (odds ratio = 0.532, $P = 0.021$). Increasing preoperative ACD was associated with high optimal vaulting (551 and 750 μm), relative to that observed the mid optimal vaulting group (odds ratio = 6.340, $P = 0.034$).

Conclusions: Myopic eyes with greater preoperative ACD, larger pupil size, and longer AL are predisposed to higher postoperative vaulting following 12.6-mm V4c ICL implantation. Therefore, the extremes of these parameters should be considered when choosing V4c ICL size.

Keywords: 12.6-mm V4c implantable collamer lenses, Postoperative vaulting, Preoperative pupil size, Anterior chamber depth, Axial length

Background

The implantable collamer lens (ICL), a posterior chamber phakic intraocular lens, effectively correct moderate to high myopia [1, 2]. In addition, the ICL has been reported to be safe and effective for the long-term correction of refractive errors in highly myopic eyes, for which laser vision surgery is not appropriate [3]. Albeit its outstanding benefit, postoperative complications have been reported [4–6]. Most of these complications are associated with vaulting of the lens (i.e., distance between the posterior surface of the ICL and the anterior surface of the crystalline lens). High vaulting conditions lead to increased intraocular pressure and inflammation by causing mechanical contact between the ICL and iris [6, 7]. Pigment dispersion, iris atrophy, secondary glaucoma, and formation of metabolic cataracts have also been associated with high vaulting conditions [8, 9]. Low

* Correspondence: tikim@yuhs.ac
[2]The Institute of Vision Research, Department of Ophthalmology, Yonsei University College of Medicine, Seoul, South Korea
Full list of author information is available at the end of the article

vaulting conditions have been reported to induce mechanical contact between the ICL and crystalline lens and cause inadequate aqueous circulation in the perilenticular space. Mechanical contact between the ICL (posterior surface) and crystalline lens (anterior surface), as well as impaired circulation of aqueous humor, are considered to play a crucial role in the development of anterior subcapsular cataracts [2, 4, 10].

The recently introduced Visian V4c ICL (STAAR Surgical Company, Monrovia, CA, USA) has been designed with a 360-μm central hole (aquaport) allowing aqueous humor to flow without the need for an iridotomy [11]. The presence of the central hole does not significantly affect the position of the ICL when comparing the V4c ICL and V4b ICL implants [12]. Recent studies have suggested that optimal ICL vaulting ranges from 250 to 750 μm [13–15]. ICL sizing based on sulcus-to-sulcus (STS) diameter, white-to-white (WTW) diameter, and anterior chamber depth (ACD) has been established as the gold standard for achieving optimal vaulting [13, 16, 17]. However, values at the low end of this range (250 μm) may be associated with peripheral crystalline lens contact, while values at the high end of this range (750 μm) may be associated with synechial angle closure. Thus, both optimal vaulting status and the extent of vaulting achieved within the optimal range may be relevant to the selection of ICL size.

Therefore, the present study aimed to analyze factors that influence vaulting in 12.6-mm V4c ICL implanted eyes that had achieved optimal vaulting between 250 and 750 μm. Only one size of V4c ICL was used for the analysis to eliminate any confounding effects of size.

Methods

Ethical approval for the present retrospective study was obtained from the Institutional Review Board of Yonsei University College of Medicine, Seoul, South Korea (4–2016-0357). The study adhered to the tenets of the Declaration of Helsinki and followed good clinical practice.

Inclusion criteria for the present study were as follows: (i) age 20–45 years; (ii) presence of myopia with a manifest refraction spherical equivalent (MRSE) between – 4.00 and – 20.00 diopters (D); (iii) astigmatism between 0.00 and – 5.00 D; (iiii) eyes that had underwent the implantation of 12.6-mm V4c ICL using standardized techniques performed by one surgeon (DSYK) between August 2013 and February 2016 and achieved optimal vaulting within the range of 250 and 750 μm. Among total 293 eyes, 7 eyes (3%) showed vaulting smaller than 250 μm and 32 eyes (11%) showed vaulting larger than 750 μm. Patients were excluded from the analysis if they had keratoconus, previous ocular or intraocular surgery, acute or chronic corneal infection (bacterial and fungal), corneal inflammation (keratitis, herpes zoster, ocular herpes, and Stevens-Johnson syndrome), glaucoma, cataract, uveitis, retinal detachment,

macular degeneration (age-related and myopic), an endothelial cell density < 2000 cells/mm^2, or an ACD from the endothelium < 2.8 mm. One eye from each patient was included in the analysis using randomization table.

All patients underwent complete ophthalmic examinations, including uncorrected and corrected distance visual acuity (Snellen lines), manifest refraction with the cross-cylinder technique following retinoscopy, slit-lamp microscopy (Haag-Streit, Gartenstadtstrasse, Köniz, Switzerland), tonometry (noncontact tonometer; NT-530, Nidek Co., Ltd., Aichi, Japan), autokeratometry (ARK-530A; Nidek Co., Ltd.), automated pupillometry (VIP-200; Neuroptics Inc., Irvine, CA, USA), noncontact specular microscopy (SP-3000P, Topcon Corporation, Tokyo, Japan), ultrasound pachymetry for measurement of central corneal thickness via contact method, A-scan ultrasonography, Visante optical coherence tomography (OCT; Carl Zeiss Meditec AG, Jena, Germany) for measurement of ACD (vertical distance from the central corneal endothelium to the anterior lens capsule) and horizontal WTW, and fundus examination. Ultrasound biomicroscopy (UBM) was performed to measure the horizontal STS diameter after instillation of proparacaine (Alcaine; Alcon, Fort Worth, TX, USA) under standard room lighting conditions. An independent physician performed all ultrasound biomicroscopy examinations using the UBM equipped with a 50 MHz transducer.

Six months after implantation, the central vaulting of the ICL over the crystalline lens was measured in the non-accommodative state using the Visante OCT. Central vaulting was defined as the distance between the posterior surface of the ICL and the anterior surface of the crystalline lens at the center of the implant. Each measurement was performed three times by one physician, and the average of the three measurements was used in the analysis. A non-accommodative state was ensured by asking patients to avoid visual display terminal equipment or books for at least 3 h before examinations [18]. Measurements were taken while the patient fixated on a collimated light-emitting diode (focus at infinity) in a room with a luminance of 2 lux [19].

Surgical procedure

The surgery was performed through a 3.0-mm clear superior corneal incision after dilation of the pupil with 0.5% phenylephrine and 0.5% tropicamide (Mydrin-P, Santen Pharmaceutical Co. Ltd., Osaka, Japan) under topical anesthesia. The anterior chamber was filled with 1% sodium hyaluronate (Healon; Abbott Medical Optics, Santa Ana, CA, USA), which was removed completely by manual irrigation and aspiration at the end of surgery. Emmetropia was the target refraction in all cases. The ICL was then inserted using an injector cartridge and correctly positioned. The V4c ICL power calculations were performed according to the manufacturer's guidelines using a modified vertex formula [20]. Following surgery, a topical antibiotic (Vigamox; Alcon Laboratories) and loteprednol etabonate 0.5% (Lotemax; Bausch & Lomb, Rochester, NY, USA) were applied four times a day for one week. After the first week, loteprednol etabonate 0.5% was replaced with 0.1% fluorometholone (Flumetholon; Santen Pharmaceutical). All eye drops were continued four times a day for one month.

Statistical analysis

The Kolmogorov-Smirnov test was used to confirm the normality of the data. Simple regression analyses and stepwise multiple regression analyses were performed to investigate the association between the amount of vaulting at 6 months after surgery and several preoperative variables. The dependent variable was the central vaulting of the ICL over the crystalline lens using the Visante OCT. Independent variables included patient age, gender, preoperative MRSE, pupil size, WTW, STS, ACD, and axial length (AL). Analysis of variance (ANOVA) followed by Bonferroni post hoc testing were performed to examine differences among subgroups, which were based on the extent of postoperative vaulting (250 to 450 μm: low optimal vaulting; 451 to 550 μm: mid optimal vaulting; and 551 and 750 μm: high optimal vaulting). Multinomial logistic regression analysis was performed to ascertain the effects of age, gender, preoperative manifest refraction spherical equivalent (MRSE), pupil size, WTW, STS, ACD, and AL on vaulting outcomes. Statistical analyses were performed using SPSS version 22.0 software (IBM Corp., Armonk, NY, USA). A *p*-value less than 0.05 was considered statistically significant.

Results

The mean patient age was 28.2 ± 5.1 (range 20–44) years, and 71% (168/236) of the patients were females. Table 1 summarizes the baseline clinical characteristics of the 236 patients and descriptive data for preoperative variables. The mean ICL power was − 11.2 ± 2.2 (range − 5.5 to − 18.0) D. The mean central vaulting of the ICL at 6 months after surgery was 519.0 ± 112.8 μm (range 250–740). All surgeries were uneventful, and no intraoperative complications were noted. No contact between the ICL and crystalline lens was observed at either the center or periphery of the implant in any patient during the follow-up period.

Table 2 shows the simple regression analysis results between postoperative vaulting and eight variables. There was significant association between postoperative vaulting and preoperative pupil size (*P* = 0.004), and between postoperative vaulting and preoperative ACD (*P* < 0.001). According to Table 3 showing the results of the stepwise multivariate regression analysis, the explanatory variables relevant to vaulting were preoperative ACD (*P* < 0.001,

Table 1 Baseline clinical characteristics of the study eyes (236 eyes)

Characteristics	Mean ± SD	Range
Age (yrs)	28.2 ± 5.1	20 to 44
Gender (male/female) (%)	29/71	
Laterality (right/left) (%)	48/52	
Preoperative CDVA (Snellen lines)	0.97 ± 0.09	1.00 to 1.20
Preoperative sphere (D)	−8.48 ± 2.28	−3.50 to −16.75
Refractive cylinder (D)	−1.41 ± 0.84	−4.75 to 0.00
Preoperative MRSE (D)	−9.19 ± 2.36	−4.00 to − 19.13
Preoperative pupil size (mm)	7.16 ± 0.64	4.70 to 8.60
Preoperative WTW (mm)	11.46 ± 0.28	10.85 to 12.80
Preoperative STS (mm)	11.65 ± 0.26	10.81 to 12.22
Preoperative ACD (mm)	3.35 ± 0.20	2.88 to 3.89
Preoperative AL (mm)	27.18 ± 1.16	23.88 to 30.82
Preoperative ECD (cells/mm^2)	3018.4 ± 301.0	2229 to 3747

CDVA corrected distance visual acuity, *MRSE* manifest refraction spherical equivalent, *D* diopters, *WTW* white-to-white, *STS* sulcus-to-sulcus, *ACD* anterior chamber depth, *AL* axial length, *ECD* endothelial cell density, *SD* standard deviation

standardized partial regression coefficient [β] = 0.305), preoperative pupil size (*P* < 0.001, β = 0.218), and preoperative AL (*P* = 0.006, β = 0.171). The multiple regression equation was expressed as follows: central vaulting (μm) = − 0.784 + (0.171 × preoperative ACD) + (0.038 × preoperative pupil size) + (0.017 × preoperative AL). The standardized partial regression coefficient was calculated to determine the magnitude of the influence of each variable. Thus, preoperative ACD was the most relevant variable, followed by preoperative pupil size and AL (Table 3). Higher central vaulting was observed in eyes with greater preoperative ACD, larger pupil size, or longer AL.

We also performed subgroup analyses according to degree of postoperative vaulting. We observed a significant difference in pupil size between the low optimal vaulting and mid optimal vaulting groups (*P* = 0.031), and

Table 2 Simple regression analysis result between the postoperative vaulting and eight variables

	R^2	P
Age (yrs)	0.012	0.092
Gender	0.003	0.370
MRSE (D)	0.011	0.103
Preoperative pupil size (mm)	0.036	0.004
Preoperative WTW (mm)	0.001	0.813
Preoperative STS (mm)	0.008	0.169
Preoperative ACD (mm)	0.072	< 0.001
Preoperative AL (mm)	0.015	0.057

MRSE manifest refraction spherical equivalent, *D* diopters, *WTW* white-to-white, *STS* sulcus-to-sulcus, *ACD* anterior chamber depth, *AL* axial length

Table 3 Results of stepwise multiple regression analysis to select variables relevant to central vaulting in 12.6-mm V4c implantable collamer lens implanted eyes with postoperative optimal range of vaulting

Variables	Partial regression coefficient (B)	Standardized partial regression coefficient (β)	P	R^2
			< 0.001	0.144
Preoperative ACD (mm)	0.171	0.305	< 0.001	
Preoperative pupil size (mm)	0.038	0.218	< 0.001	
Preoperative AL (mm)	0.017	0.171	0.006	
Constant	−0.784			

Variables in the table are ordered according to the strength of the contribution, which was based on the standardized partial regression coefficient (β)
ACD anterior chamber depth, AL axial length

between the low optimal vaulting and high optimal vaulting groups ($P = 0.002$, Fig. 1). Significant differences in ACD were also observed between the low optimal vaulting and high optimal vaulting groups ($P = 0.010$) (Table 4 and Fig. 1). Similar to findings observed for ACD, our results suggested that smaller pupil diameters were associated with low optimal vaulting values. Multinomial logistic regression analysis revealed that low preoperative pupil size was associated with low optimal vaulting (odds ratio = 0.532, $P = 0.021$, low vaulting vs mid vaulting), and that increasing preoperative ACD was associated with high optimal vaulting (odds ratio = 6.340, $P = 0.034$, mid vaulting vs high vaulting).

Discussion

In the present study, we demonstrated that preoperative ACD, followed by preoperative pupil size and preoperative AL, significantly influenced postoperative vaulting following 12.6-mm V4c ICL implantation in eyes that had achieved optimal vaulting within the range of 250–750 μm. Our findings are consistent with those of a recent study in which stepwise multiple regression analysis of patient age, preoperative refraction, WTW, horizontal and vertical STS, ACD, AL, keratometric readings, and

ICL power revealed that ACD was the only factor significantly associated with vaulting in eyes that had undergone implantation of V4c ICL [21]. This previous study included 39 eyes of 39 patients that had undergone implantation with wide range of V4c ICL overall diameters (12.1-mm, 12.6-mm, 13.2-mm, or 13.7-mm) [21]. In recent study identifying factors associated with the unexpected vaulting in eyes that had undergone implantation of V4c ICL, authors concluded that smaller sized ICL should be considered in patients with shallow ACD [22]. Postoperative vaulting was also associated with preoperative ACD, WTW, and horizontal and vertical STS in eyes that had undergone implantation of a V4 or V4c ICL [16]. In that study, the presence of a central hole and the size of the implanted V4 or V4c ICL did not significantly influence postoperative vaulting. Furthermore, in a previous study that aimed to identify ocular and lens parameters predictive of vaulting after ICL implantation, eyes with a shallower ACD and/or a smaller WTW exhibited significantly lower postoperative vaulting [23]. In our study, because ICL size was limited to only 12.6-mm, the WTW and STS were relatively less important factors predictive of vaulting when compared with the ACD.

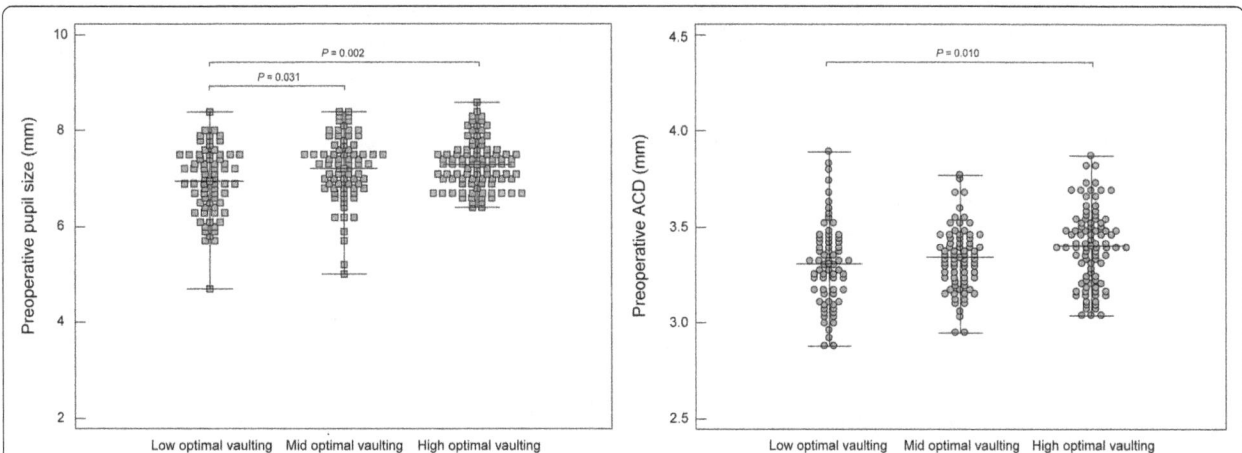

Fig. 1 Subgroup analyses according to degree of postoperative vaulting. Low optimal vaulting, 250 to 450 μm; mid optimal vaulting, 451 to 550; high optimal vaulting, 551 and 750 μm. ACD = anterior chamber depth. Error bars represent range

Table 4 Subgroup analysis of preoperative clinical factors in 12.6-mm V4c implantable collamer lens implanted eyes with postoperative optimal range of vaulting according to degree of postoperative vaulting

Characteristics	250 to 450 μm (n = 70)	451 to 550 μm (n = 75)	551 and 750 μm (n = 91)	P
Age (yrs)	29.3 ± 5.7	27.8 ± 5.4	27.6 ± 4.3	0.076
Preoperative MRSE (D)	−8.79 ± 1.90	−9.28 ± 2.24	− 9.41 ± 2.74	0.237
Preoperative pupil size (mm)	6.95 ± 0.70[a,b]	7.22 ± 0.67[a]	7.29 ± 0.50[b]	0.002
Preoperative WTW (mm)	11.47 ± 0.29	11.46 ± 0.29	11.44 ± 0.26	0.874
Preoperative STS (mm)	11.64 ± 0.30	11.61 ± 0.25	11.68 ± 0.24	0.251
Preoperative ACD (mm)	3.31 ± 0.22[c]	3.34 ± 0.17	3.40 ± 0.20[c]	0.010
Preoperative AL (mm)	26.98 ± 1.02	27.19 ± 1.15	27.32 ± 1.25	0.184

MRSE manifest refraction spherical equivalent, D diopters, WTW white-to-white, STS sulcus-to-sulcus, ACD anterior chamber depth, AL axial length
[a] $P = 0.031$ (two-way ANOVA, Bonferroni post hoc test)
[b] $P = 0.002$ (two-way ANOVA, Bonferroni post hoc test)
[c] $P = 0.010$ (two-way ANOVA, Bonferroni post hoc test)

Several previous studies have reported that changes in pupil size in response to certain stimuli, such as photopic light exposure or during accommodation, are associated with postoperative vaulting [24–26]. In a previous study, we demonstrated that pupil constriction in response to photopic light exposure creates an antero-posterior vector via iris constriction, in which the iris exerts pressure on the ICL [23]. Because the V4C ICL has a central hole, pressure equilibrium is quickly achieved between the anterior and posterior surfaces of the ICL, facilitating this process (fountain effect of aquaport). In other words, the net effect of pushing the ICL closer to the crystalline lens is produced, subsequently decreasing central vaulting. Furthermore, in a recent study of early postoperative changes in vaulting and pupil size in eyes that had undergone V4c ICL implantation, the authors reported a significant association between the changes in vaulting and those in pupil size from 1 day to 1 month postoperatively, concluding that pupil movement significantly influences postoperative vaulting [21]. These results indicate that postoperative vaulting is influenced by status of the anterior chamber. In the present study, we demonstrated that, once ICL size has been determined based on STS and WTW measurements, preoperative pupil size significantly influences postoperative vaulting. We speculate that, in association with changes in aqueous humor dynamics via the central hole in the V4c ICL, preoperative pupil size may influence circumstances at the anterior region of the eye, especially the region between the posterior cornea and anterior crystalline lens surface. Smaller pupils may exert greater pressure on the ICL than larger pupils, consequently decreasing vaulting. Indeed, our findings demonstrated that smaller preoperative pupil size was associated with low optimal vaulting, relative to values observed in the mid optimal vaulting group (odds ratio = 0.532, $P = 0.021$). Therefore, once ICL size has been determined based on preoperative ACD, AL, WTW, and STS measurements, surgeons should also consider preoperative pupil size when predicting vaulting outcomes.

Preoperative AL was significantly associated with postoperative vaulting in Stepwise multiple regression analysis. To the best of our knowledge, no previous reports have suggested that preoperative AL significantly influences postoperative vaulting. Considering that ACD is positively correlated with AL in both eyes with normal and long AL, preoperative AL may be relevant to postoperative vaulting [27].

The present study has several limitations, including its retrospective design and a relatively short follow-up duration of 6 months. However, to our knowledge, our study is the first to investigate the relationship between postoperative vaulting and preoperative pupil size in 12.6-mm V4c ICL implanted eyes with optimal range of vaulting between 250 and 750 μm. Further study investigating the effect of preoperative pupil size on aqueous humor dynamics in V4c ICL implanted eyes is warrant.

Conclusions

Our findings demonstrate that, among the studied variables, preoperative ACD most significantly influenced postoperative vaulting in 12.6-mm V4c ICL implanted eyes with optimal range of vaulting, followed by preoperative pupil size and AL. Therefore, surgeons should take into account preoperative ACD, pupil size, and AL when considering implantation of a 12.6-mm V4c ICL, particularly in patients exhibiting extreme values, for whom size adjustments may be required.

Abbreviations
ACD: Anterior chamber depth; AL: Axial length; ICL: Implantable collamer lenses; MRSE: Manifest refraction spherical equivalent; STS: Sulcus-to-sulcus; WTW: White-to-white

Funding
This research was partially supported by Basic Science Research Program through the National Research Foundation of Korea (NRF) funded by the Ministry of Education, Science and Technology (NRF-2016R1A2B4009626) and by research fund of Catholic Kwandong University International St. Mary's Hospital (CKU-201701530001). The funding agencies had no role in the design or conduct of this study; collection, management, analysis, or interpretation of the data; preparation, review, or approval of the manuscript; or in the decision to submit the manuscript for publication.

Authors' contributions
Design of the study (HL, DSYK, JYC, BJH, EKK, KYS, TIK); Conduct of the study (HL, DSYK, JYC, BJH, TIK); Collection, management, analysis, and interpretation of the data (HL, DSYK, JYC, BJH, EKK, KYS, TIK); Preparation of the manuscript (HL, DSYK, EKK, KYS, TIK); Review or approval of the manuscript (HL, DSYK, JYC, BJH, EKK, KYS, TIK).

Competing interests
Dr. Kang is consultant to Avedro Inc. and SCHWIND eye-tech-solutions. The remaining authors have no proprietary or financial interest in the materials presented herein.

Author details
[1]Department of Ophthalmology, International St. Mary's Hospital, Catholic Kwandong University College of Medicine, Incheon, South Korea. [2]The Institute of Vision Research, Department of Ophthalmology, Yonsei University College of Medicine, Seoul, South Korea. [3]Eyereum Eye Clinic, Seoul, South Korea. [4]Corneal Dystrophy Research Institute, Department of Ophthalmology, Yonsei University College of Medicine, Seoul, South Korea.

References
1. Igarashi A, Shimizu K, Kamiya K. Eight-year follow-up of posterior chamber phakic intraocular lens implantation for moderate to high myopia. Am J Ophthalmol. 2014;157(3):532–9. e531
2. Sanders DR, Doney K, Poco M. United States Food and Drug Administration clinical trial of the implantable Collamer Lens (ICL) for moderate to high myopia: three-year follow-up. Ophthalmology. 2004;111(9):1683–92.
3. Alfonso JF, Fernandez-Vega L, Lisa C, Fernandes P, Gonzalez-Meijome JM, Montes-Mico R. Collagen copolymer toric posterior chamber phakic intraocular lens in eyes with keratoconus. J Cataract Refract Surg. 2010; 36(6):906–16.
4. Schmidinger G, Lackner B, Pieh S, Skorpik C. Long-term changes in posterior chamber phakic intraocular collamer lens vaulting in myopic patients. Ophthalmology. 2010;117(8):1506–11.
5. Gonvers M, Bornet C, Othenin-Girard P. Implantable contact lens for moderate to high myopia: relationship of vaulting to cataract formation. J Cataract Refract Surg. 2003;29(5):918–24.
6. Alfonso JF, Lisa C, Abdelhamid A, Fernandes P, Jorge J, Montes-Mico R. Three-year follow-up of subjective vault following myopic implantable collamer lens implantation. Graefes Arch Clin Exp Ophthalmol. 2010; 248(12):1827–35.
7. Pineda-Fernandez A, Jaramillo J, Vargas J, Jaramillo M, Galindez A. Phakic posterior chamber intraocular lens for high myopia. J Cataract Refract Surg. 2004;30(11):2277–83.
8. Brandt JD, Mockovak ME, Chayet A. Pigmentary dispersion syndrome induced by a posterior chamber phakic refractive lens. Am J Ophthalmol. 2001;131(2):260–3.
9. Sanders DR. Anterior subcapsular opacities and cataracts 5 years after surgery in the visian implantable collamer lens FDA trial. J Refract Surg. 2008;24(6):566–70.
10. Alfonso JF, Lisa C, Fernandez-Vega L, Almanzar D, Perez-Vives C, Montes-Mico R. Prevalence of cataract after collagen copolymer phakic intraocular lens implantation for myopia, hyperopia, and astigmatism. J Cataract Refract Surg. 2015;41(4):800–5.
11. Huseynova T, Ozaki S, Ishizuka T, Mita M, Tomita M. Comparative study of 2 types of implantable collamer lenses, 1 with and 1 without a central artificial hole. Am J Ophthalmol. 2014;157(6):1136–43.
12. Kamiya K, Shimizu K, Ando W, Igarashi A, Iijima K, Koh A. Comparison of vault after implantation of posterior chamber phakic intraocular lens with and without a central hole. J Cataract Refract Surg. 2015;41(1):67–72.
13. Choi KH, Chung SE, Chung TY, Chung ES. Ultrasound biomicroscopy for determining visian implantable contact lens length in phakic IOL implantation. J Refract Surg. 2007;23(4):362–7.
14. Guell JL, Morral M, Kook D, Kohnen T. Phakic intraocular lenses part 1: historical overview, current models, selection criteria, and surgical techniques. J Cataract Refract Surg. 2010;36(11):1976–93.
15. Kojima T, Maeda M, Yoshida Y, Ito M, Nakamura T, Hara S, Ichikawa K. Posterior chamber phakic implantable collamer lens: changes in vault during 1 year. J Refract Surg. 2010;26(5):327–32.

16. Seo JH, Kim MK, Wee WR, Lee JH. Effects of white-to-white diameter and anterior chamber depth on implantable collamer lens vault and visual outcome. J Refract Surg. 2009;25(8):730–8.
17. Lovisolo CF, Reinstein DZ. Phakic intraocular lenses. Surv Ophthalmol. 2005; 50(6):549–87.
18. Lee H, Kang DS, Ha BJ, Choi M, Kim EK, Seo KY, Kim TI. Effect of accommodation on vaulting and movement of posterior chamber Phakic lenses in eyes with implantable Collamer lenses. Am J Ophthalmol. 2015; 160(4):710–6. e711
19. Lee H, Kang SY, Seo KY, Chung B, Choi JY, Kim KS, Kim TI. Dynamic vaulting changes in V4c versus V4 posterior chamber Phakic lenses under differing lighting conditions. Am J Ophthalmol. 2014;158(6):1199–204. e1191
20. Sanders DR, Vukich JA, Doney K, Gaston M, Implantable Contact Lens in Treatment of Myopia Study G. U.S. Food and Drug Administration clinical trial of the implantable contact Lens for moderate to high myopia. Ophthalmology. 2003;110(2):255–66.
21. Chen X, Miao H, Naidu RK, Wang X, Zhou X. Comparison of early changes in and factors affecting vault following posterior chamber phakic implantable Collamer Lens implantation without and with a central hole (ICL V4 and ICL V4c). BMC Ophthalmol. 2016;16(1):161.
22. Nam SW, Lim DH, Hyun J, Chung ES, Chung TY. Buffering zone of implantable Collamer lens sizing in V4c. BMC Ophthalmol. 2017;17(1):260.
23. Alfonso JF, Fernandez-Vega L, Lisa C, Fernandes P, Jorge J, Montes Mico R. Central vault after phakic intraocular lens implantation: correlation with anterior chamber depth, white-to-white distance, spherical equivalent, and patient age. J Cataract Refract Surg. 2012;38(1):46–53.
24. Du C, Wang J, Wang X, Dong Y, Gu Y, Shen Y. Ultrasound biomicroscopy of anterior segment accommodative changes with posterior chamber phakic intraocular lens in high myopia. Ophthalmology. 2012;119(1):99–105.
25. Lindland A, Heger H, Kugelberg M, Zetterstrom C. Changes in vaulting of myopic and toric implantable collamer lenses in different lighting conditions. Acta Ophthalmol. 2012;90(8):788–91.
26. Kamiya K, Shimizu K, Igarashi A, Ishikawa H. Evaluation of pupil diameter after posterior chamber phakic intraocular lens implantation. Eye. 2010;24(4): 588–94.
27. Chen H, Lin H, Lin Z, Chen J, Chen W. Distribution of axial length, anterior chamber depth, and corneal curvature in an aged population in South China. BMC Ophthalmol. 2016;16(1):47.

18

Quantitative proteomic analysis of aqueous humor from patients with drusen and reticular pseudodrusen in age-related macular degeneration

Je-Hyun Baek[1†], Daehan Lim[2†], Kyu Hyung Park[3], Jae-Byoung Chae[2], Hyoik Jang[2], Jonghyun Lee[4] and Hyewon Chung[2*]

Abstract

Background: To identify novel biomarkers related to the pathogenesis of dry age-related macular degeneration (AMD), we adopted a human retinal pigment epithelial (RPE) cell culture model that mimics some features of dry AMD including the accumulation of intra- and sub-RPE deposits. Then, we investigated the aqueous humor (AH) proteome using a data-independent acquisition method (sequential window acquisition of all theoretical fragment ion mass spectrometry) for dry AMD patients and controls.

Methods: After uniformly pigmented polarized monolayers of human fetal primary RPE (hfRPE) cells were established, the cells were exposed to 4-hydroxy-2-nonenal (4-HNE), followed by Western blotting, immunofluorescence analysis and ELISA of cells or conditioned media for several proteins of interest. Data-dependent acquisition for identification of the AH proteome and SWATH-based mass spectrometry were performed for 11 dry AMD patients according to their phenotypes (including soft drusen and reticular pseudodrusen [RPD]) and 2 controls (3 groups).

Results: Increased intra- and sub-RPE deposits were observed in 4-HNE-treated hfRPE cells compared with control cultures based on APOA1, cathepsin D, and clusterin immunoreactivity. Additionally, the differential abundance of proteins in apical and basal chambers with or without 4-HNE treatment confirmed the polarized secretion of proteins from hfRPE cells. A total of 119 proteins were quantified in dry AMD patients and controls by SWATH-MS. Sixty-five proteins exhibited significantly altered abundance among the three groups. A two-dimensional principal component analysis plot was generated to identify typical proteins related to the pathogenesis of dry AMD. Among the identified proteins, eight proteins, including APOA1, CFHR2, and CLUS, were previously considered major components or regulators of drusen. Three proteins (SERPINA4, LUM, and KERA proteins) have not been previously described as components of drusen or as being related to dry AMD. Interestingly, the LUM and KERA proteins, which are related to extracellular matrix organization, were upregulated in both RPD and soft drusen.

Conclusions: Differential protein expression in the AH between patients with drusen and RPD was quantified using SWATH-MS in the present study. Detailed proteomic analyses of dry AMD patients might provide insights into the in vivo biology of drusen and RPD.

Keywords: Age-related macular degeneration, Complement, Drusen, Reticular pseudodrusen, SWATH-MS

* Correspondence: hchung@kuh.ac.kr
†Je-Hyun Baek and Daehan Lim contributed equally to this work.
[2]Department of Ophthalmology, Konkuk University School of Medicine, Konkuk University Medical Center, 120-1 Neungdong-ro, Gwangjin-gu, Seoul, Republic of Korea
Full list of author information is available at the end of the article

Background

Age-related macular degeneration (AMD) is the progressive degeneration of the retinal pigment epithelium (RPE), retina, and choriocapillaris observed among elderly people and is one of the leading causes of blindness worldwide [1–3]. AMD is mainly divided into a dry (atrophic) subtype (80–90%) and a wet (neovascular) subtype (10–20%). A hallmark of neovascular AMD is choroidal neovascularization (CNV) with subsequent development of subretinal fluid accumulation, hemorrhage, exudation, and scarring, which can lead to the loss of vision. Currently, vision loss and blindness from neovascular AMD is largely treatable, with the advent of antiangiogenic drugs that mainly target vascular endothelial growth factor (VEGF). With the introduction of anti-VEGF intravitreal injections, the incidence of legal blindness attributable to wet AMD has decreased by 50% in some countries [3, 4].

However, the molecular mechanisms underlying dry AMD remain largely unknown; there is no proven treatment for dry AMD or its progression to geographic atrophy (GA) or for neovascular AMD. Dry AMD is a disease with various phenotypes, such as drusen and reticular pseudodrusen (RPD). Drusen, which represent the major phenotype of AMD, are focal extracellular deposits located between the RPE and Bruch's membrane (BM) that are associated with the development and progression of AMD [5, 6]. By contrast, RPD, first described in 1990 by Mimoun et al. [7], are located between the RPE and outer retina, as shown by recently evolving imaging techniques and histological studies [5]. Although the pathogenesis of RPD remains unknown, they have been recognized as an additional phenotype of AMD since they have been associated with an increased risk of progression to late forms of AMD, such as neovascular AMD and/or GA [5, 8–10]; therefore, they contribute to loss of vision by inducing atrophy in the outer retina [11].

The occurrence of RPD in Sorsby fundus dystrophy and pseudoxanthoma elasticum has been demonstrated recently [11–13], suggesting that the pathophysiology of RPD might parallel that of these diseases; dysfunction of the choroid-BM-RPE complex might be associated with the development of RPD. In the case of Sorsby fundus dystrophy, mutations in the tissue inhibitor of metalloproteinase-3 (TIMP3) gene could lead to the formation of abnormal deposits between BM and RPE and thus functionally impair the choroid-BM-RPE complex, resulting in atrophy and CNV [12]. Additionally, in the pseudoxanthoma elasticum, damage to BM leads to the development of RPD [11]. The RPE cell is a highly polarized cell type that produces and secretes proteins onto its basolateral and apical surfaces, meeting differential demands on either side of the photoreceptors and choriocapillaris and holding a large majority of the secreted proteins on the basolateral side [14, 15]. Many proteins are preferentially secreted by either the apical or basolateral surface, and their incorrect localization/function may lead to retinal degeneration.

In a previous study, we profiled and characterized the whole proteome of exosomes obtained from the aqueous humor (AH) of patients with neovascular AMD and compared the differential abundance of selected proteins in ARPE-19 cell cultures exposed to oxidative stress [16, 17]. However, neither proteomic analysis of AH from patients with dry AMD nor the pathogenic implications of dry AMD have yet been reported, mainly due to the difficulty in obtaining AH samples from dry AMD patients and the high-tech proteomic methods required to analyze the very small quantities of precious AH samples.

In the present study, to gain insight into the pathogenesis and characteristics of dry AMD and understand the underlying disease mechanisms, we first introduced a primary human fetal RPE (hfRPE) cell polarized culture model and examined the relative abundance of secreted proteins from hfRPE cells exposed to oxidative stress. Then, we investigated the AH proteome of dry AMD patients according to their phenotypes using a data-independent acquisition method (sequential window acquisition of all theoretical fragment ion mass spectrometry [SWATH-MS], a specialized high-resolution mass spectrometric technique providing quantitative accuracy and reproducibility).

Methods

Primary hfRPE cell culture and the measurement of transepithelial resistance

Primary hfRPE cells purchased from Lonza Biologics (catalog number: 194987, Lonza, Basel, Switzerland) were grown and maintained in RtEGM™ BulletKit® medium with supplements (catalog numbers: 00195406 and 00195407, respectively, Lonza) at 37 °C under 5% CO_2. The cells were seeded onto Matrigel (catalog number: 356230, Corning, NY, USA)-precoated cell culture inserts at 4.6×10^4 cells per well (Transwell 0.4-μm pores, polyester membranes; catalog number: 3450, Corning) using 24-mm-diameter inserts. The medium was changed every 2 to 3 days. Only fresh passage 1 cells were used in the experiments, when they exhibited transepithelial resistance (TER) > 500 $\Omega \cdot cm^2$ and were confluent, with a uniform hexagonal morphology and mature pigmentation, at 6 to 8 weeks after seeding. Confluent monolayers of hfRPE cells with stable TER were treated with 50 or 100 μM 4-hydroxy-2-nonenal (4-HNE) for 24 h to induce oxidative stress.

TER was measured as described previously [18, 19]. Briefly, TER was measured in a cell culture hood immediately within 3 min after the removal of hfRPE cells from the cell incubator when hfRPE cells were confluent with uniform pigmentation, 6 to 8 weeks after seeding. Epithelial Voltohmmeter (EVOM, World Precision Instruments,

FL, USA) electrodes were first washed with 70% ethanol and then with PBS. Net TERs were calculated from five independent measurements by subtracting the background resistance values of the blank, Matrigel-coated filter and culture medium from the measured resistance values ($\Omega \cdot cm^2$) for each treated condition of hfRPE cells.

Immunofluorescence and Western blotting

For immunofluorescence (IF) assays, monolayers of hfRPE cells cultured on Transwell permeable inserts were fixed with 4% paraformaldehyde (PFA) overnight. Flat mounts of fixed hfRPE cell cultures or 10-μm cryosections were washed three times in PBS and fixed in 4% PFA for 15 min. Next, the samples were permeabilized with PBST (0.1% Triton X-100 in PBS) for 5 min and blocked with blocking solution (5% BSA in PBS) for 1 h at room temperature, followed by incubation overnight at 4 °C with the primary antibodies (Table S1 in Additional file 1). The samples were then washed three times with PBS, incubated for 1 h at room temperature with the secondary antibodies (Table S1 in Additional file 1) and stained with DAPI (1:3000) in PBS for 10 min. Microphotographs were obtained using a fluorescence microscope (Scope A1, Carl Zeiss MicroImaging, Inc., oberkochen, Germany).

For Western blot analysis, 4-HNE-treated hfRPE cells from each set of conditions were lysed in radioimmunoprecipitation assay (RIPA) buffer (Thermo Scientific, MA, USA) containing protease inhibitors (Sigma-Aldrich, MO, USA) and pepstatin A (Sigma). The extracted protein sample was quantitated with a standard bicinchoninic acid (BCA) protein assay. Twenty-microgram protein samples were denatured by adding 1× sample buffer and loaded into the lanes of a 10% Tris-glycine SDS gel. The loaded proteins were subsequently electroblotted onto polyvinylidene difluoride (PVDF) membranes and blocked with 5% skim milk for 1 h at room temperature. Thereafter, the membranes were incubated overnight at 4 °C with primary antibodies (Table S2 in Additional file 1). After overnight incubation, the membranes were incubated for 1 h at room temperature with secondary antibodies (Table S2 in Additional file 1). The membranes were exposed using a luminescent image analyzer (LAS-4000, Fujifilm, Tokyo, Japan). Finally, each membrane was stripped and probed with a loading control antibody.

ELISA analysis of conditioned media

The conditioned media of hfRPE cells treated with 4-HNE or serum-free media for 24 h were collected. The levels of VEGF-A (catalog number: DVE00; R&D Systems, MN, USA), PEDF (catalog number: PED613; BioProducts MD, LLC, MD, USA), and complement factor H (CFH) (catalog number: HK342–02; Hycultbiotech, Uden, Netherlands) in conditioned media from hfRPE cells were quantitatively assessed using a sandwich ELISA kit. All procedures were performed according to the manufacturer's protocol. The dilution factors of the conditioned media from hfRPE cells were 20-fold for VEGF-A, 5000-fold for PEDF, and 1-fold for CFH. Color intensities were measured using a microplate reader (Molecular Devices, CA, USA). The standard ranges were 15.6–1000 pg/mL for VEGF-A, 0.03–1.00 ng/mL for PEDF, and 3.9–250 ng/mL for CFH. Triplicate samples were used in all assays. Inter- and intra-assay variation was 4.1% and 6%, respectively.

Patients and AH sample collection

AH samples were collected at the Department of Ophthalmology, Konkuk University Medical Center, Seoul, Korea, and at the Department of Ophthalmology, Seoul National University Bundang Hospital, Seongnam, Korea. From January 1, 2014, to December 31, 2015, 13 patients undergoing cataract surgery were enrolled in this study. Among these individuals, 11 patients with dry AMD exhibited either drusen or RPD without GA. Two patients presented no retinal diseases, including dry AMD. Patients with other ophthalmic diseases (e.g., glaucoma, uveitis, or progressive retinal disease) or uncontrolled systemic diseases (e.g., uncontrolled diabetes mellitus), or who had undergone laser or intraocular surgery were excluded. All 13 patients underwent routine senile cataract surgery for visual rehabilitation. The extent of the cataracts in each individual corresponded to the patient's age. The clinical data from the patients and controls are summarized in Table 1 and Fig. 1.

All AH samples were obtained immediately before cataract surgery. The collection of all samples was performed using standard sterile procedures, and AH samples were obtained via anterior chamber paracentesis using a 30-gauge needle. No complications were encountered after paracentesis of the anterior chamber. AH samples (100–150 μl) were placed in safe-lock microcentrifuge tubes (1.5 mL), immediately frozen at − 80 °C and stored until analysis. The study followed the guidelines of the Declaration of Helsinki, and informed written consent was obtained from all patients and control subjects. The procedure for AH collection was approved by the Institutional Review Board of Konkuk University Medical Center, Seoul, Korea.

Depletion of abundant proteins in the AH and fractionation of the AH proteome

Abundant proteins in the AH (e.g., albumin and immunoglobulin G [IgG]) were depleted with Pierce™ Top 12 Abundant Protein Depletion Spin Columns (catalog number: 85165; Thermo Scientific); these

Table 1 Summary of the demographic characteristics of dry age-related macular degeneration patients and control subjects

Property	Sample Set 1: DDA[a] in AH[b]	Sample Set 2: SWATH-MS[c] in AH		
	Dry AMD[d]	Dry AMD		Control
		Drusen	RPD[e]	
No. of AH samples	7	2	2	2
Age (mean ± SD, years)	74.6 ± 7.5	73.5 ± 4.9		74.5 ± 1.5
Sex (men:women)	3:4	0:4		0:2
Diabetes mellitus (No.)	2	1		0
Hypertension (No.)	3	1		1

[a]*DDA* data-dependent acquisition, [b]*AH* aqueous humor, [c]*SWATH-MS* sequential window acquisition of all theoretical fragment ion mass spectrometry, a specialized high-resolution mass spectrometric technique providing quantitative accuracy and reproducibility, [d]*AMD* age-related macular degeneration, [e]*RPD* reticular pseudodrusen

proteins included α1-acid glycoprotein, fibrinogen, α1-antitrypsin, haptoglobin, α2-macroglubulin, IgA, albumin IgG, apolipoprotein A-I, IgM, apolipoprotein A-II, and transferrin. From each AH sample, a 90-μL aliquot was applied to a depletion spin column and processed according to the manufacturer's protocol. Both the flow-through and eluent were subjected to SDS-PAGE, and the protein bands were then excised, sliced into pieces and digested via an in-gel digestion method.

Fractionation and AH protein digestion

To generate a comprehensive AH proteome library for SWATH-MS analysis, AH samples were processed in multiple ways (Fig. 2): with or without depletion; with in-solution digestion or in-gel digestion; and with protein- (PLRP-S column) or peptide-level fractionation (high-pH fractionation). All proteins obtained following the depletion process (each eluent and flow-through fraction) in SDS-PAGE gels were divided into 8 gel bands and digested into peptides via an in-gel digestion

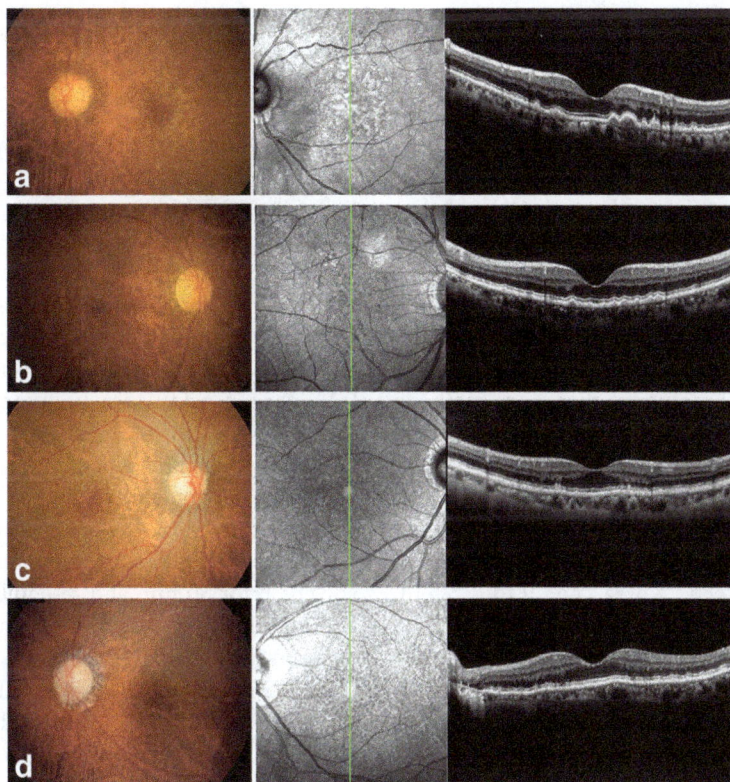

Fig. 1 Color fundus photos (left) and optical coherence tomography images (right) from patients with drusen or reticular pseudodrusen (RPD) (patients with dry age-related macular degeneration in Sample Set 2 in Table 1). (**a**) A 71-year-old woman with Drusen, (**b**) an 80-year-old woman with Drusen, (**c**) a 76-year-old woman with RPD, (**d**) a 67-year-old woman with RPD

Aqueous Humor (AH) Protein Profiling
: DDA (Data-Dependent Acquisition) Analysis-LC-MS/MS

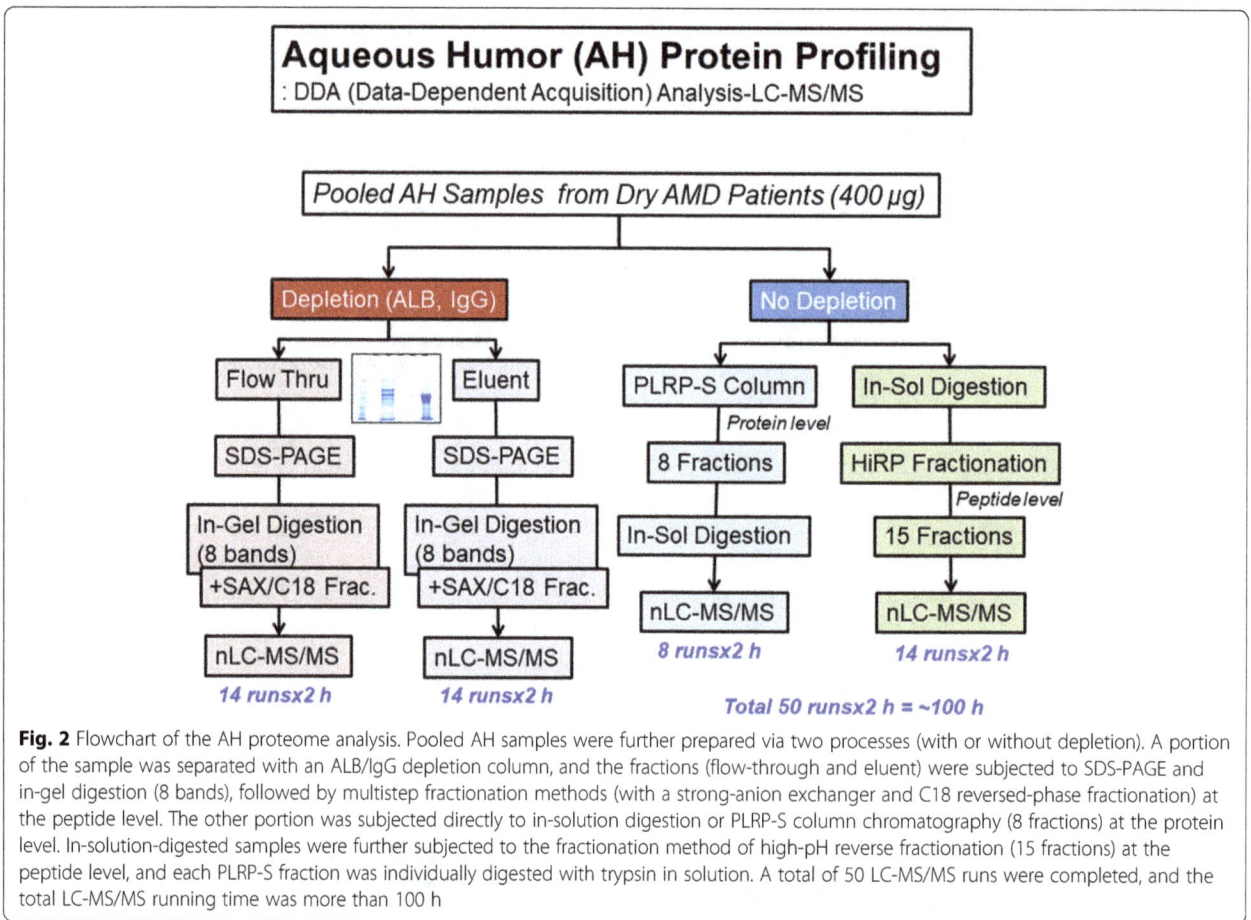

Fig. 2 Flowchart of the AH proteome analysis. Pooled AH samples were further prepared via two processes (with or without depletion). A portion of the sample was separated with an ALB/IgG depletion column, and the fractions (flow-through and eluent) were subjected to SDS-PAGE and in-gel digestion (8 bands), followed by multistep fractionation methods (with a strong-anion exchanger and C18 reversed-phase fractionation) at the peptide level. The other portion was subjected directly to in-solution digestion or PLRP-S column chromatography (8 fractions) at the protein level. In-solution-digested samples were further subjected to the fractionation method of high-pH reverse fractionation (15 fractions) at the peptide level, and each PLRP-S fraction was individually digested with trypsin in solution. A total of 50 LC-MS/MS runs were completed, and the total LC-MS/MS running time was more than 100 h

method. In-gel digestion was performed as previously reported [20]. Additionally, for the top 12 abundant protein-depleted samples (7 AMD patients), further fractionation steps were carried out to reduce proteome complexity (14 strong cation exchange fractionation steps and C18 desalting steps). Alternatively, the pooled AH samples that did not undergo depletion were separated with PLRP-S resin, and each fraction was digested through in-solution digestion methods after drying completely. In-solution digestion was performed as previously reported [21]. The AH protein samples were also digested via in-solution digestion methods without any fractionation. In addition, all peptides were fractionated with a DK-Tip C18 HiRP Fractionation kit (Diatech Korea co. Ltd., Seoul, Korea), as per the manufacturer's manual. Briefly, dried peptide samples were resuspended in 100 mM ammonium formate buffer (pH 10), loaded into an equilibrated DK-Tip C18 HiRP tip with 50 mM ammonium formate buffer (pH 10), washed with 50 µL of 50 mM ammonium formate buffer (pH 10), and then serially eluted with 50 µL of 50 mM ammonium formate buffer with acetonitrile solvent (0, 6, 12, 16, 18, 24, 30, 60%).

Data-dependent acquisition for protein identification and SWATH-MS

A Triple-TOF™ 5600+ (AB Sciex, Concord, Canada) instrument was utilized for all the experiments as described previously [22]. Briefly, the instrument was coupled with an Eksigent NanoLC-2D+ with nanoFlex cHiPLC system (0.075 mm × 15 cm column) for identification and quantification. Solvent A was composed of 0.1% formic acid/water (v/v), and solvent B was composed of 0.1% formic acid/100% acetonitrile (v/v). Peptide samples were separated in an analytical column with a linear gradient of 2% solvent B to 35% solvent B over 30 min at a flow rate of 400 nL/min. The Chip nano-LC column was regenerated by washing with 60% solvent B for 50 min and re-equilibrated with 2% solvent B for 10 min. For the data-dependent acquisition (DDA) experiment, a Triple-TOF™ 5600+ mass spectrometer was used at 250 ms for survey scans (TOF-MS) and at 150 ms for automated MS/MS scans for the top 20 ions. The MS/MS triggering criteria for parent ions were as follows: precursor intensity> 135 counts, charge state> 1, with the dynamic exclusion option (exclusion time: 15 s). For SWATH-MS-based experiments, the Triple-TOF™ 5600+ mass spectrometer was used in looped product ion mode, with 20 Da/mass windows (each SWATH window exhibited a 1 Da overlap) in the range of 400 to 1000 Da: Experiment 1: MS1 scan (400~ 1600 Da); Experiment 2: 400~ 420 Da; Experiment 3: 419~ 440 Da... Experiment 31: 979~ 1000 Da. The collision energy for each window was determined based on the appropriate collision energy for a two-charged ion centered on the window, with a spread of 15 eV. An accumulation time of 100 ms was used for each fragment ion scan and for the survey scans (total duty cycle of 3.1 s in high-sensitivity mode).

Database searching

All spectra generated from the DDA experiment were searched with the MS-GF+ (University of California, San Diego, USA; version Beta v9872) searching algorithm against a simple modified version of the UniProt human protein sequence database (UP000005640_9606_cRAP_AbSeq.fasta: a total of 429,526 protein entries including various antibody sequences and commonly contaminated proteins) with the following search parameters: full tryptic digestion, precursor ion tolerance< 50 ppm, fragment ion mass tolerance< 0.5 Da, fixed modifications for cysteine (+ 57 Da for carbamidomethylation) and biological modifications/artifacts such as methionine oxidation (+ 16 Da).

Criteria for protein identification

Scaffold (version 4.4.6, Proteome Software Inc., Portland, OR) was used to validate the MS/MS-based peptide and protein identifications. The peptide identifications were accepted if they could be established at greater than 82.0% probability to achieve a false discovery rate (FDR) of less than 1.0% with the Scaffold Local FDR algorithm. Protein identifications were accepted if they could be established at greater 5.0% probability to achieve an FDR of less than 1.0% and contained at least 2 identified peptides. Protein probabilities were assigned by the Protein Prophet algorithm [23]. Proteins that contained similar peptides and could not be differentiated based on MS/MS analysis alone were grouped to satisfy the principles of parsimony. Proteins sharing significant peptide evidence were grouped into clusters. Proteins were annotated with GO (Gene ontology) terms from gene_association.goa_human (downloaded 2014/1/28) [24].

Proteome data analysis

For SWATH-MS data, all raw data (wiff files) were converted by ProteoWizard software (Version 3.0.6965) into the mz5 format. Transition settings were as follows: MS1 filtering was performed for three isotope peaks in centroid mode with 30 ppm accuracy; MS/MS filtering for three isotope peaks was performed in centroid mode with 50 ppm accuracy. The retention time window was considered to be within 10 min of the MS/MS identification period. Extracted data were manually confirmed

considering the retention time and rank order of peak intensities from both the library spectrum and the SWATH spectrum. Perseus™ software was used for further data processing, visualization, principal component analysis (PCA), and other statistical analyses.

Results

In vitro primary hfRPE cell culture model under oxidative stress

We established a primary hfRPE cell culture model exposed to 4-HNE, one of the major oxidants generated via lipid peroxidation in the retina [25, 26]. This model mimics the in vivo environment of the RPE in patients with dry AMD, although other major oxidation products in the retina are related to the pathogenesis of AMD (Fig. 3).

To evaluate whether the hfRPE cell culture system can mimic and represent the clinical pathologic environment of the RPE in AMD, showing differential apical and basal protein secretion upon oxidative stress, we established an hfRPE Transwell culture system and evaluated monolayer formation by hexagonal, highly pigmented RPE cells and measured their TER. As previously described [18, 27], porous membrane inserts in Transwell cultures generate two compartments: the apical chambers correspond to the retinal-facing side of the RPE (RPD exist in this upper compartment), and the basal chambers correspond to the choroidal-facing side of the RPE (drusen exist in this lower compartment). Monolayers of RPE cells on Transwell plates were treated with 1, 5, 25, 50, or 100 μM 4-HNE for 24 h. No cytotoxicity was observed until the 24 h 50 μM 4-HNE treatment (data not shown). The amount of pigmentation and the immunofluorescence of the tight junction protein ZO-1 showed no significant changes between the hfRPE cells treated with 50 μM 4-HNE for 24 h and those treated under control conditions (Fig. 3a). A high level of TER (500–600 $\Omega \cdot cm^2$) was also maintained in the RPE cell cultures exposed to 50 μM 4-HNE for 24 h (Fig. 3b). Expression of the epithelial marker E-cadherin and the mesenchymal marker vimentin in hfRPE cells exposed to 4-HNE showed that the epithelial characteristics of hfRPE cells were maintained in the RPE cell cultures exposed to 50 μM 4-HNE for 24 h (Fig. 3c). Then, we identified increased intra- and sub-RPE deposits in the RPE cells exposed to 4-HNE compared to the control cells based on the immunoreactivity of APOA1, cathepsin D, and clusterin, all of which are well-established drusen components [27, 28] (Fig. 3d and e). The change in the level of CFH expression was not significant as shown by both IF and Western blotting.

Construction of the AH spectral library

Aqueous samples were processed in multiple ways, as indicated in the Methods and in Fig. 2. Protein-level

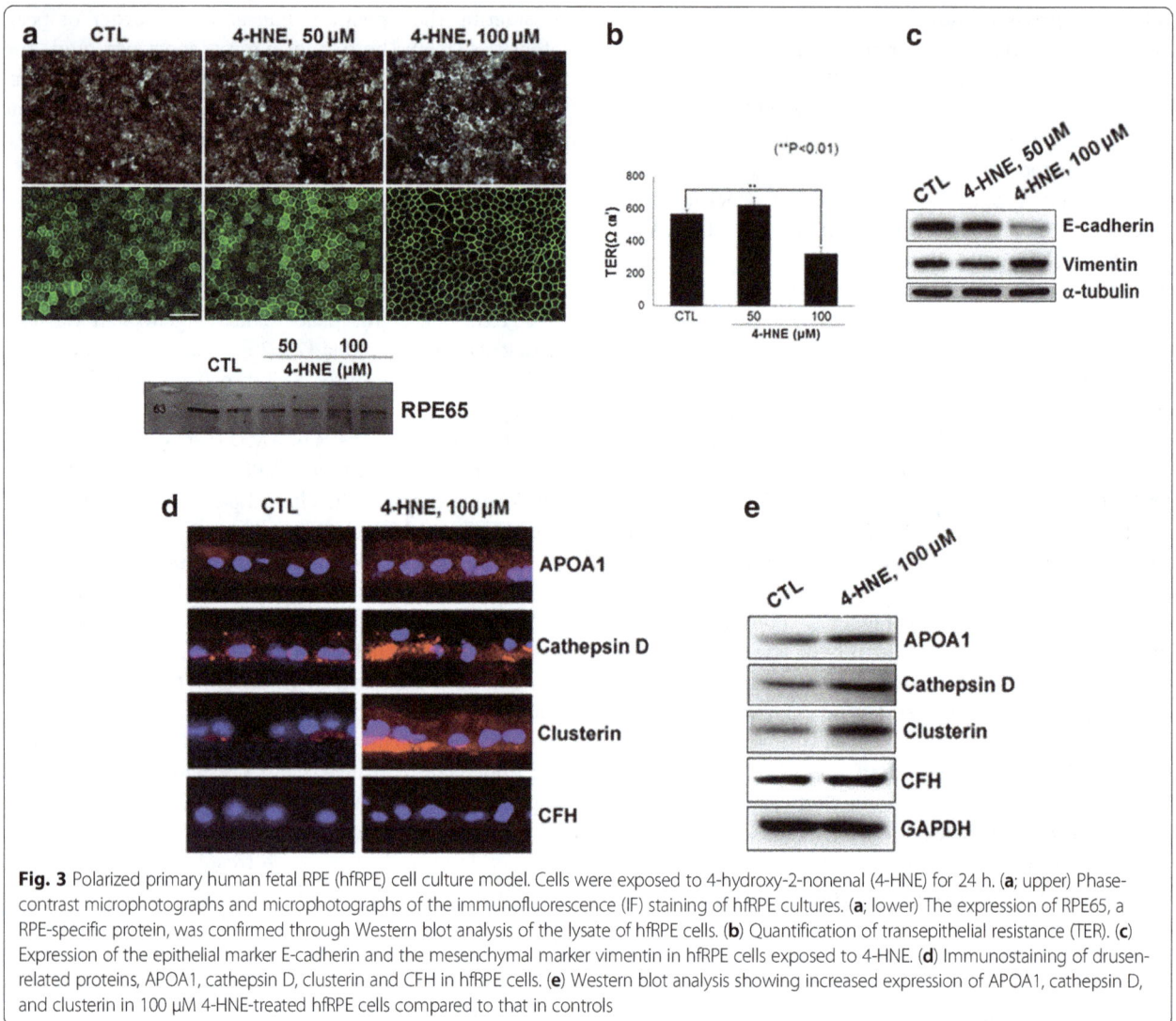

Fig. 3 Polarized primary human fetal RPE (hfRPE) cell culture model. Cells were exposed to 4-hydroxy-2-nonenal (4-HNE) for 24 h. (**a**; upper) Phase-contrast microphotographs and microphotographs of the immunofluorescence (IF) staining of hfRPE cultures. (**a**; lower) The expression of RPE65, a RPE-specific protein, was confirmed through Western blot analysis of the lysate of hfRPE cells. (**b**) Quantification of transepithelial resistance (TER). (**c**) Expression of the epithelial marker E-cadherin and the mesenchymal marker vimentin in hfRPE cells exposed to 4-HNE. (**d**) Immunostaining of drusen-related proteins, APOA1, cathepsin D, clusterin and CFH in hfRPE cells. (**e**) Western blot analysis showing increased expression of APOA1, cathepsin D, and clusterin in 100 μM 4-HNE-treated hfRPE cells compared to that in controls

separation (SDS-PAGE after depletion or PLRP-S column treatment) showed a slightly greater number of identified proteins than that achieved by peptide-level separation through high-pH reverse-phase separation. All fractionation and depletion procedures resulted in the identification of a total of 1010 proteins (383 protein groups) in a modified UniProt protein sequence database, including various immunoglobulin sequences (protein and peptide FDR < 1%, ≥two peptides per protein). When various immunoglobulins and other contaminant proteins were excluded, 329 AH proteins (260 clusters) and 3776 peptides were identified. The number of identified mass spectra was 41,903 (FDR < 1%). Among the uniquely identified peptides, the number of components in the spectral library constructed with Skyline software was 6818, which included redundant peptides with different charge states, retention times, and translational modifications.

Repertoire of the in vivo AH proteome from patients

Gene Ontology analysis of the identified AH proteins showed high percentages of extracellular proteins (185 proteins, 51.5%) and membrane proteins (101 proteins, 28.1%) other than the identified antibodies, which were classified as cytoplasmic proteins (36.8%), plasma membrane proteins (21.2%), and extracellular matrix proteins (10.6%). The percentage of all extracellular and membrane proteins reached 65.4% (Fig. 4). The AH proteins contained a high percentage of endogenous antibodies (67.4% of the total proteins). The identified AH proteins included 9 apolipoproteins (APOA1, APOA2, APOA4, APOD, APOE, APOH, APOL1, Clusterin and APOM), 17 complement components (C1q, C1r, C1s, C3, C4A, C5, C6, C7, C8α, C8β, C8γ, C9, D, H, HR1, HR2, and I), 9 proteases, 3 follistatin-related proteins (1, 4, and 5), 5 inter-alpha-trypsin inhibitor heavy chain proteins (H1, H2, H3, H4, and H5), 2 metalloproteinase inhibitors

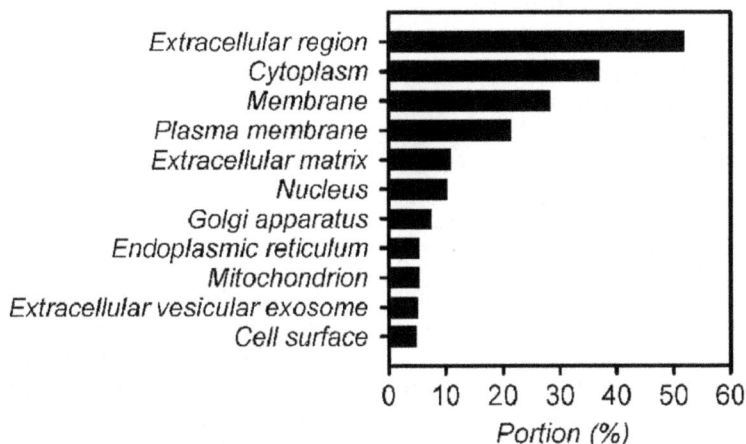

Fig. 4 Gene ontology analysis (localization) of the aqueous humor (AH) proteome of dry AMD patients with drusen and reticular pseudodrusen (RPD)

(TIMP1, TIMP2), and 2 retinol-binding proteins (RBP3 and 4). The sequence coverage of RBP3 and RBP4 was 49 and 57%, respectively. Several growth factors were also identified: PEDF, TGFBI, MEGF8, LTBP2, HGFL, HGFAC, GDF8, and 4 insulin-like growth factor-binding proteins (2, 6, 7, and ALS).

Quantitative analysis of the in vivo AH proteome of patients using SWATH-MS

Based on the AH spectral library, the abundance of each AH protein was extracted from SWATH-MS data for the control (no AMD), drusen patient, and RPD patient samples. The peak processing data acquired from limited clinical samples resulted in the quantification of 119 of 329 proteins (36.2%, Table S3 in Additional file 2). ANOVA (p-value< 0.05) showed that 65 proteins presented significantly altered abundance (54.2% of total proteins) among the three groups (control, drusen and RPD). To identify typical proteins related to pathogenesis, we performed 2D-plot analysis of the abundance ratios of the proteins with statistical significance (drusen versus control and RPD versus control) and then performed PCA with the abundance of all quantified proteins (Fig. 5a). As shown in Fig. 5b, most proteins were not prominently altered (73.3%). Eight proteins exhibited 2-fold higher abundance in both the drusen and RPD patients than in the healthy controls (APOA1, KRT79, FSTL5, LACRT, LUM, DSP, SERPINA4, and KERA). In contrast, VCAN and 18 proteins showed a 2-fold lower abundance in both the drusen and RPD patients (e.g., IGHV3–13, and SPP1). Five proteins showed a 2-fold higher abundance in the RPD group but were decreased in the drusen group (e.g.,

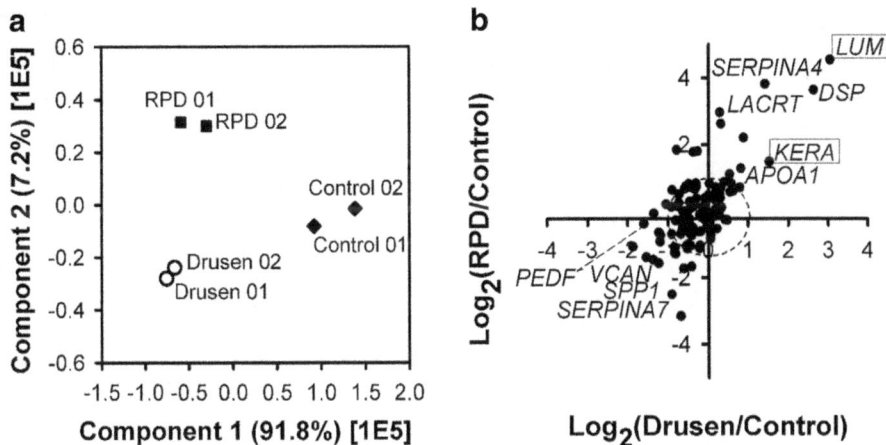

Fig. 5 (a) Principal component analysis (PCA) of quantified AH proteins from drusen, RPD, and healthy control samples. (b) 2D-plot of the relative abundance of AH proteins quantified from drusen and RPD patients versus healthy controls. Upregulated proteins are shown in the upper right quadrant and downregulated proteins in the lower left quadrant for both drusen and RPD samples. The dashed line indicates the boundary of changes in abundance according to the 2-fold criterion. Proteins indicated with boxes are new biomarker candidates in dry AMD patients

CPAMD8, ALDH3A1). Fig. 5b shows that the LUM, KERA, and VCAN proteins were differentially expressed in both the RPD and drusen groups. While LUM and KERA were upregulated, VCAN was downregulated. PEDF was downregulated in both the drusen and RPD groups but only showed a statistically significant decrease in the drusen group. Interestingly, few proteins were also observed in outlier areas (the second and fourth quadrants of Fig. 5b), indicating upregulation in the drusen group and downregulation in the RPD group or downregulation in the drusen group and upregulation in the RPD group.

Comparison of key components secreted from hfRPE cells and AH in the context of AMD pathogenesis

The AH proteins from patients with drusen and RPD were further compared with the samples from the healthy controls in terms of relative abundance (Table 2). For these samples, each protein ratio was shown on a log 2 scale: drusen or RPD against the control in AH samples. The differential expression of APOA1 and clusterin in polarized RPE cells with or without 4-HNE treatment was well correlated with the changes in relative abundance observed in the SWATH-MS analysis shown in Table 2: APOA1 was increased in both the drusen and RPD samples, and clusterin was increased in the RPD sample (Fig. 3d and e).

We then tested selective proteins from the hfRPE cell culture media and compared the changes in abundance from the differentially expressed protein (DEP) list (RPD versus control: SWATH-MS analysis) with those from the hfRPE culture media (with versus without 4-HNE treatment: ELISA). In control cultures and cultures exposed to 50 μM 4-HNE for 24 h, the total protein concentration in the conditioned media from the basal chamber was higher than that in the media from the apical chamber (the ratios of the apical to basal concentrations were 0.85 and 0.88, respectively), consistent with previous reports that a large majority of proteins are secreted in the basolateral direction [14, 15]. However, in the cultures exposed to 100 μM 4-HNE for 24 h, the total protein concentration in the conditioned media from the apical chamber was higher than that in the media from the basal chamber (the ratio of the apical to basal concentration was 1.08; Fig. 6). In conjunction with the decreases in TER, ZO-1 immunoactivity, and the expression of the epithelial marker E-cadherin in cultures exposed to 100 μM 4-HNE for 24 h (Fig. 3a, b, and c), the difference in the total protein concentration between the apical and basal chambers suggested that polarized epithelial cells might lose their polarity and cell-cell adhesions and acquire the mesenchymal characteristics of motility and invasiveness.

Among the 11 proteins listed in Table 2, the relative abundance of PEDF and CFH was compared between the AH samples from patients and the RPE cell culture media samples (Fig. 6). The level of PEDF decreased both apically and basally in the cultures exposed to oxidative stress compared to that in the control cultures, whereas the ratio of the protein concentrations secreted by the apical and basal chambers was reversed in the cultures treated with 100 μM 4-HNE compared to that in the control cultures. The apical/basal protein concentration ratios were 2.59 and 1.83 in the control cultures and the cultures exposed to 50 μM 4-HNE for 24 h, respectively; the apical/basal ratio was 0.27 in the cultures exposed to 100 μM 4-HNE for 24 h. The level of CFH

Table 2 Comparison of changes in protein abundance

Gene Name	# of Total Spectral Counts	Fold Change by Quantitative SWATH-MS Analysis		
		AH (Drusen)	AH (RPD)	Comments
APOA1	300	+ 0.82	+ 1.28	Drusen marker
APOA4	149	+ 0.22	− 0.53	Lipid metabolism
CFHR2	10	− 1.20	− 0.92	Lipid metabolism
CTSD	101	0.00	− 0.53	Autophagolysosomal
SERPINA4	46	+ 1.42	+ 3.82	Antiangiogenesis
LUM	39	+ 3.05	+ 4.54	Extracellular matrix, Regulation of transcription
KERA	3	+ 1.52	+ 1.48	Extracellular matrix, Keratan (Cornea)
CLUS	93	− 0.74	+ 0.25	Clearance of cellular debris
PEDF	407	− 1.36	− 0.07	Neurotrophic property
PTGDS	239	− 0.51	− 1.09	Neuromodulator
TIMP1	20	− 0.88	− 1.06	EMT[a] marker

[a]EMT epithelial-mesenchymal transition

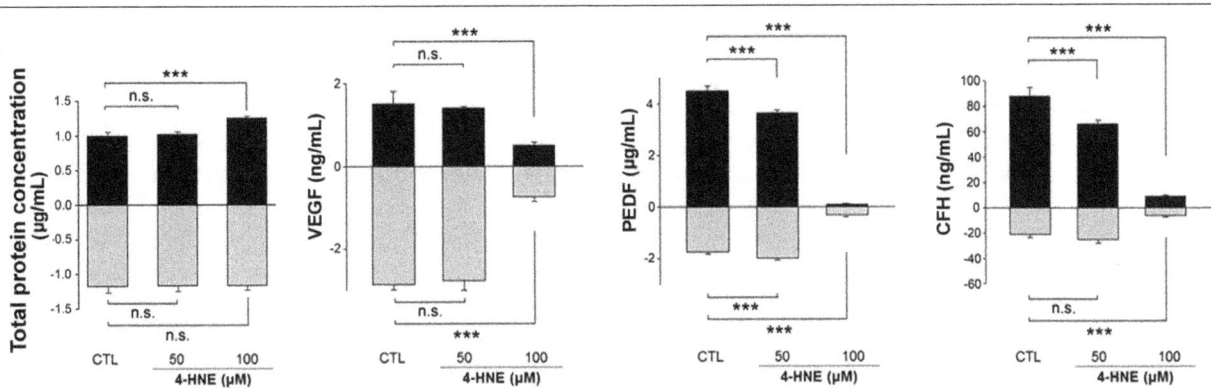

Fig. 6 Differential secretion of selected proteins in hfRPE cell cultures. Total protein concentrations in conditioned media from apical and basal baths (left end). To confirm the biological activity of VEGF, PEDF, and CFH, apical or basal media were collected at 24 h and then analyzed using ELISAs (the rest three graphs). The amount of VEGF protein in the basal media was higher than that in the apical media (2.86 ng/mL vs. 1.51 ng/mL) and was greatly decreased by 100 µM 4-HNE treatment (0.74 ng/mL vs. 0.51 ng/mL). PEDF secretion on the apical side was higher than that on the basal side (4.51 µg/mL vs. 1.74 µg/mL), and the level of PEDF was significantly decreased in a dose-dependent manner at 24 h (0.086 µg/mL and 0.32 µg/mL, in apical and basal baths treated with 100 µM 4-HNE). The ratio of the PEDF concentrations secreted in the apical and basal chambers was reversed in cultures treated with 100 µM 4-HNE. The apical/basal ratios were 2.59 and 1.83 in control cultures and cultures exposed to 50 µM 4-HNE for 24 h; the apical/basal ratio was 0.27 in cultures exposed to 100 µM 4-HNE for 24 h. The level of CFH showed similar changes: it decreased both apically and basally in cultures exposed to oxidative stress compared to control cultures. The apical/basal ratios were 4.19 and 2.64 in control cultures and cultures exposed to 50 µM 4-HNE for 24 h, respectively; the apical/basal ratio was 1.41 in cultures exposed to 100 µM 4-HNE for 24 h

showed similar changes: it was decreased both apically and basally in the cultures exposed to oxidative stress compared to the level in the control cultures. The apical/basal ratios were 4.19 and 2.64 in the control cultures and the cultures exposed to 50 µM 4-HNE for 24 h, respectively; the apical/basal ratio was 1.41 in the cultures exposed to 100 µM 4-HNE for 24 h.

Discussion

In the current study, we first investigated the AH proteome of dry AMD patients using a data-independent acquisition method (SWATH-MS), according to patient phenotype. We introduced an hfRPE culture model under oxidative stress that mimics an abnormal proteomic status reflecting AMD and used conventional methods (e.g., ELISA, IF, and WB) to confirm that a set of disease-associated candidate proteins was differentially expressed in polarized hfRPE cell cultures.

Drusen-related pathogenic environment in dry AMD mimicked by a polarized RPE cell culture model and quantitative proteomics

In the current study, we introduced an hfRPE cell culture model with a proteome that resembles the proteome of the AH from patients with drusen and RPD. Eight of eleven proteins with differential abundance between the controls and dry AMD patients in SWATH-MS analysis (Table 2) were previously considered to be major components or regulators in drusen [27, 28]. Among these proteins, APOA1, CTSD, and CLUS were found to be elevated via IF and WB analysis

in the RPE cell cultures treated with 4-HNE compared to the levels in the control cultures. In all the patient AH samples, various immunoglobulins were identified, which accounted for one-third of the total protein abundance (based on spectral counts). This high abundance of endogenous immunoglobulins detected in AH has also been observed in other body fluids (e.g., blood), suggesting that immunologic dysregulation is one of the major pathogenic mechanisms of dry AMD. Complement factor H, one of the most important soluble (secretory) complement regulatory proteins and a major inhibitor of alternative pathways providing protection against harmful complement activation [29], was decreased in both the AH from patients with drusen and RPD and the conditioned media from both apical and basal baths of cells exposed to oxidative stress in the present study. In a previous histologic study using AMD donor eyeballs, CFH immunoreactivity was identified in drusen, the sub-RPE space, along Bruch's membrane, and in the walls of choriocapillaris [30]. While some authors have reported decreased CFH expression in Bruch's membrane/choroid complexes in cases of both early AMD and geographic atrophy [31], others have found no difference in the amount of CFH proteins in Bruch's membrane/choroid tissue samples from AMD patients and controls [32]. Reduced expression of CFH has been observed in senescent or oxidative stressed RPE cell lines (ARPE-19 cells) [33, 34] suggesting that degenerative RPE cells might not be capable of synthesizing complement regulators for self-preservation under conditions of a dysregulated complement pathway;

however, the changes in the intracellular expression level of CFH have not been described in RPE from donor eyeballs or polarized hfRPE cultures. Thus, we speculate that secreted CFH, regardless of its intracellular expression level in RPE, decreases during the progression of AMD, leading to the accumulation sub-RPE deposits [35]. Various oxidation products, including advanced glycation end products such as carboxymethyllysine and reactive aldehydes such as carboxyethylpyrrole, malondialdehyde, and 4-HNE, have been shown to accumulate in the retina and cause damage to the retina during the progression of degeneration, as observed during AMD [36–38]; thus, all the phenotypes and pathologies of the RPE observed in vivo cannot be recapitulated by the application of any single agent to a culture system in vitro. However, we were able to demonstrate the compensatory role of our in vitro culture system, which reflects proteomics data from dry AMD patients, in the present study.

The RPE cell is a highly polarized cell types that produces and secretes proteins onto at basolateral and apical surface, meeting differential demands on either side of the photoreceptors and choriocapillaris and holding a large majority of secreted proteins on the basolateral side [14, 15]. In the RPE cultures exposed to oxidative stress in the present study, however, the ratios of secreted proteins between chambers corresponding to the basal and apical surfaces were reversed; the total protein concentrations in the conditioned media from the apical and basal chambers in the in vitro culture model exposed to oxidative stress were different (apical>basal) from those in the control cultures (basal>apical). Likewise, each AH sample (control, drusen, and RPD) exhibited a different total protein concentration (RPD > drusen>control). Epithelial-mesenchymal transition (EMT) is a complicated phenomenon through which polarized epithelial cells lose their polarity and cell-cell adhesions and acquire the mesenchymal characteristics of motility and invasiveness [39, 40]. Thus, it is plausible that a dysfunctional or stressed RPE cell may lose its polarity and increasingly misdirectionally secrete proteins onto the apical surface rather than onto the basolateral surface, resulting in accumulation in the subretinal space (forming RPD) rather than in the sub-RPE space. We speculate that different locations or subtypes of material deposition are associated with different statuses of the RPE, especially the maintenance of proper polarity. In terms of their composition, drusen and RPD have been shown to share several common components, including membranous vesicles, vitronectin, CFH, and apolipoproteins [6, 41–43]; however, their lipid composition is distinct, with a higher concentration of unesterified cholesterol being found in RPD [44–46].

New candidate drusen markers

Among the 11 proteins from the AH of dry AMD patients listed in Table 2, SERPINA4, LUM, and KERA have not been described among the components of drusen and have not been previously related to dry AMD, although SERPINA4 and LUM have been reported to be elevated in the retina in an ultraviolet (UV)-induced rat model of AMD [47]. The expression level of SERPINA4 in patients with drusen was also higher than that in healthy controls. One of the serine protease inhibitors, SERPINA4-like PEDF (Synonym: SERPINF1), plays a role as a potent negative regulator of angiogenesis. Interestingly, the LUM and KERA proteins were upregulated in both RPD and drusen. These two proteins are well-known for their roles in keratan sulfate proteoglycan (PG) biosynthesis in the cornea [48]. KERA has also been reported as a noncorneal keratan sulfate, such as fibromodulin, that contributes to retinal damage and repair [49] and as sulfated lactosamine, which is a common component of cell surface and extracellular glycoproteins [49]. A small amount of KERA has been found to exist in many other tissues, including the brain [50], thus suggesting its potential active role in the cellular processes of tissues. The known molecular functions of LUM or biological processes related to LUM include the regulation of transcription from the polymerase II promoter [47], collagen binding, extracellular matrix organization and the inflammatory response [51]. LUM has also been identified as a biomarker of UV toxicity associated with disruption of the interphotoreceptor matrix, indicating a role of LUM in photoreceptor cell dysfunction [47].

Although the precise role of PGs in AMD has not yet been fully investigated, the roles of heparan sulfate PG (HSPG) and chondroitin sulfate PG (CSPG) in the thickening of Bruch's membrane in early AMD have been demonstrated [52]. Roles of PGs in complement regulation have also been suggested; for example, HSPG in Bruch's membrane provides binding sites for CFH [53]. Further research is needed to explore the specific roles of lumican in the development and progression of AMD because lumican is found in RPE microvilli in addition to the cornea [54]. Thus, we propose these three proteins as new biomarkers for drusen.

Conclusions

In conclusion, the detailed proteomic analysis of dry AMD patients using SWATH-MS conducted in this study suggests a possible molecular link between in vivo disease processes and different AMD phenotypes and thus provides insights into the in vivo biology of drusen and RPD.

Abbreviations

AH: aqueous humor; AMD: age-related macular degeneration;
BCA: bicinchoninic acid; BM: Bruch's membrane; CFH: complement factor H;
CNV: choroidal neovascularization; CSPG: chondroitin sulfate PG;
EMT: epithelial-mesenchymal transition; GA: geographic atrophy;
hfRPE: human fetal RPE; HSPG: heparan sulfate PG; IF: Immunofluorescence;
PFA: paraformaldehyde; PG: proteoglycan; PVDF: polyvinylidene difluoride;
RIPA: radioimmunoprecipitation assay; RPD: reticular pseudodrusen;
RPE: retinal pigment epithelium; SWATH-MS: sequential window acquisition
of all theoretical fragment ion mass spectrometry; TER: transepithelial
resistance; TIMP3: tissue inhibitor of metalloproteinase-3; UV: ultraviolet;
VEGF: vascular endothelial growth factor

Acknowledgments

Funding

This research was supported by the National Research Foundation of Korea
(NRF) funded by the Ministry of Science and ICT (NRF-
2017R1E1A1A01073964).

Authors' contributions

HC and JHB designed the study protocol and conducted the study as
supervisors. JHB, DL, JBC, and HJ conducted experiments and statistical
analysis. HC, JHB, and DL drafted the manuscript. HC, KHP, and JL revised the
manuscript. All authors read and approved the final manuscript.

Competing interests

The authors report no conflicts of interest. The authors alone are responsible
for the content and writing of the paper.

Author details

[1]R&D Center for Clinical Mass Spectrometry, Seegene Medical Foundation,
Seoul 04805, South Korea. [2]Department of Ophthalmology, Konkuk University
School of Medicine, Konkuk University Medical Center, 120-1 Neungdong-ro,
Gwangjin-gu, Seoul, Republic of Korea. [3]Department of Ophthalmology,
Seoul National University College of Medicine, Seoul National University
Bundang Hospital, Seongnam 13620, South Korea. [4]Department of
Ophthalmology, Ilsan Paik Hospital, Inje University College of Medicine,
Goyang 10380, South Korea.

References

1. Bressler NM, Bressler SB, Congdon NG, Ferris FL, Friedman DS, Klein R, et al. Potential public health impact of age-related eye disease study results: AREDS report no. 11 Arch Ophthalmol. 2006.
2. Rofagha S, Bhisitkul RB, Boyer DS, Sadda SR, Zhang K. Seven-year outcomes in ranibizumab-treated patients in ANCHOR, MARINA, and HORIZON: a multicenter cohort study (SEVEN-UP). Ophthalmology. 2013.
3. Bloch SB, Larsen M, Munch IC. Incidence of legal blindness from age-related macular degeneration in Denmark: year 2000 to 2010. Am J Ophthalmol. 2012.
4. Mitchell P, Bressler N, Doan QV, Dolan C, Ferreira A, Osborne A, et al. Estimated cases of blindness and visual impairment from neovascular age-related macular degeneration avoided in Australia by ranibizumab treatment. PLoS One. 2014.
5. Alten F, Eter N. Current knowledge on reticular pseudodrusen in age-related macular degeneration. Br J Ophthalmol. 2015.
6. Hageman GS, Luthert PJ, Victor Chong NH, Johnson LV, Anderson DH, Mullins RF. An integrated hypothesis that considers drusen as biomarkers of immune-mediated processes at the RPE-Bruch's membrane interface in aging and age-related macular degeneration. Prog Retin Eye Res. 2001.
7. Mimoun G, Soubrane G, Coscas G. Macular drusen. J Fr Ophtalmol. 1990;13:511–30.
8. Hogg RE, Silva R, Staurenghi G, Murphy G, Santos AR, Rosina C, et al. Clinical characteristics of reticular pseudodrusen in the fellow eye of patients with unilateral neovascular age-related macular degeneration. Ophthalmology. 2014;121:1748–55.
9. Kovach JL, Schwartz SG, Agarwal A, Brantley MA, Pan SS, Haines JL, et al. The relationship between reticular Pseudodrusen and severity of AMD. Ophthalmology. 2016;123:921–3.
10. Zhou Q, Daniel E, Maguire MG, Grunwald JE, Martin ER, Martin DF, et al. Pseudodrusen and incidence of late age-related macular degeneration in fellow eyes in the comparison of age-related macular degeneration treatments trials. Ophthalmology. 2016;123:1530–40.
11. Gliem M, Hendig D, Finger RP, Holz FG, Charbel Issa P. Reticular pseudodrusen associated with a diseased bruch membrane in pseudoxanthoma elasticum. JAMA Ophthalmol. 2015;133:581–8.
12. Gliem M, Muller PL, Mangold E, Bolz HJ, Stohr H, Weber BHF, et al. Reticular Pseudodrusen in Sorsby fundus dystrophy. Ophthalmology. 2015;122:1555–62.
13. Alten F, Heiduschka P, Clemens CR, Eter N. Exploring choriocapillaris under reticular pseudodrusen using OCT-angiography. Graefes Arch Clin Exp Ophthalmol. 2016;254:2165–73.
14. Kay P, Yang YC, Paraoan L. Directional protein secretion by the retinal pigment epithelium: roles in retinal health and the development of age-related macular degeneration. J Cell Mol Med. 2013;17:833–43.
15. Gangalum RK, Atanasov IC, Zhou ZH, Bhat SP. AlphaB-crystallin is found in detergent-resistant membrane microdomains and is secreted via exosomes from human retinal pigment epithelial cells. J Biol Chem. 2011;286:3261–9.
16. Kang G-Y, Bang JY, Choi AJ, Yoon J, Lee W-C, Choi S, et al. Exosomal proteins in the aqueous humor as novel biomarkers in patients with neovascular age-related macular degeneration. J Proteome Res. 2014;13:581–95.
17. Lee H, Choi AJ, Kang G-Y, Park HS, Kim HC, Lim HJ, et al. Increased 26S proteasome non-ATPase regulatory subunit 1 in the aqueous humor of patients with age-related macular degeneration. BMB Rep. 2014;47:292–7.
18. Sonoda S, Spee C, Barron E, Ryan SJ, Kannan R, Hinton DR. A protocol for the culture and differentiation of highly polarized human retinal pigment epithelial cells. Nat Protoc. 2009;4:662–73.
19. Ablonczy Z, Dahrouj M, Tang PH, Liu Y, Sambamurti K, Marmorstein AD, et al. Human retinal pigment epithelium cells as functional models for the RPE in vivo. Invest Ophthalmol Vis Sci. 2011;52:8614–20.
20. Seong KM, Baek J-H, Yu M-H, Kim J. Rpn13p and Rpn14p are involved in the recognition of ubiquitinated Gcn4p by the 26S proteasome. FEBS Lett. 2007;581:2567–73.
21. Baek J-H, Kim H, Shin B, Yu M-H. Multiple products monitoring as a robust approach for peptide quantification. J Proteome Res. 2009;8:3625–32.
22. Lee W-K, Baek J-H, Ryoo S, Gyu Yu Y. SWATH-based Comparative Proteomic Analysis of the Mycobacterium bovis BCG-Korea Strain. 2014.
23. Nesvizhskii AI, Keller A, Kolker E, Aebersold R. A statistical model for identifying proteins by tandem mass spectrometry. Anal Chem. 2003;75: 4646–58. https://doi.org/10.1021/ac0341261.
24. Ashburner M, Ball CA, Blake JA, Botstein D, Butler H, Cherry JM, et al. Gene ontology: tool for the unification of biology. The Gene Ontology Consortium Nat Genet. 2000;25:25–9.
25. Schutt F, Bergmann M, Holz FG, Kopitz J. Proteins modified by malondialdehyde, 4-hydroxynonenal, or advanced glycation end products in lipofuscin of human retinal pigment epithelium. Invest Ophthalmol Vis Sci. 2003;44:3663–8.
26. Tanito M, Elliott MH, Kotake Y, Anderson RE. Protein modifications by 4-hydroxynonenal and 4-hydroxyhexenal in light-exposed rat retina. Invest Ophthalmol Vis Sci. 2005;46:3859–68.
27. Johnson LV, Forest DL, Banna CD, Radeke CM, Maloney MA, Hu J, et al. Cell culture model that mimics drusen formation and triggers complement activation associated with age-related macular degeneration. Proc Natl Acad Sci U S A. 2011;108:18277–82.
28. Crabb JW, Miyagi M, Gu X, Shadrach K, West KA, Sakaguchi H, et al. Drusen proteome analysis: an approach to the etiology of age-related macular degeneration. Proc Natl Acad Sci U S A. 2002;99:14682–7.

29. Anderson DH, Mullins RF, Hageman GS, Johnson LV. A role for local inflammation in the formation of drusen in the aging eye. Am J Ophthalmol. 2002;134:411–31.

30. Gehrs KM, Jackson JR, Brown EN, Allikmets R, Hageman GS. Complement, age-related macular degeneration and a vision of the future. Arch Ophthalmol (Chicago, Ill 1960). 2010;128:349–58.

31. Bhutto IA, Baba T, Merges C, Juriasinghani V, McLeod DS, Lutty GA. C-reactive protein and complement factor H in aged human eyes and eyes with age-related macular degeneration. Br J Ophthalmol. 2011;95:1323 LP–1330 http://bjo.bmj.com/content/95/9/1323.abstract.

32. Yuan X, Gu X, Crabb JS, Yue X, Shadrach K, Hollyfield JG, et al. Quantitative proteomics: comparison of the macular Bruch membrane/choroid complex from age-related macular degeneration and normal eyes. Mol Cell Proteomics. 2010;9:1031–46.

33. Marazita MC, Dugour A, Marquioni-Ramella MD, Figueroa JM, Suburo AM. Oxidative stress-induced premature senescence dysregulates VEGF and CFH expression in retinal pigment epithelial cells: implications for age-related macular degeneration. Redox Biol. 2016;7:78–87.

34. Zhang Y, Huang Q, Tang M, Zhang J, Fan W. Complement factor H expressed by retinal pigment epithelium cells can suppress neovascularization of human umbilical vein endothelial cells: an in vitro study. PLoS One. 2015;10:e0129945.

35. Weismann D, Hartvigsen K, Lauer N, Bennett KL, Scholl HPN, Charbel Issa P, et al. Complement factor H binds malondialdehyde epitopes and protects from oxidative stress. Nature. 2011;478:76–81.

36. Ethen CM, Reilly C, Feng X, Olsen TW, Ferrington DA. Age-related macular degeneration and retinal protein modification by 4-hydroxy-2-nonenal. Invest Ophthalmol Vis Sci. 2007;48:3469–79.

37. Kurien BT, Scofield RH. Autoimmunity and oxidatively modified autoantigens. Autoimmun Rev. 2008;7:567–73.

38. Kauppinen A, Niskanen H, Suuronen T, Kinnunen K, Salminen A, Kaarniranta K. Oxidative stress activates NLRP3 inflammasomes in ARPE-19 cells--implications for age-related macular degeneration (AMD). Immunol Lett. 2012;147:29–33.

39. Grassi G, Di Caprio G, Santangelo L, Fimia GM, Cozzolino AM, Komatsu M, et al. Autophagy regulates hepatocyte identity and epithelial-to-mesenchymal and mesenchymal-to-epithelial transitions promoting snail degradation. Cell Death Dis. 2015;6:e1880.

40. Lamouille S, Xu J, Derynck R. Molecular mechanisms of epithelial-mesenchymal transition. Nat Rev Mol Cell Biol. 2014;15:178–96.

41. Sivaprasad S, Bird A, Nitiahpapand R, Nicholson L, Hykin P, Chatziralli I. Perspectives on reticular pseudodrusen in age-related macular degeneration. Surv Ophthalmol. 2016;61:521–37.

42. Khan KN, Mahroo OA, Khan RS, Mohamed MD, McKibbin M, Bird A, et al. Differentiating drusen: Drusen and drusen-like appearances associated with ageing, age-related macular degeneration, inherited eye disease and other pathological processes. Prog Retin Eye Res. 2016;53:70–106.

43. Rudolf M, Malek G, Messinger JD, Clark ME, Wang L, Curcio CA. Sub-retinal drusenoid deposits in human retina: organization and composition. Exp Eye Res. 2008;87:402–8.

44. Greferath U, Guymer RH, Vessey KA, Brassington K, Fletcher EL. Correlation of histologic features with in vivo imaging of reticular Pseudodrusen. Ophthalmology. 2016;123:1320–31.

45. Curcio CA, Messinger JD, Sloan KR, McGwin G, Medeiros NE, Spaide RF. Subretinal drusenoid deposits in non-neovascular age-related macular degeneration: morphology, prevalence, topography, and biogenesis model. Retina. 2013;33:265–76.

46. Curcio CA, Presley JB, Malek G, Medeiros NE, Avery DV, Kruth HS. Esterified and unesterified cholesterol in drusen and basal deposits of eyes with age-related maculopathy. Exp Eye Res. 2005;81:731–41.

47. Kraljevic Pavelic S, Klobucar M, Sedic M, Micek V, Gehrig P, Grossman J, et al. UV-induced retinal proteome changes in the rat model of age-related macular degeneration. Biochim Biophys Acta. 2015;1852:1833–45.

48. Funderburgh JL. Keratan sulfate: structure, biosynthesis. and function Glycobiology. 2000;10:951 8.

49. Ali SAM, Hosaka YZ, Uehara M. Expression of small leucine-rich proteoglycans in the developing retina and kainic acid-induced retinopathy in ICR mice. J Vet Med Sci. 2011;73:439–45.

50. Krusius T, Finne J, Margolis RK, Margolis RU. Identification of an O-glycosidic mannose-linked sialylated tetrasaccharide and keratan sulfate oligosaccharides in the chondroitin sulfate proteoglycan of brain. J Biol Chem. 1986;261:8237–42.

51. Nikitovic D, Papoutsidakis A, Karamanos NK, Tzanakakis GN. Lumican affects tumor cell functions, tumor-ECM interactions, angiogenesis and inflammatory response. Matrix Biol. 2014;35:206–14.

52. Al Gwairi O, Thach L, Zheng W, Osman N, Little PJ. Cellular and molecular pathology of age-related macular degeneration: potential role for proteoglycans. J Ophthalmol. 2016; 2016:2913612.

53. Keenan TDL, Pickford CE, Holley RJ, Clark SJ, Lin W, Dowsey AW, et al. Age-dependent changes in heparan sulfate in human Bruch's membrane: implications for age-related macular degeneration. Invest Ophthalmol Vis Sci. 2014;55:5370–9.

54. Bonilha VL, Bhattacharya SK, West KA, Sun J, Crabb JW, Rayborn ME, et al. Proteomic characterization of isolated retinal pigment epithelium microvilli. Mol Cell Proteomics. 2004;3:1119–27.

19

Safety and efficacy of transpupillary silicone oil removal in combination with micro-incision phacoemulsification cataract surgery: comparison with 23-gauge approach

Wei Xu[*][†], Weijing Cheng[†], Hua Zhuang, Jian Guo and Guoxing Xu

Abstract

Background: To evaluate safety and efficacy of transpupillary silicone oil removal combined with micro-incision phacoemulsification cataract surgery, and to compare results of transpupillary with 23-gauge three-port vitrectomy approach.

Methods: Consecutive cases that underwent silicone oil removal using either transpupillary or three-port approach in combination with micro-incision phacoemulsification cataract surgery were retrospectively reviewed. The main outcome measures were postoperative detachment rate, silicone oil residuals, best corrected visual acuity (BCVA) and intraocular pressure (IOP).

Results: A total of 64 cases were included, 19 in transpupillary and 45 in three-port. Postoperative detachment rate within 3 months in transpupillary versus three-port was 15.8% versus 4.4% ($p = 0.14$), Silicone oil residuals was $7.4 \pm 3.2\%$ versus $7.1 \pm 2.8\%$ (transpupillary vs. three-port, $p = 0.71$). Preoperative versus postoperative BCVA (logMAR) was 1.49 ± 0.61 versus 1.42 ± 0.61 in transpupillary approach ($p = 0.28$) and 1.53 ± 0.48 versus 1.45 ± 0.57 in three-port approach ($p = 0.11$). Transpupillary approach resulted in lower IOP at postoperative day 2 (12.2 ± 2.3 mmHg vs. 13.5 ± 2.2 mmHg, $p < 0.05$), while postoperative follow-up at 1 month revealed no significant difference ($p = 0.21$).

Conclusions: Transpupillary silicone oil removal combined with micro-incision phacoemulsification cataract surgery is less invasive and can be an alternative in some circumstances.

Keywords: Silicone oil removal, Micro-incision cataract surgery, Vitrectomy, Postoperative detachment, Endotamponade

Background

Silicone oil is frequently used as endotamponade in vitrectomy for some complicated cases such as giant retinal tears [1], traumatic endophthalmitis [2], and diabetic tractional detachment [3], which provides a clear view of the fundus in comparison with gas and inhibits postoperative vitreous hemorrhage [4]. However, complications including glaucoma, cataract, band keratopathy, emulsification of

silicone oil and possible neural toxicity restrict it from a permanent vitreous substitute [5]. A number of vitreous substitutes have been investigated, but there are still barriers before clinical application [6]. Silicone oil removal is required according to post surgery follow-up. Attempt has been made to improve efficacy of and minimize surgical injury during silicone oil removal [7]. Potential complications should not be ignored. One of the most concerned complications due to silicone oil removal is postoperative retinal redetachment. Although efforts have been made to reduce percentage of detachment after silicone oil removal, the incidence reported varies from 3.5 to 13.2% [8,

* Correspondence: ocuweixu@gmail.com
[†]Wei Xu and Weijing Cheng contributed equally to this work.
Department of Ophthalmology, First Affiliated Hospital of Fujian Medical University, No. 20 Chazhong Road, Fuzhou 350005, China

9]. In the present study, we compared a transpupillary sclerotomy-free approach of silicone oil removal with standard three-port vitrectomy approach in terms of postoperative detachment rate, silicone oil residuals, visual acuity and intraocular pressure and so on.

Methods

This retrospective study was approved by the Ethic Board of the First Affiliated Hospital of Fujian Medical University and complied with the tenets of the Declaration of Helsinki. Written informed consent was obtained from all individuals. Self-paid patients that underwent silicone oil-extraction combined with micro-incision phacoemulsification and intraocular lens implantation between May 2015 and April 2017 and had a minimum follow-up of 3 month were included. These patients previously underwent pars plana vitrectomy and silicone oil (Oxane® 5700; Bausch & Lomb, Rochester, USA) tamponade due to different incidence, while postoperative follow-up revealed fully attachment of retina and present of complicated cataract. Patients were fully informed regarding the difference between transpupillary approach and three-port vitrectomy approach to select a procedure at their own decision. The outcome measures were mean surgical duration, rate of postoperative detachment, silicone oil residuals in vitreous cavity, best corrected visual acuity (BCVA) and intraocular pressure (IOP).

In transpupillary approach, a standard phacoemulsification was performed and Viscoat® (Alcon, Fort Worth, USA) was injected into the anterior chamber followed by posterior capsulotomy. Infusion tip was plugged into corneal side incision and maintain irrigation height at 110 cm. Silicone oil was manually removed through an 18-gauge catheter system (BD, Suzhou, China) which was inserted directly into vitreous cavity via corneal main incision and posterior capsular hole. A 10 ml syringe was connected to the catheter system to actively aspirate silicone oil out. Intraocular lens was implanted into capsular bag followed by a gentle irrigation/aspiration step to remove Viscoat® and possible silicone oil residuals in the anterior chamber. Cases with intraocular lens implanted in sulcus were excluded.

In three-port vitrectomy approach, 23-gauge vitrectomy incisions were made after standard phacoemulsification and intraocular lens implantation. Infusion site was made in the inferotemporal quadrant, and intraocular manipulation sites were made in the superonasal and superotemporal quadrants for silicone oil extraction and illuminator. Silicone oil was actively removed under Stellaris™ PC machine (Bausch & Lomb, Rochester, USA). After extraction of the oil, retinal inspection was performed using Resight® viewing system (Carl Zeiss, Jena, Germany). Endolaser and epiretinal membrane peeling were performed when retinal break and epiretinal membrane were found.

Statistical analysis was performed using SPSS software for Windows version 16.0 (SPSS Inc., Chicago, IL, USA). Postoperative detachment rates between the two approaches were tested by Chi-square test. Visual acuity was converted to logMAR values, including hand motion and counting fingers as previously described [10]. Vitreous cavity was demarcated in binarized ultrasonic image. Silicone oil remnants were calculated and presented as percentage of total white area in the demarcated region using Image J. Descriptive statistics were presented as mean ± SD. The threshold for statistical significance was defined as p-value < 0.05.

Results

A total of 64 consecutive cases were reviewed in this study. Demographic data of the patients was shown in Table 1. Gender ratios (male/female) were 10/9 in transpupillary approach and 23/22 in 23-gauge vitrectomy approach, respectively. The average age of the patients underwent silicone oil removal was 55.1 ± 7.0 years in transpupillary approach in contrast with 54.0 ± 11.9 years in 23-gauge approach. Among these cases, rhgematogenous retinal detachment is the most frequent cause that resulted in previous vitrectomy combined with silicone oil tamponade. The percentages were 63.2 and 77.8% (transpupillary vs. 23-gauge). Other causes include diabetic retinopathy, traumatic proliferative retinopathy and endophthalmitis. In the transpupillary group, patients had a mean duration of silicone oil tamponade for 8.0 ± 3.6 months, while in the 23-gauge group the mean duration was 6.5 ± 1.8 months.

A significant difference in mean axial length was identified between transpupillary approach and 23-gauge approach, which was 24.5 ± 1.0 mm versus 23.9 ± 0.8 mm (p < 0.05). Transpupillary approach took shorter surgical duration than 23-gauge approach. The mean time required were 53.6 ± 8.2 min and 58.8 ± 9.5 min, respectively

Table 1 Demographic data of patients

	Transpupillary	23-gauge
Mean Age (years)	55.1 ± 7.0	54.0 ± 11.9
Gender		
Male	10	23
Female	9	22
Previous Diagnosis		
RRD	12 (63.2%)	35 (77.8%)
DRP	3 (15.8%)	6 (13.3%)
Traumatic PVR	3 (15.8)	3 (6.7%)
Endophthalmitis	1 (5.2%)	1 (2.2%)
Mean Duration of Tamponade (months)	8.0 ± 3.6	6.5 ± 1.8

RRD rhgematogenous retinal detachment, *DRP* diabetic retinopathy, *PVR* proliferative vitreous retinopathy

($p < 0.05$, Table 2). In 23-gauge approach, 4 cases (8.9%) underwent endolaser coagulation and 3 cases (6.7%) underwent epiretinal membrane peeling. By contrast, these intraocular manipulations were infeasible in transpupillary approach. No significance in preoperative IOP was identified between transpupillary and 23-gauge method (13.2 ± 2.1 mmHg vs. 12.8 ± 1.8 mmHg, $p = 0.14$). Intraocular pressure at postoperative day 2 was lower in patients underwent transpupillary silicone oil removal than those using standard method (12.2 ± 2.3 mmHg vs. 13.5 ± 2.2 mmHg, $p < 0.05$). Postoperative follow-up revealed no significant difference in IOP between transpupillary and 23-gauge approach 1 month post-surgery (12.7 ± 3.4 mmHg vs. 13.8 ± 2.2 mmHg, $p = 0.21$). However, a consecutive record of postoperative IOP was not available.

Three patients got detachment within 3 months in transpupillary approach. The postoperative detachment rate was 15.8%. By comparison, detachment within 3 months only occurred on two patients in 23-gauge approach. The postoperative detachment rate was 4.4%. However, statistical analysis failed to test significant difference regarding detachment rates between the two approaches ($p = 0.14$, Chi-Square test). Data of the postoperative retinal detachment cases were shown in Table 3. These patients underwent silicone oil reinjection. Anterior chamber silicone oil frequently appeared in one patient during follow-up. This patient previously underwent transpupillary silicone oil removal. Preoperative and postoperative BCVA were defined as the latest BCVA before silicone oil removal and BCVA at the last follow-up visit. Preoperative and postoperative BCVA in transpupillary approach were 1.49 ± 0.61 and 1.42 ± 0.61 without significance ($P = 0.28$). In 23-gauge approach the data was 1.53 ± 0.48 versus 1.45 ± 0.57, without significance either ($P = 0.11$). Silicone oil

Table 2 Clinical details and surgical outcomes between two approaches

	Transpupillary	23-gauge
Axial Length (mm)	24.5 ± 1.0*	23.9 ± 0.8
Surgical Duration (min)	53.6 ± 8.2*	58.8 ± 9.5
IOP (mmHg)		
Preoperative	13.2 ± 2.1	12.8 ± 1.8
POD2	12.2 ± 2.3*	13.5 ± 2.2
POM1	12.7 ± 3.4	13.8 ± 2.2
BCVA (LogMAR)		
Preoperative	1.49 ± 0.61	1.53 ± 0.48
Postoperative	1.42 ± 0.61	1.45 ± 0.57
Silicone oil residuals (%)	7.4 ± 3.2	7.1 ± 2.8

IOP intraocular pressure, *POD2* postoperative day 2, *POM1* postoperative month 1, *BCVA* best corrected visual acuity
*$P < 0.05$

remnants were evaluated by ultrasonic image and appeared as percentages (Fig. 1). The percentages of silicone oil residuals in transpupillary versus 23-gauge approach were 7.4 ± 3.2% versus 7.1 ± 2.8% ($P = 0.71$).

Discussion

Complications of silicone oil removal include recurrent retinal detachment, vitreous hemorrhage, postoperative hypotony, macular edema, etc. In this study, we compared the incidence of silicone oil removal related complications in two different removal approaches. Transpupillary silicone oil removal combined with cataract surgery has been reported previously with an infusion cannula connected to balanced salt solution [11]. But in this study we provide a sclerotomy-free way to extracted silicone oil with minimum injury in contrast to traditional three-port sclerotomy method. In addition, silicone oil removal from the anterior chamber allows administration of topical anesthesia which avoids the risk of eye ball perforation, retrobulbar hemorrhage and optic nerve injury. This less invasive procedure requires less intraoperative and postoperative monitoring, hence makes it an economical way [12]. The average cost for a patient undergoing silicone oil removal in this approach is 30% less than traditional three-port approach. However, Silicone oil removal using three-port sclerotomy enables intraoperative intervention against new retinal breaks or epiretinal membranes, resulting in a lower rate of postoperative detachment. The rate of retinal detachment after oil removal is much lower in the traditional three-port approach, although not significant statistically. It is worthwhile to note that sclerotomy introduces potential break in the peripheral retina which cannot be identified without scleral indentation. Irrigation fluid may penetrate into subretinal space through the iatrogenic break and develop postoperative retinal detachment.

When fluid penetrates through retinal breaks into subretinal space, liquid-filled vitreous cavity tends to maintain lower pressure. Lower IOP may induce vascular dilation or even rupture in retina and choroid. Therefore, postoperative hypotony is often related to vitreous hemorrhage and recurrent retinal detachment. Early postoperative hypotony is also a risk factor for choroidal detachment [13]. In this study, silicone oil removal from the anterior chamber resulted in relatively lower IOP early post-surgery. Postoperative detachment rate in transpupillary approach is higher compared with standard three-port approach, even though without statistical significance. We considered lower postoperative IOP as a potential risk for detachment, but the current data is not enough to illustrate a correlation between postoperative IOP and detachment rate. Interestingly, lower postoperative IOP is not linked to vitreous hemorrhage as no incidence existed in transpupillary approach.

Table 3 Details in cases of postoperative retinal detachment

Case	Previous diagnosis	Duration of tamponade (months)	Approach of removal	Endolaser or ERM peeling	Surgical duration (minutes)	Onset of postoperative detachment (weeks)
1	RRD	8	Transpupillary	No	55	2
2	RRD	6	Transpupillary	No	60	4
3	DRP	6	Transpupillary	No	61	8
4	RRD	3	23G	laser	56	5
5	RRD	5	23G	No	67	4

RRD rhgematogenous retinal detachment, *DRP* diabetic retinopathy, *PVR* proliferative vitreous retinopathy, *23G* 23-gauge three-port approach

Complicated cataract frequently develops in eye with silicone oil tamponade. A combined cataract surgery is often required before silicone oil removal. In some cases, posterior capsular opacity may impede silicone oil removal though scleral port. Hence posterior capsulotomy is required before a standard oil removal procedure. Silicone oil tends to flow into the anterior chamber in this circumstance. By comparison, transpupillary approach overcomes this weakness while providing an effective and less invasive way. Previous reported transpupillary silicone oil removal approaches have already concerned on efficiency and safety [14], but the incision was larger than what we did. In this study, we were able to remove silicone oil through limbal incision at a size suitable for micro-incision cataract surgery. Reduced incision will provide better visual outcome with minimum astigmatism. However, transpupillary

method is only applicable to cases with complicated cataract. In cases with artificial or clear lens, traditional three-port method is required.

Surgical duration and silicone oil residuals in vitreous cavity are two indexes regarding the efficiency of a procedure. Although manual oil removal is administrated in transpupillary approach, it took shorter surgical duration than traditional three-port approach. Several factors account for this surgical time difference. In three-port technique, retinal inspection, laser coagulation and epiretinal membrane peeling took additional time. Besides, air-fluid exchange was used to ensure clearance of silicone oil, which also added to longer surgical duration. Interestingly, postoperative ultrasonic image did not reveal significant difference in silicone oil residuals between the two approaches. Silicone oil residuals appear much larger than they are in

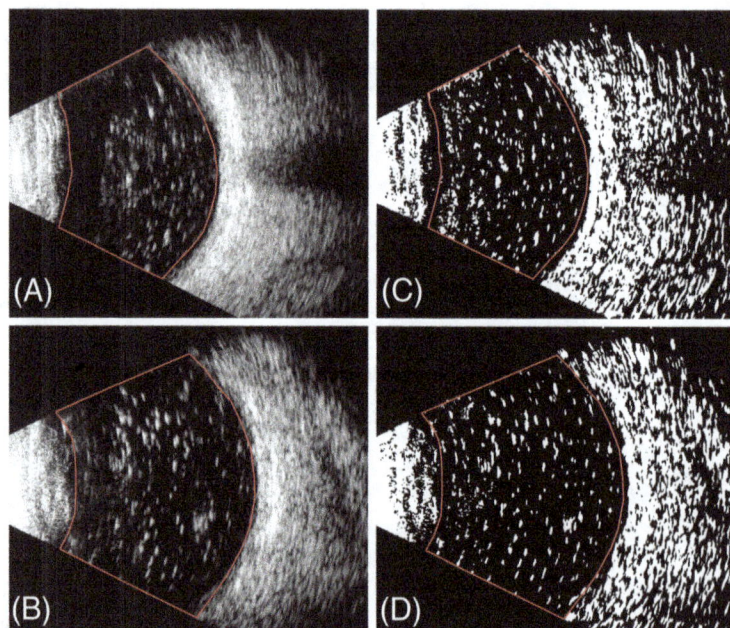

Fig. 1 Postoperative silicone oil residuals. Ultrasonic image of Silicone oil residuals were magnified due to Rayleigh scattering. Representative images of patients who underwent silicone oil removal using transpupillary approach (**a**) and 23-gauge vitrectomy approach (**b**) were shown. Images were converted using a binarization method to quantify silicone oil remnants (**c** and **d**). The selected areas were analyzed and the results were presented as percentages

ultrasonic image due to Rayleigh scattering [15], which makes quantification of the residuals possible through ultrasonic imaging. Residuals after silicone oil removal were found positively correlated with axial length using this technique [16]. However, we did not find significant difference in silicone oil residuals between groups in our study, even though significant difference in axial length was identified.

The limitation of this study lies in that this is not a randomized study. Patients were able to select a procedure at their own decision after being well informed. Due to lower cost in the transpupillary approach, patients with financial concerning tend to select a cheaper procedure. Patients requesting the cheaper operation may have worse condition which may affect the results. Cases included in transpupillary approach were much less than in traditional three-port approach, which may also affect the interpretation of the results.

Conclusion

In summary, transpupillary silicone oil removal combined with micro-incision cataract surgery is an effective and less invasive approach for the removal of silicone oil. But the infeasibility of intraoperative intervention on retina restricts selection of this surgical approach. Thoroughly preoperative inspection is required so as to reduce postoperative detachment.

Abbreviations
BCVA: Best corrected visual acuity; DRP: Diabetic retinopathy; IOP: Intraocular pressure; PVR: Proliferative vitreous retinopathy; RRD: Rhgematogenous retinal detachment

Funding
This study was supported by grants from Science and Technology Department of Fujian Province (No. 2017 J05125 and No. 2016B011), Health and Family Planning Commission of Fujian Province (No. 2017-ZQN-42) and Fujian Medical University (No. 2016QH047).

Authors' contributions
WX-study design and data collection, WC-protocol assessment and manuscript revising, HZ-study design and data collection, JG-data interpretation, GX-manuscript preparation. All authors read and approved the final manuscript.

Competing interests
The authors declare that they have no competing interests.

References
1. Berrocal MH, Chenworth ML, Acaba LA. Management of Giant Retinal Tear Detachments. J Ophthalmic Vis Res. 2017;12(1):93–7.
2. Ahmed Y, Schimel AM, Pathengay A, Colyer MH, Flynn HW Jr. Endophthalmitis following open-globe injuries. Eye (Lond). 2012;26(2):212–7.
3. Balakrishnan D, Jain B, Nayaka A, Rani PK, Mukundaprasad V, Jalali S. Role of tamponade in vitrectomy for proliferative diabetic retinopathy with vitreous hemorrhage. Semin Ophthalmol. 2016; https://doi.org/10.3109/08820538.2015.1120757.
4. Yeh PT, Yang CM, Yang CH. Distribution, reabsorption, and complications of preretinal blood under silicone oil after vitrectomy for severe proliferative diabetic retinopathy. Eye (Lond). 2012;26(4):601–8.
5. Grzybowski A, Pieczynski J, Ascaso FJ. Neuronal complications of intravitreal silicone oil: an updated review. Acta Ophthalmol. 2014;92(3):201–4.
6. Su X, Tan MJ, Li Z, Wong M, Rajamani L, Lingam G, Loh XJ. Recent progress in using biomaterials as vitreous substitutes. Biomacromolecules. 2015; 16(10):3093–102.
7. Zhang Z, Wei Y, Jiang X, Qiu S, Zhang S. A machine-independent method to have active removal of 5,000 centistokes silicone oil using plastic infusion tube and 23-gauge microcannulas. BMC Ophthalmol. 2015;15:114.
8. Choudhary MM, Saeed MU, Ali A. Removal of silicone oil: prognostic factors and incidence of retinal redetachment. Retina. 2012;32(10):2034–8.
9. Teke MY, Balikoglu-Yilmaz M, Yuksekkaya P, Citirik M, Elgin U, Kose T, Ozturk F. Surgical outcomes and incidence of retinal redetachment in cases with complicated retinal detachment after silicone oil removal: univariate and multiple risk factors analysis. Retina. 2014;34(10):1926–38.
10. Lange C, Feltgen N, Junker B, Schulze-Bonsel K, Bach M. Resolving the clinical acuity categories "hand motion" and "counting fingers" using the Freiburg visual acuity test (FrACT). Graefes Arch Clin Exp Ophthalmol. 2009; 247(1):137–42.
11. El Baha SM, Abouhussein MA, Hemeida TS. Sutureless phacoemulsification with transpupillary removal of silicone oil and intracapsular intraocular lens implantation using illuminated 23-gauge infusion system. Retina. 2011;31(2):408–12.
12. Jonas JB, Hugger P, Sauder G. Topical anesthesia for transpupillary silicone oil removal combined with cataract surgery. J Cataract Refract Surg. 2005; 31(9):1781–2.
13. Yamane S, Inoue M, Arakawa A, Kadonosono K. Early postoperative hypotony and ciliochoroidal detachment after microincision vitrectomy surgery. Am J Ophthalmol. 2012;153(6):1099–1103 e1091.
14. Assi A, Woodruff S, Gotzaridis E, Bunce C, Sullivan P. Combined phacoemulsification and transpupillary drainage of silicone oil: results and complications. Br J Ophthalmol. 2001;85(8):942–5.
15. Spaide RF, Chung JE, Fisher YL. Ultrasound detection of silicone oil after its removal in retinal reattachment surgery. Retina. 2005;25(7):943–5.
16. Shiihara H, Terasaki H, Yoshihara N, Shirasawa M, Otsuka H, Yamashita T, Yamakiri K, Sonoda S, Sakamoto T. Amount of residual silicone oil in vitreous cavity is significantly correlated with axial length. Retina. 2016;36(1):181–7.

20

Prevalence and associated factors of low vision and blindness among patients attending St. Paul's Hospital Millennium Medical College, Addis Ababa, Ethiopia

Fashe Markos Cherinet[*], Sophia Yoseph Tekalign, Dereje Hayilu Anbesse and Zewdu Yenegeta Bizuneh

Abstract

Background: Low vision and blindness are major public health problems. A vast burden of worlds visually impaired live in low-income settings especially in sub Saharan Africa. In such settings the blindness is associated with considerable disability and excess mortality, resulting in huge economic and social consequence. The main purpose of this study was to determine the prevalence and associated factors of low vision and blindness among patients at St. Paul's hospital millenium medical college.

Methods: Institution based cross sectional design study was carried out from January to April, 2017 with sample size of 904. Systematic random sampling was used to recruit the study subjects. Retrospective medical chart review was done; data was entered into and analyzed by SPSS 23. Descriptive statistics such as frequency cross tabulation and chi-square test was carried out to translate data into information. P-value less than 0.05 was considered as statistically significant.

Results: A total of 881 subjects with a response rate of 97.4% selected. The mean age of the study subjects was 44.53(SD: $\pm$ 21.85) with a range of 1–100 years. The prevalence of low vision and blindness was 91 (10.3% (95% CI: 8.2, 12.3)), and 64 (7.3 95%CI: 5.7, 9.0)) respectively. Age (p-value < 0.001), cataract (p-value = 0.002), glaucoma (p-value = 0.002) and age related macular degeneration (p-value < 0.001) were significantly associated with low vision and blindness.

Conclusion: Low vision and blindness found in this study was high. Age, cataract, glaucoma and age related macular degeneration were significantly associated with low vision and blindness. This amount of magnitude will be reduced if prevention, early diagnosis and management will be targeted towards avoidable causes of visual impairment.

Keywords: Low vision and blindness, St. Paul's hospital millennium medical college, Ethiopia

Background

In the world, the number of visually impaired is estimated to be 285 million, of whom 39 million were blind. About 82% of peoples greater than 50 years and above were blind and this indicates that the burden of visual impairment and blindness is higher on the older age groups [1]. Visual impairment includes low vision and blindness. It was defined based on visual acuity and visual field [2].

A vast burden of worlds visually impaired live in low-income settings especially in sub Saharan Africa (SSA)

[3]. Visual impairment can cause disabilities by significantly interfering with one's ability to function independently. These disabilities limit personal or socioeconomic independence and a visual handicap exists [4]. The good news is that more than two third of this visual impairment and blindness can be avoidable either by prevention and treatment [5].

According to 'vision 2020 the right to sight' plan, in 2020 preventable and avoidable causes of visual impairment and blindness will be reduced significantly to less than 0.5% in all countries or less than 1% in any community worldwide [6–9].

Ethiopia is believed to have one of the world's highest rates of blindness (1.6%) and low vision (3.7%), of which more than 80% is either treatable or preventable [2, 10–12].

* Correspondence: cheruyemark2015@gmail.com
Department of Ophthalmology, St. Paul's Hospital Millennium Medical College, Addis Ababa, Ethiopia

Low vision and blindness are believed to be common among patients in St. Paul's Hospital Millennium Medical College, though no survey was conducted in the setting. This survey was conducted with the main objective of assessing the prevalence and associated factors of low vision and blindness among patients in St. Paul's Hospital Millennium medical College (SPHMMC), Addis Ababa; Ethiopia. Thus, this evidence will help us to establish low vision and blindness rehabilitation clinic in the hospital.

Methods

Study design, setting and sampling

An institution based- cross sectional design study was conducted from January to April 2017 at SPHMMC, Tertiary Eye Care and Training Center. The center is well known college with ophthalmic medical service and ophthalmology residency training in the capital city of the country, Addis Ababa. It has been serving more than 16,000 patients with more outpatients and in some cases inpatient services per year. There are sub specialty clinics like retina, glaucoma, pediatric, oculoplasty and optometry clinics within the center. All patients come to the center have been undergoing complete eye examination including diagnostics tests. Medical, optical, laser and surgical service is the routine treatment modalities for the patients at the center. There are also one extra public and two private tertiary eye care centers in the study area. The other 10 public and 15 private secondary and primary eye centers were more focused on treating adnexal eye diseases and major surgeries like cataract and Trabeculectomy, minor surgeries and refractive services.

There was no evidence within the same study setting in which we need to consider in estimating the minimum sample size. Therefore it was considered that 50% proportion of population with visual impairment, 3% error of margin, 95% confidence interval and 10% non-respond rates were used to calculate the sample. Hence a total of 904 sample size was retrieved using single population proportion formula. The study was conducted among persons of all age groups. Study subjects were recruited from registration logbook of the clinic taking every 10th patient, the first being the 7th medical record number registered with omission of incomplete records.

Socio-demographic characteristics such as age, sex and address and clinical characteristics like Snellen visual acuity, IOP measured by non-contact air-puff tonometer, slit lamp biomicroscope and Fundus examination results including lists of all ophthalmic diagnosis written on the medical record were retrieved as their respective order. Visual acuity and IOP were measured by ophthalmic nurses while eye examinations were done by senior ophthalmologists. Visual acuity was measured by using retro-illuminated Snellen charts at 6 m and only distance one was considered; and for children less 4 years of age

HOTV cards was used. The presenting visual acuity was taken in all cases and for children less than 4 years age appropriate visual acuity equivalent recorded for analysis. Data were recorded on a customized form, and the cause of visual impairment determined from patient cards with primary diagnosis was taken for all participants with a presenting VA of less than 6/18 for each eye separately.

Operational definition

The WHO categories of visual impairment were used to define vision status for study participants. Blindness was defined as a presenting VA of less than 3/60 in the better eye. Low vision was defined as presenting VA of at least 3/60 but less than 6/18 in the better eye. Monocular visual impairment, which is not a WHO definition, was derived to represent participants who had normal or near-normal vision in the better eye (VA of at least 6/18) and visual impairment in the other eye (VA from 6/18 up to 3/60 for low vision and less than 3/60 for blindness) [13].

Data quality assurance and ethical clearance

After the survey, the investigators reviewed the forms and determined the principal disorder responsible for blindness or low vision for the participant, taking into account the main cause for each individual eye. In the instance when different causes had been identified for each eye separately in a given individual, the principal disorder was chosen to be the one that was most readily curable or, if not curable, most easily preventable. The study was conducted in accordance with declaration of Helsinki and approved by institutional review board of SPHMMC according to Ethiopian national research ethics review guideline. The privacy and confidentially of all subject was secured. The department's usual data quality control is just keeping patients' clinical profile on log book at each clinic. The data for this study was retrieved from those log-books. Institutional review board of SPHMMC stated that obtaining informed consent for participation is not applicable the study based on the secondary data.

Statistical analysis

The collected data was entered twice, carefully cleaned and analyzed using SPSS version 23 (www.ibm.com/products/spss-statistics). Descriptive statistics such as frequency distribution and central tendency measures were used to summarize the descriptive part of the study. Pearson X^2 was used to determine the factors associated with low vision and blindness [14]. P-value less than 0.05 were considered as statistically significant.

Results

A total of 881 study subjects with a response rate of 97.4% were recruited in the study. The study subjects have a mean age of 44.53(SD: ± 21.85), median of 48 with a range of 1–100 years. Among those subjects a quarter 225(25.5%) of them were in the age group of 1–26 years and about half 432(49.0%) of them were male in sex. More than three fourth 684(77.6%) of total subjects address were in urban Table 1.

Among a total study subjects, greater than four fifth 726 (82.4%) of patients have visual acuity in the range of 6/6–6/18 and more than three fourth 470 (77.9%) of patients have intraocular pressure within the range of 9–21 mmHg Table 2.

Of all study subjects about one fifth of them were presented with cataract 181 (20.5%) followed by glaucoma 158 (17.9%) and refractive error 118 (13.4%) Table 3.

A total of 155 (17.6% (95% CI: 15.2, 20.1)) subjects were visually impaired depending on the presenting visual acuity. Among the study subjects, 91 (10.3% (95% CI: 8.2, 12.3)) had low vision and 64 (7.3 95%CI: 5.7, 9.0)) blindness. One hundred sixteen (13.2% (95% CI 10.9, 15.6)) and 170(19.3% (95% CI 17.0, 22.1)) had monocular low vision and blindness respectively.

Low vision and blindness were 42(20.2%) and 34(16.3%) in age group between 63 and 100 years old respectively. Among the subjects presented with refractive error, 14 (11.9%) and 3(2.5%) had low vision and blindness whereas 1(1.4%) and 8(11.1%) traumatic patients had low vision and blindness respectively. The factors such as age (p-value < 0.001), cataract (p-value = 0.002), glaucoma (p-value = 0.002) and age related macular degeneration (p-value < 0.001) were significantly associated with low vision and blindness Table 4.

Table 1 Socio-demographic characteristics of study subjects among patients attending St. Paul's Hospital Millennium Medical College, 2017 ($n = 881$)

Variables	Frequency	Percent
Age		
1–26	225	25.5
27–48	227	25.8
49–62	221	25.1
63–100	208	23.6
Sex		
Male	432	49.0
Female	449	51.0
Address		
Urban	684	77.6
Rural	197	22.4

Table 2 Clinical Characteristics of study subjects among patients attending St. Paul's Hospital Millennium Medical College, 2017

Variables	Frequency	Percent
Visual acuity($n = 881$)		
6/6–6/18	726	82.4
6/24–3/60	91	10.3
< 3/60	64	7.3
Intraocular pressure in mmHg($n = 603$)		
< 8	3	0.5
9–21	470	77.9
> 21	130	21.6

Discussion

Visual impairment, which includes low vision and blindness, remain a public health problem that has impact on socioeconomic values and quality of life of the community. This study was targeted to determine the magnitude and factors of visual impairment under the category of low vision and blindness so that stakeholders will have evidence to plan and implement prevention and management strategies in the hospital and surrounding communities.

In the present study the prevalence of visual impairment was 155 (17.6% (95% CI: 15.2, 20.1)). This finding is higher than other studies conducted within the communities [12, 15, 16]. This indicated that hospital burden of visual impairment is the reflective of community problems. It might also revealed that the patients comes to hospital is usually after their visual function is severely

Table 3 Disease pattern of study subjects among patients attending St. Paul's Hospital Millennium Medical College, 2017 ($n = 881$)

Diseases	Frequency (%)	Presenting VA < 6/18–3/60 (%)	Presenting VA < 3/60 (%)
Cataract	181(20.5)	31(34.1)	15(23.4)
Glaucoma	158(17.9)	20(22.0)	21(23.4)
Refractive error	118(13.4)	14(15.4)	3(4.7)
Pseudophakia	111(12.6)	20(22.0)	6(9.4)
Trauma	72(8.2)	1(1.1)	8(12.5)
ARMD	29(3.3)	11(12.1)	12(18.8)
Strabismus	15(1.7)	2(2.2)	0(0.0)
DR	10(1.1)	1(1.1)	2(3.1)
HR	6(0.7)	0(0.0)	0(0.0)
Uveitis	11(1.2)	1(1.1)	2(3.1)
TCO	6(0.7)	1(1.1)	1(1.6)
NTCO	14(1.6)	2(2.2)	1(1.6)
Others	317(36.0)	1(1.1)	4(6.2)

ARMD age related macular degeneration, *DR* diabetic retinopathy, *HR* hypertensive retinopathy, *TCO* trachomatous corneal opacity, *NTCO* non-trachomatous corneal opacity

Table 4 The factors associated with low vision and blindness among patients attending St. Paul's Hospital Millennium Medical College, 2017 (n = 881)

Variables	Normal	Low vision	Blindness	X^2	p-value
Age				91.76	0.000
1–26	221(93.8%)	8(3.6%)	6(2.7%)		
27–48	210(92.5%)	10(4.4%)	7(3.1%)		
49–62	173(78.3%)	31(14.0%)	17(7.7%)		
63–100	132(63.5%)	42(20.2%)	34(16.3%)		
Sex				3.99	0.14
Male	348(80.6%)	45(10.4%)	39(9.0%)		
Female	378(84.2%)	46(10.2%)	25(5.6%)		
Address				1.38	0.50
Urban	566(82.7%)	72(10.5%)	46(6.7%)		
Rural	160(81.2%)	19(9.6%)	18(9.1%)		
Cataract				12.21	0.002
No	591(84.4%)	60(8.6%)	49(7.0%)		
Yes	135(74.6%)	31(17.1%)	15(8.3%)		
Glaucoma				12.27	0.002
No	609(84.2%)	71(9.8%)	43(5.9%)		
Yes	117(74.1%)	20(12.7%)	21(13.3%)		
Refractive error				4.66	0.1
No	625(81.9%)	77(10.1%)	61(8.0%)		
Yes	101(85.6%)	14(11.9%)	3(2.5%)		
Pseudophakia				8.40	0.02
No	641(83.2%)	71(9.2%)	58(7.5%)		
Yes	85(76.6%)	20(18.0%)	6(5.4%)		
Trauma				7.91	0.02
No	663(82.0%)	90(11.1%)	56(6.9%)		
Yes	63(87.5%)	1(1.4%)	8(11.1%)		
ARMD				84.02	0.000
No	720(84.5%)	80(9.4%)	52(6.1%)		
Yes	6(20.7%)	11(37.9%)	12(41.4%)		
Strabismus				1.28	0.53
No	713(82.3%)	89(10.3%)	64(7.4%)		
Yes	13(86.7%)	2(18.3%)	0		
DR				2.45	0.29
No	719(82.5%)	90(10.3%)	62(7.1%)		
Yes	7(70.0%)	1(10.0%)	2(20.0%)		
HR				1.29	0.53
No	720(82.3%)	91(10.4%)	64(7.3%)		
Yes	6(100%)	0	0		
Uveitis				0.97	0.38
No	718(82.5%)	90(10.3%)	62(7.1%)		
Yes	8(72.7%)	1(9.1%)	2(18.2%)		
TCO				1.15	0.56

Table 4 The factors associated with low vision and blindness among patients attending St. Paul's Hospital Millennium Medical College, 2017 (n = 881) (Continued)

Variables	Normal	Low vision	Blindness	X^2	p-value
No	722(82.5%)	90(10.3%)	63(7.2%)		
Yes	4(66.7%)	1(16.7%)	1(16.7%)		
NTCO				0.24	0.89
No	715(82.5%)	89(10.3%)	63(7.3%)		
Yes	11(78.6%)	2(14.3%)	1(7.1%)		
Others				88.05	0.000
No	414(73.4%)	90(16.0%)	60.3(10.6%)		
Yes	312(98.0%)	1(0.3%)	4(1.3%)		

ARMD age related macular degeneration, DR diabetic retinopathy, HR hypertensive retinopathy, TCO trachomatous corneal opacity, NTCO non-trachomatous corneal opacity

affected which is the common problems of low income population. It is lower than study conducted in South Africa (28.0%) and Ghana (28.2%) [17, 18]. The discrepancy observed here might be due to sampling technique in which they used non-probability sampling. The population difference and eye care service difference at the two centers might also contribute for the different proportion of visual impairment.

Among the study subjects, 91 (10.3% (95% CI: 8.2, 12.3)) had low vision and 64 (7.3 95%CI: 5.7, 9.0)) blindness. This finding indicated that the low vision and blindness is a major public health problem. In comparison to national survey result of low vision (3.7%) and blindness (1.6%) conducted 2005 in Ethiopia this finding is higher as it is hospital based unlike national survey [10]. Though 3 years left to the Vision to 2020 and 'the right to sight' goal, in this study area the burden of the low vision and blindness still high and need strengthening the prevention of avoidable causes of low vision and blindness. This result is consistent with similar study conducted in Gondar Ethiopia (15.3%) [19].

The prevalence of blindness in the study is lower than studies conducted in South Africa (10.9%) and Kenya (39.4%), higher than studies conducted in Cameroon (1.71%) but in line with study reported form Mali (5.8%) and Jordan (13.7%) [17, 20–23]. The low vision is consistent with study report from Nigeria (9.2%) and Cambodia (12%) [24, 25], but lower than South African study (16.3%) [17]. This reflects that there are a lot of factors that can contribute for geographical variations of low vision and blindness such as socio-economic difference, climatic change, gene and ethnical difference, health care service system, number of eye care givers and supportive organizations and not all of those could be investigated in the present study.

The amount of monocular low vision and blindness in this study was (13.2% (95% CI 10.9, 15.6)) and 170(19.3%

(95% CI 17.0, 22.1)) respectively. As the worst visual acuity was considered to define monocular low vision and blindness, it is expected to be higher than bilateral one. This result is higher than study done in Thailand, which reported 3.0% low vision and 4.4% blindness [26]. The discrepancy observed here might be due to different socioeconomic values and eye care seeking behaviors.

The factors associated with low vision and blindness in the current study were age ($<p < 0.001$), cataract ($p = 0.002$), glaucoma ($p = 0.002$) and age related macular degeneration ($p < 0.001$). Age was reported from different clinical and community based studies as the main risk factors for visual impairment, low vision and blindness [27, 28]. However gender was not associated with low vision or blindness like study conducted in Australia [29]. The eye conditions such as cataract, glaucoma, and age related macular degeneration were also reported as the main etiology or causes of low vision and blindness [30]. Factors such as level of education, inability to afford service cost, fear of the outcome of the surgery especially for cataract and glaucoma and cultural beliefs are some of the reason why people remain low in vision and blindness. Those diseases are among either preventable or avoidable disease if they are diagnosed and treated early.

In addition to that uncorrected refractive error, ocular trauma and Pseudophakia were also among the major causes of low vision and blindness. These finding were also reported by different studies in Ethiopia from national survey and Gurage zone [11].

There was some limitation with this study. Most importantly different associated factors were not well explored, as it was hospital based and used secondary data from patients' medical record.

Conclusion
Low vision and blindness found in this study was high. Age, cataract, glaucoma and age related macular degeneration were significantly associated with low vision and blindness. This amount of magnitude will be reduced if prevention, early diagnosis and management will be targeted towards avoidable causes of visual impairment.

Abbreviations
SPHMMC: St. Paul's Hospital Millennium Medical College; VA: Visual acuity; WHO: World Health Organization

Acknowledgments
We would like to thank SPHMMC for financial support.

Funding
The study was funded by SPHMMC and funding was for data collection, processing and write up.

Authors' contributions
SYT designed the study proposal and manage data collection, analysis and secured budget and ethical consideration. FMC developed proposal with SYT and ZYB, analyzed data with DHA and develop manuscript. DHA analyzed the data and developed manuscript with FMC. ZYB participated in proposal writing, review literatures and data collection. All authors have read and approved the final version of the manuscript.

Competing interests
The authors declare that they have no competing interests.

References
1. Pascolini D, Mariotti SPM. Global estimates of visual impairment. British J Ophthalmol. Online first published December 1, 2011 as. 2010; https://doi.org/10.1136/bjophthalmol-2011-300539.
2. Dandona L, Dandona R. Revision of visual impairment definitions in the international statistical classification of diseases. BMC Med. 2006;4:7. https://doi.org/10.1186/1741-7015-4-7.
3. Thylefors B. A simplified methodology for the assessment of blindness and its main causes. World Health Stat Q. 1987;40:129–41.
4. Frick KD, Foster A. The magnitude and cost of global blindness: an increasing problem that can be alleviated. Am J Ophthalmol. 2003;135:471–6.
5. World Health Organization VISION. The right to sight—the global initiative for the elimination of avoidable blindness. Magnitude and causes of visual impairment. Fact Sheet 282.Geneva: World Health Organization; 2020. Available: http://www.who.int/mediacentre/factsheets/fs282/en/index.html. Accessed 20 Oct 2005.
6. Thylefors B. A global initiative for the elimination of avoidable blindness. Am J Ophthalmol. 1998;125:90–3.
7. World Health Organization: Global initiative for the elimination of Avoidable blindness. WHO 2000 document WHO/PBL/97.61 Rev.2. Geneva: World Health Organization. Available: http://whqlibdoc.who.int/hq/2000/WHO_PBL_97.61_Rev.2.pdf. Accessed 20 Oct 2017.
8. World Health Organization. Strategies for the prevention of Blindness in national programmes—a primary health care approach. Geneva: World Health Organization 1997. Available: http://whqlibdoc.who.int/Publications/9241544929.pdf. Accessed 20 Oct 2005.
9. World Health Organization. Prevention of blindness and visual Impairment. 2005. Available: http://www.who.int/blindness/en/. Accessed 20 Oct 2017.
10. Berhane Y, Worku A, Bejiga A, Adamu L, Alemayehu W, Bedir A, et al. Prevalence and causes of low vision and blindness in Ethiopia 2005. Ethiop J Health Dev. 2007;21(3)
11. Melese M, Alemayehu W, Bayu S, Girma T, Hailesellasie TP, et al. Low vision and blindness in adults in Gurage zone, Central Ethiopia. Br J Ophthalmol. 2003;87(6):677–80.
12. Zerihun N, Mabey D. Blindness and low vision in Jimma zone, Ethiopia: results of population based survey. Ophthalmic Epidemiol. 1997;4:19–26.
13. World Health Organization. List of Official ICD-10 Updates Ratified October 2006. Geneva: WHO; 2006. Available from: http://www.who.int/classifications/icd/2006Updates.pdf. [Last cited on 2018 Apr 09].
14. Miller R, Siegmund D. Maximally selected chi-square statistics. Biometrics. 1982;38:11016. https://doi.org/10.2307/2529881.
15. Scheimenn JF, Inocencio F, De Lourdes Monteiro M, Andrade J, Auzemery A, Guelfi Y. Blindness and low vision in Cape Verde Islands: results of national eye survey. Ophthalmic Epidemiol. 2006;13(4):219–26.
16. Saw SM, Husain R, Gazzard GM, Koh D, Widjaja D, Tan DT. Causes of low vision and blindness in rural Indonesia. Br J Ophthalmol. 2003;87(9):1075–8.
17. Maake MM, Oduntan OA. Prevalence and causes of visual impairment in patients seen at Nkhensani hospital eye clinic, South Africa. Afr J Prm Health Care Fam Med. 2015;7(1) https://doi.org/10.4102/phcfm.v7i1.728.
18. Ansah DO. Prevalence and causes of visual impairment among patients in Juaben hospital eye clinic, Ghana. M J Opht. 2017;2(2):017.
19. Woretaw H, Shiferaw D. Prevalence and associated factors of visual impairment and blindness among at University of Gondar teaching hospital, Gondar, Northwest Ethiopia. Int J Pharm H Care Res. 2015;03(02):48–54.
20. Harrel J, Larson ND, Menza E, Mboti A. A clinic-based survey of blindness in Kenya. Community Eye Health J. 2001;14(40):68–9.
21. Eballe OA, Mvongo CE, Koki G, Moune N, Teutu C, Ellong A, et al. Prevalence and causes of blindness at a tertiary hospital in Doula, Cameroon. Clin Ophthalmol. 2011;5:1325–31.

22. Eballé AO, Boitte JP, Traoré J. Ocular disorders causing blindness in working-age outpatients: a prospective study at the African Institute of Tropical Ophthalmology (IOTA, Bamako, Mali). Santé. 2005;15(4):241–5.
23. Al-Bdour MD, All-Till ML, Abu-Khadir IB. Causes of blindness among adult Jordanians: a hospital based study. Eur J Ophthalmol. 2002;12(1):5–10.
24. Malu KN. Blindness and visual impairment in north Central Nigeria: a hospital based study. Niger Postgrad Med J. 2013;20(2):98–103.
25. Thomson I. A clinic based survey of blindness and eye disease in Cambodia. Br J Ophthalmol. 1997;81:578–80.
26. Pathanapitoon K, Ausayakhun S, Kunavisaruth P, Wattananikorn S, Ausayakhun S, Leeungurastien T, et al. Blindness and low vision in teritiary ophthalmologic center in Thailand. The importance of cytomegalovirus retinitis. Retina. 2007;27:635–40.
27. Sijuwola OO, Fasina O. Etiology of visual impairment among ophthalmic patients at federal medical center, Abeokuta, Nigeria. J west Afr Coll Surg. 2012;2(4):38–50.
28. Wang W, Chen N, Sheu M, Wang J, Hsu W, Hu Y. The prevalence and risk factors of visual impairment among the elderly in Eastern Taiwan. Kaohsiung J Med Sci. 2016;32:475–81.
29. Ramke J, Palagyi A, Naduvilath T, Du Toit R, Brian G. Prevalence and causes of visual blindness and low vision in Timor-Leste. Br J Ophthalmol. 2007; 91(9):1117–21.
30. Herse P, Gothwal VK. Survey of visual impairment in an Indian tertiary eye hospital. Indian J Ophthalmol. 1997;45(3):189–93.

21

Toxic anterior segment syndrome-an updated review

Choul Yong Park[1], Jimmy K. Lee[2] and Roy S. Chuck[2*]

Abstract

Background: Toxic anterior segment syndrome (TASS) can be a rare complication of anterior segment surgery. Here we reviewed the most recent advances in the understanding of TASS.

Methods: English articles related to TASS were retrieved from "PubMed" using the following keywords; "toxic anterior segment syndrome" or "TASS". The authors of this paper reviewed all the retrieved literature and critical findings were summarized.

Results: The onset of TASS can vary from hours to months. The clinical manifestations are also variable. The causes of TASS are broad and continue to expand and could not be elucidated in over half of the reported cases. Prompt and thorough investigation to explore the causes of TASS is critical. Surgeons should be fully aware and updated regarding possible etiologies and make ceaseless efforts to prevent TASS. This effort begins with establishing TASS prevention protocols and regularly training surgical staff. Proper cleaning of surgical instruments is critical and should follow the guidelines set by The American Society of Cataract and Refractive Surgery TASS Task Force. When TASS occurs, sharing information with other ophthalmologists and reporting new causes is crucial for the prevention of outbreaks.

Conclusions: Anterior segment surgeons should be reminded that TASS is mostly preventable by the establishment of TASS prevention protocols, regular surgical staff training and thorough adherence to recommendations for cleaning and sterilizing intraocular surgical instruments.

Keywords: Cataract, Toxic, TASS, Anterior chamber, Inflammation

Background

Toxic anterior segment syndrome (TASS) is characterized by sterile postoperative inflammation of anterior segment after intraocular surgery [1, 2]. Although TASS most often occurs after cataract surgery, it has also been reported after keratoplasty and posterior segment surgeries [3–5]. The inflammation can be mild with a minimal cellular reaction or severe enough to cause marked cornea edema and hypopyon. The onset can be acute (within days) or delayed (after several months) [1, 6]. The overall incidence of TASS was found to be 0.22% in a large case series [7]. Additionally, a significant number of reported cases have occurred as clusters of outbreaks [7–11]. In cases of severe TASS, prompt control of inflammation is essential to prevent any permanent damage to delicate ocular structures such as the corneal

endothelium, trabecular meshwork and macula. TASS frequently resembles the symptoms and signs of early postoperative bacterial endophthalmitis and therefore, makes accurate diagnosis challenging [1, 12]. While prompt initiation of oral and fortified topical antibiotics is key to the treatment of bacterial endophthalmitis, TASS usually does not respond to antibiotics and instead requires strong topical or systemic steroids for resolution. However, considering the potential detrimental and irreversible ophthalmic sequelae of bacterial endophthalmitis, most cases of unusual postoperative inflammation after cataract surgery are regarded as infectious endophthalmitis until proven otherwise.

When TASS is suspected, it is important to perform a thorough investigation to determine the causative agent. This investigation should include surgical instruments and disposable medical devices, e.g. ophthalmic viscoelastic agents, medications, surgical drapes, and sterilization

---

* Correspondence: rchuck@montefiore.org
[2]Department of Ophthalmology and Visual Sciences, Montefiore Medical Center, Albert Einstein College of Medicine, Bronx, NY, USA
Full list of author information is available at the end of the article

systems. However, even thorough clinical and laboratory investigations sometimes fail to find the causative agent in many cases of TASS [9].

By heightening professionals' awareness and understanding of TASS, new causes of TASS are reported every year. This updated information should be shared amongst ophthalmic surgeons for effective prevention of TASS. With this report, we attempt to review recent advances in the understanding of TASS. Using the PubMed search engine, the keywords "toxic anterior segment" initially retrieved 125 articles. We excluded 5 articles published before the year 2000 and then screened the title and abstract of the remaining 120 articles. A further 35 articles were excluded from this review due to being irrelevant to our topic, and 13 non-English articles were excluded. Finally, 72 articles were included in this review (see Fig. 1).

Clinical manifestations

TASS is typically characterized by unusual anterior chamber inflammation in the early postoperative period. Depending on the severity of inflammation, other symptoms may be present, such as pain, conjunctival injection or chemosis, hypopyon, corneal edema, keratic precipitates, anterior vitreous opacities, macular edema and visual deterioration [1, 6, 7, 13]. Most reported cases of TASS have been anecdotal, and therefore the clinical manifestations vary widely as shown in Table 1 [9, 10, 14–17]. However, in 2015 and 2017, two large case-series studies ($n = 251$ and $n = 147$) were conducted in Japan [8, 18]. The large sample sizes enabled the estimation of the occurrence rate of key clinical signs related to TASS (see Table 2). Anterior chamber reactions such as cell, flare and fibrin were the most common signs of TASS in these case series. Hypopyon, keratic

precipitates and vitreous opacities were found in less than a quarter of cases.

Although the onset of symptoms and involvement of vitreous was suggested as differentiating points between TASS and infectious endophthalmitis in some studies, the time before the onset of TASS is now known to vary widely [1, 8, 18]. TASS typically starts earlier (within 24 h after surgery) than infectious endophthalmitis (4–7 days after surgery). However, later onset cases are not rare. Miyake et al. reported 6 cases of late-onset TASS occurring 42 to 137 days after surgery [19]. In cases of TASS related to intraocular lens (IOL) contamination, the mean onset time from surgery to TASS was approximately 38 days [18].

Even after successful treatment, eyes with TASS can suffer significant sequelae. Avisar et al. investigated the endothelial morphology of eyes after TASS and found lower cell density, higher cell area and lower percentage of hexagonal cells [20].

Clinicians should be aware that the typical signs of TASS can be masked by strong topical steroids during the early postoperative period. Thus in some cases, TASS can manifest after discontinuation of topical steroids [21].

Etiology

Investigating the causative agent of TASS is difficult and sometimes unsuccessful. In many cases, the exact cause of TASS remains unknown even after a thorough investigation [7, 9]. Sengupta et al. reported that the etiology was not found even after a careful search in approximately 51.7% of TASS cases in their large case series (60 cases after uneventful cataract surgery) [7]. To date, the major causes implicated in TASS include inadequate cleaning of surgical instruments, contamination of surgical instrument or IOLs, and adverse drug reactions [1, 22, 23].

Surgical instrument contamination

The American Society of Cataract and Refractive Surgery (ASCRS) TASS Task Force suggested that improper cleaning of surgical instruments is the most common cause of TASS [2, 22, 24]. Inadequate flushing of hand pieces, the use of enzymatic detergents and the use of ultrasound baths were the most common factors involved in TASS, especially enzymatic detergents for cleaning instrument containing endotoxins, which are not deactivated by autoclave sterilization [1, 23, 24]. It is noteworthy that enzyme remnants still exist at the tip of surgical instruments even after vigorous flushing and rinsing [25]. These enzymes are not inactivated by heat of less than 140 °C and most Statim™ (SciCan, Canonsburg, PA) autoclaves reach temperatures of only 138 °C [26]. The dose-dependent toxicity of enzymatic

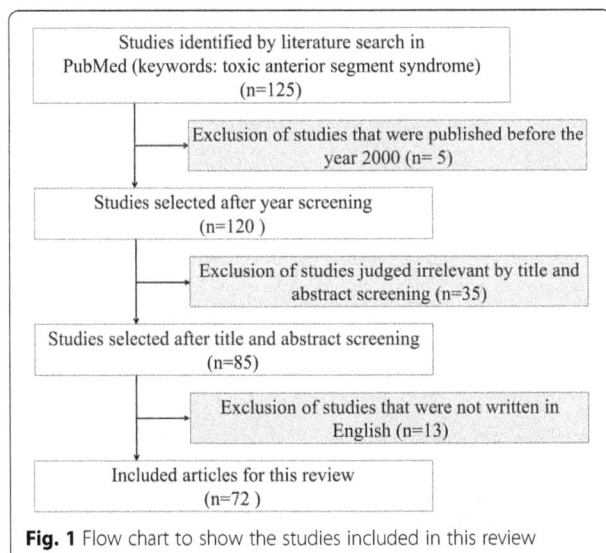

Studies identified by literature search in PubMed (keywords: toxic anterior segment syndrome) (n=125)

Exclusion of studies that were published before the year 2000 (n= 5)

Studies selected after year screening (n=120)

Exclusion of studies judged irrelevant by title and abstract screening (n=35)

Studies selected after title and abstract screening (n=85)

Exclusion of studies that were not written in English (n=13)

Included articles for this review (n=72)

Fig. 1 Flow chart to show the studies included in this review

Table 1 Summary of 15 recent case reports of toxic anterior segment syndrome

First Author (ref. no.)	Number of cases	Onset (days after the surgery)	Inciting agents	Clinical presentations	Managements (n)	Visual outcomes (n)
Miyake et al. [19]	6	42–167	IOL (ISert model 251, Hoya)	Chemosis, Ciliary injection, Decreased BCVA, Corneal edema, Anterior chamber reaction, hypopyon	Vitretomy and IOL removal (1), Capsule irrigation (2), Medical treatment only (5)	BCVA 20/100 (1), BCVA ≥20/30 (5)
Suzuki et al. [18]	251	38.44 ± 32.29 Range:0–161	IOL (ISert model 251 and 255, Hoya)	Anterior chamber reaction (99.2%), conjunctival injection (41.4%) Hypopyon (22.7%) Corneal edema (19.1%) Keratic precipitates (27.9%)	Medical treatment only (142), Surgical intervention: vitrectomy (49), IOL removal (22), chamber irrigation (51)	BCVA 0.036 ± 0.242 logMAR
Sorenson et al. [10]	10	1–7	Bacterial biofilm contamination of autoclave reservoir	Anterior chamber reaction (10), Hypopyon (3), Corneal edema (1), Anterior vitreous reaction (4)	Medical treatment only (3), Vitreous tap and intravitreal injection (7)	No light perception (1), BCVA≥20/30 (9)
Ohika et al. [8]	147	13.1 ± 16.4 Range: 1–88	IOL (Acrysof, Alcon)	Anterior chamber reaction (97.2%), Conjunctival injection (39.8%), Fibrinous inflammation (43.1%) Hypopyon (22.7%) Corneal edema (15.6%) Keratic precipitates (21.6%), Ocular pain (9.5%)	Medical treatment only (104), Surgical intervention: vitrectomy (21), IOL removal (10), chamber irrigation (33)	BCVA> 20/40 (143), BCVA≤20/40 (4)
Moyle et al. [9]	11	1	unknown	Corneal edema (11), anterior chamber reaction (10), Inflammatory plaque on IOL (5), hypopyon (3), fibrin reaction (6), mild pain (2)	Medical treatment only (11)	BCVA = 20/20 (11)
Sengupta et al. [7]	60	1	Balanced salt solution with a low pH of 6.0 (12), OVD (17), unknown (31)	Severe iridocyclitis with varying degree of corneal edema (60)	Medical treatment only (56), Vitreous tap (4)	BCVA: 0.11 ± 0.1 logMAR, range: 0–0.3 logMAR
Matsou et al. [36]	5	1	Generic trypan blue	Painless blurry vision, corneal edema, anterior chamber reaction, hypopyon and fibrin reaction	Medical treatment only (5)	BCVA: 0.82 ± 0.18 (Snellen acuity)
Bielory et al. [14]	2	1	intracameral lidocaine HCl 1% and phenylephrine 2.5% inadvertently preserved with 10% benzalkonium chloride.	Acute corneal decompensation (3)	Medical treatment only (1), Corneal transplantation for decompensated cornea (2)	BCVA = 20/20 (1), NA (1)
Althomali [38]	15	1–2	OVD	Corneal edema (15), hypopyon (8)	Medical treatment only	BCVA: count finger (2) (other retina pathology), BCVA: 20/70 (2), BCVA≥20/50 (11)
Koban et al. [16]	1	1	Inadvertent overdose of intracameral gentamicin	Hyphema, corneal edema, chemosis, hemorrhagic fibrinous reaction, Corneal decompensation	Penetrating keratoplasty after medical treatment	BCVA: 20/60
Cetinkaya et al. [54]	5	1	unknown	corneal edema (5), anterior chamber reaction (5), fibrin (3), hypopyon (3), increased intraocular pressure (3)	Penetrating keratoplasty (2)	BCVA: 20/100 (1), BCVA: 20/40 (1),

Table 1 Summary of 15 recent case reports of toxic anterior segment syndrome *(Continued)*

First Author (ref. no.)	Number of cases	Onset (days after the surgery)	Inciting agents	Clinical presentations	Managements (n)	Visual outcomes (n)
						BCVA≥20/30 (3)
Ari et al. [27]	19 (pediatric patients)	1–2	Ethylene oxide gas sterilization	Corneal edema, anterior chamber reaction,	Medical treatment only (18), Penetrating keratoplasty (1)	NA
Buzard et al. [15]	2	1	Generic trypan blue	Cornea edema, anterior chamber reaction, hypopyon	Penetrating keratoplasty (2)	NA
Maier et al. [5]	24	1–2	Contamination of corneal trephine	Graft infiltration, corneal stromal edema	Medical treatment only (24)	NA
Choi et al. [28]	15	NA	Ethylene oxide gas sterilization	Corneal edema, anterior chamber reaction, conjunctival injection, pupil irregularity, fibrin reaction	Penetrating keratoplasty (5)	BCVA≥20/200 (14), Light perception (1),

IOL intraocular lens, *BCVA* best corrected visual acuity, *NA* not available, *n* case number

detergents in corneal endothelium has previously been verified in animal models [26]. Therefore, the ASCRS Task Force on Ophthalmic Instrument Cleaning and Sterilization recommended avoiding the use of enzymatic detergents for ophthalmic instrument cleaning [24]. Additionally, ethylene oxide gas sterilization of surgical tubing lines resulted in severe TASS in 13 and 15 patients, respectively [27, 28]. Moreover, bacterial biofilm contamination of autoclave reservoirs can produce heat stable bacterial toxins continuously and contaminate surgical instruments during autoclaving [10].

Intracameral injection

Corneal endothelial toxicity and TASS are potential concerns following the intracameral injection of any pharmacologic agents. Drug components, inadvertent dilution with causative agents, preservatives, abnormal pH, or increased osmolality are all possible causes of TASS [29]. In addition, Lockington et al. found free radicals present in 19 commonly used intracameral drug preparations including phenylephrine, cefuroxime, lidocaine and bevacizumab [30]. These free radicals can induce a dose dependent cellular damage. Previously, the inadvertent use of a balanced salt solution with a low pH of

Table 2 Clinical manifestation of toxic anterior segment syndrome in large-scale outbreak studies

Clinical manifestation	Suzuki et al. [18] (n:251)	Oshika et al. [8] (n:147)	Endophthalmitis vitrectomy study [12] (n:420)
Onset after surgery (day)	38.44 ± 32.29 days Range:0–161	13.1 ± 16.4 days Range: 1–88	6 days Range: 1–63
Pain	NA	9.5%	74.3%
Blurred vision	NA	NA	94.3%
Lid swelling	NA	NA	34.5%
Injection and/or chemosis	41.4%	39.8%	82.1%
Corneal edema	19.1%	15.6%	NA
Anterior chamber fibrin reaction or membrane formation	26.7%	43.1%	NA
Anterior chamber cell and/or flare	99.2%	Cells (97.2%), flare (63.0)	NA
Hypopyon	22.7%	10.6%	85.7%
Keratic precipitates	27.9%	21.6%	NA
Anterior vitreous opacities	21.5%	23.8%	NA
Media opacity	NA	NA	99.5%
Red reflex present	NA	NA	32.0%
Macular edema or other retinal abnormalities	NA	3.8%	NA

NA not available
The last column refers clinical manifestation of endophthalmitis for the comparative purpose

6.0 resulted in 12 cases of TASS in an outbreak [7]. Recently, Bielory et al. reported that the inadvertent intracameral injection of lidocaine HCl 1% and phenyl-ephrine 2.5% preserved with 10% benzalkonium chloride resulted in severe TASS with irreversible corneal decom-pensation [14]. Koban et al. reported that inadvertent intracameral injection of a high dose (20 mg/0.5 ml) of gentamicin, prepared for subconjunctival injection, in-duced severe TASS and bullous keratopathy [16]. It is also possible that small amounts of gentamicin can access the anterior chamber through surgical incisions after subconjunctival placement [17]. Although it is de-bated, TASS after intracameral injection of cefuroxime has also been reported [31, 32]. Balanced salt solution (BSS) contamination can be another risk factor for TASS. Andonegui et al. reported five cases of TASS after using BSS prepared in a hospital pharmacy [33]. Inad-vertent seeping of ophthalmic ointment into the anterior chamber has also been implicated in causing TASS [34].

Indocyanine green dye and trypan blue for lens capsule staining

Anterior lens capsule staining with dyes such as indocya-nine green or trypan blue has generally been accepted as a safe and effective method to improve the visualization during capsulorhexis [35]. However, dye agents used for anterior capsule staining can become contaminated dur-ing the manufacturing process. Matsou et al. reported five cases of TASS and Buzard et al. reported two cases after using a generic trypan blue for capsule staining [15, 36]. Tandogan et al. investigated the toxic effect of indocyanin green in the anterior chamber of a rabbit [37]. Higher concentrations and longer exposure times have been thought to result in severe inflammation mimicking TASS.

Ophthalmic viscosurgical devices

Contamination or denaturation of ophthalmic viscosur-gical devices (OVDs) can be a potential cause of TASS. Suspicious batches of OVDs evoked 17 and 15 cases of TASS in separate studies [7, 38]. Contamination by endotoxin during manufacturing was suspected in cases where the OVDs were derived from bacterial fermenta-tion. Thus the need for guidelines for endotoxin limits in ophthalmic preparations has been proposed [38, 39].

.Traces of OVD residue attached to surgical instru-ments are sometimes not removed completely during cleaning and can denature to become toxic material. OVD denaturation can occur due to inappropriate hand-ling during shipping and storage. Recently, another large outbreak (34 cases in 2 weeks) of TASS, possibly related to OVD, was reported [40]. In this case series, utilization of new OVDs prevented further occurrence of TASS.

Intraocular lens contamination

Recently heavy metal, such as aluminum, contamination during manufacturing of IOLs was proposed as a pos-sible cause of massive (147 cases) outbreak of subacute TASS in Japan [8]. In another report, 251 cases of late onset TASS were related to a particular type of IOL [18]. Other anecdotal cases of TASS related to IOLs have also been reported [19, 41].

Patient's clinical characteristics

Patients' factors can also contribute to TASS develop-ment. Yazqan et al. investigated the systemic disease profile in TASS patients compared to controls. They found that type 2 diabetes mellitus, systemic hyperten-sion, hyperlipidemia, chronic ischemic heart disease, and chronic renal failure were significantly more common in TASS patients [42].

Evaluation for etiology

In cases of a TASS outbreak in a single institution, it is recommended that the surgical facility halts operations and immediately initiate a thorough investigation. It is important to share suspected TASS cases with other ophthalmic surgeons using the same surgical facility. By doing this, the incidence can be contained. It is also rec-ommended that outbreaks be announced to outside sur-geons in the same or different regions to share information and find any possible clues to explain re-gional outbreaks originating from IOLs or OVDs. All surgical staff members should be interviewed and any purposeful or inadvertent changes to their protocol should be investigated as shown in Fig. 2 [9].

For laboratory evaluation, aqueous tapping for micro-bial studies is recommended. Especially in severe cases of TASS, differentiating between bacterial endophthalmi-tis and TASS is a critical step in the treatment algorithm. Vitreous involvement is more common in bacterial endophthalmitis and, in this case, vitreous tapping is also necessary. However, Gram stain and culture are often negative in some infectious endophthalmitis [43]. While waiting for microbial culture and sensitivity results, any recent changes in the surgical setup such IOLs, OVDs, solutions, surgical drapes, latex gloves, moving to a new operating room, using a new sterilization system or new phacoemulsification platform should be investigated as possible sources of contamination. Consulting infection prevention teams inside the hospital can be helpful. Bacterial culture screening of operating rooms, operating tables and surgical microscopes can provide important additional information after positive microbial test re-sults. Obtaining cultures from sterilization systems is also essential for ruling out any contamination by heat stable bacterial toxins.

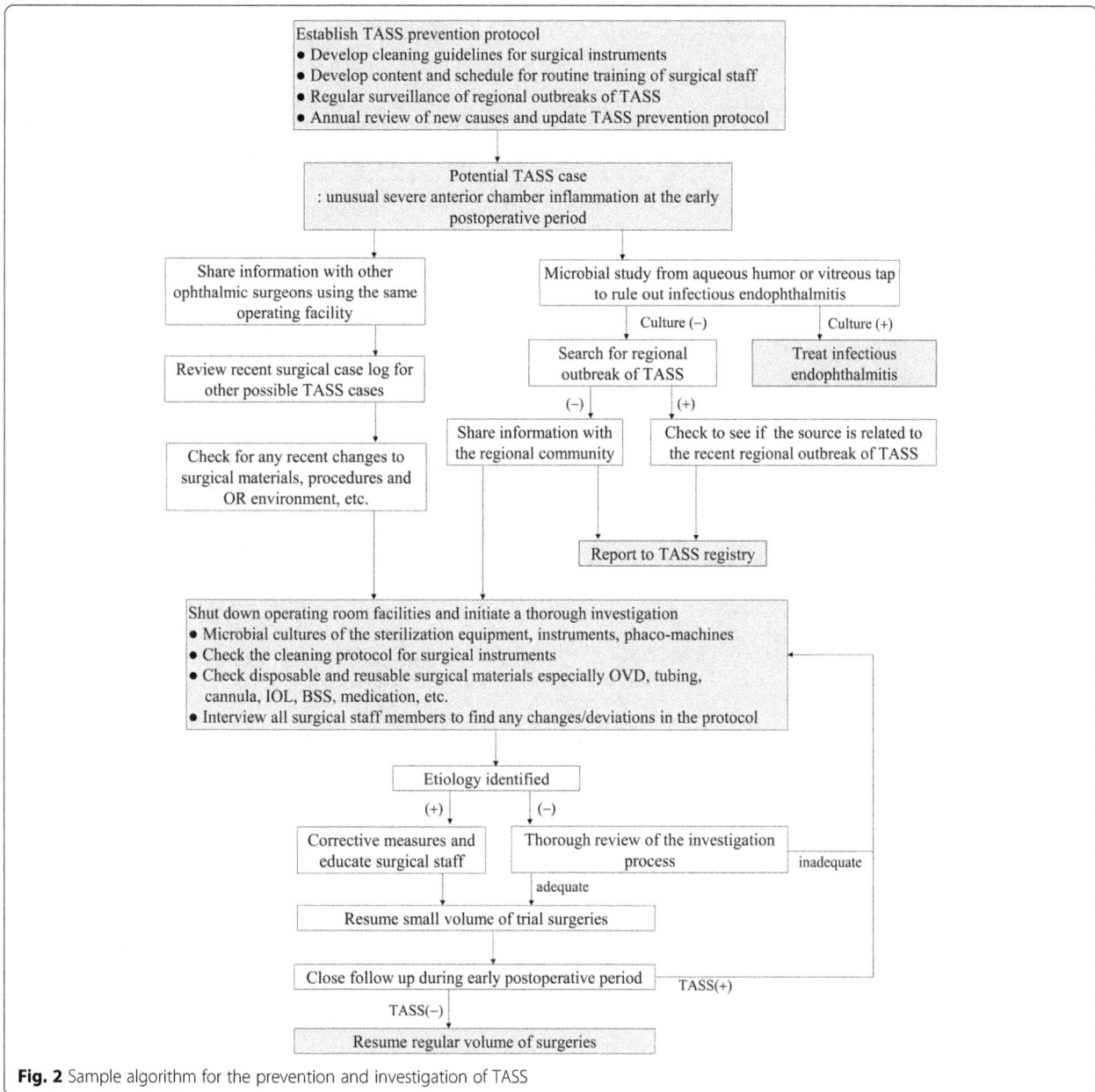

Fig. 2 Sample algorithm for the prevention and investigation of TASS

Suspected TASS cases should be reported to the TASS Registry (www.ascrs.org/tass-registry) run by the ASCRS. The website provides useful information such as TASS guidelines, a free link to the "Instrument Re-Processing and Product Questionnaire" (www.tassregistry.org/tass--combined-survey.cfm) developed by the ASCRS, and the quick link for the voluntary reporting of TASS to the Food and Drug Administration (FDA).

Prevention

The most important step for preventing TASS is raising awareness. It is very helpful to establish TASS prevention protocols and regularly train surgical staff. In the event of a

TASS outbreak, this established protocol can be a valuable guideline to determine possible etiologies.

The use of preservative-free medications is important as well. The instillation of ophthalmic ointment after cataract surgery has largely been abandoned due to the risk of TASS by inadvertent entry into the anterior chamber.

Adequate cleaning and sterilization of ophthalmic surgical instruments are crucial to prevent TASS. The ASCRS, American Academy of Ophthalmology and American Society of Ophthalmic Registered Nurses participated in the joint TASS Task Force and published guidelines on how to clean and sterilize intraocular surgical instruments to prevent TASS [44].

Table 3 Recommendations for cleaning and sterilizing intraocular surgical instruments modified from the guideline proposed by ASCRS, AAO and ASORN [44]

Ensure adequate time for thorough cleaning and sterilization of instrument

•Rigorous adherence to recommended procedures for cleaning and sterilization
•Sufficient inventory of instruments to meet surgical volume and to provide adequate time for cleaning and sterilization

Follow manufacturer's directions for use for cleaning and sterilization

Ophthalmic viscosurgical device solutions should not be allowed to dry on instruments

•Instruments should be rinsed with sterile water immediately following the use

Used instruments should be transported from the operating room in a closed container to the decontamination area

Whenever possible, use disposable instruments and/or tubing and then discard after each use.

•Do not reuse devices labeled for single use only.

Clean intraocular instruments separately from non-intraocular surgical instruments.

Avoid using enzymatic detergents for the cleaning of intraocular instruments.

•When the use of enzymatic detergents is necessary, instruments should be thoroughly rinsed with copious volumes of water to remove all detergent.

Ultrasonic cleaners should be emptied, cleaned, disinfected, rinsed and dried at least daily and preferably after each use.

Do not reuse manual cleaning tools unless designed for reuse.

•If brushes are reused, they should be designed for reuse and cleaned and treated with high-level disinfection or sterilization, preferably after each use, or at least once daily.

Rinsing should provide flow of water through or over instruments and agitation in a basin of water should not be used.

•Following thorough rinsing, instruments with lumens should be dried with forced or compressed air.

If reusable woven materials are used for draping or wrapping trays or instruments, they should be laundered thoroughly between each use to eliminate surgical compounds, debris, and cleaning agents.

Cleanliness and integrity of instruments should be verified.

Sterilization

•Glutaraldehyde is not recommended because of the toxicity of glutaraldehyde residues.
•Low temperature methods of sterilization should not be used unless validated by the instrument manufacturer.
•Regular autoclave sterilizers are preferred over Statim™ sterilizers because higher temperatures up to 190 °C can be reached.
•Verification of sterilizer function should be completed at least weekly, preferably daily.

Have a written policy in place for protocols for what happens to the instruments prior to and after each case in accordance with the manufacturer's instructions.

(Table 3) Switching to single-use disposable instruments is also an effective way to prevent contaminating instruments during cleaning and sterilization.

Treatment of TASS

Topical steroids are the mainstay treatment of TASS. In mild cases of TASS, frequent instillation (4 to 8 times per day) of a potent steroid, particularly 1% prednisolone acetate or alternatively dexamethasone 0.1% can be the initial choice of treatment [5, 9, 27, 36, 38]. Subconjunctival dexamethasone injection can be used when the effect of topical steroid is limited. In cases of severe TASS with dense fibrin and hypopyon, oral prednisolone up to 40 mg per day can be necessary to control the inflammation [19]. A topical NSAID can be added for pain control. Microbial culture can be negative in up to 30% of bacterial endophthalmitis [45]. Therefore, the combined use of broad spectrum antibiotics such as moxifloxacin is recommended, especially when the severe inflammation hinders the discrimination between TASS and bacterial endophthalmitis. In patients with severe fibrin reaction which is refractory to conventional steroid treatment, intracameral injection of recombinant tissue type plasminogen activator (25 μg/0.1 ml) can be effective [46]. Close follow up of the patient is critical to ensure that the inflammation responds to treatment. In cases where inflammation worsens with treatment, a repeat culture is recommended to rule out missed infectious endophthalmitis. Surgical interventions such as anterior chamber washout, vitrectomy or IOL removal can be performed according to the surgeon's discretion, especially if the inflammation persist despite adequate medical treatment [8]. Ohika et al. and Suzuki et al. reported 29.3% and 43.4% of TASS cases, respectively, required surgical intervention such as anterior chamber irrigation, anterior vitrectomy, vitrectomy and IOL removal in their large case series [8, 18].

Mild cases of TASS usually resolve without any complications. However, irreversible corneal endothelial damage and decompensation by uncontrolled severe TASS may require corneal transplantation. Endothelial keratoplasty is an effective way to replace decompensated corneal endothelium after severe TASS [47, 48]. Kaur et al. reported that the time interval between TASS and endothelial keratoplasty is critical for successful surgical outcomes [49]. In their report, a time interval of less than 3 months (3cases) resulted in high rate of graft failure, while 12 cases with time intervals greater than 3 months resulted in 100% successful outcomes. Therefore, the surgeon should be prudent in deciding the timing of endothelial keratoplasty. In cases of secondary glaucoma following TASS, anti-glaucoma medications and, sometimes, glaucoma surgery is needed [28, 34]. Cystoid macular edema can occur due to TASS and this may require intraocular steroids or anti-VEGF injection treatment [13].

Visual outcome

As expected, prompt diagnosis and initiation of appropriate treatment determine the visual prognosis of TASS. By quickly resolving the diagnosis and treatment, irreversible damage to the corneal endothelium, trabecular meshwork and macula can be minimized. Visual outcomes of TASS seem to be relatively good with appropriate treatment [7, 8, 18]. Sengupta et al. reported that 58 out of 60 TASS eyes achieved a best corrected visual acuity of 6/9 or better on 1 month after treatment; however, significant numbers of eyes were complicated by atrophic iris (24%), posterior capsule opacification (16%), severe anterior capsular phimosis (12.5%) and cystoid macular edema (4%) 6 months after treatment [7]. Suzuki et al. reported the visual prognosis of all patients with IOL- related TASS was good with no single case of severe visual deterioration [18]. Oshika et al. reported only 2 out of 201 TASS cases resulted in best corrected visual acuity deterioration to 20/50 and 20/100, respectively, and those were due to macular edema after TASS treatment [8].

However, it is likely that the visual outcome after TASS treatment is dependent on the etiology. TASS caused by inadvertent intracameral drug injection may result in irreversible corneal damage and poor visual prognosis. TASS related to the exposure of an intraocular instrument to glutaraldehyde (2%) resulted in irreversible corneal decompensation in 100% of affected eyes [50]. Accidental use of methylene blue for capsule staining and accidental intracameral entry of gentamicin also resulted in irreversible corneal decompensation [16, 51, 52]. Bielory et al. reported 2 out of 3 TASS cases related to the inadvertent injection of 10% benzalkonium chloride containing medication needed corneal transplantation [14]. Werner et al. reported 3 out of 8 TASS cases caused by inadvertent seeping of antibiotic-steroid ointment into the anterior chamber resulted in corneal decompensation [34].

Some TASS cases caused by gas sterilization also showed poor visual outcomes. Choi et al. and Smith et al. reported 5 out of 15 TASS cases related to ethylene oxide gas sterilization and 6 out of 10 related to plasma gas sterilization required penetrating keratoplasty due to corneal decompensation, respectively [28, 53].

Conclusions

Albeit rare, TASS can perplex ophthalmic surgeons and result in unfortunate outcomes. Whenever TASS is suspected, a thorough investigation of possible etiologies is critical, as is sharing the information with colleagues. TASS can occur anytime and unexpectedly. However, anterior segment surgeons should be aware that TASS is mostly preventable by the establishment of TASS prevention protocols, regular training, and thorough adherence to recommendations for cleaning and sterilizing intraocular surgical instruments.

Abbreviations
BSS: Balanced salt solution; IOL: Intraocular lens; OVD: Ophthalmic viscoelastic device; TASS: Toxic anterior segment syndrome

Acknowledgements
Publication of this article was supported in by a grant of the Korea Health Technology R&D Project through the Korea Health Industry Development Institute (KHIDI), funded by the Ministry of Health & Welfare, Republic of Korea (Grant number: HI-15C1653).

Funding
This work was supported in part by a grant of the Korea Health Technology R&D Project through the Korea Health Industry Development Institute (KHIDI), funded by the Ministry of Health & Welfare, Republic of Korea (Grant number: HI-15C1653).

Authors' contributions
CYP, JKL and RSC were responsible for the conception and design of this review. CYP and JKL acquired the data. CYP, JKL and RSC analyzed and interpreted the data. CYP and JKL wrote the draft. RSC and JKL revised the manuscript critically. All authors have read and approved the final manuscript.

Author details
[1]Department of Ophthalmology, Dongguk University, Ilsan Hospital, Goyang, South Korea. [2]Department of Ophthalmology and Visual Sciences, Montefiore Medical Center, Albert Einstein College of Medicine, Bronx, NY, USA.

References
1. Bodnar Z, Clouser S, Mamalis N. Toxic anterior segment syndrome: update on the most common causes. J Cataract Refract Surg. 2012;38(11):1902–10.
2. Mamalis N. Toxic anterior segment syndrome update. J Cataract Refract Surg. 2010;36(7):1067–8.
3. Sevimli N, Karadag R, Cakici O, Bayramlar H, Okumus S, Sari U. Toxic anterior segment syndrome following deep anterior lamellar keratoplasty. Arq Bras Oftalmol. 2016;79(5):330–2.
4. Moisseiev E, Barak A. Toxic anterior segment syndrome outbreak after vitrectomy and silicone oil injection. Eur J Ophthalmol. 2012;22(5):803–7.
5. Maier P, Birnbaum F, Bohringer D, Reinhard T. Toxic anterior segment syndrome following penetrating keratoplasty. Arch Ophthalmol. 2008; 126(12):1677–81.
6. Mamalis N, Edelhauser HF, Dawson DG, Chew J, LeBoyer RM, Werner L. Toxic anterior segment syndrome. J Cataract Refract Surg. 2006;32(2): 324–33.
7. Sengupta S, Chang DF, Gandhi R, Kenia H, Venkatesh R. Incidence and long-term outcomes of toxic anterior segment syndrome at Aravind eye hospital. J Cataract Refract Surg. 2011;37(9):1673–8.

8. Oshika T, Eguchi S, Goto H, Ohashi Y. Outbreak of subacute-onset toxic anterior segment syndrome associated with single-piece acrylic intraocular lenses. Ophthalmology. 2017;124:519–23.

9. Moyle W, Yee RD, Burns JK, Biggins T. Two consecutive clusters of toxic anterior segment syndrome. Optom Vis Sci. 2013;90(1):e11–23.

10. Sorenson AL, Sorenson RL, Evans DJ. Toxic anterior segment syndrome caused by autoclave reservoir wall biofilms and their residual toxins. J Cataract Refract Surg. 2016;42(11):1602–14.

11. Kutty PK, Forster TS, Wood-Koob C, Thayer N, Nelson RB, Berke SJ, Pontacolone L, Beardsley TL, Edelhauser HF, Arduino MJ, et al. Multistate outbreak of toxic anterior segment syndrome, 2005. J Cataract Refract Surg. 2008;34(4):585–90.

12. Results of the Endophthalmitis Vitrectomy Study. A randomized trial of immediate vitrectomy and of intravenous antibiotics for the treatment of postoperative bacterial endophthalmitis. Endophthalmitis Vitrectomy study group. Arch Ophthalmol. 1995;113(12):1479–96.

13. Ugurbas SC, Akova YA. Toxic anterior segment syndrome presenting as isolated cystoid macular edema after removal of entrapped ophthalmic ointment. Cutan Ocul Toxicol. 2010;29(3):221–3.

14. Bielory BP, Shariff A, Hussain RM, Bermudez-Magner JA, Dubovy SR, Donaldson KE. Toxic anterior segment syndrome: inadvertent Administration of Intracameral Lidocaine 1% and phenylephrine 2.5% preserved with 10% Benzalkonium chloride during cataract surgery. Cornea. 2017;36:621–4.

15. Buzard K, Zhang JR, Thumann G, Stripecke R, Sunalp M. Two cases of toxic anterior segment syndrome from generic trypan blue. J Cataract Refract Surg. 2010;36(12):2195–9.

16. Koban Y, Genc S, Bilgin G, Cagatay HH, Ekinci M, Gecer M, Yazar Z. Toxic anterior segment syndrome following phacoemulsification secondary to overdose of Intracameral gentamicin. Case Rep Med. 2014;2014:143564.

17. Litwin AS, Pimenides D. Toxic anterior segment syndrome after cataract surgery secondary to subconjunctival gentamicin. J Cataract Refract Surg. 2012;38(12):2196–7.

18. Suzuki T, Ohashi Y, Oshika T, Goto H, Hirakata A, Fukushita K, Miyata K, Japanese ophthalmological society HIL-REIC. Outbreak of late-onset toxic anterior segment syndrome after implantation of one-piece intraocular lenses. Am J Ophthalmol. 2015;159(5):934–939 e932.

19. Miyake G, Ota I, Miyake K, Zako M, Iwaki M, Shibuya A. Late-onset toxic anterior segment syndrome. J Cataract Refract Surg. 2015;41(3):666–9.

20. Avisar R, Weinberger D. Corneal endothelial morphologic features in toxic anterior segment syndrome. Cornea. 2010;29(3):251–3.

21. Lee SN. Mild toxic anterior segment syndrome mimicking delayed onset toxic anterior segment syndrome after cataract surgery. Indian J Ophthalmol. 2014;62(8):890–2.

22. Mamalis N. Toxic anterior segment syndrome. J Cataract Refract Surg. 2006; 32(2):181–2.

23. Cutler Peck CM, Brubaker J, Clouser S, Danford C, Edelhauser HE, Mamalis N. Toxic anterior segment syndrome: common causes. J Cataract Refract Surg. 2010;36(7):1073–80.

24. Mamalis N. Toxic anterior segment syndrome: role of enzymatic detergents used in the cleaning of intraocular surgical instruments. J Cataract Refract Surg. 2016;42(9):1249–50.

25. Tsaousis KT, Werner L, Reiter N, Perez JP, Li HJ, Guan JJ, Mamalis N. Comparison of different types of phacoemulsification tips. II. Morphologic alterations induced by multiple steam sterilization cycles with and without use of enzyme detergents. J Cataract Refract Surg. 2016;42(9):1353–60.

26. Parikh C, Sippy BD, Martin DF, Edelhauser HF. Effects of enzymatic sterilization detergents on the corneal endothelium. Arch Ophthalmol. 2002;120(2):165–72.

27. Ari S, Caca I, Sahin A, Cingu AK. Toxic anterior segment syndrome subsequent to pediatric cataract surgery. Cutan Ocul Toxicol. 2012;31(1):53–7.

28. Choi JS, Shyn KH. Development of toxic anterior segment syndrome immediately after uneventful phaco surgery. Korean J Ophthalmol. 2008; 22(4):220–7.

29. Braga-Mele R, Chang DF, Henderson BA, Mamalis N, Talley-Rostov A, Vasavada A, Committee ACC. Intracameral antibiotics: safety, efficacy, and preparation. J Cataract Refract Surg. 2014;40(12):2134–42.

30. Lockington D, Macdonald EC, Young D, Stewart P, Caslake M, Ramaesh K. Presence of free radicals in intracameral agents commonly used during cataract surgery. Br J Ophthalmol. 2010;94(12):1674–7.

31. Cakir B, Celik E, Aksoy NO, Bursali O, Ucak T, Bozkurt E, Alagoz G. Toxic anterior segment syndrome after uncomplicated cataract surgery possibly associated with intracamaral use of cefuroxime. Clin Ophthalmol. 2015;9:493–7.

32. Gardner S, Barry P, Cordoves L. Toxic anterior segment syndrome and intracameral injection of cefuroxime axetil. Clin Ophthalmol. 2015;9:1865–7.

33. Andonegui J, Jimenez-Lasanta L, Aliseda D, Lameiro F. Outbreak of toxic anterior segment syndrome after vitreous surgery. Arch Soc Esp Oftalmol. 2009;84(8):403–5.

34. Werner L, Sher JH, Taylor JR, Mamalis N, Nash WA, Csordas JE, Green G, Maziarz EP, Liu XM. Toxic anterior segment syndrome and possible association with ointment in the anterior chamber following cataract surgery. J Cataract Refract Surg. 2006;32(2):227–35.

35. Jacobs DS, Cox TA, Wagoner MD, Ariyasu RG, Karp CL, American Academy of O, ophthalmic technology assessment committee anterior segment P. Capsule staining as an adjunct to cataract surgery: a report from the American Academy of ophthalmology. Ophthalmology. 2006;113(4):707–13.

36. Matsou A, Tzamalis A, Chalvatzis N, Mataftsi A, Tsinopoulos I, Brazitikos P. Generic trypan blue as possible cause of a cluster of toxic anterior segment syndrome cases after uneventful cataract surgery. J Cataract Refract Surg. 2017;43(6):848–52.

37. Tandogan T, Khoramnia R, Uwe Auffarth G, Janusz Koss M, Young Choi C. Impact of Indocyanine green concentration, exposure time, and degree of dissolution in creating toxic anterior segment syndrome: evaluation in a rabbit model. J Ophthalmol. 2016;2016:3827050.

38. Althomali TA. Viscoelastic substance in prefilled syringe as an etiology of toxic anterior segment syndrome. Cutan Ocul Toxicol. 2016;35(3):237–41.

39. Kremer I, Levinger E, Levinger S. Toxic anterior segment syndrome following iris-supported phakic IOL implantation with viscoelastic Multivisc BD. Eur J Ophthalmol. 2010;20(2):451–3.

40. Altintas AK, Ciritoglu MY, Beyazyildi ZO, Can CU, Polat S. Toxic anterior segment syndrome outbreak after cataract surgery triggered by viscoelastic substance. Middle East Afr J Ophthalmol. 2017;24(1):43–7.

41. Kumaran N, Larkin G, Hollick EJ. Sterile postoperative endophthalmitis following HOYA IOL insertion. Eye. 2014;28(11):1382.

42. Yazgan S, Celik U, Ayar O, Ugurbas SH, Celik B, Akdemir MO, Ugurbas SC, Alpay A. The role of patient's systemic characteristics and plateletcrit in developing toxic anterior segment syndrome after uneventful phaco surgery: a case-control study. Int Ophthalmol. 2018;38(1):43–52.

43. Rahmani S, Eliott D. Postoperative Endophthalmitis: a review of risk factors, prophylaxis, incidence, microbiology, treatment, and outcomes. Semin Ophthalmol. 2018;33(1):95–101.

44. American Society of C, Refractive S, American Society of Ophthalmic Registered N, Hellinger WC, Bacalis LP, Edelhauser HF, Mamalis N, Milstein B, Masket S, Cleaning AAHTFo, et al. Recommended practices for cleaning and sterilizing intraocular surgical instruments. J Cataract Refract Surg. 2007; 33(6):1095–100.

45. Durand ML. Endophthalmitis. Clin Microbiol Infect. 2013;19(3):227–34.

46. Dotan A, Kaiserman I, Kremer I, Ehrlich R, Bahar I. Intracameral recombinant tissue plasminogen activator (r-tPA) for refractory toxic anterior segment syndrome. Br J Ophthalmol. 2014;98(2):252–5.

47. Pineda R 2nd, Jain V, Gupta P, Jakobiec FA. Descemet's stripping endothelial keratoplasty: an effective treatment for toxic anterior segment syndrome with histopathologic findings. Cornea. 2010;29(6):694–7.

48. Arslan OS, Unal M, Arici C, Gorgun E, Yenerel M, Cicik E. Descemet-stripping automated endothelial keratoplasty in eyes with toxic anterior segment syndrome after cataract surgery. J Cataract Refract Surg. 2010;36(6):965–9.

49. Kaur M, Titiyal JS, Falera R, Arora T, Sharma N. Outcomes of Descemet stripping automated endothelial Keratoplasty in toxic anterior segment syndrome after phacoemulsification. Cornea. 2017;36(1):17–20.

50. Unal M, Yucel I, Akar Y, Oner A, Altin M. Outbreak of toxic anterior segment syndrome associated with glutaraldehyde after cataract surgery. J Cataract Refract Surg. 2006;32(10):1696–701.

51. Lim AK, Ulagantheran W, Siow YC, Lim KS. Methylene blue related sterile endophthalmitis. Med J Malaysia. 2008;63(3):249–50.

52. Brouzas D, Droutsas D, Charakidas A, Malias I, Georgiadou E, Apostolopoulos M, Moschos M. Severe toxic effect of methylene blue 1% on iris epithelium and corneal endothelium. Cornea. 2006;25(4):470–1.

53. Smith CA, Khoury JM, Shields SM, Roper GJ, Duffy RE, Edelhauser HF, Lubniewski AJ. Unexpected corneal endothelial cell decompensation after intraocular surgery with instruments sterilized by plasma gas. Ophthalmology. 2000;107(8):1561–6 discussion 1567.

54. Cetinkaya S, Dadaci Z, Aksoy H, Acir NO, Yener HI, Kadioglu E. Toxic anterior-segment syndrome (TASS). Clin Ophthalmol. 2014;8:2065–9.

22

Influence of pterygium size on corneal higher-order aberration evaluated using anterior-segment optical coherence tomography

Keiichiro Minami[1]* ⓘ, Tadatoshi Tokunaga[1], Keiichiro Okamoto[2], Kazunori Miyata[1] and Tetsuro Oshika[3]

Abstract

Background: The prospective observation study aimed to evaluate changes in corneal higher-order aberrations induced by advancement of pterygium using an anterior-segment optical coherence tomography (AS-OCT) and Zernike aberration analysis.

Methods: The corneal topography of 284 eyes with primary pterygia originating from the nasal region was measured using an AS-OCT (SS-1000, Tomey). With anterior corneal elevation data, Zernike polynomial coefficients were calculated in diameters of 1.0, 3.0, and 5.0 mm, and the coma, spherical, coma-like, spherical-like, and total higher-order aberrations were obtained. Pterygium size was also measured as a ratio of positions of the pterygium end with respect to the corneal diameter and categorized in eight classes: less than 15%, 15–20%, 20–25%, 25–30%, 30–35%, 35–40%, 40–45, and 45% or larger. Increases in the aberrations were analyzed with reference to those in eyes with pterygium size < 15%.

Results: The mean age of the participants was 69.3 years, and the pterygium size ranged from 2 to 57% (mean: 28.8%). The coma aberration significantly increased when the pterygium size was 45% or larger in 1.0 and 3.0 mm diameters and over 25–30% in 5.0 mm diameter. Similar increases were found in the pterygium sizes exceeding 45, 40, and 25%, respectively, in the coma-like, spherical-like, and total higher-order aberrations. On contrast, there was no increase in the spherical aberration.

Conclusion: Increases in higher-order aberrations reflected the pterygium size, and significant aberrations were induced in 5.0 mm diameter when the end exceeded 25% of corneal diameter. The use of AS-OCT and Zernike analysis could enable objective grading of pterygium advancement based on changes in corneal optics.

Keywords: Pterygium, Anterior-segment optical coherence tomography, Zernike analysis, Higher-order aberration

Background

Pterygium, the growth of conjunctival tissue in the cornea, induces topographical irregularity. Consequently, the surface regularity index (SRI) [1, 2], higher-order irregularity (HOI) in Fourier harmonic analysis of topographic data [3, 4], and higher-order Zernike coefficients [5, 6] increase with the advancement of a pterygium. Increased

corneal irregularity leads to degradation of contrast sensitivity as well as visual impairment. Such increases could reduce the benefits of premier intraocular lens implantation [7, 8], whereas corneal irregularity has been evaluated in a particular diameter [1–6]. Hence, we modified the Fourier analysis of Placido topography data and evaluated changes in the HOI due to primary pterygia in diameters of 1.0–8.0 mm [9]. The analysis revealed steep increases in the HOI when the end of pterygium is close to the analysis diameter. With the use of this objective evaluation of corneal irregularity, the severity of pterygium could be graded [4].

* Correspondence: minami@miyata-med.ne.jp
Presented at the Association for Research in Vision and Ophthalmology annual meeting, Baltimore, May 2017
[1]Miyata Eye Hospital, 6-3 Kurahara-cho, Miyakonojo, Miyazaki 885-0051, Japan
Full list of author information is available at the end of the article

The use of anterior-segment optical coherence tomography (AS-OCT) enables accurate measurement of the anterior corneal elevation of abnormal eyes [10]. Figure 1 is topographic maps of an eye with the pterygium advancing to the center of the cornea, measured by the AS-OCT and Placido topographers. Although the pterygium surface could not be projected by Mire-ring images, the AS-OCT allowed topographic mapping without obvious defects. In the previous analysis using Placido topography [4, 5], poor quality measurements due to highly irregular surfaces were observed, resulting in incomplete topography maps. In contrast, the use of AS-OCT is more suitable for the pterygium surface. The measured AS-OCT topography could be analyzed using the Zernike polynomial expansion [11], which is more representative of optical aberrations of the cornea.

The study aimed to evaluate increases in corneal higher-order aberrations induced by advancement of pterygium using an AS-OCT and Zernike aberration analysis in multiple diameters.

Methods

The protocol of this prospective observation was approved by the ethics committee of Miyata Eye Hospital (identifier: CS-231-036), and the study adhered to the tenets of the Declaration of Helsinki. Patients who underwent pterygium excision surgery from July 2014 to December 2016 at Miyata Eye Hospital due to primary pterygium were recruited. Written informed consent for the use of clinical data was obtained from all patients before examinations. Inclusion criteria were primary pterygium originating from the nasal area without a history of any surgical treatment. Eyes that used contact lenses or had corneal diseases influencing the corneal topography such as keratoconus, primary irregular astigmatism, and corneal degeneration, were excluded.

The study comprised 284 eyes from 242 patients, and the ages of the patients ranged from 35 to 92 years (mean: 69.3 years). There were 5 pseudophakic eyes, and 68 eyes were planned for cataract surgery after pterygium excision. Preoperatively, anterior corneal topography was measured using an AS-OCT (SS-1000, Tomey). Zernike coefficients up to the sixth order were calculated from the anterior corneal elevation map data [5, 6], using the topography viewer software that was modified for calculations in diameters of 1.0 to 6.0 mm with a step of 1.0 mm (ASOCT viewer ver. 4.8.4 M3, Tomey). Coma, spherical, coma-like, spherical-like, and higher-order aberrations were obtained. The amplitude of coma aberration was calculated as an absolute amplitude of the relevant vertical and horizontal components. The coma-like and spherical-like aberrations were root mean squares (RMS) of the fourth- and sixth-order coefficients and the third- and fifth-order coefficients, respectively. Higher-order aberration was RMS of the third to sixth orders.

Ocular images were captured with a digital camera and a ratio of positions of the pterygium end with respect to the corneal diameter was obtained as pterygium size (%) [2–4]. Best corrected visual acuity (BCVA) was examined and converted to logarithm of minimum angle of resolution (logMAR) for analysis.

Statistical analysis

Pterygia normally originate on the nasal side; hence, it was supposed that asymmetry irregularity would be increased with the pterygium size. For examining this assumption, changes in the coma and spherical aberrations with the

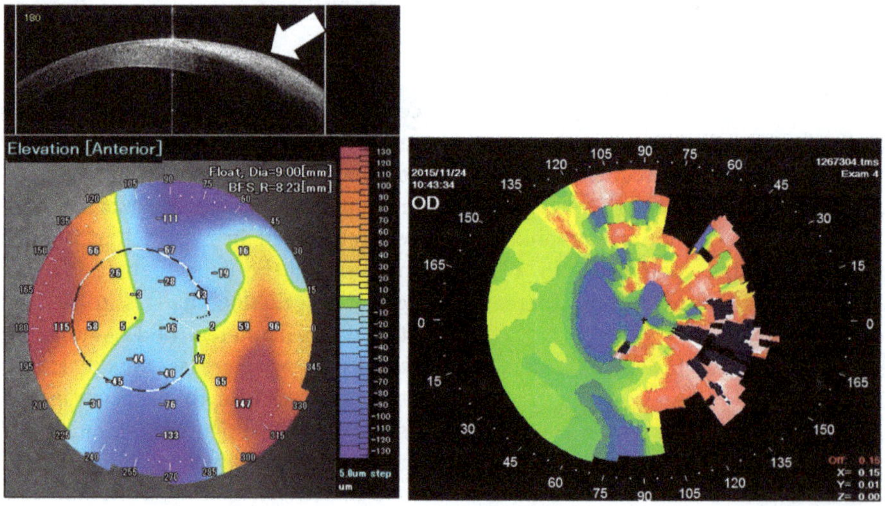

Fig. 1 Topographic maps of an eye with the pterygium measured by AS-OCT (left) and Placido (right) topographers. The use of AS-OCT allowed full topographic mapping without obvious defects while the pterygium advanced up to the corneal apex

pterygium size were compared for the diameters of 1.0, 3.0, and 5.0 mm [4]. Evaluation of a 1.0 mm diameter was considered the severest case, with a significant risk of visual function degradation. Analysis of a 3.0-mm diameter was relevant with photopic pupil diameter in adults or older adults that ranges from 2.20 to 3.77 mm [12]. This analysis diameter also has been used in conventional irregularity analysis such as SRI [1, 2]. The use of a 5.0-mm diameter was for examining the effect on the mesopic contrast sensitivity [7]. Pterygium sizes were divided into eight classes: less than 15% (< 15%), 15–20%, 20–25%, 25–30%, 30–35%, 35–40%, 40–45, and 45% or larger (≥ 45%).

When pterygium was sufficiently small and the end was not close to area of Zernike analysis, the aberration obtained should represent the corneal surface. As the pterygium end was close to the analysis area, surface irregularity induced by the advancement could increase Zernike aberrations (Fig. 2). Changes in the aberrations with the pterygium size classes were evaluated using one-way ANOVA. If the change was significant ($P < 0.05$), the differences from the values of < 15%, in which pterygium could least influence the cornea, were examined using the Dunnet multiple comparison. In addition, difference between the coma and spherical aberrations were evaluated using a paired t-test. The coma-like and spherical-like aberrations were also compared in the same manner. For the higher-order aberration, changes in the pterygium size were evaluated.

The changes in the BCVA with the pterygium sizes were examined. After excluding eyes with ocular diseases influencing visual acuity such as cataract, the BCVA for the 8 pterygium sizes were compared using the Kruskal-Wallis test following the Steel-Dwass multiple comparison.

Two-tailed $P < 0.05$ was considered a significant difference. Results are expressed as mean ± standard deviation.

Results

The mean pterygium size was 28.8 ± 10.5%, ranging from 2 to 57%. There were 18, 25, 78, 57, 28, 24, 26, and 28 eyes in the pterygium sizes of < 15%, 15–20%, 20–25%, 25–30%, 30–35%, 35–40%, 40–45%, and ≥ 45%, respectively. The mean Zernike aberrations for 1.0, 3.0, and 5.0 mm diameters are shown in Table 1. The coma aberrations were higher than the spherical aberrations in 3.0 and 5.0 mm diameters ($P < 0.001$). On the other hand, the coma-like was less than the spherical-like in diameters of 1.0 mm and vice versa in 5.0 mm. All aberrations increased with the pterygium size ($P < 0.01$, linear regression analysis) except for the spherical aberration in 5.0 mm diameter ($P = 0.083$).

Figure 3 shows changes in the coma and spherical aberrations in 1.0, 3.0, and 5.0 mm diameters with the pterygium sizes. The coma aberrations in the 1.0 and 3.0 mm diameters (lower and middle left) were significantly different from those of the pterygium size of < 15%, when the pterygium size was ≥45% ($P < 0.001$). There was significant increase with the pterygium size of 25–30% or larger ($P < 0.037$) in the 5.0 mm diameter (upper left). In the spherical aberrations (right side), such a significant increase was not found ($P > 0.05$).

Figure 4 shows changes in the coma-like and spherical-like aberrations. In both aberrations, significant difference from the pterygium size of < 15% was found when the pterygium size was ≥45% in the 1.0 mm diameter

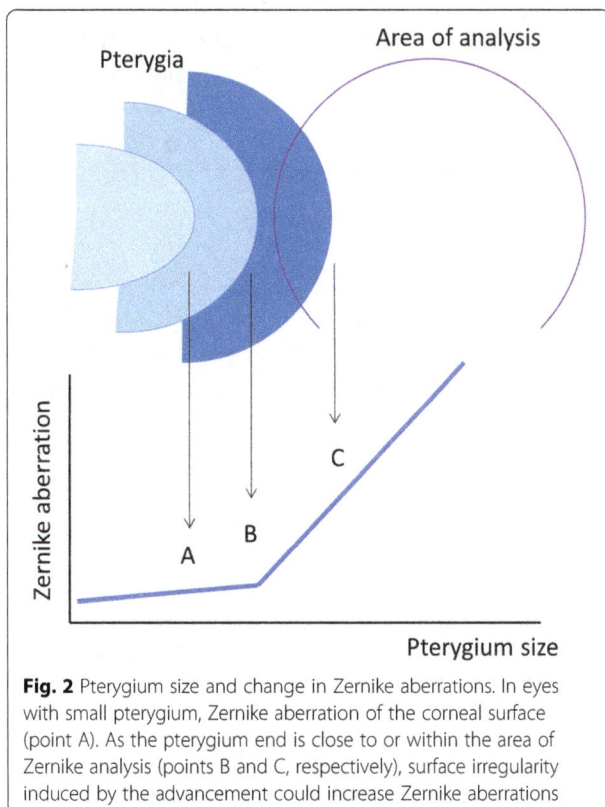

Fig. 2 Pterygium size and change in Zernike aberrations. In eyes with small pterygium, Zernike aberration of the corneal surface (point A). As the pterygium end is close to or within the area of Zernike analysis (points B and C, respectively), surface irregularity induced by the advancement could increase Zernike aberrations

Table 1 Zernike aberrations in 1.0, 3.0, and 5.0 mm diameters

Diameter	1.0 mm	3.0 mm	5.0 mm
Coma aberration (μm)	0.07 ± 0.09	0.30 ± 0.54	1.08 ± 1.21
Spherical aberration (μm)	0.10 ± 0.16	0.10 ± 0.28	−0.02 ± 0.53
P value	0.0069	< 0.001	< 0.001
Coma-like aberration (μm)[a]	0.21 ± 0.33	0.53 ± 0.89	2.43 ± 2.56
Spherical-like aberration (μm)[a]	0.27 ± 0.42	0.49 ± 0.87	1.63 ± 1.76
P value	< 0.001	0.14	< 0.001
Higher-order aberration (μm)[a]	0.35 ± 0.53	0.74 ± 1.24	2.95 ± 3.09

[a]: RMS values

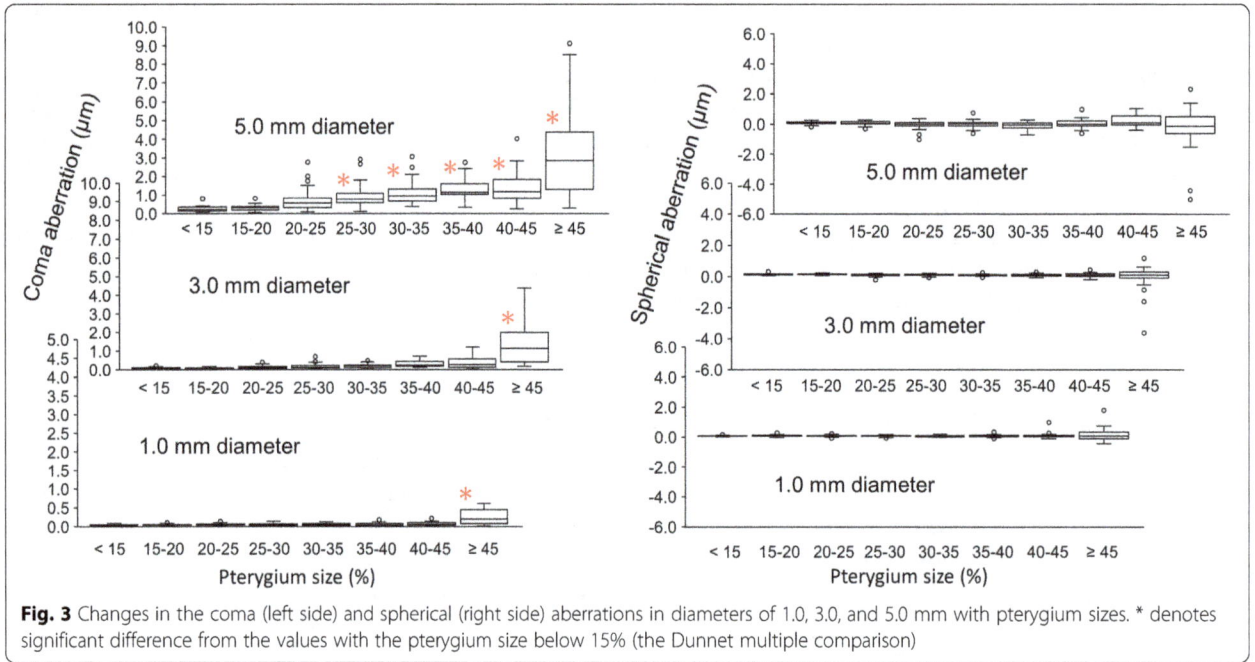

Fig. 3 Changes in the coma (left side) and spherical (right side) aberrations in diameters of 1.0, 3.0, and 5.0 mm with pterygium sizes. * denotes significant difference from the values with the pterygium size below 15% (the Dunnet multiple comparison)

($P < 0.001$) and 40–45% or larger in the 3.0 mm diameter ($P < 0.0034$). In the 5.0 mm diameter, significant increases were found with the pterygium size of 25–30% or larger ($P < 0.0033$).

Figure 5 shows changes in the higher-order aberrations. Significant differences from the pterygium size of < 15% were found in the same manner as for the coma-like and spherical-like aberrations: the pterygium

sizes of ≥45%, 40–45% or larger, and 25–30% or larger in the diameters of 1.0, 3.0, and 5.0 mm ($P < 0.001$, 0.0016, and 0.011), respectively.

The BCVA were analyzed in 201 eyes. The mean log-MAR BCVA in the pterygium sizes of < 15%, 15–20%, 20–25%, 25–30%, 30–35%, 35–40%, 40–45%, and ≥ 45% were 0.01 ± 0.29, -0.04 ± 0.13, 0.09 ± 0.35, 0.02 ± 0.13, 0.00 ± 0.14, 0.13 ± 0.28, 0.12 ± 0.25, and 0.28 ± 0.36,

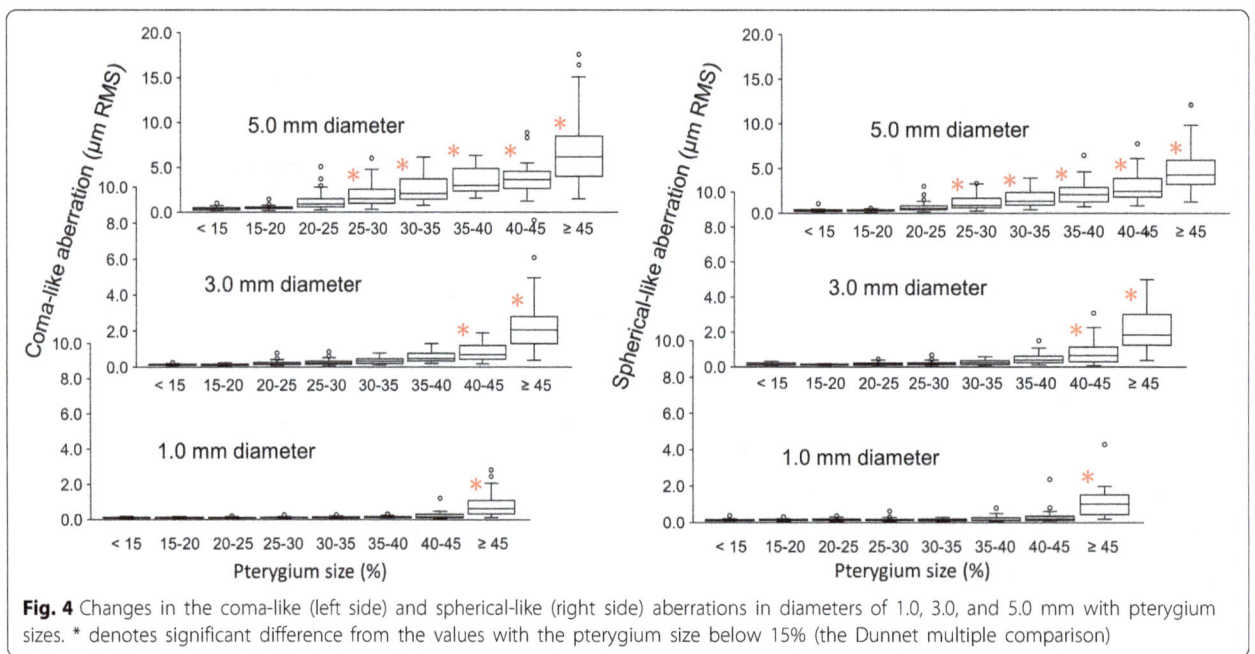

Fig. 4 Changes in the coma-like (left side) and spherical-like (right side) aberrations in diameters of 1.0, 3.0, and 5.0 mm with pterygium sizes. * denotes significant difference from the values with the pterygium size below 15% (the Dunnet multiple comparison)

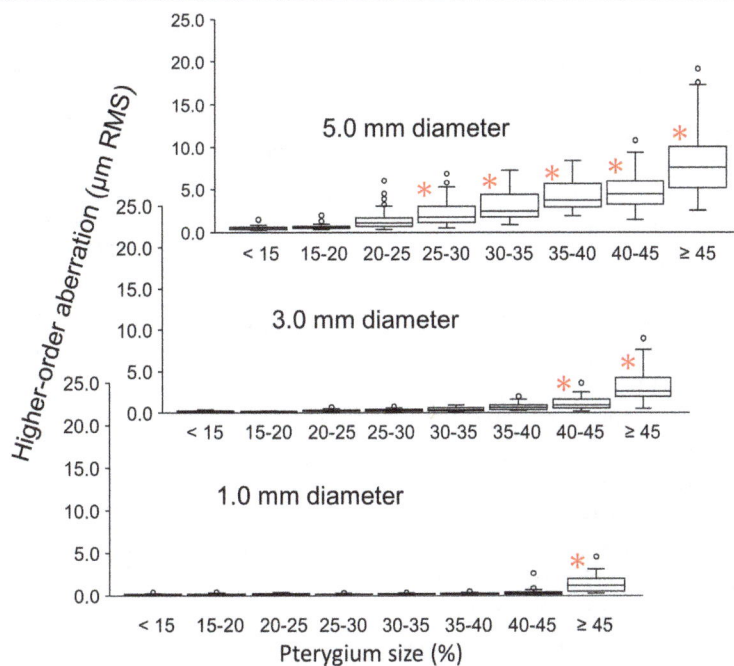

Fig. 5 Changes in the higher-order aberration in diameters of 1.0, 3.0, and 5.0 mm with pterygium sizes. * denotes significant difference from the values with the pterygium size below 15% (the Dunnet multiple comparison)

respectively. The BCVA in the pterygium size of ≥ 45% was significantly worse than the other sizes ($P > 0.01$, Steel-Dwass multiple test).

Discussion

The coma aberration showed significant increases when the pterygium size was over 45% in 1.0 and 3.0 mm diameters and 25–30% or larger in 5.0 mm diameter, whereas there was no increase in the spherical aberration. The coma-like, spherical-like, and higher-order corneal aberrations in the diameters of 1.0, 3.0, and 5.0 mm were significantly increased when the pterygium size had advanced over ≥45%, 40–45%, and 25–30%, respectively. Pesudovs et al. investigated 67 eyes before pterygium surgery, using a Placido topography, in which the mean higher-order aberrations of a 5.0 mm diameter were 0.94 ± 0.83 μm [5]. The current results were 3.1 times higher. The AS-OCT enables topography measurement for an irregular or abnormal corneal surface [10]. Hence, the current study could analyze the more severe corneal irregularity, resulting in such a difference. Evaluation of 47 preoperative eyes, using Placido and Scheimpflug imaging, resulted in higher-order aberrations of 3.06 ± 2.93 μm in a 6.0 mm diameter [6], which was close to the current results. Ozgurhan et al. reported that the coma, spherical, and higher-order aberrations were correlated with the size of the pterygium [6]. Although the definition of pterygium size and the diameter of the Zernike analysis were not the same,

similar trends were obtained in the current study, except for the spherical aberration. The current results showed no significant change in the spherical aberration, and this difference would result from ethnic difference in corneal diameter and the use of AS-OCT topographer.

Corneal irregularity of a primary pterygium was evaluated using Fourier harmonic analysis of Placido topography data within 1.0, 3.0, and 5.0 diameters, and the HOI components steeply increase at the pterygium sizes of 29.7, 21.4, and 16.5%, respectively [4]. Even though the topography measurement technology and the analysis method of corneal irregularity were different, the both results showed that increases in corneal irregularity due to pterygium advancements altered with the diameter of analysis. Hence, it could be convincing that the Zernike analysis in multiple diameters enables an objective evaluation of pterygia based on corneal optical property. From comparison of the pterygium size occurring significant increases, it was demonstrated that the current method was less sensitive to detect pterygium advancement than the previous method.

In the coma-like, spherical-like, and higher-order aberrations, significant increases occurred in the same pterygium sizes. It has been assumed that the third-order aberration mostly contributes to the pterygium size, and the difference from the higher-order aberration is relatively small [5]. The current results also showed that contributions of the coma and coma-like aberrations were higher. Whereas, the spherical-like aberration showed association with the pterygium size, although such an association was not found in the spherical aberration. It was speculated that increases in the pterygium surface (conjunctival epithelium) would increase the fourth-order Zernike coefficients, except for the spherical aberration term. Detailed analysis of the AS-OCT image is necessary to examine the influence of the pterygium surface.

A pterygium grading system was proposed using the Fourier harmonic analysis of Placido topography data [4]. The combination of the AS-OCT and Zernike analysis could detect the pterygium severity in a similar manner. The changes in the BCVA met the significant increases in the coma, coma-like, spherical-like, and higher-order aberration in 1.0 mm diameter. Hence, the ability of AS-OCT in irregular surface measurement, and the Zernike aberration expression that closely represents the optical aberrations, would be more advanced than the previous grading system [4].

There were several limitations in the current study. First, the pterygium size was evaluated in proportion to the corneal diameter. The distance between the pterygium end and the corneal apex was not measured in the current observation study. For more precise evaluation, measurement of the distance from the corneal apex is preferred [13]. Second, although the topography data was obtained with AS-OCT, there were cases in which the topography had partial defects. Although the use of AS-OCT is robust against corneal surface abnormalities [10, 14], measurement of the conjunctival surface on the pterygium is still challenging. Next, the corneal irregularity analysis method depends on the technology used for topography measurement (for example, Placido or AS-OCT). The corneal elevation map is obtained from the Mire ring image in Placido topography, so that radical scale varies with the keratometry. A steep cornea results in a dense rings image and overestimates in the radical scale. Presently, the compatibility is not confirmed.

Conclusions

The use of AS-OCT and Zernike analysis revealed that significant aberrations were induced in 5.0 mm diameter when the end exceeded 25% of corneal diameter. Such an objective evaluation of corneal higher-order aberration could enable a grading of pterygium advancement based on changes in corneal optics.

Abbreviations

AS-OCT: Anterior-segment optical coherence tomography; HOI: Higher-order irregularity; RMS: Root mean square; SRI: Surface regularity index

Acknowledgements

We thank Tomey Corporation who modified a software of the Zernike coefficient calculation for accommodating multiple diameters.

Authors' contributions

Design of the study (KIM, TO); data collection (TT, KM); statistical analysis (KIM, KO); preparation of the manuscript (KIM, TT, KO); critical revision (KM, TO). All authors read and approved the final version to be published.

Competing interests

Dr. Minami is an investigator of the patents of the software used (pending). Mr. Okamoto is an employee of Tomey corporation. Dr. Miyata is an investigator of the patents (pending), and received financial support from Tomey. For the remaining authors, none were declared.

Author details

[1]Miyata Eye Hospital, 6-3 Kurahara-cho, Miyakonojo, Miyazaki 885-0051, Japan. [2]Tomey Corporation, Nishi-ku, Nagoya, Aichi, Japan. [3]Department of Ophthalmology, Faculty of Medicine, University of Tsukuba, Tsukuba, Ibaraki, Japan.

References

1. Stern GA, Lin A. Effect of pterygium excision on induced corneal topographic abnormalities. Cornea. 1998;17:23–7.
2. Nejima R, Masuda A, Minami K, Mori Y, Hasegawa Y, Miyata K. Topographic changes after excision surgery of primary pterygia and the effect of pterygium size on topographic restoration. Eye Contact Lens. 2015;41:58–63.
3. Tomidokoro A, Oshika T, Amano S, Eguchi K, Eguchi S. Quantitative analysis of regular and irregular astigmatism induced by pterygium. Cornea. 1999;18: 412–5.
4. Miyata K, Minami K, Otani A, Tokunaga T, Tokuda S, Amano S. Proposal for a novel severity grading system for pterygia based on corneal topographic data. Cornea. 2017;36:834–40.
5. Pesudovs K, Figueiredo FC. Corneal first surface wavefront aberrations before and after pterygium surgery. J Refract Surg. 2006;22:921–5.
6. Ozgurhan EB, Kara N, Cankaya KI, Sezgin Akcay BI, Kurt T, Yilmaz I, et al. Corneal wavefront aberrations after primary and recurrent pterygium surgery. Eye Contact Lens. 2015;41:378–81.
7. Schuster AK, Tesarz J, Vossmerbaeumer U. The impact on vision of aspheric to spherical monofocal intraocular lenses in cataract surgery: a systematic review with meta-analysis. Ophthalmology. 2013;120:2166–75.
8. Schuster AK, Tesarz J, Vossmerbaeumer U. Ocular wavefront analysis of aspheric compared with spherical monofocal intraocular lenses in cataract surgery: systematic review with metaanalysis. J Cataract Refract Surg. 2015;41:1088–97.
9. Minami K, Miyata K, Otani A, Tokunaga T, Tokuda S, Amano S. Detection of increase in corneal irregularity due to pterygium using Fourier series harmonic analyses with multiple diameters. Jpn J Ophthalmol. 2018;62:342–8.
10. Nakagawa T, Maeda N, Higashiura R, Hori Y, Inoue T, Nishida K. Corneal topographic analysis in patients with keratoconus using three-dimensional anterior segment optical coherent tomography. J Cataract Refract Surg. 2011;37:1871–8.
11. Pérez-Merino P, Ortiz S, Alejandre N, Jiménez-Alfaro I, Marcos S. Quantitative OCT-based longitudinal evaluation of intracorneal ring segment implantation in keratoconus. Invest Ophthalmol Vis Sci. 2013;54:6040–51.
12. Nakamura K, Bissen-Miyajima H, Oki S, Onuma K. Pupil sizes in different Japanese age groups and the implications for intraocular lens choice. J Cataract Refract Surg. 2009;35:134–8.
13. Ha J, Cremers SL, Korchak M, Koppinger J, Martinez JA. A new automated method to grade pterygium severity using Scheimpflug imaging. Ophthalmology. 2016;123:2435–6.
14. Fukuda S, Beheregaray S, Hoshi S, Yamanari M, Lim Y, Hiraoka T, et al. Comparison of three-dimensional optical coherence tomography and combining a rotating Scheimpflug camera with a Placido topography system for forme fruste keratoconus diagnosis. Br J Ophthalmol. 2013;97:1554–9.

23

The healing effect of the collagen-glycosaminoglycan copolymer on corneal thinning

Shu-Ya Wu[1], Chien-Yi Pan[2], Elizabeth P. Shen[1], I-Shiang Tzeng[3] and Wei-Cherng Hsu[1,4*] (iD)

Abstract

Background: To study the healing processes of partial thickness wounds in the adult rabbit cornea after grafting a porous collagen-glycosaminoglycan copolymer matrix (CG).

Methods: In this study, the regeneration of surgically-induced rabbit corneal defect implanted with CG was investigated. The corneal partial thickness wound was created by 7.5 mm trephine. The wound was implanted with CG. Effects on wound healing was analyzed using clinical data on epithelial migration and corneal thickness, and histological data on collagen and alpha smooth muscle actin distribution.

Results: Compared with control group, CG induced a relatively severe inflammatory reaction in grafted cornea until the CG matrix was completely degraded. The new vessel ingrowth and stromal regeneration maintained the corneal thickness. The grafted cornea was significantly thicker ($P < 0.001$) than the control group. On day 90, the corneal opacity score of the control group was one and the grafted cornea was two.

Conclusion: CG copolymer matrix can successfully repair the damaged corneal stroma by injury, and regain its thickness. However, CG matrix induced inflammatory healing process thus causing mild corneal haziness and neovascularization.

Keywords: 3D scaffold, Collagen-glycosaminoglycan copolymer, Corneal thinning, Healing process

Background

Corneal melting with perforation is a severe, vision-threatening complication of corneal disorders such as corneal ulceration, chemical burn and autoimmune keratitis. In the acute stage, the urgent approach is to limit inflammation by directing against the cause as well as to optimize epithelial healing [1]. Furthermore, surgical procedures, including tissue adhesive [1, 2], amniotic membrane transplantation [1, 3], conjunctival flaps [1, 3], pericardial membrane graft [4], are done to temporarily maintain the integrity of the globe. In general, this involves a multistage surgery [1]. The final tectonic keratoplasty is performed to restore visual function. The surgical methods include full-thickness penetrating keratoplasty, lamellar corneal patch graft, and deep anterior lamellar keratoplasty [1, 5–8], depending on the size and location of perforation. In these procedures, it is essential to have graft material for repair of the corneal defect readily available.

Shortage of graft material for repair, particularly in developing countries, has prompted the development of bioengineered tissue alternatives. Tissue engineering relies on the use of three-dimensional porous scaffolds to provide appropriate microenvironment to induce regeneration of injured tissues and organs. The porous collagen-glycosaminoglycan copolymer matrix (CG matrix) is composed of type I collagen and chondroitin 6-sulfate. The collagen of the corneal stroma is largely type I collagen. Previous study demonstrated that CG matrix in eyes could modulate the healing procedure of conjunctival wound, reducing scarring contraction and promoting the formation of a near-normal sub-conjunctival stroma [9]. The CG matrix also serves as

* Correspondence: cyao@seed.net.tw

[1]Department of Ophthalmology, Taipei Tzu Chi Hospital, Buddhist Tzu Chi Medical Foundation, No. 289, Jianguo Rd., Xindian Dist., New Taipei City 231, Taipei, Taiwan (R.O.C.)

[4]Tzu Chi University College of Medicine, Hualien, Taiwan

Full list of author information is available at the end of the article

a three-dimensional scaffold for cell migration and proliferation on surgical bleb defect to maintain the size of bleb and repair the leakage [10, 11]. CG matrix supplies good biocompatibility on the ocular surface. Therefore, CG matrix has a potential to be used as an alternative graft material for repair of corneal thinning by suppling thicker extracelluar matrix in the wound bed. However, considering that diameter, spacing, and spatial orientation of the collage fibrils in the corneal stroma is essential for corneal transparency [12], we tested the healing effect of CG matrix on corneal thinning in a rabbit model. This study provides preliminary results for further advanced studies.

Methods
Animals and model of corneal thinning
All investigations conformed to the ARVO statement for the use of Animals in Ophthalmic and Vision Research. A drug-free, biodegradable, porous collagen matrix of 1% collagen/C-6-S copolymer (iGen) measuring 7.5 mm in diameter and 2 mm in thickness was used. The synthesis of the CG matrix was described in previous study but the type I collagen was purified from porcine skin [10]. The pores of the matrix ranged from 20 μm to 200 μm (Fig. 1). Twenty-four female New Zealand albino rabbits (Level Biotechnology Inc.) weighing 2.5–3.5 Kg were anesthetized by intramuscular injection of ketamine (35 mg/kg) and xylazine (5 mg/kg). Surgical procedures were done under surgical microscope with the eyelids held open by a spectrum. Both eyes underwent deep lamellar keratectomy (DLK) with 7.5 mm trephine to a depth of almost 1/2 the corneal thickness without damaging the corneal endothelium. The right eye served as control and was not implanted with CG matrix (ungrafted eye); while the left eye, as study group,

had CG matrix laid over the cornea bed (grafted eye). Both eyes were then covered with therapeutic soft contact lens (Purevision, Bausch & Lomb). Lateral tarsorrhaphy was performed over one-third length of the eyelids to prevent loss of contact lens.

Healing effects of CG matrix on the corneal thinning were assessed on days 3, 7, 14, 28, 60, and 90 after surgical procedures (assessment days). Animals were euthanized by intracardinal injection of sodium pentobarbital (398 mg/ml at 1.0 ml/10 lb. body weight). Immediately after euthanising, eyes were enucleated from the orbit.

Slit-lamp examination and clinical score of corneal opacity
Slit lamp examination was performed to evaluate corneal opacity on assessment days. Corneal opacity was scored using a five-point scale where 0 is no opacity, completely clear cornea; 1 is sight haziness, iris and lens visible; 2 is moderately opaque, iris and lens still detectable; 3 is severely opaque, iris and lens hardly visible; and 4 is completely opaque, with no view of iris and lens [13].

Corneal thickness measurements
In all rabbits, corneal thickness of both eyes was measured by Schiempflug photography before and after DLK on surgery day, and on assessment days. Wilcoxon signed-rank test ($P < 0.001$) was used to compare corneal thickness between pre- and post-operation, as well as between control and study eyes over time.

Histopathologic and immune staining studies
Four rabbits were euthanized on each assessment day. Close upper and lower eyelid sutures were performed to protect the cornea. Entire eye globes were harvested from the orbit and were soaked in Modified Davison's fluid for 24 h. The globes were fixed in 10% neutral

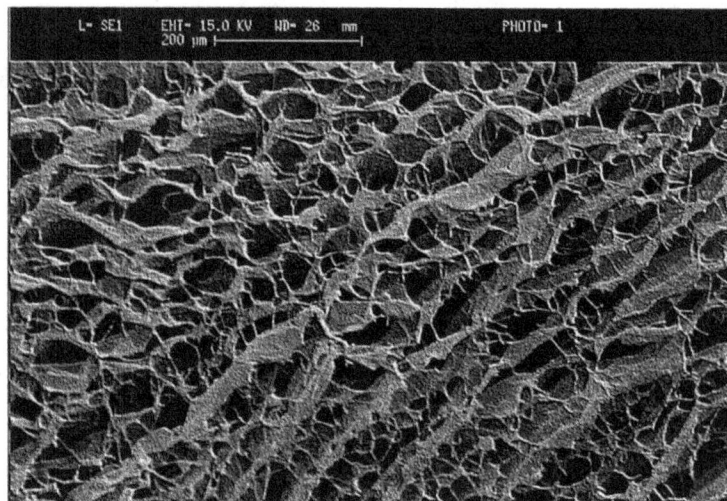

Fig. 1 Scanning electron micrograph of the collagen-glycosaminoglycan copolymer matrix implant

buffered formalin. Corneas with limbus were harvested and embedded in paraffin. The 7 μm sectioned corneas were stained with Masson's trichrome to evaluate the distribution of collagen. With Masson's trichrome stain, collagen was stained blue, cellular material stained red, and cell nuclei stained purple. Additional tissue sections were used for alpha-smooth muscle actin (α-SMA) immunocytochemistry to identify myofibroblasts [14–16].

Results

Day 3

On post-DLK day 3, the ungrafted eyes (right eyes) showed moderate corneal opacity with iris and lens detectable (corneal opacity score of 2, Fig. 2b); while corneas of grafted eyes (left eyes) were completely opaque (corneal opacity score of 4) due to CG matrix graft (Fig. 2a). Silt-lamp examinations of grafted eyes showed central cornea to be thicker than the peripheral cornea (Fig. 2a).

Histopathologic study with Masson's trichrome stain revealed acute inflammation in both groups (Fig. 2c and d). In the grafted eyes, polymorphonuclear neutrophils (PMNs), epithelial cells, and fibroblasts were found around and adherent to the CG matrix implant. In the ungrafted eyes, only PMNs and re-epithelial cells migrated and adhered to the corneal wound. The staining for α-SMA was negative in both groups.

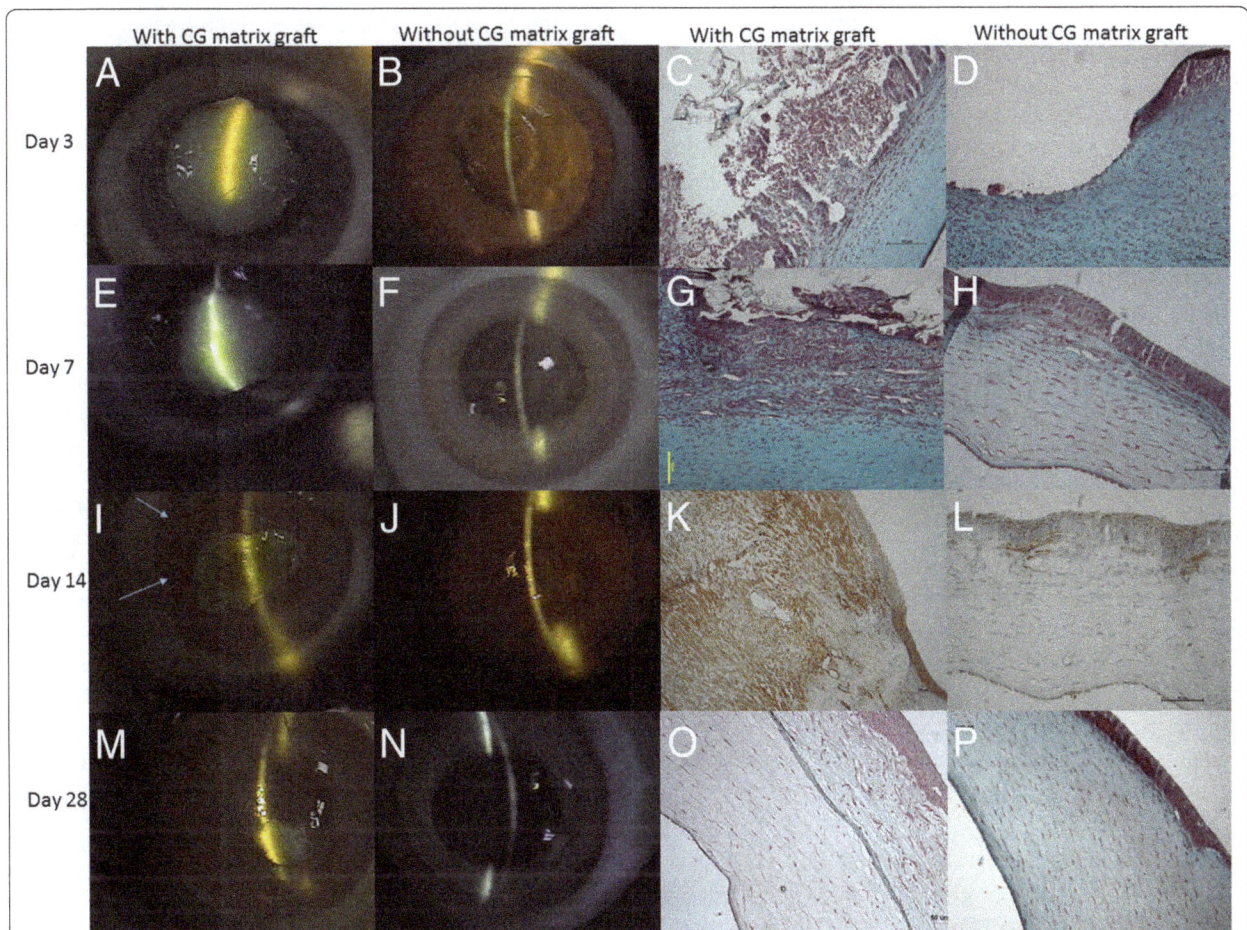

Fig. 2 Photographs of slit-lamp examination and histopathological results on day 3, 7, 14, 28 after surgery. **a** Matrix- grafted cornea (**b**) Ungrafted cornea. Masson's trichrome stain showing (**c**) massive inflammatory cells infiltration around the corneal wound with CG matrix and collagen ingrowth (blue stain). **d** only some inflammatory cell infiltration and re-epithelialization. **e** Matrix- grafted cornea with tiny vessel ingrowth (**f**) Ungrafted cornea wound margin identified by the blue arrows with edema. Masson's trichrome stain showing (**g**) predominantly fibroblasts, epithelial cells and inflammatory cells into CG matrix with collagen regeneration. **h** epithelial and stromal regeneration (100×). **i** Matrix-grafted cornea with new vessels (blue arrow) and CG matrix degradation over upper corneal wound. **j** Ungrafted cornea with reduced wound area. α-smooth muscle actin stain showing (**k**) strong positive cells over regenerative corneal stroma. **l** only some positive cells infiltrated into the regenerative stroma of the ungrafted cornea (100×). **m** CG matrix-grafted cornea with incomplete degradation and decreasing neovascularization. **n** Ungrafted cornea with near complete healing. One corneal opacity score. Masson's trichrome stain showing (**o**) irregular arrangement of new collagen deposition upon complete degradation of collagen-GAG scaffold wound with thickening the stroma thickness. **p** complete re-epithelization and wound healing

Day 7

On post-DLK day 7, the cornea of the ungrafted eyes became more opaque (corneal opacity score of 3) because of corneal edema (Fig. 2f); while the corneal opacity of the grafted eyes remained at 4 due to incomplete CG matrix degradation (Fig. 2e). With regard to histopathologic findings, the grafted eyes showed marked re-epithelial cells infiltration, and prominent deposition of collagen and fibroblast-like cells in line with stromal regeneration of corneal wound (Fig. 2g). In the ungrafted eyes, stromal regeneration and re-epithelialization were found to a lesser degree (Fig. 2h). The intensity of α-SMA staining was stronger in grafted eyes than in ungrafted eyes.

Day 14

Through slit-lamp examination, the ungrafted eyes showed clearer corneas (corneal opacity score of 2) and the re-epithelization of corneal wounds was complete (without positive Fluorescein stain) (Fig. 2j). In contrast, the corneas of grafted eyes were still opaque due to presence of CG matrix, the corneal opacity score remained at 4 (Fig. 2i); however, the periphery were healing, clearer, and had new vessels.

In the ungrafted eyes, corneal wound displayed lesser inflammatory reaction and presence of some cells positively stained with α-smooth muscle actin stain (Fig. 2l). The corneas of grafted eyes had comparatively thicker epithelial layer and strong positive cells over regenerative stroma on α-smooth muscle actin stain (Fig. 2k).

Day 28

In the ungrafted eyes, the corneal opacity score was 1 (Fig. 2n). Histologically, the wound healing process of the ungrafted eyes was deemed complete by negative α-smooth muscle actin stain and absence of inflammatory cells (Fig. 2p).

In the grafted eyes, CG matrix was still incompletely degraded, thus the corneal opacity score remained at 4 but the peripheral areas, without CG matrix, had score of 3

(Fig. 2m). Compared to post-DLK day 14, the number and diameter of new vessels decreased (Fig. 2m); and loosely organized collagen fibers and fibroblasts-like cells surrounded the partially degraded CG matrix (Fig. 3a and b).

Days 60 & 90

On post-DLK days 60 and 90, the corneas of ungrafted eyes remained clear (corneal opacity score maintained at 1) (Fig. 4b and d). On post-DLK day 60, the corneas of the grafted eyes had corneal opacity score of 3 because of scar formation though the CG matrix was completely degraded (Fig. 4a). By post-DLK day 90, corneas of grafted eyes became clearer and the score was 2 (Fig. 4c).

On post-DLK day 90, cornea of grafted eyes were obviously thicker than those of ungrafted eyes (Fig. 4e and f) but the arrangement of keratocytes showed a more randomized pattern over a superficial layer of stroma (Fig. 5).

On post-DLK day 60, grafted eyes showed presence of positively α-SMA stained cells in the stroma of the corneal wound without porous structure. There were no positively α-SMA stained cells in the ungrafted eyes (Fig. 6).

Corneal thickness measurements

Corneal thickness of the ungrafted eyes (right eyes) before DLK (mean ± SD) was 317.92 ± 20.33 μm and 158.29 ± 27.30 μm after DLK, while that of the grafted eyes were 317.44 ± 21.04 μm and 151.3 ± 31.51 μm, respectively. The difference in corneal thickness between pre-operation and post-operation was statistically significant ($P < 0.001$) in both the ungrafted and grafted eyes. Between grafted and ungrafted eyes, the post-DLK corneal thickness was not statistically significant.

The mean corneal thickness of the ungrafted eyes were 245 ± 15.59 μm, 274.5 ± 15.62 μm, 315.5 ± 6.29 μm, 311.75 ± 7.50 μm, and 307.25 ± 11.19 μm on post-DLK days 3, 7, 28, 60, and 90, respectively. The corneal thickness on post-DLK day 14 was not measured due to

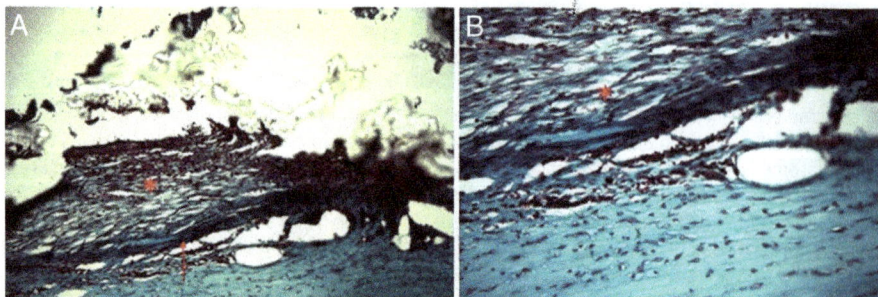

Fig. 3 Micrographs at two different magnification powers (**a**) 100× (**b**) 200× of CG matrix grafted cornea on day 28. Masson's trichrome stain showing (**a**) high cellularity and irregular collagen deposition (red star) upon corneal wound bed (red arrow) with incomplete collagen-GAG scaffold degradation (**b**) CG matrix maintaining the porous scaffold (red star)

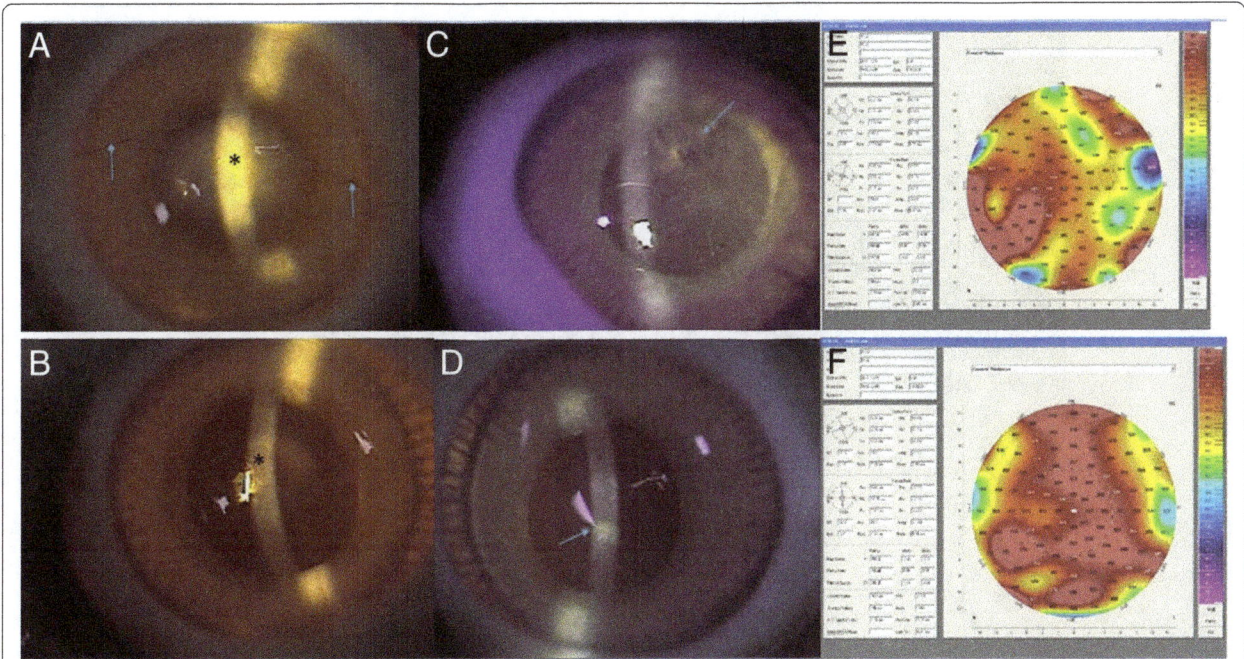

Fig. 4 Postoperative day 60, slit-lamp examination revealing (**a**) central scar formation (black star) with vessel ingrowth on matrix-grafted cornea (blue arrow), and complete CG matrix degradation (**b**) more transparent central cornea in control eye. Postoperative day 90, slit-lamp examination showing (**c**) the transparency of matrix-grafted cornea being more limpid (black star) than (**a**) the cornea on day 60, but less transparent than the ungrafted cornea (**d**). Scanning Pentacam photographs on day 90 revealing the thickness of CG matrix-grafted cornea (**e**) being thicker than the control one (**f**). The areas indicated by the arrows in Figs. **e** and (**c**) show consistent results by two different methods. The same as for Figs. (**f**) and (**d**)

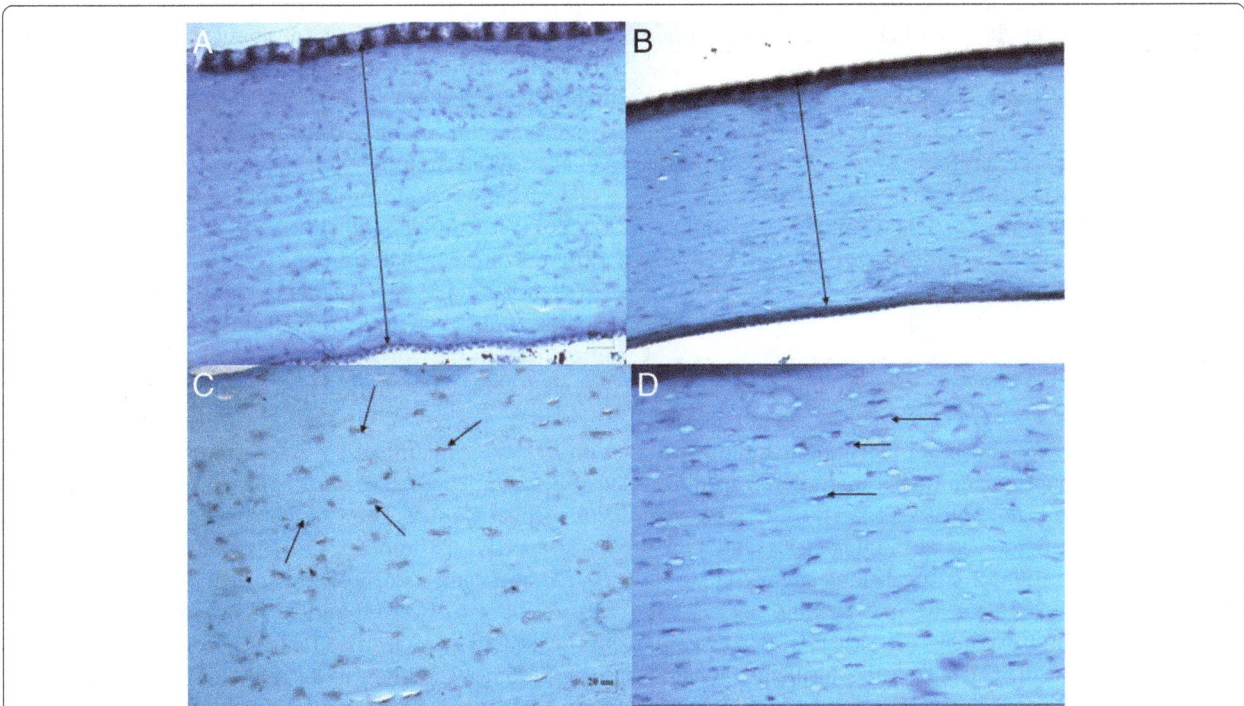

Fig. 5 The corneal thickness of collagen-GAG scaffold (**a**) is thicker than the control one (**b**) as indicated by the arrows (Masson's Trichrome stain, 100×). The arrangement of keratocytes (black arrows) in collagen-GAG scaffold treated wound are more random (**c**) than control one (**d**) as indicated by the black arrows (Masson's Trichrome stain, 200×)

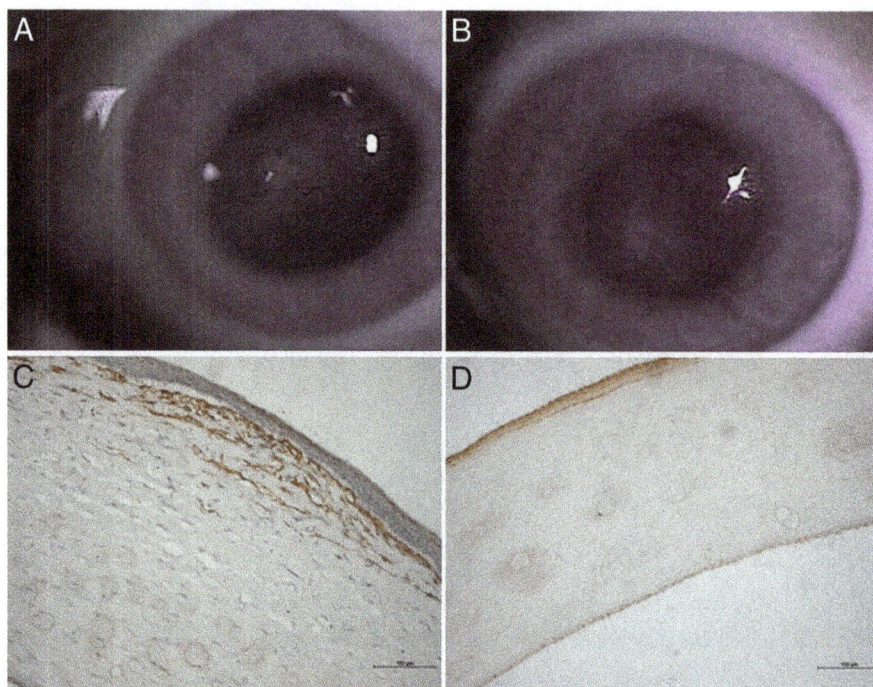

Fig. 6 External eye photographs on day 60 of (**a**) CG matrix-grafted cornea and (**b**) ungrafted cornea.α-SMA stains showing (**c**) positive cells found in the stroma of matrix-grafted cornea and (**d**) no positive cells in ungrafted cornea (100×)

corneal edema. For the grafted eyes, mean central corneal thickness was only measurable by pentacam on post-DLK day 90 at 487.25 ± 14.89 μm; on the other prior assessment days, the pentacam failed to measure the central corneal thickness due to presence of non-degraded CG matrix and opacity. The mean central corneal thickness of grafted eyes was significantly thicker ($P < 0.001$) than the ungrafted eyes on post-DLK day 90 (Fig. 7). The results and comparisons between grafted and ungrafted eyes were summarized in Table 1.

Discussion

Corneal thinning by trauma, surgery, infection, or inflammation triggers a series of corneal wound healing processes and corneal matrix remodeling, including stromal keratocyte apoptosis, epithelial migration, myofibroblast proliferation, and fibrosis [17, 27, 28]. However, these responses might lead to angiogenesis and compromise the restoration of corneal transparency [18, 19]. In addition, if incomplete wound healing persists, it could cause no improvement of corneal thickness and even perforation [20]. Currently, the ultimate management to correct stromal scarring and corneal thinning is corneal transplantation. Full or partial-thickness corneal grafts are effective means of restoring transparency and thickness, but this procedure relies on fresh donated

cadaveric cornea. Due to shortage of donor cornea, it is imperative to find viable alternatives to corneal tissue.

Type I collagen accounts for about 85% of the fibrillar collagen in human corneal stroma. In the form of heterotypic fibrils with type V collagen, type I collagen are crucial for corneal transparency [21]. The porous collagen-glycosaminoglycan copolymer matrix (type I collagen and chondroitin 6-sulfate) was designed as temporary scaffolds with stiffness that maintains corneal structure in corneal thinning, while the surrounding corneal stroma tissue regenerates and replaces the original scaffold over time. In this study, CG matrices were implanted in the corneal stroma of 24 rabbits after deep lamellar keratectomy and observed over a 90-day period thereafter. On day 3, the grafted cornea showed infiltration of acute inflammatory cells around CG matrix. On day 7, new vessels began to appear at the periphery of the corneal wound. The CG matrix degraded completely between days 28 and 60. On day 60, CG matrix disappeared and central corneal scar formation with peripheral vessels ingrowth were found. And on day 90, the cornea of the grafted eyes cleared (Table 1). From the histopathologic findings, the intensity of α-SMA staining increased progressively from 7th to the 14th day then decreased gradually overtime but remaining positive at day 60. Therefore, CG matrix induced stronger inflammatory reaction and delayed wound healing process up to the

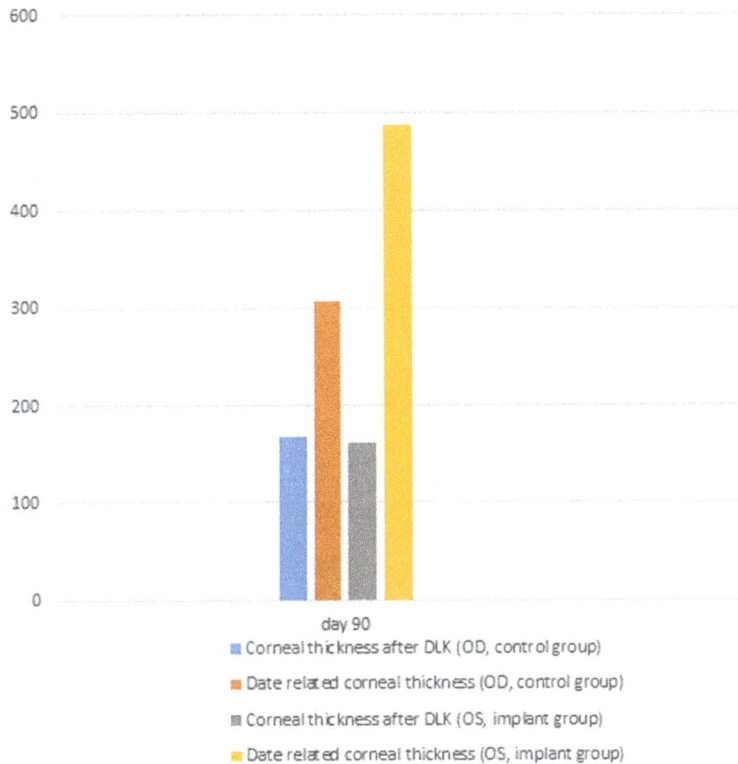

Fig. 7 Comparison of corneal thickness on day 90 after surgery

3rd month as evidenced by persistence of α-SMA stained cells [22–26].

Inflammation is a fundamental process in corneal wound healing. The infiltrating inflammatory cells and cytokines activate keratocytes differentiation into fibroblasts and myofibroblasts [22–26]. They migrate and accumulate in the provisional matrix of the wound site and secrete and deposit collagen [27, 28]. Severe inflammation might overwhelm the antiangiogenic mechanism of cornea and might give rise to a secondary ingrowth of blood vessels from the limbus into the central cornea [18, 29, 30]. Prolonged myofibroblasts activation and

Table 1 The summary of the results and comparison between collagen-glycosaminoglycan copolymer matrix grafted cornea and un-grafted cornea

	Day 3	Day 7	Day 14	Day 28	Day 60	Day 90
Corneal opacity score						
grafted cornea	4	4	4	4	3	2
un-grafted cornea	2	3	2	1	1	1
Corneal thickness						
grafted cornea(μm)	NA	NA	NA	NA	NA	487.25 ± 14.89
un-grafted cornea(μm)	245 ± 15.59	274.5 ± 15.62	NA	315.5 ± 6.29	311.75 ± 7.50	307.25 ± 11.19
Neovascularization						
grafted cornea	−	+	+	+	+	+
un-grafted cornea	−	−	−	−	−	−
α-SMA-positive cell						
grafted cornea	−	+	+	+	+	−
un-grafted cornea	−	+	+	−	−	−

NA not applicable, + positive, − negative

ongoing deposition of repair matrix would cause corneal scarring and opacification [31]. These two physiologic conditions may complicate corneal wound healing resulting to poor vision. With tissue engineered CG matrix providing the 3-dimensional porous scaffold and appropriate microenvironment to promote more fibroblast and myofibroblast repopulation, the healing processes are modified and optimized [9–11].

During the degradation of CG matrix, the patterns of cell migration and proliferation changes and the coexisting inflammation activates more fibroblasts and myofibroblasts. These keep depositing multiple elements of extracellular matrix to increase the corneal thickness [32]. By remodeling the healing stroma, and replacing the disorganized repair matrix with regular corneal extracellular matrix, a better transparency can be achieved [33, 34]. In addition, the number and the diameter of new vessels slowly decreases as the remodeling progresses [35].

In our study, the complete re-epithelization of the cornea wound on ungrafted eyes was achieved on day 14 but stroma remodeling was finished on day 28. In the grafted eyes, these results were observed on day 60 and day 90, respectively. These demonstrated that the wound healing proceeded from a proliferation phase to a stromal remodeling stage. Utsunomiya et al. in 2014 also observed the wound healing process after corneal stromal thinning shifted from an acute wound healing phase to a remodeling phase by anterior segment optical coherence tomography (OCT) [36]. The time to complete corneal wound healing in grafted eyes was influenced by the process and timing of CG matrix degradation. As a result, the intensity of corneal inflammation induced by CG matrix combined with the duration of CG degradation influenced the degree of stromal thickening, scarring and neovascularization.

CG matrix for repair of corneal thinning must be strong and implantable to maintain the corneal shape and curvature at the early stage. Additionally, the material should be able to maintain the 3-dimensional structure to support cell adhesion, migration and turnover into host extracellular matrix over time. In this study, we used soft contact lens and lateral tarsorrhaphy to anchor the CG matrix to corneal wound without further invasive procedures. This procedure minimizes disturbance of epithelium and maintains corneal shape without suturing, thereby avoids stimulation of an aggressive wound healing response. Though the main purpose of contact lens and tarsorrhaphy was to keep the CG graft in situ, they both also exerted certain pressure and compressed the CG matrix making it less prone to deformation. The CG matrix in our study was constructed by blending type I collagen with chondroitin 6-sulfate, with glutaraldehyde crosslinking. Compression test indicated that the matrix, upon compression by external force,

becomes more rigid and becomes more difficult to deform [10]. In previous study, 2 mm thickness of collagen/C-6-S copolymer was used to repair conjunctival defect and the implantation reduced contraction and promoted the formation of a nearly normal subconjunctival stroma. The matrix was almost completely degraded on day 28 [9–11]. Therefore, 2 mm thickness collagen matrix with compression molding was used to resist the external forces by tarsorrhaphy and contact lens as well as enzymatic degradation. The majority of degradation of the CG matrix occurred in the first 4 postoperative weeks. Previous studies reported degradation rates of different collagen scaffolds to be 4 to 5 weeks, similar to what we observed in our study [37–39]. Based on the histopathologic findings of this study (Fig. 3), the 3-dimensional scaffold was maintained to a certain degree without collapsing, and this allows for cell migration and proliferation to happen. At the early stage, CG matrix maintains the good crosslinking structure to maintain the original porous structure without collapsing and result in the predictable randomized collagen deposition pattern. At the later stage, degrading CG matrix became less rigid and was flattened in a more parallel way by the pressure of tarsorrhaphy on it and resulted in better corneal clarity in the grafted group than expected.

In this study, CG matrix significantly increased the thickness of the healed cornea compared with ungrafted ones on day 90 ($P < 0.001$). From histological findings, the increased thickness resulted from additional lamella of new collagen deposition. Moreover, pentacam successfully measured the true central corneal thickness of the grafted eyes due to the improved clarity of the cornea. These results demonstrated that the new collagen ingrowth can undergo further remodeling to increase the corneal transparency. Although the corneas of grafted eyes were relatively hazy compared with the ungrafted ones, CG matrix was successful as a 3-dimensional temporary scaffold for corneal regeneration to regain the corneal thickness [39]. Corneal transparency greatly depends on the organization of the type I collagen fibrils, especially their diameter and regular lamellae organization [21]. While the slow degradation of CG matrix and inflammation induced by CG matrix lead to thicker cornea, both also resulted in corneal haziness. Therefore, finding the balance between corneal thickening and corneal haziness induced by CG matrix must be overcome. The limitation of this work is that corneal healing response from injury differs based on the nature of the insults such as chemical burn [40].

This study showed the healing effect of CG matrix on corneal thinning by injury. In the future, CG matrix may be designed with a different degradation rate so as to optimize stromal regeneration, or with a different porous size, diameter and arrangement to better regulate the assembly of cornea fibrils and the organization of the extracellular matrix to maintain corneal transparency [41, 42].

Conclusion

Corneal perforation directly relates to the thickness of corneal stroma under the condition of corneal epithelial defect. Even though corneal scar formation and vessels ingrowth cause opacity of the cornea, less chance of corneal perforation is noted clinically. The 3-dimensional collagen-glycosaminoglycan scaffold offers a new micro-environment for cell migration, proliferation and differentiation but we still need to do more research to decrease the inflammation by modifying the degradation rate and create more parallel structure for corneal wound healing.

Abbreviations

3D: three-dimensional; CG: collagen-glycosaminoglycan; DLK: deep lamellar keratectomy; OCT: optical coherence tomography; PMNs: polymorphonuclear neutrophils; α-SMA: alpha-smooth muscle actin

Acknowledgements
Not applicable.

Funding
Not applicable.

Authors' contributions
SYW analyzed the data and wrote the manuscript. CYP performed the study WCH design the study, analyzed the data, and wrote the manuscript. EPS helped with acquisition of data. IST took statistics. All authors read and approved the final manuscript.

Competing interests
The authors declare that they have no competing interest.

Author details
[1]Department of Ophthalmology, Taipei Tzu Chi Hospital, Buddhist Tzu Chi Medical Foundation, No. 289, Jianguo Rd., Xindian Dist., New Taipei City 231, Taipei, Taiwan (R.O.C.). [2]Wu Chou Animal Hospital, Taipei, Taiwan. [3]Department of Research, Taipei Tzu Chi Hospital, Buddhist Tzu Chi Medical Foundation, Taipei, Taiwan. [4]Tzu Chi University College of Medicine, Hualien, Taiwan.

References
1. Jhanji V, Young AL, Mehta JS, et al. Management of corneal perforation. Surv Ophthalmol. 2011;56:522–38.
2. Weiss JL, Williams P, Lindstrom RL, et al. The use of tissue adhesive in corneal perforations. Ophthalmology. 1983;90:610–5.
3. Abdulhalim BE, Wagih MM, Gad AA, et al. Amniotic membrane graft to conjunctival flap in treatment of non-viral resistant infectious keratitis: a randomised clinical study. Br J Ophthalmol. 2015;99:59–63.
4. Alio JL, Rodriguez AE, Martinez LM. Bovine pericardium membrane (tutopatch) combined with solid platelet-rich plasma for the management of perforated corneal ulcers. Cornea. 2013;32:619–24.
5. Yokogawa H, Kobayashi A, Yamazaki N, et al. Surgical therapies for corneal perforations: 10 years of cases in a tertiary referral hospital. Clin Ophthalmol. 2014;8:2165–70.
6. Vanathi M, Sharma N, Titiyal JS, et al. Tectonic grafts for corneal thinning and perforations. Cornea. 2002;21:792–7.
7. Hanada K, Igarashi S, Muramatsu O, et al. Therapeutic keratoplasty for corneal perforation: clinical results and complications. Cornea. 2008;27:156–60.
8. Anshu A, Parthasarathy A, Mehta JS, et al. Outcomes of therapeutic deep lamellar keratoplasty and penetrating keratoplasty for advanced infectious keratitis: a comparative study. Ophthalmology. 2009;116:615–23.
9. Hsu WC, Spilker MH, Yannas IV, et al. Inhibition of conjunctival scarring and contraction by a porous collagen-glycosaminoglycan implant. Invest Ophthalmol Vis Sci. 2000;41:2404–11.
10. Hsu WC, Ritch R, Krupin T, et al. Tissue bioengineering for surgical bleb defects: an animal study. Graefes Arch Clin Exp Ophthalmol. 2008;246:709–17.
11. Chen HS, Ritch R, Krupin T, et al. Control of filtering bleb structure through tissue bioengineering: an animal model. Invest Ophthalmol Vis Sci. 2006;47:5310–4.
12. Freegard TJ. The physical basis of transparency of the normal cornea. Eye. 1997;11:465–71.
13. Shin YJ, Hyon JY, Choi WS, et al. Chemical injury-induced corneal opacity and neovascularization reduced by rapamycin via TGF-β1/ERK pathways regulation. Invest Ophthalmol Vis Sci. 2013;54:4452–8.
14. Jester JV, Petroll WM, Barry PA, et al. Expression of alpha-smooth muscle (alpha-SM) actin during corneal stroma wound healing. Invest Ophthalmol Vis Sci. 1995;36:809–19.
15. Darby I, Skalli O, Gabbiani G. alpha-smooth muscle actin is transiently expressed by myofibroblasts during experimental wound healing. Lab Investig. 1990;63:21–9.
16. Ehrlich HP. Wound closure: evidence of cooperation between fibroblasts and collagen matrix. Eye. 1988;2:149–57.
17. Torricelli AA, Santhanam A, Wu J, et al. The corneal fibrosis response to epithelial-stromal injury. Exp Eye Res. 2016;142:110–8.
18. Bourghardt Peebo B, Fagerholm P, Traneus-Röckert C, et al. Time-lapse in vivo imaging of corneal angiogenesis: the role of inflammatory cells in capillary sprouting. Invest Ophthalmol Vis Sci. 2011;52:3060–8.
19. Hassell JR, Birk DE. The molecular basis of corneal transparency. Exp Eye Res. 2010;91:326–35.
20. Liu CY, Kao WW. Corneal epithelial wound healing. Prog Mol Biol Transl Sci. 2015;134:61–71.
21. Massoudi D, Malecaze F, Galiacy SD. Collagens and proteoglycans of the cornea: importance in transparency and visual disorders. Cell Tissue Res. 2016;363:337–49.
22. Wilson SE, Mohan RR, Mohan RR, et al. The corneal wound healing response: cytokine-mediated interaction of the epithelium, stroma, and inflammatory cells. Prog Retin Eye Res. 2001;20:625–37.
23. Behm B, Babilas P, Landthaler M, et al. Cytokines, chemokines and growth factors in wound healing. J Eur Acad Dermatol Venereol. 2012;26:812–20.
24. Jester JV, Barry-Lane PA, Cavanagh HD, et al. Induction of alpha-smooth muscle actin expression and myofibroblast transformation in cultured corneal keratocytes. Cornea. 1996;15:505–16.
25. Beales MP, Funderburgh JL, Jester JV, et al. Proteoglycan synthesis by bovine keratocytes and corneal fibroblasts: maintenance of the keratocyte phenotype in culture. Invest Ophthalmol Vis Sci. 1999;40:1658–63.
26. West-Mays JA, Dwivedi DJ. The keratocyte: corneal stromal cell with variable repair phenotypes. Int J Biochem Cell Biol. 2006;38:1625–31.
27. Kuo IC. Corneal wound healing. Curr Opin Ophthalmol. 2004;15:311–5.
28. Fini ME, Stramer BM. How the cornea heals: cornea-specific repair mechanisms affecting surgical outcomes. Cornea. 2005;24:S2–S11.
29. Cursiefen C, Küchle M, Naumann GO. Angiogenesis in corneal diseases: histopathologic evaluation of 254 human corneal buttons with neovascularization. Cornea. 1998;17:611–3.

30. Bock F, Maruyama K, Regenfuss B, et al. Novel anti (lymph) angiogenic treatment strategies for corneal and ocular surface diseases. Prog Retin Eye Res. 2013;34:89–124.
31. Karamichos D, Guo XQ, Hutcheon AE, et al. Human corneal fibrosis: an in vitro model. Invest Ophthalmol Vis Sci. 2010;51:1382–8.
32. McLaughlin CR, Fagerholm P, Muzakare L, et al. Regeneration of corneal cells and nerves in an implanted collagen corneal substitute. Cornea. 2008;27:580–9.
33. Petroll WM, Kivanany PB, Hagenasr D, et al. Corneal fibroblast migration patterns during intrastromal wound healing correlate with ECM structure and alignment. Invest Ophthalmol Vis Sci. 2015;56:7352–61.
34. Raghunathan VK, Thomasy SM, Strøm P, et al. Tissue and cellular biomechanics during corneal wound injury and repair. Acta Biomater. 2017;58:291–301.
35. Mukwaya A, Lennikov A, Xeroudaki M, et al. Time-dependent LXR/RXR pathway modulation characterizes capillary remodeling in inflammatory corneal neovascularization. Angiogenesis. 2018;21:395–413.
36. Utsunomiya T, Hanada K, Muramatsu O, et al. Wound healing process after corneal stromal thinning observed with anterior segment optical coherence tomography. Cornea. 2014;33:1056–60.
37. Koulikovska M, Rafat M, Petrovski G, et al. Enhanced regeneration of corneal tissue via a bioengineered collagen construct implanted by a nondisruptive surgical technique. Tissue Eng Part A. 2015;21:1116–30.
38. Ho LT, Harris AM, Tanioka H, et al. A comparison of glycosaminoglycan distributions, keratan sulphate sulphation patterns and collagen fibril architecture from central to peripheral regions of the bovine cornea. Matrix Biol. 2014;38:59–68.
39. Liu Y, Gan L, Carlsson DJ, et al. A simple, cross-linked collagen tissue substitute for corneal implantation. Invest Ophthalmol Vis Sci. 2006;47:1869–75.
40. Ishizaki M, Zhu G, Haseba T, Shafer SS, Kao WW. Expression of collagen I, smooth muscle alpha-actin, and vimentin during the healing of alkali-burned and lacerated corneas. Invest Ophthalmol Vis Sci. 1993;34(12):3320–8.
41. Ghezzi CE, Rnjak-Kovacina J, Kaplan DL. Corneal tissue engineering: recent advances and future perspectives. Tissue Eng Part B Rev. 2015;21:278–87.
42. Murphy CM, Duffy GP, Schindeler A, et al. Effect of collagen-glycosaminoglycan scaffold pore size on matrix mineralization and cellular behavior in different cell types. J Biomed Mater Res A. 2016;104:291–304.

24

Keratometric measurements and IOL calculations in pseudophakic post-DSAEK patients

Ke Xu, Hong Qi* ⓘD, Rongmei Peng, Gege Xiao, Jing Hong, Yansheng Hao and Boping Ma

Abstract

Background: To compare different K readings in pseudophakic patients post-Descemet's stripping automated endothelial keratoplasty (DSAEK) and evaluate corresponding prediction errors in intraocular lens (IOL) power calculations.

Methods: Subjects that underwent cataract surgery and DSAEK surgery at least 3 and 6 months prior, respectively, and IOL implantation in the capsular bag were included in this study. Manifest refraction and IOL information were recorded. A Scheimpflug keratometer (Pentacam) was used for corneal measurements, including the mean anterior and posterior radii of curvature, simulated keratometer (SimK), true net power (TNP), and equivalent K reading (EKR) at the 4.0-mm zone. Conventional keratometry was acquired using the IOLMaster (K_{Master}). The four K measurements were evaluated for calculating the predicted refraction.

Results: The study included 20 eyes from 19 subjects. The ratio of the posterior to the anterior corneal radius was $74.1 \pm 3.24\%$. Comparison of the four keratometric methods (K_{Master}, SimK, EKR, and TNP) revealed statistically significant differences among all the methods besides K_{Master} and SimK. Of the four IOL calculation methods(K_{Master}, SimK, EKR and TNP method),the arithmetic prediction error of the K_{Master}, SimK, and EKR methods featured nonsignificant differences from zero($p = 0.07$, 0.19 and 0.84 respectively); the EKR method calculated the highest percentage of eyes with IOLs within the prediction error.

Conclusions: IOL calculations in post-DSAEK eyes using K_{Master}, SimK, and EKR can yield small refractive errors after surgery. The EKR (4.0-mm diameter) method was found to be the most accurate.

Keywords: Descemet's stripping automated endothelial keratoplasty, IOL, Keratometry, Pentacam

Background

Accurate assessment of the total corneal power of eyes following corneal refractive surgery is essential for determining optimal intraocular lens (IOL) power, and the difficulties in accurately evaluating corneal power after laser-assisted in situ keratomileusis (LASIK) have been well described [1, 2]. Descemet's stripping automated endothelial keratoplasty (DSAEK) procedure is a lamellar corneal surgical technique used to replace the abnormal corneal endothelium of patients with endothelial disease [3]. The literature features a dearth concerning the

proportion of DSAEK performed on phakic eyes without concomitant cataract surgery relative to the total number of DSAEK conducted. The technical advantages of DSAEK encouraged surgical intervention earlier in the course of clinical treatment, resulting in an increased number of patients presenting with clear lenses at the time of corneal intervention [4, 5]. This is particularly the case for patients with familial Fuchs dystrophy and clinically significant corneal disease that requires intervention at a relatively early age [6]. When these patients develop a clinically significant cataract post-DSAEK, changes on the posterior surface of the cornea affect the accuracy of keratometry (K) measurements and subsequent IOL power calculations. Previous studies have compared corneal power parameters after DSAEK with

* Correspondence: docqihong@163.com
Department of Ophthalmology, Beijing Key Laboratory of Restoration of Damaged Ocular Nerve, Peking University Third Hospital, 49 North Garden Road Haidian District, Beijing 100191, People's Republic of China

those of control or pre-DSAEK groups [7–11]; however, data on the accuracy of K measurements in post-DSAEK corneas and the prediction error in IOL power calculations among post-DSAEK patients is lacking.

The present retrospective study therefore aimed to compare K readings obtained with a conventional keratometer (IOLMaster) and a Scheimpflug keratometer in pseudophakic, post-DSAEK patients to evaluate prediction errors in IOL power calculations.

Methods

The present study conducted a retrospective review of 19 pseudophakic patients who underwent DSAEK at Peking University Third Hospital's Department of Ophthalmology and whose initial visit occurred between February 2016 and July 2016. The investigation was performed according to the tenets of the Declaration of Helsinki. The need for informed consent was waived and the study protocol was approved by Peking University Third Hospital Medical Science Research Ethics Committee.

Exclusion criteria included the following: history of ocular trauma, scarring, or severe edema of the corneal stroma; capsular or zonular anomalies of the lens; silicone oil in the posterior segment; diabetic macular changes; pathologic myopia; best-corrected visual acuity (BCVA) of < 20/100; and the inability to complete post-operative examinations. The present study included subjects whose cataract and DSAEK surgery needed to have been completed at least 3 and 6 months prior, respectively.

All patients underwent a routine phacoemulsification procedure and implantation of a foldable IOL in the capsular bag. Cataract surgery could occur prior to, in conjunction with, or after the performance of DSAEK, which were all performed by a single surgeon (J. Hong) according to a previously described procedure [12, 13]. The cataract surgery date, DSAEK surgery date, IOL type, and diopter information were recorded.

Patients attended regularly scheduled examinations that included evaluations of manifest refraction, uncorrected visual acuity, and BCVA; a slit-lamp examination; and anterior segment optical coherence tomography (Visante Model 1000, Carl Zeiss Meditec) to obtain total cornea and graft thickness(CT and GT,respectively) at the vertex and 2-mm points(0°, 90°, 180°, 270°). The Pentacam rotating Scheimpflug imaging system (Oculus, Wetzlar, Germany) was used for all corneal measurements: mean anterior radius of curvature, mean posterior radius of curvature, simulated keratometer reading (SimK), true net power (TNP), and equivalent K reading (EKR) at the 4.0-mm zone. The scans were repeated if the device did not issue a quality output reading of "OK." Only patients with a quality output reading of

"OK" were included in the study. Conventional K and axial length (AL) measurements were acquired by the IOLMaster (Carl Zeiss, Meditec AG, Jena, Germany) using the default settings for pseudophakic eyes.

A simplified relationship between the K readings (in diopters) and the value of the anterior corneal radius r (in millimeters) was used to calculate conventional K acquired by the IOLMaster(K_{Master}): $K_{Master} = 0.3375/r_{anterior}$. The principle of SimK from the Pentacam system used in this study is identical to the conventional keratometric method: $SimK = 0.3375/r_{anterior}$. TNP represents the sum of the anterior and posterior corneal powers [14]. This value was calculated using the following formula (1): $TNP = 0.376/r_{anterior} – 0.04/r_{posterior}$. In untreated eyes, $r_{posterior}$ can be substituted by $0.822r_{anterior}$ [15, 16]: $TNP_{untreated} = 0.3273/r_{anterior}$. EKR was advanced by Holladay and his colleagues to evaluate the total corneal power after corneal refractive surgery and was calculated using the following formula(2): $EKR = 0.376/r_{anterior} – 0.3165/r_{posterior}$ [17]. In untreated eyes, $r_{posterior}$ can be substituted by $0.822r_{anterior}$ [15, 16]: $EKR_{untreated} = 0.337496/r_{anterior}$.

The different K readings were introduced into the calculation formula attached to the IOLMaster to obtain the predicted refraction. The IOL power calculations were performed using third-generation formulas (SRK/T for AL > 26 mm, Hoffer Q for AL < 22 mm, and Holladay 1 for AL from 22 to 26 mm) as recommended by Hoffer with optimized A-constants for different implanted IOLs [18]. Predicted refraction was collected from the biometry reading of the selected IOLs. Achieved refraction was the spheroequivalent value of the manifest refraction. The arithmetic prediction error (achieved refraction minus predicted refraction), absolute error, and percentage of eyes within 0.5 D, 1.0 D, and 2.0 D were calculated. According to Chang [19], an adjustment of target refraction by 0.17 to 0.24D is required to simulate a phakic eye model. This range was calculated as the approximate mean of the hyperopic shift between the pseudophakic predicted refraction and the phakic predicted refraction. Therefore, all prediction refraction values were adjusted by a decrease of 0.2 D, the mean of 0.17 and 0.24 D.

Statistical analyses were performed using SPSS for Windows (version 16.0, SPSS, Inc.). A Student's t-test was used to evaluate the presence of significant differences in the data. The relationship between the differences in K readings and the corneal profiles was assessed via regression analysis. A p-value of < 0.05 was considered statistically significant.

Results

The present study evaluated 20 pseudophakic eyes (right, 12; left, 8) from 19 patients (five men) who had undergone DSAEK. The mean age of the patients was

70 ± 12 years (range, 38–83 years). Prior to DSAEK surgery, the cohort included six eyes with Fuch's endothelial dystrophy, six eyes with corneal endothelial decompensation of unknown etiology, and eight eyes with post-cataract or post-IOP-elevation bullous keratoplasty. Of the 20 eyes, one underwent DSAEK prior to cataract surgery, seven received DSAEK after cataract surgery, and 12 underwent the two surgeries during the same procedure. The mean postoperative times following the cataract and DSAEK surgeries were 730 days (range 183–1524 days) and 626 days (range 181–1402 days), respectively. The mean spheroequivalent value of achieved refraction was – 1.43 D (range – 6.25 to 2.13 D). The mean AL was 24.09 ± 2.87 mm (range 21.08 to 31.50 mm). AL of < 22.0 mm (Hoffer Q formula) featured in two eyes (10%); 15 eyes (75%) had an AL of 22.0–26.0 mm (Holladay 1 formula); and three eyes (15%) had an AL of > 26.0 mm (SRK/T formula). All 20 implanted IOLs were acrylic and placed in the capsular bag. The models of the IOLs were as follows: nine were Model 400, Medennium, Inc.; five, AR40e, Abbott Medical Optics, Inc.; three, YA-60BB, Hoya Corporation; one, ZCB00, Abbott Medical Optics, Inc.; one, HQ-201HEP, HexaVision SARL; and one, ZA9003, Abbott Medical Optics, Inc. The mean anterior corneal radius was 7.68 ± 0.30 mm, and that of the posterior corneal radius was 5.69 ± 0.28 mm; the ratio of the posterior to the anterior corneal radius was 74.1 ± 3.24% (range 67.8–81.8%). The mean central graft thickness was 117.25 ± 41.83 µm. The mean graft thickness at the 2-mm corneal point was 138.74 ± 46.05 µm.

Figure 1 shows the K values for each keratometric method. Comparisons among the four keratometric methods [Conventional K from the IOLMaster (K_{Master}) and SimK, EKR, and TNP from the Pentacam] revealed no statistically significant difference between K_{Master} and SimK; statistically significant differences were, however, detected among all other comparisons among the keratometric methods. K_{Master} (44.18 ± 1.50) and SimK (44.01 ± 1.71) featured the largest mean K-values, followed respectively by EKR (43.59 ± 1.72) and TNP (42.05 ± 1.77). Table 1 shows the differences in the observed K values in relation to TNP.

Table 2 shows the relationship between the corneal profile and K reading differences. There was a very strong correlation between the ratio of the posterior to the anterior corneal radius and the SimK-TNP difference ($r^2 = 0.73$, $p < 0.001$). Table 3 shows the arithmetic error and absolute error of predictions using the four K readings. Comparison of arithmetic errors using the different Ks and a paired t-test found no statistically significant difference between K_{Master} and SimK; statistically significant differences were found for all other comparisons among the keratometric methods (Fig. 2). A paired t-test revealed no statistically significant differences among the absolute errors of K_{Master}, SimK, and EKR.

Of the four IOL calculation methods [the IOLMaster-measured K and three Pentacam-measured corneal powers (SimK, EKR and TNP) inserted into the three third-generation formulas], only the arithmetic error of the TNP method was significantly different from zero (one-sample t-test, $p < 0.01$); that of the other three

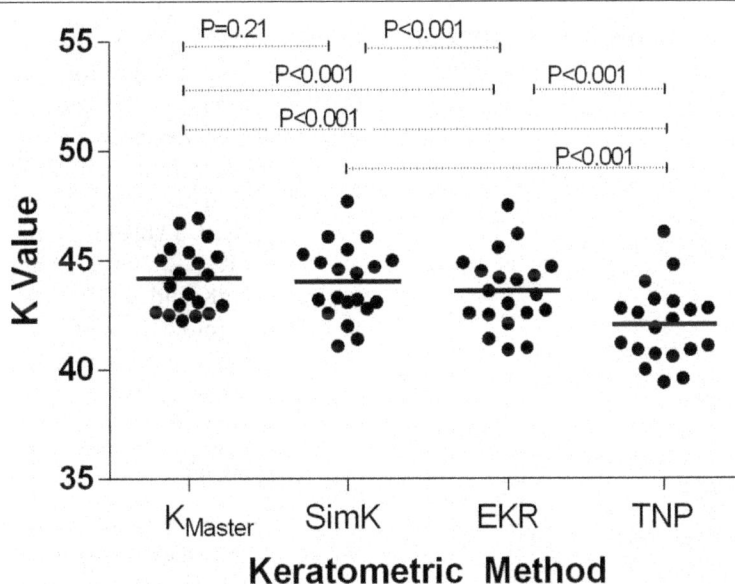

Fig. 1 Scatterplot of mean K values for the keratometric methods. Statistically significant differences were observed in all t-test pairs, except between K_{Master} and SimK. K_{Master}, conventional K obtained with the IOLMaster; SimK, simulated keratometer reading; EKR, equivalent K reading; TNP, true net power

Table 1 Mean K values of different keratometric methods and comparison between those K values and TNP

| Type of K | n | Mean(D) ± SD | Range | Difference from TNP | | |
				Mean (D) ± SD	95% CI of difference	P value
K_{Master}	20	44.18 ± 1.50	42.28 to 46.95	2.13 ± 0.61	1.85 to 2.41	< 0.001
SimK	20	44.01 ± 1.71	41.10 to 47.70	1.96 ± 0.33	1.81 to 2.11	< 0.001
EKR at 4.0 mm	20	43.59 ± 1.72	40.90 to 47.50	1.55 ± 0.27	1.42 to 1.67	< 0.001
TNP	20	42.05 ± 1.77	39.40 to 46.30	–	–	–

K_{Master} conventional K via IOLMaster, SimK simulated keratometer reading, EKR equivalent K reading, TNP true net power

methods (K_{Master}, SimK and EKR) featured nonsignificant differences with a value of zero ($p = 0.07$, 0.19, and 0.84, respectively). The percentages of eyes within 0.50, 1.00, and 2.00 D, and that exceeding 2.00 D of the prediction error of the three different methods are shown in Table 4. The EKR method featured the highest percentage values for each category and the lowest mean absolute prediction error value (0.74 ± 0.68).

Discussion

In the present study, we investigated four keratometric methods and predicted their respective post-DSAEK IOL-calculation error in pseudophakic patients. Several studies reported a hyperopic shift after DSAEK, ranging from 0.7 to 1.5 D [1, 3, 8, 9, 20, 21]. The hyperopic shift is partially explained by the meniscus-shaped configuration of the endothelial graft, which is thicker in the periphery and likely contributes to the increased curvature of the posterior surface [2, 9, 21, 22]. We found that after DSAEK, the normal physiologic relationship between the anterior and posterior surfaces, on which the conventional K measurement is based, was altered; the accuracy of the K measurement and subsequent IOL-power calculation was consequently affected. To the best of our knowledge, this is the first study to report IOL calculations in post-DSAEK patients.

Table 2 Relationship between corneal profile and K reading differences

Difference of Method	Correlated factor	r^2	P value
K_{Master} - TNP	$R_{posterior}/R_{anterior}$	0.19	0.05
	central/peripheral CT	0.24	0.03*
	central/peripheral GT	0.11	0.16
Sim K- TNP	$R_{posterior}/R_{anterior}$	0.73	< 0.001*
	central/peripheral CT	0.42	0.00*
	central/peripheral GT	0.29	0.01*
EKR at 4.0 mm - TNP	$R_{posterior}/R_{anterior}$	0.16	0.09
	central/peripheral CT	0.16	0.08
	central/peripheral GT	0.15	0.09

*K_{Master} Conventional K via IOLMaster, SimK Simulated keratometer reading, EKR Equivalent K reading, TNP True net power, R posterior mean posterior radius of the corneal curvature, R anterior mean anterior radius of the corneal curvature, CT total corneal thickness, GT corneal graft thickness. *p < 0.05*

The mean ratio of the posterior corneal radius to the anterior corneal radius of an untreated cornea is 82.2% [15, 16]. In post-DSAEK patients, we found that this ratio decreased to 74.1% (SD 3.24%), confirming that posterior lamellar grafts alter the corneal profile. When a non-uniform thickness graft, thicker in its periphery than in its center, is added to the posterior host cornea, it contributes to the reduction of the posterior corneal radius of curvature and thereby decreases the ratio of the posterior corneal radius to the anterior corneal radius. Conventional keratometry assumes that the radius of the curvature of the posterior ocular surface is 82.2% that of the anterior corneal surface. This explains the significant difference in the corneal powers detected by K_{Master} and TNP (44.18 vs. 42.05 D, $p < 0.01$), as well as by SimK and TNP (44.01 vs. 42.05 D, $p < 0.01$).

For subjects who underwent DSAEK, the ratio of the posterior to anterior corneal radii was 0.741. Hence, $r_{posterior}$ can be substituted by $0.741 r_{anterior}$ in formula1 and 2. The TNP and EKR for these subjects were calculated as follows: $TNP_{DSAEK} = 0.3220/ r_{anterior}$; $EKR_{DSAEK} = 0.3333/ r_{anterior}$. Table 5 shows the different K formulae used for the measurements obtained before and after the DSAEK; the different coefficients used in these formulae can partially account for the differences and sequence in keratometry. Previous studies on virgin eyes found that K_{Master} and SimK values were higher than those of TNP by approximately 1.13–1.43 D [23–27]. The present study observed a post-DSAEK difference of approximately 2.13 D between K_{Master} and TNP and a difference of 1.96 D between SimK and TNP; both differences are greater than those found in virgin eyes. While The coefficients in the formulae for K_{Master} and SimK did not change after DSAEK, the smaller coefficient of the TNP formula decreased after DSAEK. The latter finding may account for the change in K distance after DSAEK.

Accounting for both the anterior and posterior corneal surfaces, TNP may more accurately reflect the actual corneal refractive power than the other K values. Our regression analysis of the corneal profile and SimK-TNP difference revealed that the latter was strongly correlated with the ratio of the posterior to the anterior corneal

Table 3 Arithmetic error and absolute error of prediction using different K readings

Method	n	Arithmetic Error (D)			Absolute Error (D)		
		Mean(D) ± SD	Minimum - Maximum	Range	Mean(D) ± SD	Minimum - Maximum	Range
K_{Master}	20	0.44 ± 1.02	−1.70 to 2.32	4.02	0.89 ± 0.63	0.01 to 2.32	2.31
SimK	20	0.32 ± 1.03	−1.90 to2.32	4.22	0.82 ± 0.68	0.05 to 2.32	2.27
EKR	20	−0.05 ± 1.02	−2.40 to 1.91	4.31	0.74 ± 0.68	0.03 to 2.40	2.37
TNP	20	−1.35 ± 1.06	−3.90 to 0.76	4.66	1.42 ± 0.95	0.05 to 3.90	3.85

K_{Master} conventional K via IOLMaster, *SimK* simulated keratometer reading, *EKR* equivalent K reading, *TNP* true net power

radius ($r^2 = 0.73$, $p < 0.001$). We further found that the difference between the SimK and TNP was weakly correlated with the central/peripheral CT ($r^2 = 0.42$) and the GT ($r^2 = 0.29$). The possible reason is that measuring the thickness 2 mm from the vertex of the total cornea and graft cannot reflect the peripheral profile and, when compared with the ratio of the posterior to the anterior corneal radius (mean radius on a 3-mm ring), the latter may better reflect the corneal profile.

Despite the fact that the same principle underlies the Pentacam (SimK) and IOLMaster (K_{Master}) systems, the present study failed to observe a correlation between the keratometric power deviation (K_{Master} versus TNP) and the ratio of the posterior to the anterior corneal radius ($r^2 = 0.19$, $p > 0.05$). This may be explained by the parameters of SimK, TNP, and the ratio of the posterior to anterior corneal radius been derived from the same corneal topography system, whereas that for K_{Master} is not. Our finding that the EKR-TNP difference was not correlated with the corneal profile may be accounted for

by the following: the mean value of EKR was between those of SimK and TNP and the deviation from TNP was small.

Employing the original implanted IOL power and optical biometry, Chang et al. [19] reported that the IOL-Master predicted more hyperopic refraction in pseudophakic eyes and observed a mean hyperopic shift of approximately 0.17D to 0.24 D in the pseudophakic-predicted refraction relative to those calculated from phakia using the SRK II and SRK/T formulae. The subjects in the present study also exhibited a pseudophakic condition. To simulate the phakic eye, 0.20 D (the mean of 0.17D and 0.24 D) was subtracted from each predicted refraction to compensate for our use of third-generation IOL formulae. The arithmetic prediction errors of the IOL calculations using K_{Master}, SimK, and EKR were not significantly different from zero. Comparison of the arithmetic error of the three methods using a paired t-test revealed statistically significant differences between EKR and SimK as well as

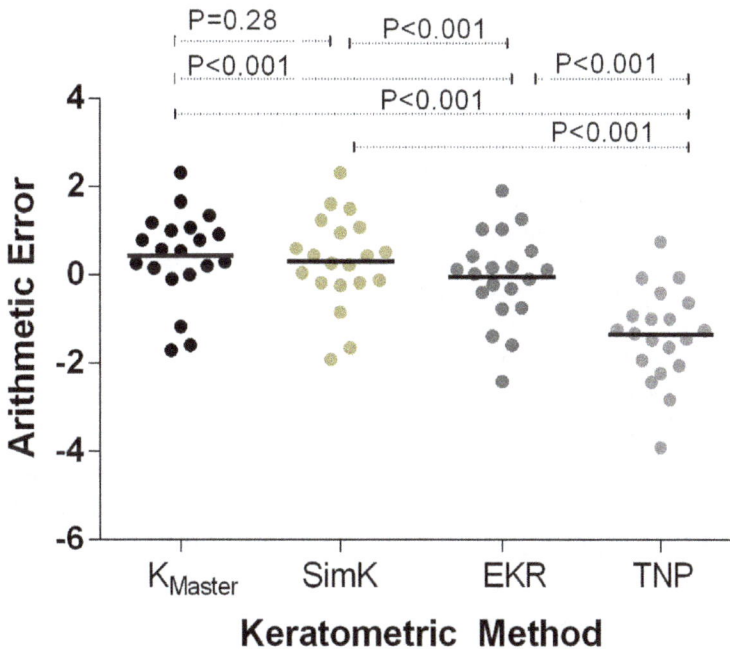

Fig. 2 Arithmetic error plot using different K reading methods. K_{Master}, conventional K obtained with the IOLMaster; SimK, simulated keratometer reading; EKR, equivalent K reading; TNP, true net power

Table 4 Percentage of eyes within 0.50 D, 1.00 D, and 2.00 D, and exceeding 2.00 D of the prediction error of the 3 different methods

Method	Prediction Error (%)			
	Within ±0.50D	Within ±1.00D	Within ±2.00D	> 2.00D
K_{Master}	30	55	95	5
SimK	45	65	95	5
EKR	50	65	95	5

K_{Master} conventional K via IOLMaster, *SimK* simulated keratometer reading, *EKR* equivalent K reading

between EKR and K_{Master}. The percentages of eyes within 0.50, 1.00, and 2.00 D, and that exceeding 2.00 D of the prediction error of the three different methods confirmed that the EKR method produced the highest percentage values for each category. Considering that the mean value of the absolute prediction error of the EKR method was the lowest (EKR, 0.74; SimK, 0.82; K_{Master} 0.89), we suggest that EKR be used in IOL calculations in post-DSAEK eyes. Benchmarks for refractive success after routine cataract surgery are reported as 85% within 1.0 D and 55% within 0.5 D of the intended refraction [28]. As 50% of patients were within 0.5 D of the predicted value, the present study demonstrates that an accuracy would be nearly achievable by using the 4.0-mm-diameter EKR.

Conventional keratometry has been noted to overestimate corneal power in patients after myopic laser refractive surgery, which may result in an undesirable, unexpectedly large hyperopic refractive error [29–31]. The present study found that the arithmetic prediction error of K_{Master} and SimK was not significantly different from zero, indicating that although LASIK and DSAEK both change the relationship between the anterior and posterior corneal refractive powers, the latter induces a smaller impact on corneal refractive power than does the former. This finding may be accounted for by the following mechanisms. (i) Unlike LASIK, changes in the corneal power after DSAEK mainly occur in the posterior cornea, which has low refractive power [9, 32]. (ii) Post-DSAEK eyes feature a graft diameter that is sufficiently large to maintain a continuous change in the central-area curvature, further allowing paracentral measurement of conventional keratometry to be conducted. (iii) Improvements in the preparation of DSAEK

grafts reduce variations in the corneal profile, thus eliminating postoperative changes in refraction.

The present investigation was subject to the limitation of a small sample size and those inherent to retrospective studies. Pseudophakic post-DSAEK eyes were evaluated, but adjustments were required to simulate phakic post-DSAEK eyes. Using EKR in a clinical scenario would therefore likely achieve less than the 50% within 0.5 D of the intended refraction. Further, although some cases indicated that intraocular surgery with appropriate precautions could be performed safely in post-DSAEK eyes, K measurements may be affected by phacoemulsification-related damage to the corneal endothelium during cataract surgery post-DSAEK [33]. Future prospective clinical studies from multiple centers will help address and attenuate these limitations.

Conclusions

The ratio of the posterior to the anterior corneal radius of curvature decreased to74.1% following DSAEK. The deviation between SimK versus TNP in post-DSAEK eyes increased and was strongly correlated with the ratio of the posterior to the anterior corneal radius of curvature. IOL calculations in post-DSAEK eyes using K_{Master} SimK, and EKR can yield small refractive errors after surgery; however, EKR (4.0-mm diameter) was found to be the most accurate.

WHAT WAS KNOWN

- Accurate assessment of the total corneal power in eyes after corneal refractive surgery is essential for determining the optimal IOL power. The difficulty in accurately evaluating corneal power after LASIK surgery is well established.
- In patients with cataracts post-DSAEK, changes in the posterior surface of the cornea will affect the accuracy of K measurements and subsequent IOL-power calculations. Little is currently known regarding the accuracy of K measurements in post-DSAEK corneas.

WHAT THIS PAPER ADDS

- For IOL calculations in post-DSAEK eyes, the use of conventional K measurements will not yield a large refractive change. A K measurement obtained using the Pentacam, which accounts for both the anterior and posterior corneal surfaces, is considered the most accurate. This study is the first to assess IOL calculations in post-DSAEK eyes.

Table 5 Different K formulas before and after DSAEK surgery

Untreated Eye	After DSAEK
$K_{Master} = 0.3375/r_{anterior}$	$K_{Master} = 0.3375/r_{anterior}$
$Sim\,K = 0.3375/r_{anterior}$	$Sim\,K = 0.3375/r_{anterior}$
$EKR_{untreated} = 0.337496/r_{anterior}$	$EKR_{DSAEK} = 0.3333/r_{anterior}$
$TNP_{untreated} = 0.3273/r_{anterior}$	$TNP_{DSAEK} = 0.3220/r_{anterior}$

Acknowledgements
We would like to thank Dr. Haikun Wang in our medical statistics department. He provided thoughtful, professional advice that helped to remedy statistical problems in our study.

Funding

This study was supported by National Natural Science Foundation of China (No.81570813). The authors have no financial or proprietary interest in a product, method, or material described herein.

Financial disclosure

No author has a financial or proprietary interest in any material or method mentioned.

Authors' contributions

K.X. – Design, drafting, data acquisition, analysis, and interpretation. H.Q.- Design drafting, data acquisition, analysis, and interpretation. R.P. – Design, drafting, data acquisition, analysis, and interpretation. G.X. – Design, drafting, and analysis. J.H. - Drafting, data acquisition, and analysis. Y.H. - Design, drafting, and data acquisition. B.M. - Design, drafting, and data acquisition. All authors read and approved the final manuscript.

Competing interests

The authors declare that they have no competing interests.

References

1. Koenig SB, Covert DJ, Dupps WJ Jr, et al. Visual acuity, refractive error and endothelial cell density six months after Descemet stripping and automated endothelial keratoplasty (DSAEK). Cornea 2007;26:670–674.
2. Rao SK, Leung CKS, Cheung CYL, et al. Descemet stripping endothelial keratoplasty: effect of the surgical procedure on corneal optics. Am J Ophthalmol. 2008;145:991–6.
3. Gorovoy MS. Descemet-stripping automated endothelial keratoplasty. Cornea. 2006;25:886–9.
4. Price FW Jr, Price MO. Descemet's stripping with endothelial keratoplasty in 200 eyes: early challenges and techniques to enhance donor adherence. J Cataract Refract Surg. 2006;32:411–8.
5. Terry MA, Shamie N, Chen ES, et al. Endothelial keratoplasty for Fuchs' dystrophy with cataract: complications and clinical results with the new triple procedure. Ophthalmology. 2009;116:631–9.
6. Afshari NA, Pittard AB, Siddiqui A, et al. Clinical study of Fuchs cornealendothelial dystrophy leading to penetrating keratoplasty: a 30-yearexperience. Arch Ophthalmol. 2006;124:777–80.
7. Covert DJ, Koenig SB. New triple procedure: Descemet's stripping and automated endothelial keratoplasty combined with phacoemulsification and intraocular lens implantation. Ophthalmology. 2007;114:1272–7.
8. Koenig SB, Covert DJ. Early results of small-incision Descemet's stripping and automated endothelial keratoplasty. Ophthalmology. 2007;114:221–6.
9. Scorcia V, Matteoni S, Scorcia GB, et al. Pentacam assessment of posterior lamellar grafts to explain hyperopization after Descemet's stripping automated endothelial keratoplasty. Ophthalmology. 2009;116:1651–5.
10. Prasher P, Muftuoglu O, Bowman RW, et al. Corneal power measurement with a rotating Scheimpflug imaging system after Descemet-stripping automated endothelial keratoplasty. J Cataract Refract Surg. 2010;36:1358–64.
11. Clemmensen K, Ivarsen A, Hjortdal J. Changes in Corneal Power After Descemet Stripping Automated Endothelial Keratoplasty. J Refract Surg. 2015;31:807–12.
12. Hong Y, Peng RM, Wang M, et al. Suture pull-through insertion techniques for Descemet stripping automated endothelial keratoplasty in Chinese phakic eyes: outcomes and complications. PLoS One. 2013;8:e61929.
13. Hong Y, Hong J, Xu YG, et al. Comment on phakic descemet stripping automated endothelial keratoplasty: prevalence and prognostic impact of postoperative cataracts. Cornea. 2013;32:217.
14. Savini G, Hoffer KJ. Pentacam HR equivalent K-reading. J Refract Surg. 2010; 26:389–91.
15. Tang M, Chen A, Li Y, et al. Corneal power measurement with Fourier-domain optical coherence tomography. J Cataract Refract Surg. 2010;36:2115–22.
16. Ho JD, Tsai CY, Tsai RJ, et al. Validity of the keratometric index: evaluation by the Pentacam rotating Scheimpflug camera. J Cataract Refract Surg. 2008;34:137–45.
17. Holladay JT, Hill WE, Steinmueller A. Corneal power measurements using scheimpflug imaging in eyes with prior corneal refractive surgery. J Refract Surg. 2009;25(10):862–8.
18. Hoffer KJ. Clinical results using the Holladay 2 intraocular lens power formula. J Cataract Refract Surg. 2000;26:1233–7.
19. Chang SW, Yu CY, Chen DP. Comparison of intraocular lens power calculation by the IOLMaster in phakic and eyes with hydrophobic acrylic lenses. Ophthalmology. 2009;116:1336–42.
20. Lee WB, Jacobs DS, Musch DC, et al. Descemet's stripping endothelial keratoplasty: safety and outcomes. A report by the American Academy of ophthalmology. Ophthalmology. 2009;116:1818–30.
21. Holz HA, Meyer JJ, Espandar L, et al. Corneal profile analysis after Descemet stripping endothelial keratoplasty and its relationship to postoperative hyperopic shift. J Cataract Refract Surg. 2008;34:211–4.
22. Bahar I, Kaiserman I, McAllum P, et al. Comparison of posterior lamellar keratoplasty techniques to penetrating keratoplasty. Ophthalmology. 2008; 115:1525–33.
23. Hua Y, Zhang X, Utheim TP, et al. Evaluation of equivalent keratometry readings obtained by Pentacam HR (high resolution). PLoS One. 2016;11: e0150121.
24. Saad E, Shammas MC, Shammas HJ. Scheimpflug corneal power measurements for intraocular lens power calculation in cataract surgery. Am J Ophthalmol. 2013;156:460–7.
25. Symes RJ, Ursell PG. Automated keratometry in routine cataract surgery: comparison of Scheimpflug and conventional values. J Cataract Refract Surg. 2011;37:295–301.
26. Symes RJ, Say MJ, Ursell PG. Scheimpflug keratometry versus conventional automated keratometry in routine cataract surgery. J Cataract Refract Surg. 2010;36:1107–14.
27. Shammas HJ, Hoffer KJ, Shammas MC. Scheimpflug photography keratometry readings for routine intraocular lens power calculation. J Cataract Refract Surg. 2009;35:330–4.
28. Gale RP, Saldana M, Johnston RL, et al. Benchmark standards for refractive outcomes after NHS cataract surgery. Eye. 2009;23:149–52.
29. Tang M, Li Y, Avila M, et al. Measuring total corneal power before and after laser in situ keratomileusis with high-speed optical coherence tomography. J Cataract Refract Surg. 2006;32:1843–50.
30. Seiler T, McDonnell P. Excimer laser photorefractive keratectomy. Surv Ophthalmol. 1995;40:89–118.
31. Seitz B, Torres F, Langenbacher A, et al. Posterior corneal curvature changes after myopic laser in situ keratomileusis. Ophthalmology. 2001;108:666–72.
32. de Sanctis U, Angeloni M, Zilio C, et al. Corneal power after Descemet stripping automated endothelial keratoplasty using microkeratome-prepared tissues. Opt Vis Sci. 2011;88:697–702.
33. Chaurasia S, Ramappa M, Sangwan V. Cataract surgery after Descemet stripping endothelial keratoplasty. Indian J Ophthalmol. 2012;60:572–4.

25

Cancer-associated retinopathy preceding the diagnosis of cancer

Florence Hoogewoud[1][*] ⓘ, Pauline Butori[1], Philippe Blanche[2] and Antoine P. Brézin[1]

Abstract

Background: The early diagnosis of cancer is of crucial importance and a key prognostic factor. Cancer-associated retinopathy (CAR) can be symptomatic prior to other manifestations directly related to malignant tumors. The aim of this study was to show that, in selected cases, ophthalmic findings are consistent enough with the diagnosis of CAR to trigger investigations aimed at detecting a previously unknown malignancy.

Methods: This was a monocentric retrospective case series performed in a tertiary referral center. Patients with a diagnosis of CAR were included. Diagnosis was based on the clinical presentation, the visual field and electroretinogram alterations. The clinical presentation, visual field testing and electroretinographic results were analyzed as well as the malignancies identified following the diagnosis of CAR. Follow-up data was collected.

Results: Four patients (two men, two women, median age 65.5 years) were included. All patients presented with posterior segment inflammation at initial presentation as well as advanced visual field loss and an extinguished electroretinogram. The best corrected decimal visual acuity was 0.8 or better in both eyes of three patients and decreased to 0.3 OD and 0.2 OS in one patient due to a bilateral macular edema. No patient had a previously known history of cancer. Once the diagnosis of CAR was made, investigations aimed at identifying a malignant tumors subsequently led to the diagnosis of two cases of small cell lung tumors, of one prostate carcinoma and of a uterine sarcoma. The treatment of CAR included plasmapheresis, systemic corticosteroids, azathioprine, cyclosporine and periocular or intraocular corticosteroid injections. In all cases the intraocular inflammation resolved, but pigment mottling, diffuse retinal atrophy, optic disc pallor and arterial narrowing were among manifestations observed during the follow-up of the patients.

Conclusion: In selected patients, findings suggestive of CAR can be useful for the early detection of a cancer.

Keywords: Cancer-associated retinopathy, Uveitis, Paraneoplastic retinopathy, Cancer

Background

Cancer-Associated Retinopathy (CAR) is a paraneoplastic, autoimmune retinopathy characterized by diffuse retinal degeneration. CAR is associated with a variety of cancers, among which small cell lung carcinoma are the most frequent [1]. Subacute visual loss and visual field constriction are the usual presenting symptoms. The malignancy associated with a CAR can be diagnosed before or after the onset of the ocular manifestations. Because CAR is rare, the descriptions of the disease are based on small series and case reports. As cancer research progresses with improved treatments and increased survival rates, the long term visual outcome of CAR can now be assessed.

The aim of this study was to highlight that in selected cases, ophthalmic findings are consistent enough with the diagnosis of CAR to trigger investigations aimed at detecting a previously unknown malignancy.

Methods

A retrospective chart review was performed of CAR patients diagnosed at Cochin University Hospital, a uveitis referral center in Paris, France, from 1994 and 2015. The diagnosis of CAR was based on the observation of an intraocular inflammation, the presence of a tubularvisual field (VF) as well as electroretinography (ERG) testing. All patients had a negative family history of retinitis pigmentosa and underwent an extensive workup to exclude other causes of uveitis. The study was performed in accordance with declaration of Helsinki and approved by

* Correspondence: fhoogewoud@gmail.com
[1]Department of Ophthalmology, National Referral Center for rare Ocular Diseases, Hôpital Cochin, APHP, Université Paris Descartes, Paris, France
Full list of author information is available at the end of the article

Table 1 Patients' baseline characteristics

Case n°	Gender	Age-range	Type of cancer	Time to diagnosis (months)	Decimal BCVA (OD/OS)	Anterior Segment inflammation	Vitritis	Periphlebitis	Macular edema	Waxy optic pallor	Arteriolar narrowing	OCT	Visual Field	ERG
1	F	61–70	Uterine Sarcoma	2	0.9/1	yes	no	yes	no	yes	yes	ORAFS	tubular	extinguished
2	M	51–60	Lung, small cell	1	0.9/1	no	yes	no	no	yes	yes	ORAFS	tubular	extinguished
3	M	71–80	Prostate adenocarcinoma	25	0.3/0.2	no	yes	no	yes	no	no	CME	tubular	extinguished
4	F	61–70	Lung, small cell	1	0.8/0.8	no	unknown	yes	no	unknown	yes	ORAFS	tubular	extinguished

BCVA Best corrected visual acuity, *OCT* Optical coherence tomography, *CME* Cystoid macular edema, *ORAFS* Outer retinal atrophy with foveolar sparing

the ethics committee of the French Society of Ophthalmology (IRB 00008855 Société Française d'Ophtalmologie IRB#1).

Results

Four patients met our inclusion criteria: two males and two females, with a median age of 65.5 years (range 58 to 71 years). Presenting complaints were a loss of visual acuity in two cases, VF constriction with photophobia in one case, visual vibrations and floaters in another. The time interval between the first symptoms and the first visit to an ophthalmologist ranges from 2 weeks to 1 month. Subsequently three out of four patients were immediately referred to us and one patient was referred 13 months later.

In all patients, the diagnosis of cancer was unknown at the time of the first ophthalmic visit and none had a significant medical history. The initial ophthalmological presentations are outlined in Table 1. Anterior chamber inflammation was absent in three cases and in the other graded 1+ OU without keratic precipitates or synechiae. Posterior segment inflammation included a 1+ vitreous haze and/or peripheral periphlebitis and one case of bilateral macular edema and papillitis. Visual fields were significantly constricted in all cases with a tubular pattern characterized by limits of the V-1 isopter within the central 30°. Two patients had a fluorescein angiography (FA) in the early course of their disease (patients 1 and 3). Both had periphlebitis and papillitis. Patient 3 had additional macular edema. Patient 4 had an FA 7 years after the onset of the disease: she had no active inflammation but a hyperfluorescence around the vessels due to a window defect caused by atrophy. On ERG, three out of four patients had no identifiable A or B waves from the background noise for all stimuli. Patient 3 presented an undistinguishable rod- and mixed-response; cone-response showed severely reduced amplitudes of the A and B waves

with normal implicit times and a conserved morphology. Three patients had a best corrected decimal visual acuity (decimal BCVA) of 0.8 or better in both eyes, with a characteristic pattern of outer retinal atrophy and foveolar sparing on OCT (Fig. 1). One patient had a decimal BCVA of 0.3 and 0.2 due to a bilateral cystoid macular edema.

A cancer was diagnosed in all four patients, with two cases of small cell lung tumor, one case of prostate carcinoma and one uterine sarcoma. The treatment prescribed to the patients included plasmapheresis and/or systemic corticosteroids and/or azathioprine and/or cyclosporine (Additional file 1). Patient 3, who presented with a macular edema and grade 1+ vitritis, was initially diagnosed as a case of idiopathic posterior uveitis and treated by periocular or intraocular corticosteroid injections.

Intraocular inflammation subsided in all patients within their follow-up, which ranged from 2 months to 10 years. Patients 3 and 4, for whom the follow-up was the longest, developed a retinitis pigmentosa-like pattern of retinal pigment spicules, diffuse peripheral retinal atrophy and arterial narrowing (Fig. 2). Within the follow-up OCT imaging showed an outer retinal atrophy with foveal sparing in 3 cases, whereas one patient had a diffuse macular atrophy in the left eye and an irreversible macular edema in the right eye.

Discussion

CAR was first defined in 1976 by Sayer et al. who described a clinical triad of photosensitivity, attenuated retinal arterioles, and visual field loss with a ring scotoma in three patients with non-ophthalmic anaplastic tumor [2]. Subsequently, various case reports have associated this syndrome with other malignancies [3, 4]. Additional clinical features have been described including extinguished ERG, waxy optic disc pallor [5, 6], and retinal vasculitis [7]. Intraocular inflammation as a manifestation of CAR has been

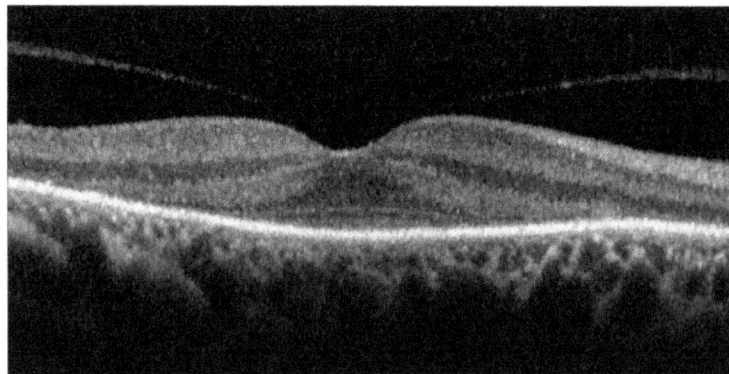

Fig. 1 Spectral-domain optical coherence tomography (Spectralis, Heidelberg Engineering, Germany) showing the loss of the external limiting membrane, of the inner segment/outer segment junction and of the outer nuclear and plexiform layers with a sparing of the foveal region

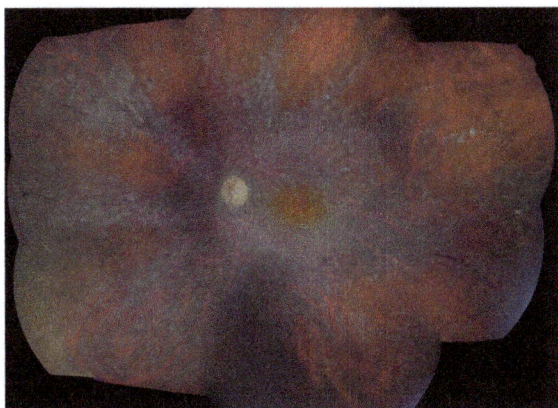

Fig. 2 Fundus photography (Digital Non-Mydriatic Retinal Camera, Canon, USA) of patient four at the last follow-up. Diffuse retinal atrophy combined with arteriolar attenuation, optic disc pallor and pigment deposits are observed

previously reported in the literature [8] and was observed in all of our cases at presentation. The intraocular inflammation can lead to an initial work-up targeted to detect other causes of uveitis, before CAR is diagnosed. Optic disc pallor was already seen at the first examination in two patients for whom the time interval between reported symptoms and diagnosis was short. This might reflect the fact that an underlining subacute inflammation might have remained unnoticed for a long time before the first symptoms. Atrophy of the outer retinal layers with foveal sparing was the most frequent OCT finding in our patients and was a helpful sign in the diagnosis of CAR [9]. After an initial inflammatory phase, late findings including retinal pigment epithelial mottling and retinal atrophy have been reported and were observed in our two patients with a long follow-up [10, 11]. In these cases the treatments used were unsuccessful to prevent a diffuse retinal atrophy with a poor visual outcome.

The pathophysiology of CAR remains incompletely understood but molecular mimicry is the generally accepted mechanism. Multiple anti-retinal antibodies have been described in CAR. The most commonly identified auto-antibody is targeted against recoverin. Photoreceptors apoptosis induced by the intravitreal injection of anti-recoverin has been shown in an experimental model [12]. Recent evidence suggests that the cellular rather the humoral immunity can play a role in the disease [13]. This would explain the large number of CAR for which auto-antibodies are not detected. The role of the auto-antibodies as an adjunctive test in the diagnosis of CAR is also controversial with an estimated sensitivity of 55.6% at presentation [5]. The specificity is also low as anti-retinal antibodies can be found in the serum of control patients. [14] Moreover, the absence of auto-antibodies has a very low negative predictive value and

the lack of a standardized methods has led to an important variability in the ability of laboratories to detect retinal auto-antibodies [15]. Although retinal auto-antibodies were not tested in our patients, their diagnosis of CAR were based on distinctive ophthalmological manifestations and led us with sufficient confidence to search for a malignancy.

Conclusion

CAR can precede the diagnosis of cancer. When CAR is recognized ophthalmologists can help their patients in referring them for a workup aimed at detecting a primary tumor.

Abbreviations

BCVA: Best-corrected visual acuity; CAR: Cancer-associated retinopathy; ERG: Electroretinogram; OCT: Optical coherence tomography; VF: Visual field

Acknowledgements
The authors acknowledge Dr. Pierre-Raphaël Rothschild for his help with this study.

Funding
No funding.

Authors' contributions
FH collected the data and wrote the manuscript, PBu and PBI collected the data and revised the manuscript and AB designed the study, analyzed the data and revised the manuscript. All authors have read and approved the manuscript.

Competing interests
The authors declare that they have no competing interests.

Author details
[1]Department of Ophthalmology, National Referral Center for rare Ocular Diseases, Hôpital Cochin, APHP, Université Paris Descartes, Paris, France. [2]Department of Internal Medicine, National Referral Center for Rare Systemic Autoimmune Diseases, Hôpital Cochin, APHP, Paris, France.

References
1. Chan JW. Paraneoplastic retinopathies and optic neuropathies. Surv Ophthalmol. 2003;48:12–38.
2. Sawyer RA, Selhorst JB, Zimmerman LE, Hoyt WF. Blindness caused by photoreceptor degeneration as a remote effect of cancer. Am J Ophthalmol. 1976;81:606–13.
3. Scott CL, Cher LM, O'Day J. Cancer associated retinopathy and non-small cell lung cancer. J Clin Neurosci Off J Neurosurg Soc Australas. 1997;4:355–7.
4. Katsuta H, Okada M, Nakauchi T, Takahashi Y, Yamao S, Uchida S. Cancer-associated retinopathy associated with invasive thymoma. Am J Ophthalmol. 2002;134:383–9.
5. Ohguro H, Yokoi Y, Ohguro I, Mamiya K, Ishikawa F, Yamazaki H, et al. Clinical and immunologic aspects of cancer-associated retinopathy. Am J Ophthalmol. 2004;137:1117–9.
6. Matsui Y, Mehta MC, Katsumi O, Brodie SE, Hirose T. Electrophysiological findings in paraneoplastic retinopathy. Graefes Arch Clin Exp Ophthalmol Albrecht Von Graefes Arch Für Klin Exp Ophthalmol. 1992;230:324–8.
7. Anastasakis A, Dick AD, Damato EM, Spry PG, Majid MA. Cancer-associated retinopathy presenting as retinal vasculitis with a negative ERG suggestive of on-bipolar cell pathway dysfunction. Doc Ophthalmol Adv Ophthalmol. 2011;123:59–63.

8. Makiyama Y, Kikuchi T, Otani A, Oishi A, Guo C, Nakagawa S, et al. Clinical and immunological characterization of paraneoplastic retinopathy. Invest Ophthalmol Vis Sci. 2013;54:5424–31.

9. Pepple KL, Cusick M, Jaffe GJ, Mruthyunjaya P. SD-OCT and autofluorescence characteristics of autoimmune retinopathy. Br J Ophthalmol. 2013;97:139–44.

10. Oohira A. Fifteen-year follow-up of patient with cancer-associated retinopathy. Jpn J Ophthalmol. 2007;51:74–5.

11. Adamus G, Amundson D, MacKay C, Gouras P. Long-term persistence of antirecoverin antibodies in endometrial cancer-associated retinopathy. Arch Ophthalmol Chic Ill 1960. 1998;116:251–3.

12. Adamus G, Machnicki M, Elerding H, Sugden B, Blocker YS, Fox DA. Antibodies to recoverin induce apoptosis of photoreceptor and bipolar cells in vivo. J Autoimmun. 1998;11:523–33.

13. Maeda A, Maeda T, Liang Y, Yenerel M, Saperstein DA. Effects of cytotoxic T lymphocyte antigen 4 (CTLA4) signaling and locally applied steroid on retinal dysfunction by recoverin, cancer-associated retinopathy antigen. Mol Vis. 2006;12:885–91.

14. Ten Berge JC, van Rosmalen J, Vermeer J, Hellström C, Lindskog C, Nilsson P, et al. Serum autoantibody profiling of patients with paraneoplastic and non-paraneoplastic autoimmune retinopathy. PLoS One. 2016;11:e0167909.

15. Faez S, Loewenstein J, Sobrin L. Concordance of antiretinal antibody testing results between laboratories in autoimmune retinopathy. JAMA Ophthalmol. 2013;131:113–5.

26

Comparison of clinical characteristics and antibiotic susceptibility between *Pseudomonas aeruginosa* and *P. putida* keratitis at a tertiary referral center: a retrospective study

Chan Ho Cho and Sang-Bumm Lee*

Abstract

Background: To compare clinical characteristics and antibiotic susceptibilities in patients with *Pseudomonas aeruginosa* (PA) and *P. putida* (PP) keratitis at a tertiary referral center in South Korea.

Methods: Forty-nine cases of inpatients with culture-proven PA and PP keratitis were reviewed retrospectively between January 1998 and December 2017. We excluded cases of polymicrobial infection. Epidemiology, predisposing factors, clinical characteristics, antibiotic susceptibilities, and treatment outcomes were compared between the PA and PP groups. The risk factors for poor clinical outcome were evaluated on the basis of the total cohort and analyzed using multivariate logistic regression.

Results: A total of 33 eyes with PA keratitis and 16 eyes with PP keratitis were included. The mean age was 47.0 years in the PA group and 59.3 years in the PP group (*p* = 0.060). Differences were observed between the PA and PP groups in hypopyon (45.5% vs 6.3%, *p* = 0.006) and symptom duration (4.3 vs 9.5 days, *p* = 0.022). The most common predisposing factor for PA was wearing contact lenses (36.4%) and that for PP was corneal trauma (62.5%). No significant differences were observed in sex, previous topical steroid use, systemic disease, or duration of hospitalization between the two groups. The PA and PP groups both demonstrated good efficacy of colistin (both 100%), tobramycin (93.3%, 100%), ceftazidime (93.9%, 87.5%), and ciprofloxacin (96.6%, 87.5%). Imipenem (100% vs 81.3%, *p* = 0.030), piperacillin (96.6% vs 75%, *p* = 0.047), and ticarcillin (85% vs 0%, *p* < 0.001) showed significantly lower efficacy in the PP group than in the PA group. A poor clinical outcome was observed in 31.2% of the PA group and 37.5% of the PP group (*p* = 0.665). The risk factors for poor clinical outcome were previous ocular surface disease (odds ratio 10.79, *p* = 0.012) and hypopyon (odds ratio 9.02, *p* = 0.024).

Conclusions: The PA group was more closely associated with younger age, wearing contact lenses, shorter symptom duration, and hypopyon, whereas the PP group was more closely associated with elderly age, corneal trauma, and decreased efficacy of the beta-lactams. Clinical outcomes were not significantly different between the two groups. Previous ocular surface disease and hypopyon were the risk factors for poor clinical outcome.

Keywords: Antimicrobial susceptibility, Contact lenses, *Pseudomonas aeruginosa*, *Pseudomonas putida*, Ulcerative keratitis

* Correspondence: sbummlee@ynu.ac.kr
Department of Ophthalmology, Yeungnam University College of Medicine,
170, Hyunchung-ro, Nam-gu, Daegu 705-717 (42415), South Korea

Background

The *Pseudomonas* species are ubiquitous gram-negative bacteria that are major opportunistic human pathogens that cause infection, including that of the cornea. *P. aeruginosa* (PA) is one of the pathogens most destructive to the eye and is a leading cause of bacterial keratitis in contact lens (CL) wearers and those with ocular injuries [1, 2]. *Pseudomonas* keratitis progresses rapidly and is characterized by infiltration of inflammatory cells and tissue destruction. It can lead to corneal perforation and subsequent loss of vision if appropriate therapy is not promptly initiated. Therefore, culture-proven diagnosis and prompt treatment of *Pseudomonas* keratitis are crucial.

Pseudomonas species other than PA are considered to be less virulent than PA. This is explained by genetic differences such as the presence of DNA associated with the synthesis of protease IV [3]. *P. putida* (PP) belongs to the fluorescent group of *Pseudomonas* species, a group of opportunistic pathogens that primarily cause nosocomial infections [4]. PP is recognized as a rare cause of systemic infections, such as sepsis, mainly observed in immunocompromised patients [4, 5]. In the field of ophthalmology, there are few reports of *P. putida* keratitis [6].

Antibiotic resistance of *Pseudomonas* species has been reported to be steadily increasing over the past several decades. For example, fluoroquinolone is the drug of choice in cases of *Pseudomonas* infection; however, increasing resistance to this drug has been observed since the 1990s [7, 8]. Recently, the incidence of multidrug-resistant PA and PP isolates has been reported; hence, it is essential to evaluate periodic antibiotic susceptibility [5, 9].

The PA and PP species belong to the same genus, but there was no clinical analysis comparing between PA and PP keratitis. Therefore, we conducted a comparative study of patients with PA and PP keratitis at a tertiary referral center in South Korea. The aim of this study is to compare epidemiology, predisposing factors, clinical characteristics, antibiotic susceptibility, and treatment outcome between PA and PP keratitis.

Methods

We conducted a retrospective, observational case series study of patients with culture-proven PA and PP keratitis at Yeungnam University Hospital in South Korea between January 1998 and December 2017. We excluded cases of polymicrobial infection and cases of outpatients. Admission decisions were based on the severity of keratitis, potential threat to vision, and need for intensive topical antimicrobial agents, and were determined by a single physician (S. B. Lee). During admission treatment, the patient was discharged if no further surgical treatment was required and complete epithelialization with sterilization were achieved.

Microbiological records and medical charts were reviewed retrospectively. We compared epidemiology, predisposing factors, clinical characteristics, antibiotic susceptibility, and treatment outcome between the PA and PP groups. Epidemiological data, including sex, age, seasonal distribution, symptom duration (defined as interval from the onset of symptoms to the time of initial presentation), and duration of hospitalization (defined as the period from admission to discharge), were reviewed. Age was divided into four subgroups (0–19, 20–39, 40–59, and ≥ 60 years). Predisposing factors, including corneal trauma, wearing CLs, previous ocular surface disease (OSD), previous ocular surgery, topical antibiotic use, topical steroid use, and underlying systemic disease, were evaluated. The categories of corneal trauma include those caused by industrial materials, foreign bodies, or vegetable matter. Clinical characteristics, including the location and size of the corneal lesion, and hypopyon were reviewed at initial presentation. Corneal lesions were divided into central and peripheral lesions according to their location on the basis on the middle point of the corneal radius. The size of the corneal lesion was based on the size of the corneal epithelial defect with estimation of the area of an equivalent rectangle. The largest linear dimension of the epithelial defect and its largest possible perpendicular within the confines of the epithelial defect were measured using the ruler of a slit lamp biomicroscope [10].

Before therapy was initiated, corneal scrapings of all cases were obtained using a No. 15 Bard-Parker knife (Aspen Surgical, Caledonia, MI, USA) after application of 0.5% proparacaine hydrochloride (Alcaine®, Alcon, Fort Worth, TX, USA) for anesthesia. Simultaneously, conjunctival swab was performed for all cases using a sterile cotton-tipped swab for thioglycolate broth. Scrapings were smeared on glass slides and Gram staining was performed. The cultured bacteria were identified using an automatic microbiological analyzer (VITEK 2 system; bioMérieux, Marcy l'Etoile, France). Antibiotic susceptibility testing was performed using the Kirby–Bauer disc diffusion method, and the minimum inhibitory concentration was determined using an automated microbiological analyzer.

All patients were treated topically with antibiotic eye drop (January 1998–October 2005: 0.5% levofloxacin, Cravit®, Santen, Osaka, Japan; November 2005–December 2017: 0.5% moxifloxacin, Vigamox®, Alcon, Fort Worth, TX, USA) with fortified topical antibiotics (2% tobramycin, 5% ceftazidime) and systemic antibiotics (second generation cephalosporins and aminoglycoside) before the microbiological results were obtained.

Treatment outcomes, including epithelial healing time, final visual acuity, complications (such as persistent epithelial defect, corneal perforation, or endophthalmitis), surgical intervention, and clinical outcome were reviewed. Presenting (initial) and final Snellen best corrected visual acuity (BCVA) scores were reviewed and converted to log-MAR scale scores. The clinical outcomes were assessed at the end of three months or at the completion of treatment and classified into three groups (good, moderate, and poor), as defined by Green [11]. Good (moderate) outcome was defined as final VA of 6/12 or better (6/18–6/60), no complications or surgical intervention, and no decrease in VA during treatment. Poor outcome was defined as final VA worse than 6/60, decrease in VA during treatment, presence of complications, or requiring surgical intervention.

The data were statistically analyzed using the Statistical Package for the Social Sciences 20.0 (IBM, Armonk, NY, USA). The chi-squared and Fisher's exact tests were used for categorical data. Independent t-tests were used for comparison of mean values. Statistical significance was defined as $p < 0.05$. The risk factors for poor clinical outcome were performed on the total cohort of PA and PP keratitis and analyzed using logistic regression. In the univariate analysis, an independent variable with $p < 0.1$ was included in the multivariate analysis, and a variable with a final $p < 0.05$ was considered a significant risk factor. This study was approved by the Institutional Review Board of the Yeungnam University Hospital, South Korea (file no. YUMC 2017–07-014) and complied with the principles outlined in the Declaration of Helsinki.

Results

During the 20-year study period, 937 inpatient cases were diagnosed clinically as bacterial keratitis, of which 383/937 (40.9%) were culture positive. *Pseudomonas* species were found in 88 of 383 positive cultures (23.0%). The most common *Pseudomonas* species was PA (46/88, 52.3%), followed by PP (25/88, 28.4%), and other *Pseudomonas* species (17/88, 19.3%). After excluding polymicrobial infection, 33 cases of PA and 16 cases of PP were included in the study.

Epidemiologic findings and predisposing factors

The epidemiology and predisposing factors are summarized in Table 1. The mean age was higher in the PP group than in the PA group with no significant difference (59.3 ± 18.9 vs 47.0 ± 24.4 years, $p = 0.060$). The most common age subgroup was the 20–30-year-old subgroup in the PA group and the ≥60-year-old group in the PP group. Symptom duration was significantly longer in the PP group than in the PA group (9.5 ± 7.8 vs 4.3 ± 3.9 days, $p = 0.022$). No significant differences were observed in sex, seasonal distribution, and duration of hospitalization between the PA and PP groups.

The most common predisposing factor for PA was wearing CLs and that for PP was corneal trauma. The ratio of wearing CLs (36.4% vs 0%, $p = 0.005$) and corneal trauma (27.3% vs 62.5%, $p = 0.018$) showed a significant difference

Table 1 Epidemiologic characteristics and predisposing factors of *Pseudomonas aeruginosa* and *P. putida* keratitis

Characteristics	P. aeruginosa (n = 33)	P. putida (n = 16)	p-value (x²-test)
Male sex	16 (48.5)	7 (43.8)	0.755
Age, mean ± SD, years	47.0 ± 24.4	59.3 ± 18.9	0.060†
Age subgroup			
0–19	2 (6.1)	1 (6.3)	1.000*
20–39	14 (42.4)	1 (6.3)	0.018*
40–59	4 (12.1)	6 (37.5)	0.060*
≥ 60	13 (39.4)	8 (50.0)	0.482
Symptom duration‡			
mean ± SD, days	4.3 ± 3.9	9.5 ± 7.8	0.022†
> 5 days	8 (24.2)	11 (68.8)	0.003
Duration of hospitalization§,			
mean ± SD, days	10.4 ± 6.4	8.6 ± 4.9	0.325†
Seasonal distribution			
Spring (Mar-May)	7 (21.2)	2 (12.5)	0.698*
Summer (Jun-Aug)	6 (18.2)	6 (37.5)	0.169*
Autumn (Sep-Nov)	15 (45.5)	3 (18.8)	0.069
Winter (Dec-Feb)	5 (15.2)	5 (31.3)	0.261*
Predisposing factors			
Corneal trauma	9 (27.3)	10 (62.5)	0.018
Contact-lens wear	12 (36.4)	0 (0.0)	0.005*
Previous OSD#	7 (21.2)	6 (37.5)	0.304*
Previous ocular surgery¶	5 (15.2)	3 (18.8)	1.000*
Previous topical antibiotics use	12 (36.4)	8 (50.0)	0.362
Previous topical steroid use	5 (15.2)	0 (0.0)	0.158*
Systemic disease**	10 (30.3)	7 (43.8)	0.354
No apparent cause	8 (24.2)	4 (25.0)	1.000*

SD standard deviation, *OSD* ocular surface disease

Values indicate numbers (proportion) unless otherwise noted

*The p-value was calculated using Fisher's exact test

†The p-value was calculated using independent *t*-test

‡Interval from the onset of symptoms to the time of initial presentation

§The period from admission to discharge

#*P. aeruginosa* group included necrotizing scleritis (two cases), exposure keratopathy (two cases), neurotrophic keratopathy (one case), bullous keratopathy (one case), and previous corneal ulcer (one case); *P. putida* group included exposure keratopathy (two cases), pseudophakic bullous keratopathy (one case), leukoma adherence (one case), herpetic keratitis (one case), and recurrent erosion syndrome (one case)

¶*P. aeruginosa* group included cataract surgery (four cases) and pars plana vitrectomy due to proliferative diabetic retinopathy (one case); *P. putida* group included cataract surgery (two cases) and Ahmed valve implantation due to neovascular glaucoma (one case)

**P. aeruginosa* group included hypertension only (four cases), diabetes mellitus (three cases), cardiovascular abnormality with hypertension (two cases), and cardiovascular abnormality only (one case). *P. putida* group included hypertension only (three cases), diabetes mellitus with hypertension (one case), hepatitis B with hypertension (one case), rheumatoid arthritis (one case), and atrial septal defect (one case)

between the PA and PP groups. The ratio of previous OSD (37.5% vs 21.2%, $p = 0.304$) was higher in the PP group than in the PA group, with no significant difference. The details of previous OSD and previous ocular surgery are described in the Table 1. No significant differences were observed between the PA and PP groups in the ratio of previous ocular surgery, previous topical antibiotic use, previous topical steroid use, or systemic diseases.

Clinical characteristics at initial presentation and treatment outcome (Table 2)

Both PA and PP groups had more central corneal lesions, with no significant difference between the two groups. No significant differences were observed in epithelial defect size between the PA and PP groups when the reference was ≥ 5 mm^2. Hypopyon was significantly higher in the PA group than in the PP group (45.5% vs 6.3%, $p = 0.006$).

Table 2 Clinical characteristics and treatment outcomes of *Pseudomonas aeruginosa* and *P. putida* keratitis

Characteristics	P. aeruginosa (n = 33)	P. putida (n = 16)	p-value (x^2-test)
Central lesion[‡]	24 (72.7)	12 (75.0)	1.000*
Epithelial defect size ≥5 mm^2	21 (63.6)	9 (56.3)	0.619
Hypopyon	15 (45.5)	1 (6.3)	0.006
Epithelial healing time ≥ 10 days	20 (60.6)	9 (56.3)	0.771
Complications**	5 (15.2)	3 (18.8)	1.000*
Surgical treatment[++]	5 (15.2)	2 (12.5)	1.000*
Presenting BCVA[§]			
mean ± SD, logMAR	1.66 ± 0.95	1.53 ± 1.10	0.675[†]
< 0.1, Snellen	20 (62.5)	9 (56.3)	0.676
Final BCVA[§]			
mean ± SD, logMAR	0.98 ± 1.12	1.09 ± 1.22	0.760[†]
< 0.1, Snellen	9 (28.1)	6 (37.5)	0.509
Decreased BCVA[#§]	8 (25.0)	5 (31.3)	0.735*
Clinical outcome[§¶]			
Good	11 (34.4)	7 (43.8)	0.527
Moderate	11 (34.4)	3 (18.8)	0.328*
Poor	10 (31.2)	6 (37.5)	0.665

BCVA best corrected visual acuity, *logMAR* logarithm of the minimum angle of resolution, *SD* standard deviation
Values indicate numbers (proportion) unless otherwise noted
*The p-value was calculated using Fisher's exact test
[†]The p-value was calculated using independent t-test
[‡]Corneal lesion is located within the 1/2 radius from the center of the cornea
**Complicated cases in P. aeruginosa group were persistent epithelial defect (two cases), impending corneal perforation (two cases), and progression of infection (one case); those in P. putida group was persistent epithelial defect (three cases)
[++]Surgical treatment cases in P. aeruginosa group were amniotic membrane transplantation (three cases), tarsorrhaphy (one case), and evisceration (one case); those in P. putida group was amniotic membrane transplantation (two cases)
[§]Total n = 48: One young child in the P. aeruginosa group who could not read letters was excluded
[#]Cases of final BCVA worsened from presentation
[¶]The clinical outcomes were assessed at the end of three months or at the completion of treatment and classified into three groups, as defined by Green [11].

More than half of the patients in both PA and PP groups had more than 10 days of epithelial healing time. There were no significant differences in the ratio of complications and surgical treatment between the PA and PP groups. All complicated cases in the PA group and two of three complicated cases in the PP group required surgical intervention. The details of complicated cases and surgical treatment cases are described in the Table 2.

In both PA and PP groups, final BCVAs improved significantly compared to presenting BCVAs ($p = 0.006$, $p = 0.018$, respectively). Mean presenting BCVAs, mean final BCVAs, the ratio of final BCVAs < 0.1 (snellen), and the ratio of decreased BCVAs at final visit were not significantly different between the PA and PP groups. The ratio of poor clinical outcome was 31.2% in the PA group and 37.5% in the PP group, with no statistically significant difference ($p = 0.665$).

Antimicrobial susceptibility

The antibiotic susceptibility of both groups is shown in Table 3. Imipenem (100% vs 81.3%, $p = 0.030$) and piperacillin (96.6% vs 75%, $p = 0.047$) were significantly more effective in the PA group than in the PP group. Ticarcillin (85% vs 0%, $p < 0.001$) and ticarcillin/clavulanate (74.1% vs 0%, $p < 0.001$) were relatively effective against PA, but both were ineffective against PP. Colistin, tobramycin, meropenem, ceftazidime, ciprofloxacin, and levofloxacin showed good effectiveness in both PA and PP group.

Risk factor analysis of poor clinical outcomes

In the univariate logistic regression analysis, previous OSD, previous ocular surgery, nonuse of CLs, age of ≥50 years, epithelial healing time (≥10 days), and hypopyon were significant variables (all, $p < 0.1$). The multivariate logistic regression analysis of the significant variables revealed that previous OSD (odds ratio [OR] 10.79, 95% confidence interval [CI] 1.67–69.76, $p = 0.012$) and hypopyon (OR 9.02, 95% CI 1.33–61.25, $p = 0.024$) were statistically significant risk factors for poor clinical outcome (Table 4).

Discussion

The proportion of gram-negative bacteria among total bacterial keratitis has been increasing recently. Tam et al. reported that the proportion of gram-negative bacterial keratitis increased from 19% in 2000–2003 to 30% in 2012–2015 [12]. *Pseudomonas* species has continued to be the most common isolate of gram-negative bacterial keratitis; the proportion varies among countries, ranging from 10% of cases in North America [12–14], 24.4% in Taiwan [15], 32.5% in South Korea [16], and up to 52% in South India [17].

PP is a relatively rare pathogen of corneal infection and has been rarely reported. This study includes the

Table 3 Antibiotics susceptibility of *Pseudomonas aeruginosa* and *P. putida* keratitis during the 1998–2017 period

Antibiotics	P. aeruginosa (n = 33)	P. putida (n = 16)	p-value (x^2-test)
Beta-lactams			
Ticarcillin	17/20 (85.0)	0/7 (0.0)	< 0.001*
Tic/clav	20/27 (74.1)	0/16 (0.0)	< 0.001
Piperacillin	28/29 (96.6)	12/16 (75.0)	0.047*
Pip/tazo	18/19 (94.7)	12/16 (75.0)	0.156*
Carbenicillin	10/14 (71.4)	–	–
Amp/sul	0/17 (0.0)	0/12 (0.0)	–
Cefotaxime	0/28 (0.0)	1/16 (6.3)	0.364*
Ceftazidime	31/33 (93.9)	14/16 (87.5)	0.588*
Cefepime	30/31 (96.8)	15/16 (93.8)	1.000*
Aztreonam	16/29 (55.2)	1/16 (6.3)	0.001
Imipenem	33/33 (100.0)	13/16 (81.3)	0.030*
Meropenem	28/28 (100.0)	14/16 (87.5)	0.127*
Aminoglycosides			
Amikacin	30/33 (90.9)	16/16 (100.0)	0.541*
Gentamicin	30/33 (90.9)	15/16 (93.8)	1.000*
Tobramycin	14/15 (93.3)	7/7 (100.0)	1.000*
Netilmicin	2/2 (100.0)	3/4 (75.0)	1.000*
Isepamicin	2/2 (100.0)	3/4 (75.0)	1.000*
Fluoroquinolones			
Ciprofloxacin	28/29 (96.6)	14/16 (87.5)	0.285*
Levofloxacin	6/7 (85.7)	6/7 (85.7)	1.000*
Others			
Pipemidic acid	3/4 (75.0)	–	–
Tigecycline	2/16 (12.5)	1/9 (11.1)	1.000*
TMP/SMX	0/28 (0.0)	0/16 (0.0)	–
Colistin	18/18 (100.0)	15/15 (100.0)	–

Tic/clav = ticarcillin/clavulanate;
Pip/tazo = piperacillin/tazobactam; Amp/sul = ampicillin/sulbactam;
TMP/SMX = trimethoprim/sulfamethoxazole
Values are presented as n1/n2 (%), where n1 is the number of isolates with susceptibility and n2 is the number of tested isolates
*The p-value was calculated using Fisher's exact test

largest number (16 eyes) of culture-proven PP keratitis. PP is known to be found in soil and water and is a rare source of human infection, causing nosocomial infections particularly in immunocompromised patients [18]. In this study, differences in epidemiologic and predisposing factors between the PA and PP group were identified. Compared to the PA group, the PP group had slightly higher ratio of compromised condition such as older age, previous OSD, and underlying systemic diseases, but with no statistically significant.

Many studies have reported wearing CLs as a common predisposing factor of bacterial keratitis [19, 20]. The close relationship between PA keratitis and CL wearing is well-known [21, 22]. In contrast, the studies of the association of PP keratitis with wearing CLs are rare reported, with only a case study of PP identified in orthokeratology-related cases [6]. In this study, CL wearing was the most common predisposing factor in the PA group, but there was no association between the PP group and CL wearing. The reason for the low detection of PP in CL wearing is not yet known, and further studies of the association between the PP and CL wearing are needed in the future.

The mean age of the PP group was higher than that of the PA group. In this study, we found that wearing CL was mainly restricted to younger ages, with all CL wearers aged < 50 years. When the CL wearers were excluded (PA 21 cases, PP 16 cases), the mean age showed no significant difference between the PA and PP groups (61.1 ± 18.9 vs 59.3 ± 18.9 years, p = 0.772).

The long interval of symptom duration is associated with delayed diagnosis and treatment, which has been reported to affect treatment outcomes. Fong et al. reported that delayed diagnosis and treatment of *Pseudomonas* keratitis may lead to subsequent failure of medical therapy with serious complications [23]. The mean symptom duration was longer in the PP group than in the PA group; even when the cases with CL wearers were excluded, the mean symptom duration was still longer in the PP group than in the PA group (9.5 ± 7.8 vs 5.5 ± 4.3 days, p = 0.077). In

Table 4 Risk factors for poor clinical outcome* in *Pseudomonas* keratitis[†] (univariate and multivariate logistic regression analysis[‡])

Variables	Univariate analysis			Multivariate analysis		
	OR	95% CI	p-value	OR	95% CI	p-value
Hypopyon	3.57	0.98–12.97	0.053	9.02	1.33–61.25	0.024
Epithelial healing time ≥ 10 (days)	4.91	1.17–20.62	0.030	–	–	–
Age ≥ 50 (years)	5.57	1.33–23.44	0.019	4.85	0.74–31.68	0.099
Nonuse of CLs	7.86	0.91–67.57	0.060	–	–	–
Previous ocular surgery	9.00	1.56–51.95	0.014	6.48	0.72–58.65	0.097
Previous OSD	16.11	3.38–76.76	< 0.001	10.79	1.67–69.76	0.012

CI confidence interval, CL contact lens, OSD ocular surface disease, OR odds ratio
*The clinical outcomes were assessed at the end of three months or at the completion of treatment and classified into three groups, as defined by Green [11].
[†]Total cohort of *P. aeruginosa* and *P. putida* keratitis, total n = 48: One young child in the *P. aeruginosa* group who could not read letters was excluded
[‡]Multivariate logistic regression analysis was performed using the backward-conditional method for the factors with a p-value < 0.1 in univariate logistic regression analysis

univariate analysis, symptom duration was identified as a significant factor for poor clinical outcome in the PA group (OR 1.26, 95% CI 1.01–1.57, $p = 0.044$) and was nonsignificant in the PP group (OR 1.11, 95% CI 0.95–1.30, $p = 0.188$). These results seem to be related to the characteristics of the PA keratitis showing rapid progression of corneal lesion from the early stage of keratitis and were interpreted that PP keratitis showed relatively slow progression compared to PA.

Among the clinical characteristics, hypopyon was significantly more common in the PA group than in the PP group, and no significant differences were observed in location of the corneal lesions or epithelial defect sizes between the two groups. When the cases with CL wearers were excluded, hypopyon was still more common in the PA group than in the PP group (57.1% vs 6.3%, $p = 0.001$); central lesion (76.2% vs 75%, $p = 1.000$) and epithelial defect size > 5 mm^2 (71.4% vs 56.2%, $p = 0.338$) were nonsignificant. These results show that the clinical characteristics of PA keratitis are more severe than those of PP, even if the CL wearers group is excluded. These results can be explained by difference in virulence among *Pseudomonas* species [3]. The virulence of the PA is known to be due to proteases (alkaline protease, elastase A, and elastase B) and exotoxins, which actively digest corneal proteins and result in the degradation of the proteoglycan matrix [2, 24–26]. However, the associated corneal virulence factors including exotoxins and a secreted protease are absent in the PP [1, 2, 27].

Antibiotic susceptibility must be analyzed in relation to regional characteristics. In a study comparing the susceptibility of PA to ciprofloxacin, gentamicin, and cephalosporins by country, ciprofloxacin and gentamicin exhibited low resistance of under 10% in most countries for the period of 1990–2003. However, in India study resistance to ciprofloxacin reached 30% and resistance to gentamicin reached 46% (1992–2003 period). The ceftazidime resistance ranged from 0 to 14% by country [28]. In our study, ciprofloxacin, gentamicin, and ceftazidime demonstrated less than 10% of resistance in PA.

Decreased antibiotic susceptibility of PP to beta-lactams was observed in this study. Many other studies also reported beta-lactam resistance of PP in nosocomial infection [5, 29]. One of the resistance mechanisms reported was that clinical isolates of PP produce metallo-beta-lactamases, conferring resistance to beta-lactams such as carbapenems [30]. Among beta-lactams, the susceptibility of PP to cefepime (93.8%) and ceftazidime (87.5%), commonly used antibiotics for the treatment of bacterial keratitis, was relatively good in this study.

Because PA species is a more virulent than PP species, the clinical characteristics of the PA keratitis are expected more rapid progression and more severe clinical findings, and show worse outcome than PP keratitis. However, in this study, poor clinical outcome was observed at a similar rate between the PA and PP groups. Even when the cases with CL wearers were excluded, the ratio of poor clinical outcome was similar between the PA and PP group (45.0% vs 37.5%, $p = 0.741$). This result may be related to the higher ratio of previous OSD and elderly age in the PP group than that of PA group, which are risk factors for poor clinical outcome. In addition, this result show that the PP species can also be a causative pathogen of severe keratitis. Therefore, clinicians should pay attention to the clinical significance of PP keratitis in patients with these factors.

The significant risk factors for poor clinical outcome were previous OSD and hypopyon. Several studies have reported previous OSD as prognostic factors of bacterial keratitis [11, 31]. It is thought that the treatment outcomes of patients with previous OSD could be affected by the preexisting disease itself. Hypopyon in bacterial keratitis comprises sterile leukocytic exudate that is associated with severe inflammation. A relationship has been reported between hypopyon and treatment outcome; Lavinsky et al. found that the degree of hypopyon was significantly related to the length of hospital stay and worse visual outcome in patients admitted for bacterial keratitis [32].

Our study had some limitations. First, this study was retrospective and had a limited number of included cases. Second, the included patients were confined to inpatients in a tertiary referral center and might have had more severe symptoms compared with outpatients or those at a primary medical clinic. Therefore, the results of this study are limited to those of patients at tertiary hospitals. Third, this study was performed at a single center; therefore, our results may not represent nationwide data of South Korea. A future study using multicenter data is required. Despite these limitations, this study provides epidemiological data, predisposing factors, clinical characteristics, and antibiotic susceptibility of PP which is a rare pathogen causing bacterial keratitis. Another strength of this study is that it enabled the assessment of clinical characteristics of monomicrobial infection by excluding factors associated with other pathogens in polymicrobial infection.

Conclusions

In conclusion, PA keratitis was more closely associated with young age and CL wear, and PP keratitis was more closely associated with elderly age and corneal trauma. The efficacy of beta-lactams in the PP group was lower than that in the PA group. The PA group had shorter symptom duration and more severe clinical characteristics, such as hypopyon, than the PP group, but the clinical outcomes were not significantly different between the two groups. The risk factors for poor clinical outcomes of *Pseudomonas* keratitis were previous OSD and hypopyon. This study provides information on the differences in clinical characteristics and antibiotic susceptibility between patients with PA and PP keratitis in South Korea.

Abbreviations

BCVAs: Best corrected VAs; CI: Confidence interval; CL: Contact-lens; OR: Odds ratio; OSD: Ocular surface disease; PA: *Pseudomonas aeruginosa*; PP: *Pseudomonas putida*; VA: Visual acuity

Authors' contributions

CHC literature research, drafting, language editing, critical revision and final approval of manuscript. SBL patient interaction, patient diagnosis, language editing, critical revision, and final approval of manuscript. All authors read and approved the final manuscript.

Competing interests

The authors declare that they have no competing interests.

References

1. Traidej M, Caballero AR, Marquart ME, Thibodeaux BA, O'Callaghan RJ. Molecular analysis of Pseudomonas aeruginosa protease IV expressed in Pseudomonas putida. Invest Ophthalmol Vis Sci. 2003;44(1):190–6.
2. Thibodeaux BA, Caballero AR, Marquart ME, Tommassen J, O'Callaghan RJ. Corneal virulence of Pseudomonas aeruginosa elastase B and alkaline protease produced by Pseudomonas putida. Curr Eye Res. 2007;32(4):373–86.
3. Caballero A, Thibodeaux B, Marquart M, Traidej M, O'Callaghan R. Pseudomonas keratitis: protease IV gene conservation, distribution, and production relative to virulence and other Pseudomonas proteases. Invest Ophthalmol Vis Sci. 2004;45(2):522–30.
4. Yoshino Y, Kitazawa T, Kamimura M, Tatsuno K, Ota Y, Yotsuyanagi H. Pseudomonas putida bacteremia in adult patients: five case reports and a review of the literature. J Infect Chemother. 2011;17(2):278–82.
5. Kim SE, Park SH, Park HB, Park KH, Kim SH, Jung SI, Shin JH, Jang HC, Kang SJ. Nosocomial Pseudomonas putida bacteremia: high rates of Carbapenem resistance and mortality. Chonnam Med J. 2012;48(2):91–5.
6. Ying-Cheng L, Chao-Kung L, Ko-Hua C, Wen-Ming H. Daytime orthokeratology associated with infectious keratitis by multiple gram-negative bacilli: Burkholderia cepacia, Pseudomonas putida, and Pseudomonas aeruginosa. Eye Contact Lens. 2006;32(1):19–20.
7. Garg P, Sharma S, Rao GN. Ciprofloxacin-resistant Pseudomonas keratitis. Ophthalmology. 1999;106(7):1319–23.
8. Chaudhry NA, Flynn HW Jr, Murray TG, Tabandeh H, Mello MO Jr, Miller D. Emerging ciprofloxacin-resistant Pseudomonas aeruginosa. Am J Ophthalmol. 1999;128(4):509–10.
9. Vazirani J, Wurity S, Ali MH. Multidrug-resistant Pseudomonas aeruginosa keratitis: risk factors, clinical characteristics, and outcomes. Ophthalmology. 2015;122(10):2110–4.
10. Mukerji N, Vajpayee RB, Sharma N. Technique of area measurement of epithelial defects. Cornea. 2003;22(6):549–51.
11. Green MD, Apel AJ, Naduvilath T, Stapleton FJ. Clinical outcomes of keratitis. Clin Exp Ophthalmol. 2007;35(5):421–6.
12. Tam ALC, Cote E, Saldanha M, Lichtinger A, Slomovic AR. Bacterial keratitis in Toronto: a 16-year review of the microorganisms isolated and the resistance patterns observed. Cornea. 2017;36(12):1528–34.
13. Pachigolla G, Blomquist P, Cavanagh HD. Microbial keratitis pathogens and antibiotic susceptibilities: a 5-year review of cases at an urban county hospital in North Texas. Eye Contact Lens. 2007;33(1):45–9.
14. Peng MY, Cevallos V, McLeod SD, Lietman TM, Rose-Nussbaumer J. Bacterial keratitis: isolated organisms and antibiotic resistance patterns in San Francisco. Cornea. 2018;37(1):84–7.
15. Gupta PC, Ram J. Shifting trends in bacterial keratitis in Taiwan: a 10-year review in a tertiary-care hospital. Cornea. 2016;35(9):e26.
16. Cho EY, Lee SB. Gram-negative bacterial keratitis: a 15-year review of clinical aspects. J Korean Ophthalmol Soc. 2015;56(10):1479–88.
17. Bharathi MJ, Ramakrishnan R, Shivakumar C, Meenakshi R, Lionalraj D. Etiology and antibacterial susceptibility pattern of community-acquired bacterial ocular infections in a tertiary eye care hospital in South India. Indian J Ophthalmol. 2010;58(6):497–507.
18. Bogaerts P, Huang TD, Rodriguez-Villalobos H, Bauraing C, Deplano A, Struelens MJ, Glupczynski Y. Nosocomial infections caused by multidrug-resistant Pseudomonas putida isolates producing VIM-2 and VIM-4 metallo-beta-lactamases. J Antimicrob Chemother. 2008;61(3):749–51.
19. Ng AL, To KK, Choi CC, Yuen LH, Yim SM, Chan KS, Lai JS, Wong IY. Predisposing factors, microbial characteristics, and clinical outcome of microbial keratitis in a tertiary Centre in Hong Kong: a 10-year experience. J Ophthalmol. 2015;2015:769436.
20. Bourcier T, Thomas F, Borderie V, Chaumeil C, Laroche L. Bacterial keratitis: predisposing factors, clinical and microbiological review of 300 cases. Br J Ophthalmol. 2003;87(7):834–8.
21. Tam C, Mun JJ, Evans DJ, Fleiszig SM. The impact of inoculation parameters on the pathogenesis of contact lens-related infectious keratitis. Invest Ophthalmol Vis Sci. 2010;51(6):3100–6.
22. Liesegang TJ. Contact lens-related microbial keratitis: part II: pathophysiology. Cornea. 1997;16(3):265–73.
23. Fong CF, Tseng CH, Hu FR, Wang IJ, Chen WL, Hou YC. Clinical characteristics of microbial keratitis in a university hospital in Taiwan. Am J Ophthalmol. 2004;137(2):329–36.
24. Tang A, Caballero AR, Marquart ME, O'Callaghan RJ. Pseudomonas aeruginosa small protease (PASP), a keratitis virulence factor. Invest Ophthalmol Vis Sci. 2013;54(4):2821–8.
25. Twining SS, Kirschner SE, Mahnke LA, Frank DW. Effect of Pseudomonas aeruginosa elastase, alkaline protease, and exotoxin a on corneal proteinases and proteins. Invest Ophthalmol Vis Sci. 1993;34(9):2699–712.
26. Wretlind B, Pavlovskis OR. The role of proteases and exotoxin a in the pathogenicity of Pseudomonas aeruginosa infections. Scand J Infect Dis Suppl. 1981;29:13–9.
27. Udaondo Z, Molina L, Segura A, Duque E, Ramos JL. Analysis of the core genome and pangenome of Pseudomonas putida. Environ Microbiol. 2016;18(10):3268–83.
28. Willcox MD. Review of resistance of ocular isolates of Pseudomonas aeruginosa and staphylococci from keratitis to ciprofloxacin, gentamicin and cephalosporins. Clin Exp Optom. 2011;94(2):161–8.
29. Molina L, Udaondo Z, Duque E, Fernandez M, Molina-Santiago C, Roca A, Porcel M, de la Torre J, Segura A, Plesiat P, et al. Antibiotic resistance determinants in a Pseudomonas putida strain isolated from a hospital. PLoS One. 2014;9(1):e81604.
30. Lombardi G, Luzzaro F, Docquier JD, Riccio ML, Perilli M, Coli A, Amicosante G, Rossolini GM, Toniolo A. Nosocomial infections caused by multidrug-resistant isolates of Pseudomonas putida producing VIM-1 metallo-beta-lactamase. J Clin Microbiol. 2002;40(11):4051–5.
31. Morlet N, Minassian D, Butcher J. Risk factors for treatment outcome of suspected microbial keratitis. Ofloxacin Study Group Br J Ophthalmol. 1999;83(9):1027–31.
32. Lavinsky F, Avni-Zauberman N, Barequet IS. Clinical characteristics and outcomes of patients admitted with presumed microbial keratitis to a tertiary medical center in Israel. Arq Bras Oftalmol. 2013;76(3):175–9.

27

Incidence of myopia and biometric characteristics of premyopic eyes among Chinese children and adolescents

Lan Li[1], Hua Zhong[2], Jun Li[3], Cai-Rui Li[4*] and Chen-Wei Pan[5*]

Abstract

Background: To determine the one-year incidence and progression rates of myopia and its association with baseline ocular biometric parameters in school-based samples of children and adolescents in China.

Methods: Two thousand four hundred thirty two grade 1 and 2346 grade 7 students living in the southwest part of China participated in the baseline survey. After 1 year, 2310 (95.0%) grade 1 and 2191 (93.4%) grade 7 students attended the follow-up examination. Refractive error was measured after cycloplegia using the same autorefractor and by the same optometrists in the baseline and follow-up examination. Myopia was defined as spherical equivalent of less than − 0.50 diopter.

Results: The overall one-year incidence of myopia was 33.6% (95% confidence interval [CI]: 31.7–35.5) among grade 1 students and 54.0% (95% CI: 51.5–56.5) for grade 7 students. The one-year myopia progression rate was − 0.97 D (95% CI: -1.22 to − 0.71) in grade 1 students and − 1.02 D (95% CI: -1.07 to − 0.96) in grade 7 students. Per mm increase in baseline axial lengths increased the risk of myopia onset by 28% among grade 1 students and 22% among grade 7 students after 1 year. The incidence rates of myopia were found to be higher in grade 7 students with thinner premyopic lenses.

Conclusions: The incidence and progression rates of myopia were very high in Chinese children and adolescents in recent years. Premyopic eyes were characterized with longer axial lengths and thinner lenses. These data had considerable implications for formulating myopia prevention strategies in China.

Keywords: Myopia, Incidence, Axial length, Epidemiology

Background

Myopia is a major cause of reduced vision among children and adolescents [1–4]. Multiethnic studies have provided initial evidence supporting that the prevalence of myopia varies among different ethnic groups and individuals of Chinese ancestries are always reported to have a higher prevalence of myopia compared with other ethnic groups living in the same areas [5–7]. This observed ethnic differences might be attributable to Chinese specific cultures which highly emphasize on early educational achievements and passing exams [3].

In epidemiology, prevalence is an estimate on disease burdens while incidence describes how rapidly the disease develops. While the prevalence of myopia has been extensively reported in children and adolescents of Chinese ancestries [8–16], few studies have addressed the incidence of myopia in this ethnic group. The landmark epidemiologic study on myopia in Chinese children, the Singapore Cohort Study of the Risk Factors for Myopia (SCORM), have reported the 3-year cumulative incidence of myopia among Chinese children aged 7 to 9 years in Singapore [17]. Considering the different country-specific environmental exposures and schooling systems which might have significant impacts on myopia onset and progression, the findings from Singapore Chinese living outside China could not be directly extrapolated to Chinese children in China. The Anyang

* Correspondence: lcrbrett@163.com; pcwonly@gmail.com
[4]Department of Ophthalmology, the First Affiliated Hospital of Dali University, 32 Mangyong Road, Dali 671003, China
[5]School of Public Health, Medical College of Soochow University, 199 Ren Ai Road, Suzhou 215123, China
Full list of author information is available at the end of the article

Childhood Eye Study on children living in the central areas of China indicated that mean change in refractive error per year was – 0.48 diopter (D) [18]. However, China is a large country with various cultures in different areas. Thus, data regarding myopia incidence and progression rates in Chinese children are far from conclusive.

More importantly, refractive status is physiologically determined by biometric parameters such as axial length (AL), corneal power (CP), anterior chamber depth (ACD) and lens thickness (LT) [19]. Although quite a few studies have analyzed the data on the refractive associations with biometric parameters, most of them are cross-sectional and cannot reflect the biometric characteristics before the onset of myopia [20–24]. Understanding the characteristics of premyopic eyes are important from a disease prevention perspective.

In this study, we reported the one-year incidence and progression rates of myopia and their associations with baseline ocular biometric parameters in school-based samples of Chinese children and adolescents in the southwestern part of China.

Methods

Study population

The Mojiang Myopia Progression Study is a school-based cohort study aiming to longitudinally observe the onset and progression of myopia in school-aged children in rural China. The study included two cohorts: elementary school grade 1 students and middle school grade 7 students. Elementary school grade 1 students would be followed until they entered middle schools and middle school grade 7 students would be followed until they entered high schools. Such a study design would facilitate the follow up of the cohorts and possibly reduce the loss-to-follow-up rate considering the current Chinese schooling system. The baseline survey was conducted in 2016 and the first follow up visit was conducted in 12 months. Mojiang, a small county located in Southwestern China with a population of 0.36 million and an area of 5312 km^2, was chosen as the study site due to its relatively stable demographic structure and similar socioeconomic status to the average of rural China. The compulsory schooling system is well executed in Mojiang with an enrollment rate of 99% for elementary and middle schools in 2014. Thus, school-based samples in Mojiang are highly representative of the local population and could be regarded as population-based sample.

All the grade 1 students from elementary schools and grade 7 students from middle schools in Mojiang were invited to participate in the study. For the baseline survey, the students roster was obtained from each school's principal to ascertain the eligibility of the study

participants, that is, he or she should have been living in Mojiang for at least 1 year and planned to live there for at least 4 years. A cell phone message was sent to the parents to explain the nature of the study and invite them to participate in the study. For those who didn't agree to participate or didn't respond, telephone interview was made to let them better understand the nature of the study and the importance of their children's vision development. If the parents could not be reached by cell phone message or telephone, home visits were made. In the end of the study, a total of 2432 (90.2%) grade 1 students and 2346 (93.5%) grade 7 students participated in the baseline survey. After 1 year, 2310 (95.0%) grade 1 students and 2191 (93.4%) grade 7 students successfully attended the one-year follow-up examination.

Ethics committee approval was obtained from the Institutional Review Board of Kunming Medical University. We carried out the study according to the tenets of the Declaration of Helsinki involving human participants and the approved guidelines. Additionally, we obtained written informed consents from at least one parent or legal guardian of each participant.

Refractive error and ocular biometry measurement

The protocols for measuring refractive error and ocular biometry were the same between the baseline and follow-up visit. Each participant's refractive status was measured before and after cycloplegia using an autorefractor (RM-8000; Topcon Corp., Tokyo, Japan) by optometrists or trained technicians. For cycloplegia, each participant was first administered two drops of 1% cyclopentolate (Alcon) after a 5-min interval. Thirty minutes later, a third drop was administered if pupillary light reflex was still present or the pupil size was less than 6.0 mm. The first five valid readings of autorefraction were used and averaged using vector methods to generate a single estimate of refractive error. All five readings should be at most 0.50 D apart in both the spherical and cylinder components. Myopia was defined as spherical equivalent (SE) less than – 0.50D. An IOL Master (Carl Zeiss Meditec AG, Jena, Germany) was used to measure ocular biometric parameters including AL, CP and ACD. LT was measured by using Lenstar LS900 (Haag-Streit Koeniz, Switzerland). Three repeated reading were obtained and averaged before cycloplegia.

Questionnaires

The questionnaires used in this study were similar to many previous myopia epidemiologic studies on Chinese children. The questionnaires were filled up by the parents or legal guardians of the children. We collected detailed information regarding socioeconomic status, parental education, parental history of myopia, medical history, time spent on reading and writing, time spent on watching TV, time spent on playing computers and outdoor activities.

Statistical analysis

The incidence rate of myopia was defined as the proportion of participants in whom myopia developed during the 1-year follow-up period among those without myopia at the baseline examination. Myopia progression rate was defined as the refraction at the baseline examination subtracted from that at the follow-up examination among those with myopia at the baseline visit. Logistic regression models were established to calculate odds ratios (ORs) and 95% confidence intervals (CIs), using incident myopia as the outcome measure and various baseline ocular biometric parameters as exposures. Univariate analysis was performed first and multivariate analysis was additionally performed adjusting for myopia-related variables including gender, height, parental myopia, time for nearwork and time spent outdoors. Because the refractive error and biometric data from both eyes were similar, only the results from the right eye are presented. Statistical analysis was performed using a statistical software package (SPSS for Windows, version 18.0; Chicago, IL).

Results

Totally, 2310 grade 1 students and 2191 grade 7 students who attended the follow-up examination were included in this analysis. The distributions of SEs and ALs of the cohorts are shown in Figs. 1 and 2. No differences were observed in the distribution of gender and baseline refraction of participants who remained in the study in the follow-up visit and who were lost to follow-up in both cohorts. There were 2377 grade 1 students and 1653 grade 7 students who were not myopic at baseline (SE < – 0.5 D). Table 1 depicts the one-year incidence of myopia by age and gender in both cohorts. The overall one-year incidence of myopia was 33.6% (95% CI: 31.7–35.5) among grade 1 students and 54.0% (95% CI: 51.5–56.5) for grade 7 students. The incidence rates of myopia were higher in girls than in boys but the gender differences were not statistically significant among grade 1 students (P = 0.33).

There were 51 grade 1 students and 646 grade 7 students who were myopic at baseline. The progression rates of myopia among those who had already been myopic at baseline are shown in Table 2. The one-year myopia progression rate was – 0.97 D (95% CI: -1.22 to – 0.71) in grade 1 students and – 1.02 D (95% CI: -1.07 to – 0.96) in grade 7 students. There were no gender differences in myopia progression rates between boys and girls in both cohorts (P = 0.76 for grade 1 students and P = 0.87 for grade 7 students). The proportions of individuals with myopia progression rates of more than – 1.0 D were 41.8% among grade 1 students and 45.5% among grade 7 students. The proportion of individuals with myopia progression rates of more than – 2.0 D were 12.7%

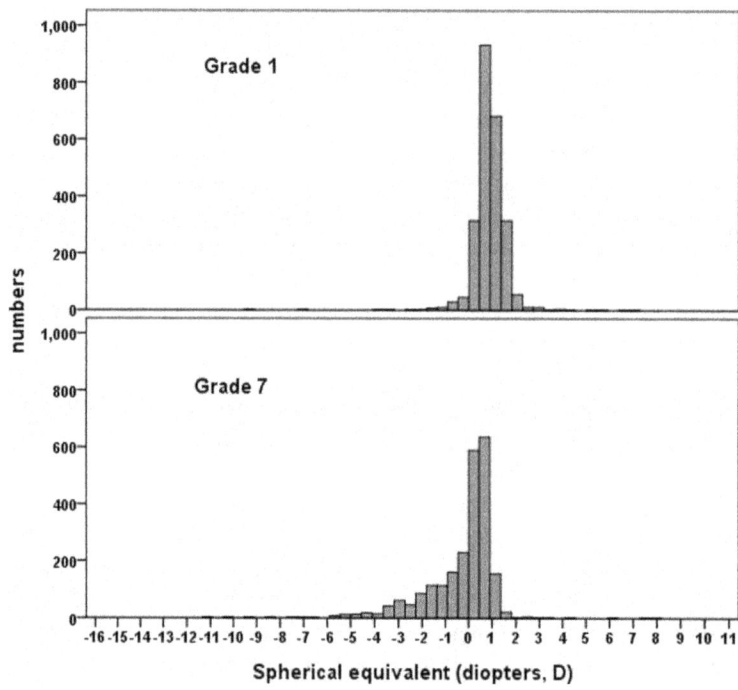

Fig. 1 Distributions of baseline refractive error in grade 1 and 7 students

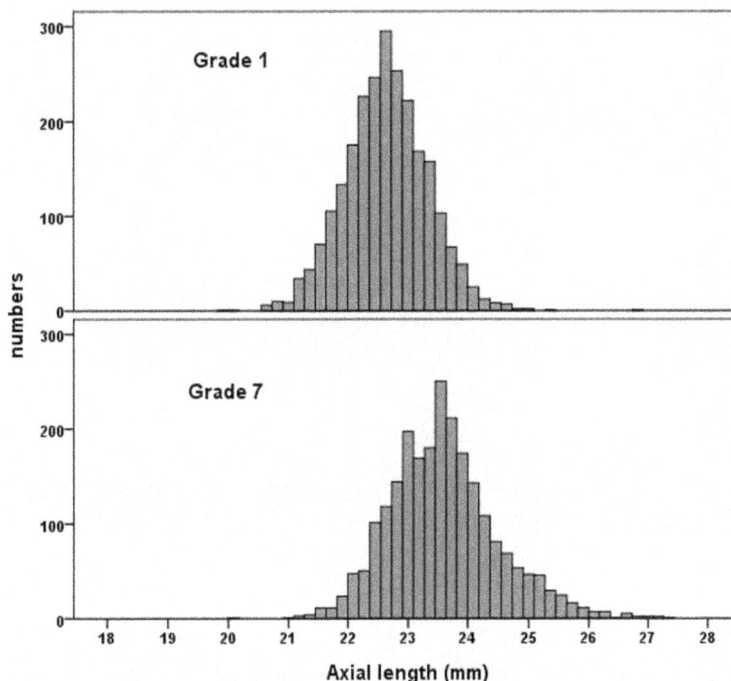

Fig. 2 Distributions of baseline axial length in grade 1 and 7 students

among grade 1 students and 6.1% among grade 7 students. Myopia progression rates did not differ significantly in students with and without myopia at baseline (P for grade 1 students = 0.67, P for grade 7 students = 0.32).

Table 3 shows the biometric characteristics of premyopic eyes in both cohorts. In this analysis, incident myopia was treated as the outcome variable while baseline ocular biometric parameters were treated as exposures. We found that longer ALs were associated with higher risks of myopia in both cohorts. Per mm increase in baseline ALs increased the risk of myopia onset by 28% among grade 1 students (OR = 1.28) and 22% among grade 7 students (OR = 1.22) after 1 year in univariate analysis. Similarly, more hyperopic refractive errors at

baseline were associated with lower risks of myopia in both cohorts. The incidence rates of myopia were found to be higher in grade 1 students with thinner premyopic lenses. These associations between baseline biometric parameters and myopia incidence remained significant, even after controlling for myopia-related variables such as gender, height, parental myopia, near work and time outdoors. Myopia-related lifestyles such as near work and time outdoors were not associated with incident myopia or myopia progression in this study. (all $P > 0.10$).

Discussion

Our study indicated that the incidence of myopia was very high in Chinese children and adolescents in recent

Table 1 Incidence of myopia among grade 1 and 7 students

	Population at risk (N)	n	Incidence (%)	95% confidence interval	P*
Grade 1					
All	2377	798	33.6	31.7–35.5	
Boys	1317	431	32.7	30.2–35.3	0.33
Girls	1060	367	34.6	31.8–37.5	
Grade 7					
All	1545	834	54.0	51.5,56.5	
Boys	866	415	47.9	44.6,51.3	< 0.001
Girls	679	419	61.7	58.0,65.4	

*Comparing boys with girls

Table 2 Progression rates of myopia among grade 1 and 7 students

	N	Progression rate		% with change> − 1.0 D			% with change> − 2.0 D		
		Mean	95% CI	N	%	95% CI	N	%	95% CI
Grade 1 students									
With myopia	51	−0.97	− 1.22,-0.71	23	41.8	28.4, 55.3	7	12.7	3.6, 21.8
Boys	26	−1.01	− 1.33,-0.68	12	46.2	25.9, 66.7	4	15.4	0.5, 30.2
Girls	25	−0.93	−1.34,-0.51	11	37.9	19.1, 56.7	3	10.3	0.0, 22.1
P		0.76			0.54			0.58	
Without myopia	2259	−1.29	−1.33, − 1.19	1340	56.4	54.4, 58.4	379	15.9	14.5, 17.4
Boys	1253	−1.23	− 1.28, − 1.18	714	54.2	51.5, 56.9	190	14.4	12.5, 16.3
Girls	1006	−1.36	− 1.42, − 1.29	626	59.1	56.1, 62.0	189	17.8	15.5, 20.1
P		0.002			0.02			0.02	
With myopia									
-0.5~ − 1.0 D	34	−0.97	−1.24,-0.69	18	50.0	32.8, 67.2	4	11.1	0.3, 21.9
< −1.0 D	17	−0.96	−1.55,-0.38	5	26.3	4.5, 48.1	3	15.8	0.0, 33.9
P		0.99			0.09			0.62	
Grade 7 students									
With myopia	646	−1.02	−1.07, −0.96	315	45.5	41.7, 49.2	42	6.1	4.3, 7.8
Boys	249	−1.02	−1.12, −0.93	117	42.4	36.8, 48.3	18	6.5	3.6, 9.5
Girls	397	−1.01	−1.08, −0.95	198	47.5	42.7, 52.3	24	5.8	3.5, 8.0
P		0.87			0.19			0.68	
Without myopia	1545	−1.20	−1.25, −1.16	1014	65.6	63.3, 68.0	163	10.6	9.0, 12.1
Boys	866	−1.17	−1.22, − 1.12	562	64.9	61.7, 68.1	83	9.6	7.6, 11.6
Girls	679	−1.25	−1.31, − 1.18	452	66.6	63.0, 70.1	80	11.8	9.4, 14.2
P		0.08			0.49			0.16	
With myopia									
-0.5~ − 1.0 D	175	−0.97	−1.09, −0.85	97	55.4	48.0, 62.9	11	6.3	2.7, 9.9
-1.01~ − 2.0 D	229	−0.95	−1.07, −0.83	109	47.6	41.1, 54.1	15	6.6	3.3, 9.8
< −2.0 D	242	−0.92	−1.08, − 0.77	109	45.0	38.7, 51.4	16	6.6	3.5, 9.8
P		0.93			0.10			0.99	

D diopters *CI* confidence interval

years. Approximate 30% of the grade 1 students and 50% of the grade 7 students became myopic just 1 year after they had entered primary and secondary schools. Myopia also progressed rapidly among myopic Chinese school students with the annual progression rate of being about − 1.0D. We also found that premyopic eyes were characterized with longer ALs and thinner LTs. Our study had considerable implications for formulating myopia prevention strategies in China.

The incidence rate of myopia in our study could be compared with other reports in different populations. An early study (published in 2002) in the mainland of China reported that the annualized incidence rates of myopia (SE < − 0.5D) were only 1.6% in 5-year-olds and 10.7% in 12-year-olds. [25] In Chinese children in Hong Kong (published in 2004), the annualized incidence rates were 13.1% in 7-year-olds, 14.8% in 8-year-olds, and 15.0% in 9-year olds. [26] In a report published in 2005, the 3-year cumulative incidence rates of myopia were 47.7, 38.4 and 32.4% among Singapore Chinese children aged 7, 8 and 9 years, respectively. Compared with these estimates published more than 10 years ago, the incidence of myopia observed in our study was much higher. The differences might be attributable to the changes in environmental exposures between generations, including a more competitive educational system and less time spent outdoors in recent years. For example, Chinese cultures emphasizes on outstanding academic achievements and the college entrance examination in China is extremely competitive in recent years. Chinese school students are at the preparation stage of this examination when they just enter secondary schools. This situation has been resulting in a sedentary lifestyle combined with large amounts of time on

Table 3 Biometric characteristics of premyopic eyes among grade 1 and 7 students

Baseline biometric characteristics	Grade 1 students				Grade 7 students			
	Univariate		Multivariate-adjusted[a]		Univariate		Multivariate-adjusted[a]	
	OR (95% CI)	P	OR (95% CI)	P	OR (95% CI)	P	OR (95% CI)	P
AL (per mm increase)	1.28 (1.13, 1.46)	< 0.001	1.93 (1.24,2.30)	0.004	1.22 (1.06, 1.41)	0.005	1.51 (1.28,1.77)	< 0.001
LT (per mm increase)	0.55 (0.35, 0.87)	0.01	0.67 (0.45,0.92)	0.02	0.78 (0.45,1.36)	0.38	0.67 (0.38, 1.18)	0.17
ACD (per mm increase)	0.92 (0.63, 1.34)	0.67	0.70 (0.21,2.27)	0.55	1.44(0.94,2.22)	0.10	1.39 (1.22,3.04)	0.005
CP (per diopter increase)	0.95 (0.90,1.01)	0.11	0.86 (0.71, 1.05)	0.14	1.05 (0.98, 1.13)	0.20	0.99 (0.92,1.07)	0.78
SE (per diopter increase)	0.48 (0.40,0.58)	< 0.001	0.61 (0.36, 0.99)	0.04	0.12 (0.09,0.16)	< 0.001	0.13 (0.09,0.18)	< 0.001

AL axial length, LT lens thickness, ACD anterior chamber depth, CP corneal power, SE spherical equivalent, OR odds ratio, CI confidence interval
[a]Controlling for gender, height, parental myopia, near work and time outdoors

reading and writing and less time outdoors [27]. In addition, the development of modern digital products such as computers, smart mobile phones and IPads may also explained the high incidence of myopia among Chinese children, though the harmful impacts of these modern digital products on vision health need to be further clarified. Besides the variations in educational pressures and the use of modern digital products, other population-wide changes in environmental and lifestyle factors such as climate, diet, sleep may also be taken into consideration. Although there have not been sufficient data addressing the potential impacts of these changes on myopia, one can only speculate which of these factors, if any, might be effective. For instance, it was reported that Chinese children who had higher saturated fat and cholesterol intake tended to have longer ALs [28]. It is likely that children may take more food with more saturated fat and cholesterol in recent years with the development of economy in China.

We observed some gender differences in myopia progression rates. For example, baseline SE were comparable between boys and girls in grade 1 students but myopic progression in non-myopic participants was significantly greater in girls during 1 year. Myopic incidence was also found to be greater in girls (47.9% vs 61.7%) in grade 7 students. This differences might be explained by the gender differences in time outdoors, as girls usually spent less time outdoors compared with boys.

In this study, we also described biometry characteristics of premyopic eyes. We found that premyopic eyes were characterized with longer ALs and thinner lenses. These findings indicated that abnormal growth of eyeballs might have taken place before the onset of myopia. Children and adolescents who had a certain eye size or shape such as excessively long eyes and thinner lenses might be more susceptible to myopia. We also found that thinner lens was associated with a higher myopia incidence in grade 1 but not in grade 7 students. It was likely that older students might have less variations in

lens thickness compared with younger ones, resulting in a loss in statistical power to detect a significant association. More efforts are needed to compare eye growth during different phases of refractive development and risk models should be established to predict myopia formation based on ocular biometric parameters and lifestyle risk factors in Chinese children. The information would be valuable to guide clinical management and prevention of myopia in school children.

The public health implications in the observed trend of development of early myopia during the early years in primary or secondary schools in China is considerable. Nowadays, myopia is not a exclusive public health concern in urban Asian communities such as Shanghai, Taiwan, Hong Kong and Singapore. The situation seems to be even worse in areas of mainland China where area-level socioeconomic status are relatively lower. Thus, myopia prevention strategies must be adjusted to balance the allocation of health resources between the "old" and "new" myopia epidemic areas. More vision screening programs incorporated with health education and promotion programs may be launched to detect early myopia and to update current prescriptions of spectacle in schools. Routine screening of ocular biometry among school-aged children are recommended.

Strengths of our study included the school-based sample, longitudinal design, and high follow-up rate. The measurement of refraction and biometric data also followed standardized protocols which facilitated the inter-study comparisons. We were also aware of the limitations of the study. First, the follow-up period was relatively short. We would continue follow up these two cohorts in the future. Second, the data of our study may not be generalizable to all children in China considering the large variations in environmental exposures and cultures in different parts of China. Last but not least, when interpreting these results, one should also bear in mind that the refractive error data were obtained from autorefraction techniques and may be susceptible to measurement errors. In this study, we had tried our best to minimize this measurement error by taking the average of five measurements for each estimate of SEs and by measuring refractive error using the same equipment and by the same optometrists in the baseline and follow-up examinations.

Conclusions

In conclusion, nowadays the incidence and progression rates of myopia are high in Chinese school students. Pre-myopic students with longer ALs and thinner LTs are more prone to develop myopia. These data are crucial to clinicians and public health practitioners regarding health care planning and intervention.

Abbreviations
AL: Axial length; CI: Confidence interval; D: Diopters; OR: Odds ratio; SE: Spherical equivalent

Funding
This study was funded by the National Natural Science Foundation of China under grant no. 81773449 and grant no. 81560169. The funders had no role in study design, data collection and analysis, decision to publish, or preparation of the manuscript.

Authors' contributions
HZ and CWP designed the study. LL, HZ, JL, CRL and CWP performed the research. LL and CWP analyzed the data and wrote the paper. HZ supervised the study. All authors read and approved the final manuscript.

Competing interests
The authors declare that they have no competing interests.

Author details
[1]Department of Ophthalmology, the First People's Hospital of Kunming City, Kunming, China. [2]Department of Ophthalmology, the First Affiliated Hospital of Kunming Medical University, Kunming, China. [3]Department of Ophthalmology, the Second People's Hospital of Yunnan Province, Kunming, China. [4]Department of Ophthalmology, the First Affiliated Hospital of Dali University, 32 Mangyong Road, Dali 671003, China. [5]School of Public Health, Medical College of Soochow University, 199 Ren Ai Road, Suzhou 215123, China.

References
1. Pan CW, Chen X, Gong Y, Yu J, Ding H, Bai J, Chen J, Zhu H, Fu Z, Liu H. Prevalence and causes of reduced visual acuity among children aged three to six years in a metropolis in China. Ophthalmic Physiol Opt. 2015;

2. Sun HP, Li A, Xu Y, Pan CW. Secular trends of reduced visual acuity from 1985 to 2010 and disease burden projection for 2020 and 2030 among primary and secondary school students in China. JAMA Ophthalmol. 2015; 133(3):262–8.

3. Morgan I, Rose K. How genetic is school myopia? Prog Retin Eye Res. 2005; 24(1):1–38.

4. Morgan IG, Ohno-Matsui K, Saw SM. Myopia. Lancet. 2012;379(9827): 1739–48.

5. Pan CW, Zheng YF, Anuar AR, Chew M, Gazzard G, Aung T, Cheng CY, Wong TY, Saw SM. Prevalence of refractive errors in a multiethnic Asian population: the Singapore epidemiology of eye disease study. Invest Ophthalmol Vis Sci. 2013;54(4):2590–8.

6. Tan CS, Chan YH, Wong TY, Gazzard G, Niti M, Ng TP, Saw SM. Prevalence and risk factors for refractive errors and ocular biometry parameters in an elderly Asian population: the Singapore longitudinal aging study (SLAS). Eye (Lond). 2011;25(10):1294–301.

7. Pan CW, Klein BE, Cotch MF, Shrager S, Klein R, Folsom A, Kronmal R, Shea SJ, Burke GL, Saw SM, et al. Racial variations in the prevalence of refractive errors in the United States: the multi-ethnic study of atherosclerosis. Am J Ophthalmol. 2013;155(6):1129–38. e1121

8. Lam CSY, Lam CH, Cheng SCK, Chan LYL. Prevalence of myopia among Hong Kong Chinese schoolchildren: changes over two decades. Ophthal Physl Opt. 2012;32(1):17–24.

9. Li SM, Liu LR, Li SY, Ji YZ, Fu J, Wang Y, Li H, Zhu BD, Yang Z, Li L, et al. Design, methodology and baseline data of a school-based cohort study in Central China: the Anyang childhood eye study. Ophthalmic Epidemiol. 2013;20(6):348–59.

10. Wu JF, Bi HS, Wang SM, Hu YY, Wu H, Sun W, Lu TL, Wang XR, Jonas JB. Refractive error, visual acuity and causes of vision loss in children in Shandong, China. The Shandong children eye study. PLoS One. 2013;8(12): e82763.

11. Sun J, Zhou J, Zhao P, Lian J, Zhu H, Zhou Y, Sun Y, Wang Y, Zhao L, Wei Y, et al. High prevalence of myopia and high myopia in 5060 Chinese university students in shanghai. Invest Ophthalmol Vis Sci. 2012;53(12):7504–9.

12. Guo K, Yang d Y, Wang Y, Yang XR, Jing XX, Guo YY, Zhu D, You QS, Tao Y, Jonas JB. Prevalence of myopia in schoolchildren in Ejina: the Gobi Desert children eye study. Invest Ophthalmol Vis Sci. 2015;56(3):1769–74.

13. Ma Y, Qu X, Zhu X, Xu X, Zhu J, Sankaridurg P, Lin S, Lu L, Zhao R, Wang L, et al. Age-specific prevalence of visual impairment and refractive error in children aged 3-10 years in shanghai, China. Invest Ophthalmol Vis Sci. 2016;57(14):6188–96.

14. He M, Zeng J, Liu Y, Xu J, Pokharel GP, Ellwein LB. Refractive error and visual impairment in urban children in southern China. Invest Ophthalmol Vis Sci. 2004;45(3):793–9.

15. You QS, Wu LJ, Duan JL, Luo YX, Liu LJ, Li X, Gao Q, Wang W, Xu L, Jonas JB, et al. Prevalence of myopia in school children in greater Beijing: the Beijing childhood eye study. Acta Ophthalmol. 2014;92(5): e398–406.

16. Qian DJ, Zhong H, Li J, Niu Z, Yuan Y, Pan CW. Myopia among school students in rural China (Yunnan). Ophthalmic Physiol Opt. 2016;36(4):381–7.

17. Saw SM, Tong L, Chua WH, Chia KS, Koh D, Tan DT, Katz J. Incidence and progression of myopia in Singaporean school children. Invest Ophthalmol Vis Sci. 2005;46(1):51–7.

18. Li SM, Li H, Li SY, Liu LR, Kang MT, Wang YP, Zhang F, Zhan SY, Gopinath B, Mitchell P, et al. Time outdoors and myopia progression over 2 years in Chinese children: the Anyang childhood eye study. Invest Ophthalmol Vis Sci. 2015;56(8):4734–40.

19. Brown NP, Koretz JF, Bron AJ. The development and maintenance of emmetropia. Eye (Lond). 1999;13(Pt 1):83–92.

20. Lim LS, Saw SM, Jeganathan VS, Tay WT, Aung T, Tong L, Mitchell P, Wong TY. Distribution and determinants of ocular biometric parameters in an Asian population: the Singapore Malay eye study. Invest Ophthalmol Vis Sci. 2010;51(1):103–9.

21. Ojaimi E, Rose KA, Morgan IG, Smith W, Martin FJ, Kifley A, Robaei D, Mitchell P. Distribution of ocular biometric parameters and refraction in a population-based study of Australian children. Invest Ophthalmol Vis Sci. 2005;46(8):2748–54.

22. Xie R, Zhou XT, Lu F, Chen M, Xue A, Chen S, Qu J. Correlation between myopia and major biometric parameters of the eye: a retrospective clinical study. Optom Vis Sci. 2009;86(5):E503–8.

23. He M, Huang W, Li Y, Zheng Y, Yin Q, Foster PJ. Refractive error and biometry in older Chinese adults: the Liwan eye study. Invest Ophthalmol Vis Sci. 2009;50(11):5130–6.

24. Pan CW, Wong TY, Chang L, Lin XY, Lavanya R, Zheng YF, Kok YO, Wu RY, Aung T, Saw SM. Ocular biometry in an urban Indian population: the Singapore Indian eye study (SINDI). Invest Ophthalmol Vis Sci. 2011;52(9):6636–42.

25. Zhao J, Mao J, Luo R, Li F, Munoz SR, Ellwein LB. The progression of refractive error in school-age children: Shunyi district, China. Am J Ophthalmol. 2002;134(5):735–43.

26. Fan DS, Lam DS, Lam RF, Lau JT, Chong KS, Cheung EY, Lai RY, Chew SJ. Prevalence, incidence, and progression of myopia of school children in Hong Kong. Invest Ophthalmol Vis Sci. 2004;45(4):1071–5.

27. Ji CY, Chen TJ. Empirical changes in the prevalence of overweight and obesity among Chinese students from 1985 to 2010 and corresponding preventive strategies. Biomed Environ Sci. 2013;26(1):1–12.

28. Lim LS, Gazzard G, Low YL, Choo R, Tan DT, Tong L, Yin Wong T, Saw SM. Dietary factors, myopia, and axial dimensions in children. Ophthalmology. 2010;117(5):993–7. e994

28

Visual acuity improvement after phacoemulsification cataract surgery in patients aged ≥90 years

Taku Toyama[1], Takashi Ueta[2,3]* ⓘ, Masato Yoshitani[1], Rei Sakata[1] and Jiro Numaga[1]

Abstract

Background: Visual acuity (VA) outcomes after phacoemulsification cataract surgery in the very elderly (≥90 years) compared to those in younger patients remain unclear till date.

Methods: We retrospectively investigated 138 (group 1) and 152 (group 2) eyes in patients aged ≥90 and < 80 years, respectively, with senile cataracts who underwent phacoemulsification and intraocular lens implantation between 2014 and 2016. Four highly experienced ophthalmic surgeons performed the procedures. Intra- and post-operative complications were compared between the two groups. To investigate the effectiveness of cataract surgery in improving best-corrected VA (BCVA) at 1 and 3 months postoperatively, multiple regression analysis was performed with variables of age, cataract grades, sex, and history of diabetes mellitus (DM) and hypertension.

Results: The intra- and post-operative complication rates were similar between the two groups. After adjusting for the difference in cataract grades, multiple regression analysis indicated that BCVA improvement was equally favorable in both groups at 1 and 3 months postoperatively but was less favorable in patients with a history of DM at 3 months postoperatively ($P = 0.042$).

Conclusion: Phacoemulsification in patients aged ≥90 years improves VA as effectively and safely as it does in younger patients, at least when performed by experienced surgeons.

Keywords: Cataract, Phacoemulsification, Visual acuity, Surgical outcomes

Background

Senile cataract is the most common cause of visual acuity (VA) loss in the elderly population, and it also impairs the overall quality of life. Significant cataract is considered to affect approximately 50% people by their 70s and 100% by their 90s [1]. Impaired VA in the elderly is associated with decreased capability for daily activities, decreased social functioning, and limited life expectancy [2–5].

As healthcare systems have prevailed, and surgical devices and techniques have advanced, phacoemulsification has been performed safely in many elderly patients, such as those aged ≥90 years. However, it is true that more challenges exist in the cataract surgery for such patients including harder cataract, shallower anterior chamber, smaller pupil size, higher rates of exfoliation syndrome, weaker Zinn's zonule, and insufficient cooperation during surgery [6]. Evidence regarding visual outcomes after cataract surgery in such elderly patients remains limited.

Therefore, we evaluated the VA outcomes of cataract surgery in patients aged ≥90 years compared to those in younger patients.

Methods

Patients

The institutional review board of Tokyo Metropolitan Geriatric Hospital and Institute of Gerontology approved this retrospective study (certificate approval number: R15–54). We searched records of patients aged ≥90 years

* Correspondence: ueta-tky@umin.ac.jp
[2]Department of Ophthalmology, Graduate School of Medicine and Faculty of Medicine, The University of Tokyo, 7-3-1, Hongo, Bunkyo-ku, Tokyo 113-8655, Japan
[3]Department of Ophthalmology, Center Hospital of the National Center for Global Health and Medicine, 1-21-1 Toyama Shinjyuku-ku, Tokyo 162-8655, Japan
Full list of author information is available at the end of the article

who underwent cataract surgery between January 2014 and December 2016 at Tokyo Metropolitan Geriatric Hospital; we identified 232 eyes of 145 patients who underwent phacoemulsification. The cataracts had caused VA impairment with unacceptable glare, diplopia, and/or reduced quality of vision. Comprehensive ophthalmic examinations were conducted pre- and post-operatively; best-corrected VA (BCVA), intraocular pressure, slit-lamp microscopy, and dilated-pupil fundu-scopic examination. Lens status was recorded as the pictures of slit-lamp microscopy as well as the descriptions. Optical coherence tomography was conducted to evaluate macular edema/thickening when deemed necessary by the physician.

A patient was excluded because comprehensive ophthalmic examinations were not feasible owing to a significant decline in his cognitive function. Another patient was excluded because he had undergone combined trabeculotomy. Additionally, 14 eyes were excluded because of ocular comorbidities that affected VA, including age-related macular degeneration in 4, branch retinal vein occlusion (BRVO) in 4, central retinal vein occlusion (CRVO) in 3, corneal opacity in 2, and advanced glaucoma in 1. One eye per each patient was enrolled in this study. If both the eyes were eligible, the first operated eyes were enrolled. As a result, 138 eyes of 138 patients aged ≥90 years were included in the study (group 1).

During the same 3-year period, 2566 cataract surgeries were performed in patients aged < 80 years. Because the age group was the most predominant for senile cataract surgery, it was regarded as the control group for the purpose of this study. Data on 80 consecutive eyes in each year from 2014 to 2016 were retrieved for the control group (158 patents, 240 eyes). Six eyes were excluded because of ocular comorbidities that affected VA, including BRVO in 3, CRVO in 1, diabetic macular edema in 1, and amblyopia in 1. One eye per each patient was enrolled so that the control group (group 2) consisted of 152 eyes of 152 patients aged < 80 years.

Cataract surgery

Phacoemulsification with intraocular lens (IOL) implantation was performed using topical anesthesia with or without additional sub-Tenon anesthesia. All operations were performed by four highly experienced attending ophthalmologists. The procedures were identical in all patients. Using the INFINITI Vision System (Alcon, Inc., Fort Worth, TX, USA), a small 2.4-mm incision was made followed by continuous tear capsulotomy, hydrodissection, phacoemulsification, and insertion of the IOL. Post operative treatment consisted of topical combination levofloxacin, betamethasone, and nepafenac eye drops for 4 weeks, followed by nepafenac eye drop for

another 2 months. The SRK/T formula was used to calculate lens power. Five IOL models were used in group 1 (HOYA 255 [Hoya Surgical Optics, Chino Hills, CA, USA] in 48 eyes, Alcon MN60AC in one, Alcon SN60WF in 57, Alcon SN6AT in 11, and HOYA XY1 in 21), and four IOL models in group 2 (HOYA 255 in 88 eyes, Alcon SN60WF in 57, Alcon MN60AC in one, and Alcon SN6AT in six).

Data extraction

BCVA improvement at 1 and 3 months postoperatively was the primary outcome measure in our study. Data on cataract grade, age, sex, baseline BCVA, medical history of diabetes mellitus (DM) and hypertension (HT), ocular comorbidities, and intra- and post-operative complications were extracted. Decimal VA values were converted into the logarithm of the minimum angle of resolution (logMAR) for analysis.

Statistical analysis

Statistical analysis was performed using EZR software, version 1.37 (Saitama Medical Center, Jichi Medical University, Saitama, Japan) [7]. Univariate analysis for numeric and categorical data was performed with Student's t test and Fisher's exact test, respectively. Multivariate analyses to determine factors affecting postoperative VA and its improvement from preoperative VA were performed using a multiple regression model with standard least-squares. $P < 0.05$ was considered statistically significant.

Results

Patient characteristics are shown in Table 1. Mean age ± standard deviation (SD) was 92.2 ± 2.3 (range, 90–101) and 72.3 ± 5.6 (range, 52–79) years in groups 1 and 2, respectively, and there were 40/98 and 54/98 male/female patients, respectively. The male/female balance was not statistically different between the groups ($P = 0.26$). A history of DM was noted in 16 (11.6%) and 30 (19.7%) patients, respectively ($P = 0.076$) and a history of HT in 92 (66.7%) and 67 (44.1%), respectively ($P < 0.001$).

Severity of cataract was graded using the Lens Opacities Classification System III (LOCS III) cataract grade classification [8] (Table 1). As expected, the eyes in group 1 had more severe nuclear opacity compared to the eyes in group 2 ($P < 0.001$, Fig. 1). However, there was no significant difference in severity of cortical ($P = 0.164$) and posterior ($P = 0.192$) cataract between the groups (Table 1).

Preoperative BCVA (mean ± SD) was worse in group 1 than in group 2 (0.70 ± 0.60 vs. 0.40 ± 0.47 logMAR, respectively; $P < 0.001$; Table 1). Postoperative BCVA (mean ± SD) also was worse in group 1 than group 2 at 1 and 3 months postoperatively (0.11 ± 0.13 vs. -0.01

Table 1 Characteristics of the enrolled eyes

	Group 1 (≥90 years old)	Group 2 (< 80 years old)	P Value
Eyes (patients)	138	152	
Age, Mean ± SD (range)	92.3 ± 2.3	72.3 ± 5.6	< 0.001*
Male/female	40/98	54/98	0.259
Systemic comorbidities			
DM, patients (%)	16(11.6%)	30(19.7%)	0.0761
HT, patients (%)	92(66.7%)	67(44.1%)	< 0.001*
LOCS III Grading (Nuclear cataract)			< 0.001*
1	0	0	
2	9	33	
3	63	88	
4	49	24	
5	10	4	
6	7	3	
LOCS III Grading (Cortical cataract)			0.164
1	27	12	
2	58	77	
3	45	57	
4	8	6	
LOCS III Grading (Posterior cataract)			0.192
1	100	100	
2	13	14	
3	14	21	
4	8	15	
5	3	2	
Preoperative BCVA, logMAR ± SD	0.70 ± 0.60	0.46 ± 0.50	< 0.001*
Postoperative BCVA, logMAR ± SD			
1 month	0.11 ± 0.13	−0.01 ± 0.12	< 0.001*
3 months	0.11 ± 0.12	− 0.01 ± 0.11	< 0.001*

SD standard deviation
*Statistically significant *P* values

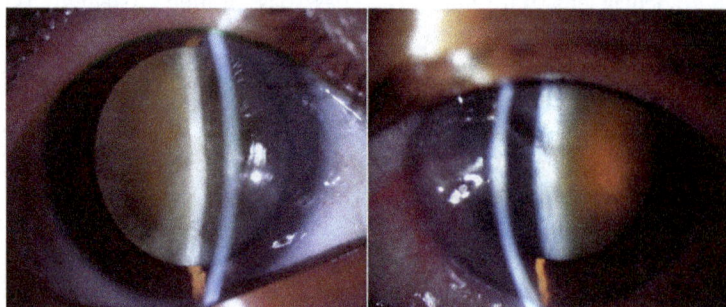

Fig. 1 Representative pictures of higher grade cataracts in patients ≥90 years old

± 0.12 and 0.11 ± 0.12 vs. − 0.01 ± 0.11 logMAR for 1 and 3 months, respectively; $P < 0.001$; Table 1).

Intraoperative complication rates were low in both groups (Table 2). In group 1, anterior capsular tear occurred in four eyes (2.9%), posterior capsule perforation in one (0.72%), and Zinn's zonular dialysis in two (1.4%). In group 2, anterior capsular tear occurred in three eyes (2.0%), Zinn's zonular dialysis in one (0.66%), and wound burning in one (0.66%). Anterior vitrectomy was necessary in one eye with posterior capsule perforation in group 1. In total, the intraoperative complication rate was not significantly different between groups 1 (5.0%) and 2 (3.3%; $P = 0.56$).

Postoperative complication rates are shown in Table 3. In group 1, IOP elevation requiring topical treatments occurred in three eyes (2.2%), corneal epithelial damage in three (2.2%), and cystoid macular edema in one (0.72%). In group 2, IOP elevation occurred in seven eyes (4.6%) and corneal epithelial damage in one (0.66%). One eye in group 2 needed yttrium-aluminum-garnet laser posterior capsulotomy by 3 months postoperatively (0.66%). Totally, the postoperative complication rate was not significantly different between groups 1 (5.1%) and 2 (5.9%; $P = 0.80$; Table 3).

To understand the effect of phacoemulsification on VA in the different age groups, postoperative BCVA improvement was analyzed using a multiple regression model with explanatory variables comprising the different age groups, male/female balance, cataract grades, and history of DM and HT (Tables 4 and 5). As expected, higher grades in nuclear, cortical, and posterior cataracts were related to significantly larger BCVA improvement postoperatively (Tables 4 and 5). After adjusting for differences in cataract grades and other confounders, analysis showed that postoperative BCVA improvement in group 1 was as good as that in group 2 at 1 (Table 4) and 3 (Table 5) months. Male/female balance and history of HT did not have an effect. History of DM had no effect on BCVA improvement after 1 month (Table 4) but negatively affected BCVA improvements by 0.14 logMAR at 3 months postoperatively ($P = 0.049$; Table 5).

Table 2 Intraoperative complications

	Group 1 (≥90 years old)	Group 2 (< 80 years old)	P value
Anterior capsule tear	4 (2.9%)	3 (2.0%)	
Posterior capsule perforation	1 (0.72%)	0 (0%)	
Zinn's zonular dialysis	2 (1.4%)	1 (0.66%)	
Wound burning	0 (0%)	1 (0.66%)	
Total	7 (5.0%)	5 (3.3%)	0.56

Table 3 Postoperative complications

	Group 1 (≥90 years old)	Group 2 (< 80 years old)	P value
IOP elevation	3 (2.2%)	7 (4.6%)	
Corneal epithelial disorder	3 (2.2%)	1 (0.66%)	
PCO	0 (0%)	1 (0.66%)	
CME	1 (0.72%)	0 (0%)	
Total	7 (5.1%)	9 (5.9%)	0.80

IOP intraocular pressure, *PCO* posterior capsule opacity, *CME* cystoid macular edema

Discussion

With advancement in surgical techniques and technologies, phacoemulsification in patients aged > 90 years has not been rare. However, visual outcomes postoperatively in this age group have remained unclear to date. We investigated a relatively large number of eyes in patients aged ≥90 years and elucidated how older age could affect VA outcomes after phacoemulsification compared to younger patients.

In the literature, several studies have evaluated effects of age on postoperative VA after cataract surgery, but not specifically after phacoemulsification. Some studies have shown that patients aged > 80 years had a significantly higher risk of failure to achieve postoperative VA better than 0.67 [9] or 6/12 [10]. Another study also indicated that patients aged > 90 years had a higher risk of poor VA outcome [11]. Another study of 37 patients aged ≥90 years also found that postoperative VA was worse with increasing age [12]. On the other hand, one study indicated that not age itself, but ocular comorbidities were responsible for the worse VA outcome in the very elderly population [6]. A limitation of these studies is that they were conducted a relatively long time ago, and their conclusions were based on surgeries performed before 2000. At that time, a significant number of cases had been treated with extracapsular cataract extraction (23% [11], 48% [9]) rather than phacoemulsification. A more recent report found no difference in postoperative VA between 31 eyes of patients aged ≥90 years and 70 eyes of patients aged < 90 years [13]. Other recent studies also have shown favorable VA outcomes after cataract surgery in patients aged ≥90 years, though without comparison to younger patients [14, 15]. Another limitation is that these previous studies have used postoperative VA as an outcome measure, but not improvement in postoperative VA. In our study both pre- and postoperative VA was significantly worse in the older patients as indicated in previous literature; however, the postoperative VA improvement was equally favorable in younger and older patients.

The features of cataract surgery in the very elderly include systemic/ocular comorbidities, impaired cognitive function, higher-grade cataract, risk of capsule rupture

Table 4 Multiple regression analysis on variables potentially predicting BCVA improvement 1 month after surgery

	Estimate, logMAR (95%CI)	P value
Group 1 (≥90 years old)	−0.014 (− 0.099–0.072)	0.76
Male	−0.014 (− 0.099–0.072)	0.75
DM	− 0.034 (− 0.14–0.074)	0.54
HT	0.017 (− 0.063–0.098)	0.67
LOCS III (Nuclear Cataract, vs grade 2)		
3	0.19 (0.076–0.31)	0.0013*
4	0.37 (0.24–0.50)	< 0.001*
5	0.95 (0.74–1.2)	< 0.001*
6	2.0 (1.8–2.2)	< 0.001*
LOCS III (Cortical Cataract, vs grade 1)		
2	0.13 (0.0041–0.26)	0.043*
3	0.28 (0.15–0.41)	< 0.001*
4	0.65 (0.45–0.86)	< 0.001*
LOCS III (Posterior Cataract, vs grade 1)		
2	0.19 (0.046–0.33)	0.0096*
3	0.35 (0.23–0.47)	< 0.001*
4	0.74 (0.59–0.89)	< 0.001*
5	1.5 (1.1–1.8)	< 0.001*

CI confidence interval
*Statistically significant *P* value

Table 5 Multiple regression analysis on variables potentially predicting BCVA improvement 3 month after surgery

	Estimate, logMAR (95%CI)	P value
Group 1 (≥90 years old)	−0.060(− 0.17 to 0.048)	0.28
Male	0.039(−0.081 to 0.16)	0.52
DM	−0.14(− 0.27 to − 0.0053)	0.042*
HT	− 0.0087(− 0.11 to 0.095)	0.87
LOCS III (Nuclear Cataract, vs grade 2)		
3	0.25(0.095 to 0.40)	0.0016*
4	0.42(0.25 to 0.58)	< 0.001*
5	1.03(0.79 to 1.3)	< 0.001*
6	1.8(1.5 to 2.2)	< 0.001*
LOCS III (Cortical Cataract, vs grade 1)		
2	0.19(0.014 to 0.36)	0.034*
3	0.36(0.18 to 0.53)	< 0.001*
4	0.80(0.55 to 1.0)	< 0.001*
LOCS III (Posterior Cataract, vs grade 1)		
2	0.22(0.042 to 0.39)	0.015*
3	0.37(0.21 to 0.53)	< 0.001*
4	0.78(0.58 to 0.98)	< 0.001*
5	1.8(1.3 to 2.3)	< 0.001*

CI confidence interval
*Statistically significant *P* value

and dialysis, postoperative infection, and corneal edema. Our results suggested that when performed by experienced surgeons who are able to manage these risks using current techniques and devices, phacoemulsification cataract surgery is safe and effective even in patients aged ≥90 years.

In 2012, Mutoh et al. [13] reported similar rates of intraoperative complications in patients aged ≥90 years compared to those aged < 90 years, whereas in 2000, Berler et al. [16] reported significantly higher rates of intraoperative complications in patients aged ≥88 years compared to those aged < 88 years. In both studies, enrolled patients had undergone phacoemulsification. Our results are consistent with the more recent report by Mutoh et al. [13] and suggested that the development of surgical instruments and techniques in recent years has contributed to intraoperative safety for the very elderly patients undergoing phacoemulsification.

Postoperative complications in the very elderly compared to younger patients have not been clear in the literature. In 2004, Syam et al. [15] reported on postoperative complications after cataract surgery in patients aged > 96 years. In that study, phacoemulsification was performed in 30 eyes and extracapsular extraction in four, and the rate of postoperative complications was 11.8% (postoperative uveitis in two eyes and incarceration of iris paracentesis wound in two). They concluded that cataract surgery can be performed even in the very elderly. In our study, there was no statistical difference in the frequency of postoperative complications between younger and older patients (5.9% vs. 5.1%: *P* = 0.8). However, it should be noted that very elderly patients often needed help from family members for postoperative care, including eye drops and follow-up visits.

In our study, a history of DM significantly affected BCVA improvement at 3 months postoperatively, which is consistent with previous findings [11]. Other studies also indicated that diabetic patients without diabetic retinopathy have a thicker macula after cataract surgery [17, 18]. The increase in macular thickness is considered to occur 3 to 6 months after cataract surgery, which might explain why we found the effect of DM history on VA improvement at 3 months but not at 1 month postoperatively. In addition, another study reported that after cataract surgery, the mean interval between surgery and the first recording of postoperative macular edema was 39.5 days, and this was found in 4% of diabetic patients [19].

A limitation of our study was the retrospective nature based on data from a single hospital. All surgeries were performed by experienced surgeons, and our conclusions might not be true for less experienced surgeons. Relatively short follow-up duration might be another limitation, and extended follow-up might have clarified more post-surgical complications including posterior capsule opacity and lens dislocation. In addition, VA was the outcome measures in our study; however, other outcome measures, including contrast sensitivity and quality of life, also would be important for future studies.

Conclusions

The present study has addressed for the first time BCVA improvement in the very elderly (i.e., ≥90 years old) after phacoemulsification cataract surgery, and our multivariate analyses have indicated its similar effectiveness and safety to younger patients.

Abbreviations
BCVA: Best-corrected VA; BRVO: Branch retinal vein occlusion; CRVO: Central retinal vein occlusion; DM: Diabetes mellitus; HT: Hypertension; IOL: Intraocular lens; logMAR: Logarithm of the minimum angle of resolution; SD: Standard deviation; SE: Standard error; VA: Visual acuity

Acknowledgements
None.

Funding
None.

Authors' contributions
Conception and design (TT, TU, RS, JN); data acquisition (TT, MY); analysis (TT, MY); drafting manuscript (TT); critical revision (TU, RS, JN); supervision (TU, JN); final approval (TT, TU, MY, RS, JN).

Competing interests
The authors declare that they have no competing interests.

Author details
[1]Department of Ophthalmology, Tokyo Metropolitan Geriatric Hospital and Institute of Gerontology, 35-2, Sakae-cho, Itabashi-ku, Tokyo 173-0015, Japan. [2]Department of Ophthalmology, Graduate School of Medicine and Faculty of Medicine, The University of Tokyo, 7-3-1, Hongo, Bunkyo-ku, Tokyo 113-8655, Japan. [3]Department of Ophthalmology, Center Hospital of the National Center for Global Health and Medicine, 1-21-1 Toyama Shinjyuku-ku, Tokyo 162-8655, Japan.

References
1. McCarty CA, Keeffe JE, Taylor HR. The need for cataract surgery: projections based on lens opacity, visual acuity, and personal concern. Br J Ophthalmol. 1999;83:62–5.
2. Rubin GS, Bandeen-Roche K, Huang GH, Munoz B, Schein OD, Fried LP, et al. The association of multiple visual impairments with self-reported visual disability: SEE project. Invest Ophthalmol Vis Sci. 2001;42:64–72.
3. Branch LG, Horowitz A, Carr C. The implications for everyday life of incident self-reported visual decline among people over age 65 living in the community. Gerontologist. 1989;29:359–65.
4. Lee PP, Spritzer K, Hays RD. The impact of blurred vision on functioning and well-being. Ophthalmology. 1997;104:390–6.
5. Klein R, Klein BE, Moss SE. Age-related eye disease and survival. The Beaver Dam Eye Study. Arch Ophthalmol. 1995;113:333–9.
6. Lundstrom M, Stenevi U, Thorbum W. Cataract surgery in the very elderly. J Cataract Refract Surg. 2000;26:408–14.
7. Kanda Y. Investigation of freely available easy-to-use software 'EZR' for medical statistics. Bone Marrow Transplant. 2013;48:452–8.
8. Chylack LT Jr, Wolfe JK, Singer DM, Leske MC, Bullimore MA, Bailey IL, et al. The lens opacities classification system III. The longitudinal study of cataract study group. Arch Ophthalmol. 1993;111(6):831–6.
9. Norregaard JC, Hindsberger C, Alonso J, Bellan L, Bernth-Petersen P, Black C, et al. Visual outcomes of cataract surgery in the United States, Canada, Denmark, and Spain. Report from the international cataract surgery outcomes study. Arch Ophthalmol. 1998;116:1095–100.
10. Westcott MC, Tuft SJ, Minassian DC. Effect of age on visual outcome following cataract extraction. Br J Ophthalmol. 2000;84:1380–2.
11. Desai P, Minassian DC, Reidy A. National cataract surgery survey 1997-8: a report of the results of the clinical outcomes. Br J Ophthalmol. 1999;83:1336–40.
12. Monestam E, Wachmeister L. Impact of cataract surgery on the visual ability of the very old. Am J Ophthalmol. 2004;137:145–55.
13. Mutoh T, Isome S, Matsumoto Y, Chikuda M. Cataract surgery in patients older than 90 years of age. Can J Ophthalmol. 2012;47:140–4.
14. Michalska-Małecka K, Nowak M, Gościniewicz P, Karpe J, Słowińska-Łożyńska L, Łypaczewska A, et al. Results of cataract surgery in the very elderly population. Clin Interv Aging. 2013;8:1041–6.
15. Syam PP, Eleftheriadis H, Casswell AG, Brittain GP, McLeod BK, Liu CS. Clinical outcome following cataract surgery in very elderly patients. Eye (Lond). 2004;18:59–62.
16. Berler DK. Intraoperative complications during cataract surgery in the very old. Trans Am Ophthalmol Soc. 2000;98:127–30.
17. Stunf Pukl S, Vidović Valentinčič N, Urbančič M, Irman Grčar I, Grčar R, Pfeifer V, et al. Visual acuity, retinal sensitivity, and macular thickness changes in diabetic patients without diabetic retinopathy after cataract surgery. J Diabetes Res. 2017. https://doi.org/10.1155/2017/3459156.
18. Katsimpris JM, Petropoulos IK, Zoukas G, Patokos T, Brinkmann CK, Theoulakis PE. Central foveal thickness before and after cataract surgery in normal and in diabetic patients without retinopathy. Klin Monatsbl Augenheilkd. 2012;229:331–7.
19. Chu CJ, Johnston RL, Buscombe C, Sallam AB, Mohamed Q, Yang YC. Risk factors and incidence of macular edema after cataract surgery a database study of 81984 eyes. Ophthalmology. 2016;123:316–23.

29

Single-step Transepithelial photorefractive keratectomy in the treatment of mild, moderate, and high myopia: six month results

Lei Xi[1], Chen Zhang[2] and Yanling He[3]*

Abstract

Background: To evaluate the safety, efficacy, and the refractive outcomes of single-step transepithelial photorefractive keratectomy (TransPRK) for the correction of mild, moderate, and high myopia.

Methods: This study consecutively recruited 32 high myopic eyes, 32 mild myopic and 32 moderate myopic eyes. Eyes with myopia that had undergone TransPRK treatment. Pre- and post-operative visual and refractive data, corneal Higher Order Aberration (HOA) as well as safety and efficacy indices were analyzed at 6 months postoperatively.

Results: Six months after TransPRK, the manifest refraction spherical equivalent (SE) was not significantly between high myopia group and moderate myopia group ($p = 0.636$). No eyes lost ≥2 lines of corrected distant visual acuity (CDVA) in high myopic eyes. The uncorrected distance visual acuity (UDVA) was significantly higher in low and moderate myopia groups than the high myopia group ($P < 0.001$; $P = 0.002$). The CDVA was not significantly different between moderate and high myopia groups ($P = 0.057$). There was no significant difference in mean safety index between high myopia group (1.01 ± 0.14) and mild myopia group (1.08 ± 0.15) ($P > 0.05$). The mean safety index was significantly higher in the moderate myopia group (1.16 ± 0.23) than in the high myopia group (1.01 ± 0.14) ($P = 0.002$). The efficacy index was significantly higher in the moderate myopia group (1.05 ± 0.20) than in the high myopia group (0.89 ± 0.17) ($P = 0.02$), and there was no significant difference between the high myopia group (0.89 ± 0.17) and the low myopia group (0.96 ± 0.16) ($P = 0.14$).

Conclusions: The mean safety index was over 1.0 in the three groups. TransPRK showed acceptable safety and efficacy in the moderate myopic eyes, as well as mild and high myopic eyes. High myopic eyes got very similar refractive results with moderate myopic eyes six months postoperatively. The safety and efficacy indexes were not significantly different between the high myopia group and the low myopia group.

Keywords: Transepithelial photorefractive keratectomy, Myopia, TransPRK

Background

Transepithelial photorefractive keratectomy (TransPRK) is becoming increasingly popular in the treatment of myopia. TransPRK has a higher laser cutting frequency than traditional PRK. The unique feature of this technique is that it removes the corneal epithelium and stroma in a single step with one ablation profile. Its advantages include flap free, minimal trauma to the eye and without flap-related complications [1]. Moreover, the corneal biomechanics are less affected than other refractive procedures, including Small Incision Lenticule Extraction (SMILE) [2]. Also it allows reoperation. Previous studies have demonstrated that TransPRK is safe, predictable and effective in the correction of myopia and myopic astigmatism [3–6]. A study showed that TransPRK and femtosecond-assisted laser in situ keratomileusis (LASIK) share similar refractive outcomes in myopia correction [7]. Another study found that

* Correspondence: heyanling2002@sohu.com
[3]Department of Ophthalmology, Peking University People's Hospital, Xizhimen South Street 11, Xi Cheng District, Beijing 100044, China
Full list of author information is available at the end of the article

TransPRK using SmartPulse Technology (SPT) provides significant accelerated healing and visual rehabilitation than without SPT [8]. However, there is a lack of comparative data on the safety, efficacy and refractive outcomes between low to moderate myopic eyes and high myopic eyes after TransPRK surgery.

This prospective clinical study evaluated the early visual acuity, refractive error and efficacy outcomes of TransPRK in different ranges of myopic eyes with low (< 2D) astigmatism.

Methods

Patient population and study design
This study enrolled patients consecutively between October 2016 and March 2017 at the Department of Ophthalmology at Peking University. Patients were divided into three groups: low myopia (≤ – 3.00D), moderate myopia (– 3.00D to – 6.00D) and high myopia (≥ – 6.00 D) [9]. All the patients provided informed consent. The study followed the tenets of the Declaration of Helsinki and institutional review board.

Patient enrolment criteria
Inclusion criteria were as follows: age over 18 years with stable refraction for at least 12 months, corrected distance visual acuity (CDVA) of at least 20/25, cylinder refraction lower than 2.0 diopter (D), discontinued contact lens use for at least 1 month, free of ocular disease and estimated postoperative corneal stromal bed thickness of more than 350 μm.

Preoperative examination
Preoperative examination included slit-lamp examination, intraocular pressure measurement, corneal epithelium assessment by fluorescein staining, tear breakup time, Schirmer I test, UDVA and CDVA, corneal topography (Optikon SpA, Rome, ITALY), pentacam scheimpflug topography (Oculus, Wetzlar, Germany), manifest and cycloplegic refraction, ultrasound pachymetry and fundus examination.

Surgical technique
All surgeries were performed by a single surgeon using the SCHWIND Amaris 500E excimer laser platform (SCHWIND eye-tech-solutions GmbH, Kleinostheim, Germany). The ablation algorithm was calculated using ORK-CAM software. For each treatment, the epithelium thickness profile that 55 μm centrally and 65 μm peripherally based on the population statistic. The target refraction was emmetropia in all eyes. After surgery, the cornea was irrigated with a cool balanced salt solution and a soft bandage contact lens was applied for three to four days. Patients were instructed to use 0.5% levofloxacin (Cravit; Santen, Inc.) four times a day for one week and 0.1% fluorometholone (Allergan, Inc.) eye drops four times a day, then tapered progressively over the following four months.

Safety and efficacy
The safety index is defined as the ratio of postoperative CDVA/preoperative CDVA. The efficacy index is defined as the ratio of postoperative UDVA/preoperative CDVA.

Corneal wavefront aberration measurement
Corneal wavefront aberration were measured by a rotating Scheimpflug Camera (Pentacam; Oculus). The examinations were made in a dark room in the morning. Higher order aberrations (HOAs) of the cornea with a 6.0-mm analysis diameter were calculated separately from the total cornea preoperatively and 6 months postoperatively.

Statistical analysis
Data were analyzed using SPSS 20.0 (SPSS Inc., Chicago, IL, USA). The one-way analysis of variance (ANOVA) was used to compare the differences between the study groups. LSD was performed in the analysis. Differences with a p value of 0.05 or less were considered statistically significant. Pearson correlation test was used to analyze the correlation between the attempted SE refraction and the achieved SE refraction.

Results
A total of 96 eyes were included in this study. Each group included 32 eyes. All eyes completed the six-month follow-up. The patients' characteristics were shown in Table 1.

Visual acuity
Table 2 shows the preoperative variables of patients. The logMAR CDVA was not significantly different between

Table 1 Demographic characteristics of study patients

Group	Patients/eyes	Gender	Mean age	Age range
Low myopia	21/32	16 women, 5 men	30.76 ± 5.17	20–37
Moderate myopia	18/32	15 women, 3 men	29.11 ± 5.17	19–37
High myopia	21/32	11 women, 10 men	30.57 ± 4.43	23–38

Age is expressed as mean years±SD; Low myopia vs Moderate myopia P = 0.301; Low myopia vs High myopia P = 0.901; Moderate myopia vs High myopia P = 0.360

Table 2 Preoperative Variables of Patients

	Low myopia (Mean ± SD)	Moderate myopia (Mean ± SD)	High myopia (Mean ± SD)	F (P)	P
					*<0.001
Sphere (D)	−1.25 to −3.00	−3.25 to −5.50	−6.00 to −7.50	349.29 (<0.001)	†<0.001
	−2.43 ± 0.57	−4.16 ± 0.72	−6.39 ± 0.50		‡<0.001
					*0.296
Cylinder (D)	0.00 to −1.75	0.00 to −1.75	0.00 to −1.75	2.332 (0.103)	†0.27
	−0.70 ± 0.46	−0.56 ± 0.54	−0.88 ± 0.58		‡0.033
					*0.02
SE refraction (D)	−1.25 to −3.625	−3.25 to −6.25	−6.00 to −8.00	262.51 (<0.001)	†<0.001
	−2.78 ± 0.65	−4.43 ± 0.85	−6.85 ± 0.61		‡<0.001
					*<0.001
UDVA (logMAR)	0.30 to 1.30	0.70 to 1.50	0.80 to 1.50	32.22 (<0.001)	†<0.001
	0.77 ± 0.21	0.97 ± 0.19	1.18 ± 0.20		‡<0.001
					*0.002
CDVA (logMAR)	0.00 to −0.20	0.00 to −0.20	0.00 to −0.20	5.01 (<0.001)	†0.198
	−0.128 ± 0.063	−0.075 ± 0.072	−0.103 ± 0.07		†0.067

SE = spherical equivalent refraction, UCVA = uncorrected visual acuity, CDVA = corrected distance visual acuity
Data are expressed as means±SD. *Low myopia vs Moderate myopia. †Low myopia vs High myopia. ‡Moderate myopia vs High myopia

the high myopia group and the low group ($P = 0.198$), and between the high group and the moderate group ($P = 0.067$). After six months, 100% of low myopia and moderate myopia had a UDVA of logMAR (20/20) or better, 94% of high myopia eyes had a UDVA of logMAR (20/20) or better (Fig. 1). There was no significant difference between the high myopia group and the moderate myopia group in the CDVA ($P = 0.057$) (Table 3). The best corrected visual acuity of patients with low myopia, moderate myopia and high myopia is greater than logMAR (20/20). Figure 2 shows the change of Snellen lines of logMAR CDVA. No eye lost 2 or more lines of CDVA.

Refractive results and accuracy
Table 3 shows the postoperative refraction. The spherical equivalent refraction (SE) was not significantly different between the high myopia group and the moderate myopia group ($P = 0.636$). The postoperative UDVA was lower in the high myopia group than in low to moderate myopia groups ($P < 0.001$; $P = 0.002$). The postoperative SE was shown in Fig. 3. 65.7% of eyes had SE within ±0.50D in the high myopia group, 78.1% and 87.5% in the low and moderate myopia groups. After 6 months, 90.6% of eyes had between 0.00 and 0.50D of astigmatism in the low myopia group, as compared with 87.5% in the moderate group and 71.9% in the high myopia group (Fig. 4).

The correlation between attempted and achieved SE datas were shown in Fig. 5 ($R^2 = 0.81$ for low myopia, $R^2 = 0.80$ for moderate myopia and $R^2 = 0.67$ for high myopia). 4% of the eyes were overcorrected in the low myopia and the high myopia group. 16% of the eyes were overcorrected in the moderate myopia group.

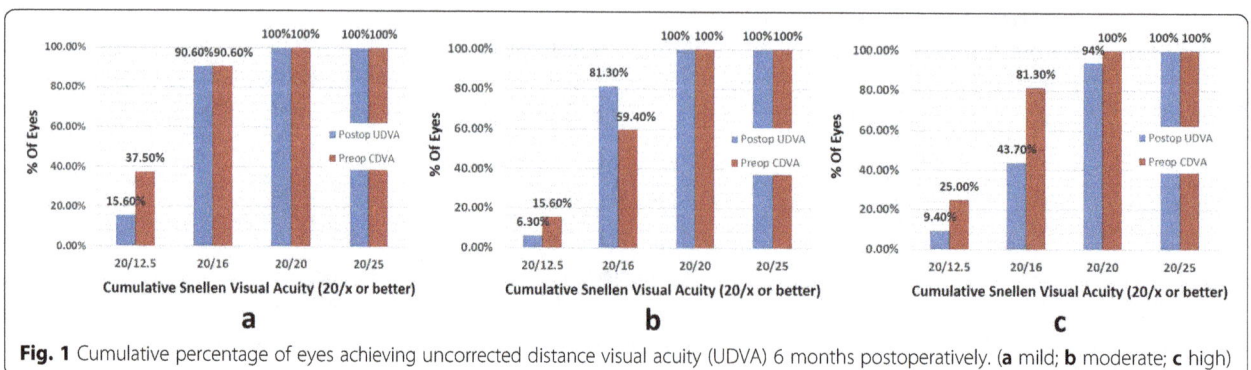

Fig. 1 Cumulative percentage of eyes achieving uncorrected distance visual acuity (UDVA) 6 months postoperatively. (**a** mild; **b** moderate; **c** high)

Table 3 Postoperative Variables of Patients

	Low myopia (Mean ± SD)	Moderate myopia (Mean ± SD)	High myopia (Mean ± SD)	F (P)	P
Sphere (D)	0.00 to −0.75	−0.75 to 1.25	−0.50 to 1.00	12.10 (<0.001)	*<0.001 †<0.001
	−0.32 ± 0.23	0.19 ± 0.54	0.28 ± 0.51		‡0.406
Cylinder (D)	0.00 to −0.75	0.00 to −1.00	0.00 to −1.00	0.98 (0.378)	*0.705 †0.079
	−0.32 ± 0.23	−0.34 ± 0.23	−0.43 ± 0.27		‡0.196
SE refraction (D)	−0.25 to 1.125	−0.875 to 1.00	−1.00 to 0.875	3.45 (0.036)	*0.015 †0.048
	0.30 ± 0.33	0.02 ± 0.51	0.07 ± 0.52		‡0.636
UDVA (logMAR)	−0.20 to 0.00	−0.20 to 0.00	−0.20 to 0.10	8.65 (<0.001)	*0.408 †<0.001
	−0.106 ± 0.05	−0.09 ± 0.05	−0.047 ± 0.076		‡0.002
CDVA (logMAR)	−0.20 to 0.00	−0.20 to 0.00	−0.20 to 0.00	5.43 (0.006)	*0.18 †0.001
	−0.159 ± 0.056	−0.138 ± 0.066	−0.106 ± 0.072		‡0.057

SE = spherical equivalent refraction, UCVA = uncorrected visual acuity, CDVA = corrected distance visual acuity. Data are expressed as Means±SD. *Low myopia vs Moderate myopia. †Low myopia vs High myopia. ‡Moderate myopia vs High myopia

Safety and efficacy

The mean safety index was over 1.0 in the three groups (Fig. 6). The safety index was not significantly different between the high myopia group (1.01 ± 0.14) and the low myopia group (1.08 ± 0.15) (P > 0.05). The moderate myopia group (1.16 ± 0.23) was significantly higher than the high myopia group (P = 0.002).

The efficacy index was 0.96 ± 0.16 in the low myopia group, 1.05 ± 0.20 in the moderate myopia group, and 0.89 ± 0.17 in the high myopia group. The differences in efficacy index between the high myopia group and the low myopia were not statistically significant (P = 0.14). However, the moderate myopia group was significantly higher than high myopia group (P = 0.002).

Corneal HOAs

The preoperative Corneal HOAs were not significantly different between the three groups. After six months,

Table 4 showed that the high myopic corneal HOAs (1.07 ± 0.26) were significantly higher than low myopic corneal HOAs (0.64 ± 0.20) (P<0.001) and moderate myopic corneal HOAs (0.75 ± 0.20) (P < 0.001).

Discussion

This study demonstrated that one-step TransPRK could correct low to high myopia effectively. Six months after surgery, there was a significant improvement in UDVA, SE and astigmatism in the low, moderate and high myopia groups. More than 95% of the treated eyes were within ±1.00D of the intended target refraction. No eye lost two or more lines of CDVA.

Nearly 80% of the eyes in the low and moderate myopia groups and 65% of eyes in the high myopia group reached within ±0.50D of SE by six months after the operation. Previous clinical studies [3, 4, 10–13] have reported acceptable visual and refractive outcomes after TransPRK.

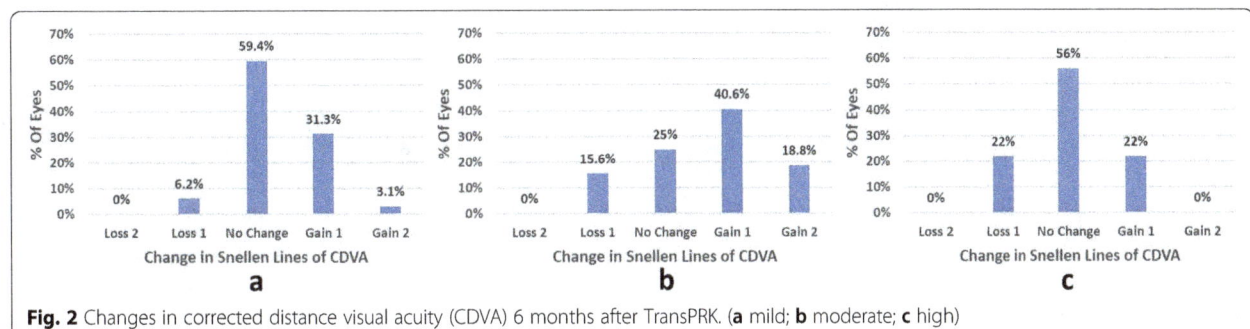

Fig. 2 Changes in corrected distance visual acuity (CDVA) 6 months after TransPRK. (**a** mild; **b** moderate; **c** high)

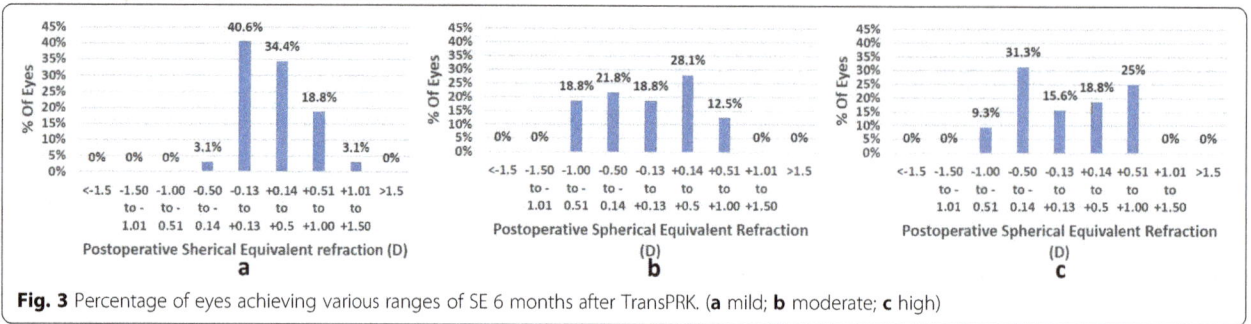

Fig. 3 Percentage of eyes achieving various ranges of SE 6 months after TransPRK. (**a** mild; **b** moderate; **c** high)

However, most of these studies concentrated on low and moderate myopia or high myopia only. In this study, we analyzed our results in different groups of myopia.

In our study, 100% of low and moderate myopia eyes achieved a UDVA of 20/20 or better six months after the operation, while 94% of the high myopia eyes achieved a UDVA of 20/20 or better. Our results are comparable to the previous studies of TransPRK [3, 5, 7] and small-incision lenticule extraction. [14, 15] We found a statistically significant difference in postoperative UDVA between the low and moderate myopia groups versus the high myopia group. The reason may be the increased HOAs of the cornea postoperatively or the changes of high myopia fundus preoperatively. However, there was no significant difference in the CDVA between the moderate myopia group and the high myopia group. This indicated that TransPRK for high myopia was safe.

In our high myopia group, 65.7% of eyes were within ±0.50D and 100% of eyes were within ±1.0D of the intended SE refraction six months postoperatively. Our results agreed to some extent with other studies. Antonios et al. [3] found that 81.3% and 96.6% were within ±0.50D and ± 1.0D in high myopia patients 12 months postoperatively. Aslanides et al. [13] reported 91.4% and 97.1% were within ±0.50D and ± 1.0D by using Mitomycin C (MMC) therapy for the prevention of haze. They got accurate results than us within ±0.50D. There were

no significant differences in the SE within ±1.0D. We found a difference between the attempted and the achieved SE correction in the three groups, with a tendency of overcorrection. The overcorrection may be related to corneal dehydration during surgery. The longer time possibly increases dehydration of the corneal stroma [1]. We suppose that the ablation of TransPRK should be modified in our future work.

In terms of safety, the mean safety index was greater than 1.0 in the three groups. The highest safety index was seen in the moderate myopia group in our study. In the low myopia group, 93.8% of eyes had no change or better CDVA postoperatively. In the moderate myopia group, 15.6% of eyes lost one line of CDVA and more than a half of eyes gained one or two lines of CDVA postoperatively. While in high myopia group, 22% of eyes lost one line CDVA. However, no statistically significant difference was found in the postoperative CDVA between the moderate and high myopia groups. The loss of the BCVA may be caused by the increase of the HOAs on the cornea postoperatively. Our results are more or less similar to other studies of refractive surgeries. Antonios R et al. [3] reported that 81.3% of high myopia eyes were between±0.50D after the treatment of TransPRK. Serrao S et al. [16] reported the safety index of the high myopia eyes treated by PRK was 0.81 one year postoperatively. Ikeda T et al. [17] found 77% of high myopic eyes showed no change or gain in CDVA

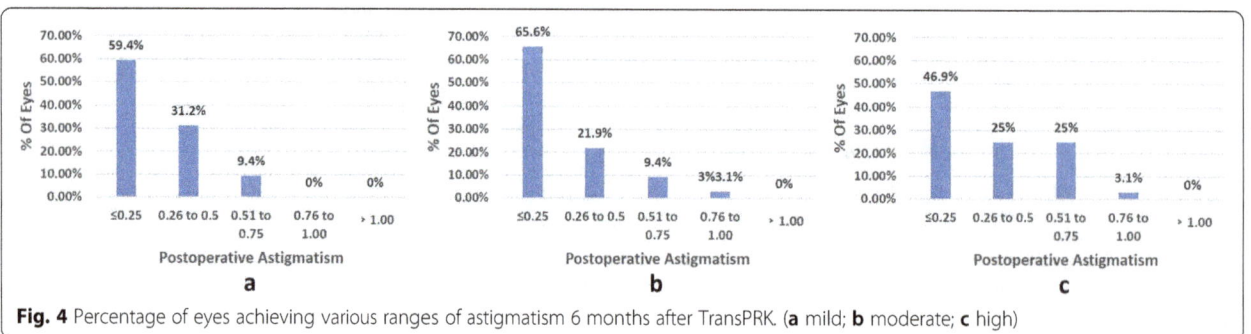

Fig. 4 Percentage of eyes achieving various ranges of astigmatism 6 months after TransPRK. (**a** mild; **b** moderate; **c** high)

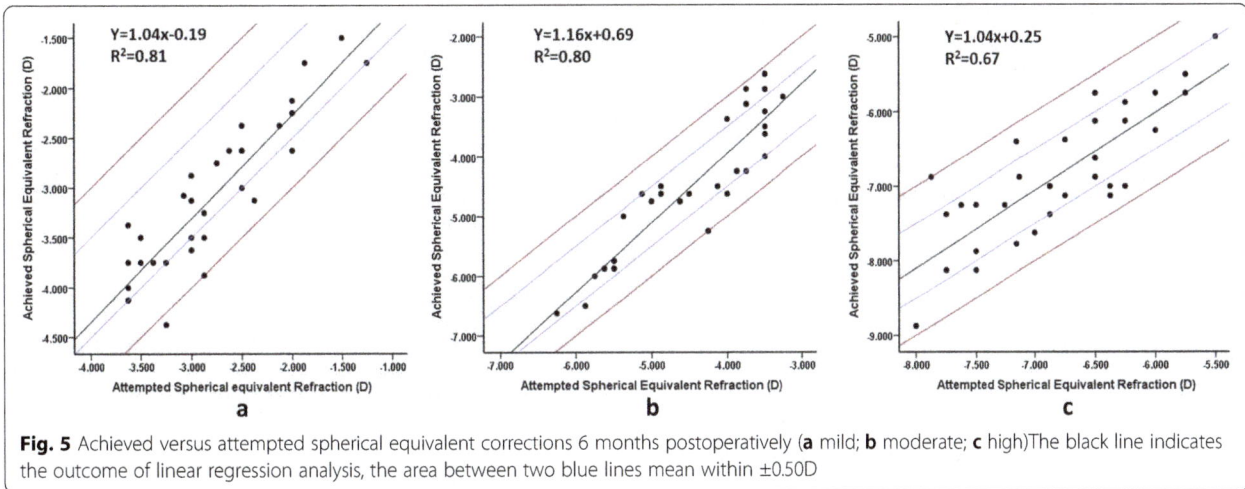

Fig. 5 Achieved versus attempted spherical equivalent corrections 6 months postoperatively (**a** mild; **b** moderate; **c** high)The black line indicates the outcome of linear regression analysis, the area between two blue lines mean within ±0.50D

one year after LASIK. Torky MA et al. [14] found that 88.2% of high myopic eyes got the SE within±0.50D by SMILE surgery six months postoperatively. Similarly, Jin HY et al. [18] found that 87% of high myopic eyes got the SE within±0.50D by SMILE surgery .

Moreover, the efficacy and UDVA were improved significantly in each group. The highest efficacy index was seen in the moderate myopia group. No differences in efficacy were found between the high myopia group and the low myopia group. The study indicates that TransPRK is effective for moderate myopia, as well as mild and high myopia. The single-step ablation profile targets 55 μm centrally and 65 μm peripherally, using theoretical simulations for the scope of ablation optical zone (OZ). Different patients showed different corneal epithelial thicknesses. Mild myopia patients may be more influenced by the difference between the surgical setting of corneal thickness and actual corneal thickness.

Corneal HOA changes were evaluated in this study. We found a significant increase in total corneal HOAs after surgery. Previous studies had reported that HOAs were related to the shadows, halos and night vision glare [19, 20]. The high myopia group showed significantly higher corneal HOAs than the low and moderate myopia groups. One study found that an RMS value of HOAs less than 1.0 had no noticeable effect on the clarity of retinal image, while blur could be seen with 1.0 to 1.5 μm of wavefront aberrations [21]. This may cause the decreased CDVA and UDVA in high myopia group postoperatively.

In conclusion, our data shows that TransPRK is a safe and effective surgical option in mild to high myopia. A

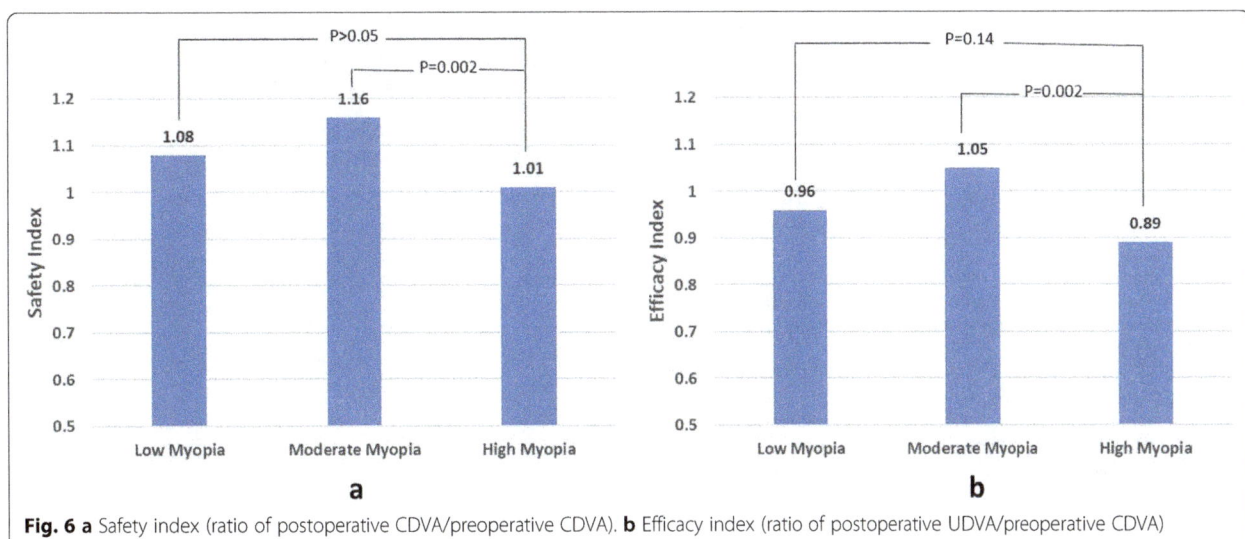

Fig. 6 a Safety index (ratio of postoperative CDVA/preoperative CDVA). **b** Efficacy index (ratio of postoperative UDVA/preoperative CDVA)

Table 4 Summary of corneal HOAs preoperatively and six months postoperatively

	Preoperation	F (P)	P	Postoperation	F (P)	P
Low myopia	0.39 ± 0.11	2.18 (0.119)	*0.808	0.64 ± 0.20	33.21 (<0.001)	*0.058
Moderate myopia	0.40 ± 0.12		†0.058	0.75 ± 0.20		†<0.001
High myopia	0.45 ± 0.14		‡0.098	1.07 ± 0.26		‡<0.001

Data are expressed as Means±SD. *Low myopia vs Moderate myopia. †Low myopia vs High myopia. ‡Moderate myopia vs High myopia

large sample size and long-term results are needed in furture studies.

Conclusions

TransPRK is a safe and effective surgical option in the treatment of mild and moderate myopia, and showed acceptable safety and efficacy in high myopia.

Abbreviations

CDVA: corrected distance visual acuity; HOAs: higher order wavefront aberrations; LASIK: laser in situ keratomileusis; MMC: Mitomycin C; OZ: optical zone; SE: spherical equivalent; SPT: SmartPulse Technology; TransPRK: Transepithelial photorefractive keratectomy; UDVA: uncorrected distance visual acuity

Funding

This study was not supported by any research grants.

Authors' contributions

Study concept and design (LX, YLH, CZ); collection, management, analysis, and interpretation of data (LX, CZ, YLH); and preparation, review, or approval of the manuscript (YLH, CZ, LX). All authors read and approved the final manuscript.

Competing interests

The authors declare that they have no competing interests

Author details

[1]Department of Ophthalmology, Peking University International Hospital, Beijing, China. [2]Tianjin Medical University Eye hospital, Tianjin Medical University Eye Institute, School of Optometry and Ophthalmology, Tianjin, China. [3]Department of Ophthalmology, Peking University People's Hospital, Xizhimen South Street 11, Xi Cheng District, Beijing 100044, China.

References

1. Fadlallah A, Fahed D, Khalil K, Dunia I, Menassa J, El Rami H, et al. Transepithelial photorefractive keratectomy: clinical results. J Cataract Refract Surg. 2011;37(10):1852–7.
2. Wu W, Wang Y. The Correlation Analysis between Corneal Biomechanical Properties and the Surgically Induced Corneal High-Order Aberrations after Small Incision Lenticule Extraction and Femtosecond Laser In Situ Keratomileusis. J Ophthalmol. 2015;2015:758196.
3. Antonios R, Abdul Fattah M, Arba Mosquera S, Abiad BH, Sleiman K, Awwad ST. Single-step transepithelial versus alcohol-assisted photorefractive keratectomy in the treatment of high myopia: a comparative evaluation over 12 months. Br J Ophthalmol. 2017;101(8):1106–12.
4. Adib-Moghaddam S, Soleyman-Jahi S, Salmanian B, Omidvari AH, Adili-Aghdam F, Noorizadeh F, et al. Single-step transepithelial photorefractive keratectomy in myopia and astigmatism: 18-month follow-up. J Cataract Refract Surg. 2016;42(11):1570 8.
5. Kaluzny BJ, Cieslinska I, Mosquera SA, Verma S. Single-step Transepithelial PRK vs alcohol-assisted PRK in myopia and compound myopic astigmatism correction. Medicine (Baltimore). 2016;95(6):e1993.
6. Luger MH, Ewering T, Arba-Mosquera S. Consecutive myopia correction with transepithelial versus alcohol-assisted photorefractive keratectomy in contralateral eyes: one-year results. J Cataract Refract Surg. 2012 Aug;38(8):1414–23.
7. Luger MH, Ewering T, Arba-Mosquera S. Myopia correction with transepithelial photorefractive keratectomy versus femtosecondLassisted laser in situ keratomileusis: one-year case-matched analysis. J Cataract Refract Surg. 2016;42(11):1579–87.
8. Aslanides IM, Kymionis GD. Trans advanced surface laser ablation (TransPRK) outcomes using SmartPulse technology. Cont Lens Anterior Eye. 2017;40(1):42–6.
9. Li L, Cheng GPM, Ng ALK, Chan TCY, Jhanji V, Wang Y. Influence of Refractive Status on the Higher-Order Aberration Pattern After Small Incision Lenticule Extraction Surgery. Cornea. 2017 Aug;36(8):967–72.
10. Stojanovic A, Chen S, Chen X, Stojanovic F, Zhang J, Zhang T, et al. One-Step Transepithelial Topography-Guided Ablation in the Treatment of Myopic Astigmatism. PLoS One. 2013;8(6):e66618.
11. Naderi M, Jadidi K, Mosavi SA, Daneshi SA. Transepithelial Photorefractive Keratectomy for Low to Moderate Myopia in Comparison with Conventional Photorefractive Keratectomy. J Ophthalmic Vis Res. 2016;11(4):358–62.
12. Yildirim Y, Olcucu O, Alagoz N, Agca A, Karakucuk Y, Demirok A. Comparison of visual and refractive results after transepithelial and mechanical photorefractive keratectomy in myopia. Int Ophthalmol. 2018;38(2):627–33.
13. Aslanides IM, Georgoudis PN, Selimis VD, Mukherjee AN. Single-step transepithelial ASLA (SCHWIND) with mitomycin-C for the correction of high myopia: long term follow-up. Clin Ophthalmol. 2014;9:33–41.
14. Torky MA, Alzafiri YA. Visual and refractive outcomes of small-incision lenticule extraction in mild, moderate, and high myopia: six- month results. J Cataract Refract Surg. 2017;43(4):459–65.
15. Chan TC, Yu MC, Ng A, Wang Z, Cheng GP, Jhanji V. Early outcomes after small incision lenticule extraction and photorefractive keratectomy for correction of high myopia. Sci Rep. 2016;6:32820.
16. Serrao S, Lombardo G, Ducoli P, Lombardo M. Long-term corneal wavefront aberration variations after photorefractive keratectomy for myopia and myopic astigmatism. J Cataract Refract Surg. 2011;37(9):1655–66.
17. Ikeda T, Shimizu K, Igarashi A, Kasahara S, Kamiya K. Twelve-year follow-up of lase in situ Keratomileusis for moderate to high myopia. Biomed Res Int. 2017;2017:9391436.
18. Jin HY, Wan T, Wu F, Yao K. Comparison of visual results and higher-order aberrations after small incision lenticule extraction (SMILE): high myopia vs. mild to moderate myopia. BMC Ophthalmol. 2017;17(1):118.
19. Yamane N, Miyata K, Samejima T, Hiraoka T, Kiuchi T, Okamoto F, et al. Ocular higher-order aberrations and contrast sensibility after conventional laser in situ keratomileusis. Invest Ophthalmol Vis Sci. 2004s;45(11):3986–90.

30

Factors related to survival outcomes following orbital exenteration: a retrospective, comparative, case series

Orapan Aryasit*[iD], Passorn Preechawai, Chakree Hirunpat, Orasa Horatanaruang and Penny Singha

Abstract

Background: Orbital exenteration is a disfiguring procedure that aims to achieve local control. It is commonly a part of the management of malignant orbital tumor which is a life-threatening condition. It is necessary to determine predictive factors associated with overall survival (OS) following orbital exenteration.

Methods: This was a retrospective, comparative, case series of 39 patients with malignant tumors who underwent orbital exenteration. Patient records were reviewed for age, clinical presentation, preoperative visual acuity (VA), tumor size, surgical margin, tumor invasiveness, recurrent disease, and status of distant metastasis. Kaplan-Meier curves were used to assess OS and event-free survival (EFS). The predictive factors related to OS were identified using multivariate analysis.

Results: The mean age was 62.9 years (range, 5.5 to 89.7 years), 68.4% presented with VA < 20/400. The mean size of all tumors was 32 ± 18 mm. Distant metastasis at diagnosis was reported in 11 patients (28.2%). Twenty-two patients died during follow-up. The median OS and EFS were 3.89 years and 3.01 years, respectively. The predictive factors for worse OS on multivariate analysis were preoperative VA < 20/400 (adjusted hazard ratio [aHR] 4.67, $P = 0.003$), tumor size larger than 20 mm (aHR 3.14, $P = 0.022$,) and positive distant metastasis at diagnosis (aHR 15.31, $P < 0.001$).

Conclusions: The prognostic factors for poor survival outcome following orbital exenteration were a preoperative VA < 20/400, tumor size > 20 mm, and distant metastasis at diagnosis mostly due to patient negligence.

Keywords: Orbital exenteration, Predictive factor, Metastasis, Overall survival

Background

Orbital exenteration is a disfiguring procedure which removes all of the orbital contents including the periosteum and eyelids with or without the orbital bone. Modern exenteration was first described by George Bartisch in 1583 (cited by Goldberg et al. [1]). A number of diseases require orbital exenteration to achieve local control; for example, destructive tumors that have spread to the orbit, lacrimal gland malignancies, and fungal infections. About 50% of exenteration cases originate from the eyelids or periocular skin [1, 2].

Most publications on predictive factors associated with survival outcomes following orbital exenteration were reported from developed countries. Wong et al. reported

that survival was significantly more closely related to the histopathological diagnosis (mostly basal cell carcinoma) than surgical margins [3]. Otherwise, positive final surgical margin had a poor prognosis in patients who underwent orbital exenteration for advanced periorbital skin cancer [4]. In addition, bone erosion and perineural invasion were the predictive factors for poor survival of orbital exenteration [4, 5].

The goal of our study was to examine the predictive factors related to overall survival (OS) following orbital exenteration in patients with malignancy. We considered the following factors that could predict survival: age, presenting symptoms and their duration, preoperative visual acuity (VA), tumor size (greatest dimension of the lesion in millimeters), histopathological diagnosis, surgical margin, tumor invasiveness (lymphovascular, perineural, bony), recurrent disease, and status of metastasis.

* Correspondence: all_or_none22781@hotmail.com
Department of Ophthalmology, Faculty of Medicine, Prince of Songkla University, 15, Kanjanavanich Rd, Kohong, Hat Yai, Songkhla 90110, Thailand

Methods

Study design

This retrospective study included patients admitted for total or extended orbital exenteration performed between January 2006 and February 2016 at Songklanagarind Hospital which is a major tertiary-care center and university hospital in southern Thailand. Approval was obtained from the Ethics Committee of the Faculty of Medicine, Prince of Songkla University, and this study adhered to the tenets of the Declaration of Helsinki. We excluded patients with non-malignancy who underwent orbital exenteration.

Data collection

Patient records were reviewed for age, gender, presenting symptoms and their duration, preoperative VA after referral from a primary or secondary care center, indication for surgery, tumor origin, tumor size, histopathological diagnosis, surgical margin, tumor invasiveness (lymphovascular, perineural, bony), status of distant metastasis, surgical complications, recurrent disease, date of death (if applicable), and cause of death of deceased patients. We defined a large tumor as > 20 mm in greatest dimension. Poor preoperative VA was defined as < 20/400 using the WHO blindness classification [6] as a potential predictive factor affecting OS.

Statistical analysis

Data were analyzed using Stata Statistical Software (STATA MP 14.1. StataCorp LP). Event-free survival (EFS) was measured from the date of orbital exenteration to recurrent disease or death due to any cause. OS was defined as the date of orbital exenteration until last follow-up or death. Patients without an event or death were censored at the time of last known follow-up or May 1, 2017. VA loss, large tumor, extraocular muscle involvement, tumor invasiveness, unclear surgical margin, recurrent disease, and distant metastasis at diagnosis were the factors used in the Kaplan Meier analysis with a confidence interval [7]. The log-rank test was used to potentially predict a poor prognosis for OS. The Mann-Whitney U test was also used for the statistical analysis.

Multivariate models were constructed including minimal sets of adjustment variables indicated by a directed acyclic graph using DAGitty Version 3.0 (Johannes Textor, Utrecht University, The Netherlands) to minimize bias in the estimation. The causal diagram between the variables of interest and covariables was created based on causal assumptions, and the total effect of influencing survival was reported. Cox proportional hazards models were used to analyze the predictive factors for survival outcomes following orbital exenteration. A P value < 0.05 was considered to indicate statistical significance.

Results

Patient data and histopathologic diagnosis

From a total of 41 patients who underwent orbital exenteration over the study period, only 2 patients were excluded: 1 invasive aspergillosis and 1 mucormycosis. Thirty-nine patients (21 males, 18 females) were enrolled in the study with a mean age of 62.9 ± 20.4 years (range, 5.5 to 89.7 years). Fourteen different tumors were identified (Table 1). The most common tumor origins in the exenterated patients were the conjunctiva and the eyelids. In addition, 14 patients (9 males and 5 females) with a mean age of 67.1 years were diagnosed with squamous cell carcinoma. The most common presenting symptoms and signs were restriction of extraocular movement (74.4%), followed by blurry vision (68.4%), mass (66.7%), and eye pain (41.0%). Eleven patients with distant metastasis had blurry vision (81.8%) and eye pain (45.5%).

The preoperative VA was equal to or better than 20/400 in 12, less than 20/400 to light perception in 13, no light perception in 13, and no data available in 1 case. The mean tumor size was 32 ± 18 mm (range, 10 to 100 mm), and mean duration of presenting symptoms was 67.9 weeks (range, 4.3 weeks to 6.0 years). Five patients had regional nodal metastasis at initial diagnosis. Distant metastases were detected in 11 patients (liver in 3, brain in 2, lung in 2, bone in 2, and multiple sites in 2) that consisted of 3 squamous cell carcinomas, 3 malignant melanomas, 3 adenoid cystic carcinomas, 1 retinoblastoma, and 1 apocrine carcinoma. The median sizes of tumor in the non-metastasis group versus metastasis group were 27.5 mm and 35 mm, respectively, but the difference between the groups was not statistically significant

Table 1 Tissue origin and histological diagnosis of 39 exenterated cases

Origin	Histological diagnosis	Number of cases
Conjunctiva	Squamous cell carcinoma	11
	Malignant melanoma	1
	Mucoepidermoid carcinoma	1
Eyelid	Squamous cell carcinoma	3
	Sebaceous cell carcinoma	3
	Basal cell carcinoma	2
	Malignant melanoma	2
	Adenocarcinoma	2
Lacrimal gland	Adenoid cystic carcinoma	5
	Adenocarcinoma	1
Globe	Choroidal melanoma	2
	Retinoblastoma	2
Orbit	Malignant fibrous histiocytoma	3
	Apocrine carcinoma	1

(P = 0.332). Of the 39 patients, 32 patients had neglected their disease, 4 had delayed initial diagnosis, and only 3 underwent primary treatment before orbital exenteration.

Treatment modalities and outcome

Of the 39 patients, 31 underwent total orbital exenteration and 8 underwent extended orbital exenteration. Six patients underwent additional resection: 2 parotidectomies, 1 neck node dissection, 1 craniofacial surgery, 1 maxillectomy, 1 ethmoidectomy, and 1 lateral rhinectomy. The orbital reconstructions involved 23 skin grafts, 12 bare bones, and 4 local flaps. Ten patients received only postoperative radiation, 7 received combined chemoradiation, and 1 received only chemotherapy.

Seven patients experienced recurrence at the mean time of 34.7 weeks (range, 10.4 weeks to 1.38 years) with a mean follow-up time of 3.1 years (range, 1.6 months to 12.0 years). Seventeen patients were living and 22 had died. Deaths in 3 patients were unrelated to the tumor. The median OS and EFS of all exenterated patients were 3.89 years and 3.01 years, respectively. The Kaplan-Meier estimates for OS at 1, 3, and 5 years were 69.1%, 50.5%, and 41.1%, respectively (Fig. 1a). The EFS at 1, 3, and 5 years were 66.6%, 47.5%, and 37.8%, respectively (Fig. 1b).

The log-rank test was used to identify variables significantly associated with OS (Table 2). The prognostic factors that could significantly predict inferior survival outcome in our study using univariate analysis were preoperative VA < 20/400 (P = 0.018), tumor size > 20 mm (P = 0.032), distant metastasis at diagnosis (P < 0.001), and recurrent disease (P = 0.043).

A clear surgical margin was obtained in 25 cases (64.1%). Of these, 4 cases had regional nodal metastasis and 6 had distant metastasis at initial diagnosis. Fourteen patients were reported to have an unclear surgical margin (6/6 lacrimal gland, 3/4 orbit, 3/13 conjunctiva, 2/12 eyelid). The OS rates for clear surgical margins at 1

and 5 years were 68.0% and 35.3%, respectively. We also analyzed the OS for unclear surgical margins at 1 and 5 years and the results were 71.4% and 39.1%, respectively.

The 1-year and 5-year OS rates were 91.7% and 68.8%, respectively, for patients with preoperative VA ≥ 20/400 which were superior compared with VA < 20/400 (Fig. 2a). The Kaplan-Meier estimates for OS for tumor size > 20 mm at 1 and 5 years were 65.4% and 27.6%, respectively, whereas for tumor size ≤ 20 mm at 1 and 5 years, the OS estimates were 76.2% and 67.7%, respectively (Fig. 2b). Patients with distant metastasis at diagnosis had an inferior OS (24.2% and 0% at 1 and 5 years, respectively) in comparison with patients without distant metastasis (91.3% and 62.8% at 1 year and 5 years, respectively) (Fig. 2c). Recurrent disease was significantly associated with worse OS (Fig. 2d).

Multivariate analysis of OS revealed three predictive factors that were independently related to survival outcome following orbital exenteration: preoperative VA < 20/400 (adjusted hazard ratio [aHR] 4.67, 95% confidence interval [CI] 1.27 to 17.12, P = 0.003), tumor size > 20 mm (aHR 3.14, 95% CI 1.06 to 9.32, P = 0.022), and positive distant metastasis at diagnosis (aHR 15.31, 95% CI 4.25 to 55.19, P < 0.001) (Table 3).

The OS rates of 14 patients with squamous cell carcinoma at 1, 3, and 5 years were 78.6%, 50.3%, and 25.1%, respectively. Distant metastasis at initial diagnosis and recurrent disease were significantly associated with worse OS of squamous cell carcinoma patients using the log-rank test (P = 0.001 and P = 0.020, respectively).

Discussion

This 10-year study found malignancies in 39 of 41 patients (95.1%) who underwent an orbital exenteration. These results were similar to previously published data [8–11]. Before 1990, the most common histopathologic

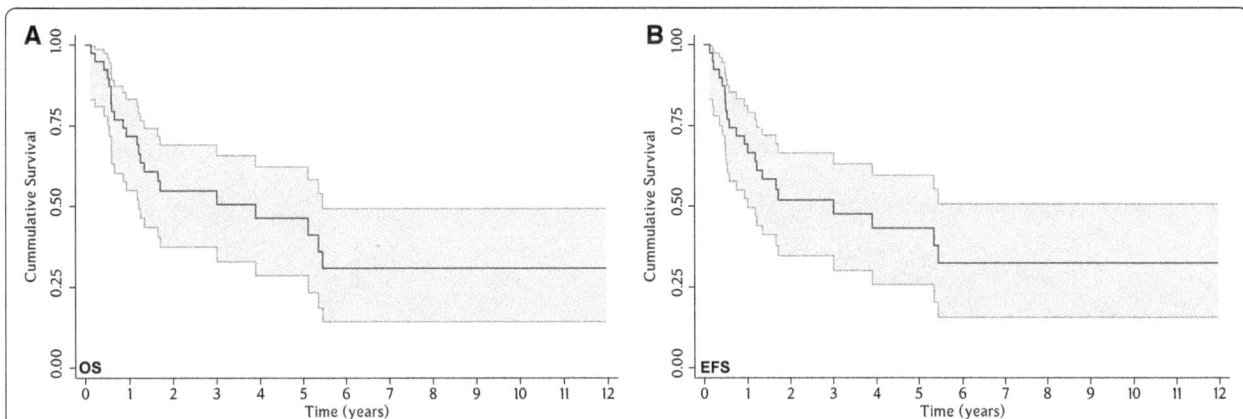

Fig. 1 Kaplan-Meier survival analysis for 39 cases: (a) Overall survival (OS). (b) Event-free survival (EFS). The shaded areas represent 95% confidence interval (CI)

Table 2 Univariate analysis for various factors related to overall survival (OS)

Characteristic	survival					P value
	n/N	Median survival time (years)	1 year (%)	3 years (%)	5 years (%)	
Overall rate	22/39	3.89	69.1	50.5	41.2	
Gender						
Male	11/21	5.11	71.4	60.3	46.5	0.269
Female	11/18	1.34	66.2	19.3	19.3	
Mean age (years)						
≤ 63	11/18	1.65	55.0	40.1	30.0	0.516
> 63	11/21	5.35	76.2	51.9	41.5	
Mean duration of presenting symptom (weeks)						
≤ 67.9	16/26	3.89	65.2	51.8	41.5	0.967
> 67.9	6/13	1.70	69.2	48.5	48.5	
Restriction of extraocular movements						
No	4/10	5.35	90.0	75.0	56.0	0.093
Yes	18/29	1.65	58.0	36.2	29.0	
Mass						
No	6/13	5.35	69.2	29.7	29.7	0.965
Yes	16/26	3.01	69.2	49.0	37.8	
Eye pain on presentation						
No	13/23	3.01	69.6	55.8	42.5	0.646
Yes	9/16	3.89	68.8	40.1	20.1	
VA						
≥ 20/400	3/12	10.1	91.7	68.8	68.8	0.018*
< 20/400	18/26	1.65	57.4	38.1	30.5	
Tumor size						
≤ 20 mm	4/13	11.95	76.2	67.7	67.7	0.032*
> 20 mm	18/26	1.65	65.4	41.4	27.6	
Histopathologic diagnosis						
Non-squamous cell carcinoma	15/25	3.01	63.8	43.8	37.6	0.528
Squamous cell carcinoma	7/14	5.35	78.6	50.3	25.1	
Tumor origin						
Lid	6/12	3.01	83.3	44.4	22.2	0.660
Lacrimal, globe, and orbit	8/14	0.85	50.0	40.0	40.0	
Conjunctiva	8/13	5.11	69.2	52.8	39.6	
Surgical margins						
Unclear margin	7/14	5.45	71.4	52.1	39.1	0.597
Clear margin	15/25	3.89	68.0	44.1	35.3	
Tumor invasiveness (lymphovascular, perineural, bony)						
No	15/29	3.89	65.5	48.6	41.7	0.453
Yes	7/10	3.01	80.0	40.0	20.0	
Status of metastasis						
No distant metastasis	9/23	5.45	91.3	70.6	62.8	< 0.001*
Regional nodal metastasis	3/5	3.01	60.0	60.0	0.0	
Distant metastasis	10/11	0.59	24.2	0.0	0.0	

Table 2 Univariate analysis for various factors related to overall survival (OS) *(Continued)*

Characteristic	survival						P value
	n/N	Median survival time (years)	1 year (%)	3 years (%)	5 years (%)		
Adding resection							
No	18/33	3.89	63.5	47.9	41.9		0.815
Yes	4/6	3.01	83.3	33.3	0.0		
Radiation							
No	12/22	3.89	72.7	52.0	36.4		0.579
Yes	10/17	5.11	64.7	37.8	37.8		
Chemotherapy							
No	16/31	3.89	77.3	53.5	41.3		0.197
Yes	6/8	0.65	37.5	18.8	18.8		
Recurrent disease							
No	16/32	5.35	74.9	55.5	44.1		0.043*
Yes	6/7	0.85	28.6	0.0	0.0		

n deceased patients, *N* total patients, *VA* Visual acuity, **P value < 0.05*

diagnosis in patients requiring orbital exenteration was basal cell carcinoma (23.1% to 35.5%) [12–14]. Of note, an increasing trend was reported in the cases of squamous cell carcinoma due to globe or periorbital invasion that could not be managed by a simple surgical excision which comprised 32.3% to 38.4% of all exenterated patients [10, 15, 16].

Our study also reported the most common indication for orbital exenteration was squamous cell carcinoma in 34.1% (conjunctiva in 11 and eyelid in 3). We found a low proportion of basal cell carcinoma (5.1%). Ali et al. reported that ocular surface squamous neoplasia (44.4%) and sebaceous gland carcinoma (18.5%) were the most common indications for orbital exenteration in India [17]. Ocular surface squamous neoplasia is predominant in Asian and African countries because of chronic sun exposure and agricultural occupations [18, 19]. Of the 14 squamous cell carcinoma patients in our report, 64.3% were males. Demographic data of the current study also suggested a male predominance and the mean

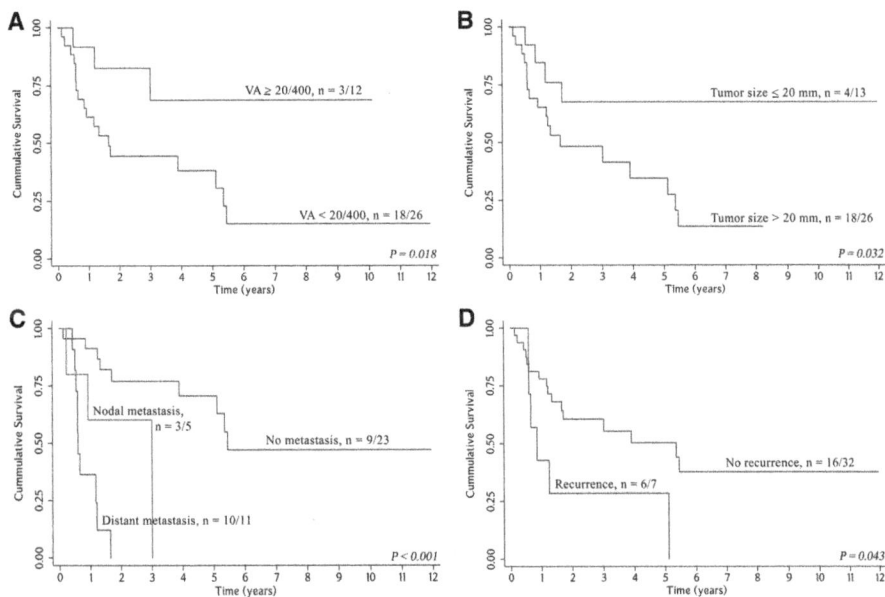

Fig. 2 Kaplan-Meier survival analysis for each group: (**a**) Overall survival (OS) for patients with VA ≥20/400 versus VA < 20/400 (**b**) OS for patients with tumor size ≤20 mm versus tumor size > 20 mm. (**c**) OS for patients with no distant metastasis, regional nodal metastasis versus distant metastasis. (**d**) OS for patients with or without recurrent disease

Table 3 Multivariate analysis of predictors associated with overall survival (OS) showing total effect

Variable	Minimally sufficient adjustment set	Exposure variable: Level	Adjusted Hazard Ratio (95% CI)	P value
Mean age (years)		≤ 63	1	
		> 63	0.75 (0.33, 1.75)	0.519
Mean duration of presenting symptom (weeks)	- Histopathologic diagnosis	≤ 67.9	1	
		> 67.9	1.19 (0.41, 3.45)	0.751
Restriction of extraocular movements	- Mean duration of presenting symptom	No	1	
	- Tumor invasiveness	Yes	2.39 (0.71, 7.98)	0.199
	- Tumor origin			
Mass		No	1	
		Yes	1.02 (0.40, 2.64)	0.965
Eye pain on presentation	- Histopathologic diagnosis	No	1	
		Yes	1.40 (0.56, 3.48)	0.476
VA	- Mean age	≥ 20/400	1	
	- Histopathologic diagnosis	< 20/400	4.67 (1.27, 17.12)	0.003*
	- Tumor origin			
	- Tumor size			
Tumor size	- Mean duration of presenting symptom	≤ 20 mm	1	
	- Histopathologic diagnosis	> 20 mm	3.14 (1.06, 9.32)	0.022*
Histopathologic diagnosis	- Mean age	Non-squamous cell	1	
	- Tumor origin	Squamous cell	0.58 (0.15, 2.30)	0.435
Tumor origin		Lid	1	
		Lacrimal, globe, and orbit	1.57 (0.54, 4.59)	0.674
		Conjunctiva	1.09 (0.37, 3.16)	
		Conjunctiva	1	
		Lacrimal, globe, and orbit	1.44 (0.53, 3.91)	
Surgical margins		Clear margin	1	
		Unclear margin	0.78 (0.32, 1.94)	0.593
Tumor invasiveness (lymphovascular, perineural, bony)		No	1	
		Yes	1.41 (0.57, 3.48)	0.466
Status of metastasis	- Mean duration of presenting symptom	Negative	1	
	- Histopathologic diagnosis	Regional nodal metastasis	3.32 (0.76, 14.52)	< 0.001*
	- Tumor size	Distant metastasis	15.31 (4.25, 55.19)	
Adding resection	- Tumor invasiveness	No	1	
	- Recurrent disease	Yes	0.57 (0.15, 2.23)	0.403
	- Surgical margins			
Radiation	- Status of metastasis	No	1	
	- Surgical margins	Yes	1.27 (0.45, 3.56)	0.654
Chemotherapy	- Status of metastasis	No	1	
		Yes	1.76 (0.63, 4.93)	0.298
Recurrent disease		No	1	
		Yes	2.62 (0.99, 6.91)	0.070

CI confidence interval, LR likelihood ratio, VA Visual acuity, *P value < 0.05

age of nearly 70 years in those patients with squamous cell carcinoma corresponded to the findings of prior studies [20, 21]. Our study revealed a low rate of basal cell carcinoma in association with orbital exenteration. This might be due to the fact that basal cell carcinoma is a less aggressive tumor and the patient usually has time to recognize it.

Interestingly, we revealed that tumor-related survival was significantly better for patients with a preoperative VA ≥20/400 than for patients with a VA < 20/400. In addition, the common clinical presentation in our study was blurry vision which presented in nearly 70%. Therefore, preoperative VA was one of the predictive factors related to OS. A possible reason for this is the origin of the tumor (i.e. the globe). For example, retinoblastoma and choroidal melanoma, which invade the sclera and involve the optic nerve or the orbit, are associated with a low rate of survival in spite of orbital exenteration [22–25]. A second reason is that malignant tumors of periorbital structures that affect the vision are typically invasive and highly aggressive in behavior. Even though the patient may have mild visual impairment in case of partial globe or optic nerve involvement, we recommend performing an orbital exenteration before the tumor advances further.

Although we were able to achieve local control with clear surgical margins in 25 patients (64.1%), 10 of these patients had positive metastasis at initial diagnosis (4 patients had regional nodal metastasis [2 squamous cell carcinomas and 2 malignant melanomas] and 6 had distant metastasis [3 malignant melanomas, 2 squamous cell carcinomas, and 1 retinoblastoma]). Notably, we confirmed that the clear surgical margin group had a high rate of nodal or distant metastasis at diagnosis (40%). The log-rank test revealed that clear versus unclear surgical margins did not show statistical significance in terms of OS ($P = 0.597$). Since a high proportion of metastasis was found in patients with clear surgical margins, we propose that micrometastasis occurred prior to orbital exenteration. However, surgical margins play an important role in controlling the site of the malignant tumors. Mouriaux et al. also reported that surgical margins significantly affected the control of local recurrence, which was not related to survival [15]. On the other hand, Gerring et al. reported that an unclear surgical margin was the only factor associated with a poor prognosis on multivariate analysis in patients undergoing orbital exenteration due to advanced periorbital non-melanoma skin cancer [4]. For the unclear surgical margin cases, adjuvant radiotherapy or chemotherapy or both increased the surgical cure rate [9, 10, 26]. Tumor invasiveness (lymphovascular, perineural, bony) was also not associated with a poor survival outcome which was contrary to the findings of previous studies [8, 27]. However, it is important to recognize that our study had too few cases to detect statistical significance.

In this current study, tumor size greater than 20 mm at presentation was considered a large tumor and this significantly affected OS. Several studies of eye cancer also reported that larger tumor size posed a risk of local recurrence or metastasis which was possibly associated with the inferior survival outcome [28, 29]. Therefore, patient awareness and education is important to detect the disease in the early stage and receive proper management.

Distant metastasis at diagnosis is defined following the tumor-node-metastasis staging system and is associated with a poor overall prognosis. Therefore, distant metastasis was a predictive factor that helped estimate survival in our study, in which 11 of the 39 orbital exenterations had distant metastasis at diagnosis. The OS rates of the metastasis group were 81.8% and 24.2% at 6 months and 1 year, respectively. All patients with distant metastasis at diagnosis died within 1.65 years. The design of our study did not compare the OS between the patients who received only palliative chemoradiation without an orbital exenteration and the patients who underwent an orbital exenteration and adjuvant chemoradiation. Although orbital exenteration has the surgical goal of complete excision, it can improve local control to eliminate aggressive growth in the cases of a very large tumor and eye pain. However, in the metastasis group, the surgeon should discuss the choices of reconstruction and probably prefer a more conservative surgery.

The 5-year OS rate of all patients in our study was 41.2%. This was lower compared to those of other studies because most of our patients in our study presented with large squamous cell carcinomas which pointed to patient negligence in treating the problem [2, 8, 30].

One prior study revealed the OS rate of non-basal cell carcinoma (mostly, squamous cell carcinoma) at 5 years was 58% [3]. However, in the advanced age group with periorbital squamous cell carcinoma, the 1-year OS rate was only 50.5% [21]. The current study reported the OS rate of squamous cell carcinoma patients at 5 years which was also low (25.1%). The possibility of death due to the histopathologic diagnosis was higher among squamous cell carcinoma patients who had distant metastasis at diagnosis or the recurrent disease or both.

A limitation of our study was its retrospective design. However, orbital exenteration is a rare procedure. During the study period, we performed only 4 cases per year in our institution. Therefore, conducting a prospective study would be difficult. Additionally, the short follow-up time limited our ability to identify the real number of cases with a local recurrence. The follow-up time needed is more than 3 years. Furthermore, this study included various histological types of tumors. Although, our study reported the OS of squamous cell carcinoma patients and two predictors that were significantly associated with worse prognosis, we were not able to classify the predictive factors affecting survival outcome for each histological type due to the small number of patients. The strength of this study is the information that it provides on predictive factors related to survival outcome of exenterated patients who have advanced tumors.

Conclusions

In summary, orbital exenteration can control local malignant tumors, but it is questionable in the treatment of cases with distant metastasis. The most common indication in our study was squamous cell carcinoma of the conjunctiva. Poor preoperative VA, larger tumor size, and distant metastasis were significantly associated with worse OS. Although a clear surgical margin was not related to survival, we recommend performing a clear surgical margin procedure and treating the early-stage disease, including cases with a small tumor size. The information on potential factors to predict OS may support patient counseling and the most effective treatment modality.

Abbreviations

aHR: adjusted hazard ratio; CI: confidence interval; DAG: directed acyclic graph; EFS: event-free survival; LR: likelihood ratio; OS: overall survival; SD: standard deviation; VA: visual acuity

Acknowledgements

The research was supported by grant from Faculty of Medicine, Prince of Songkla University. We would like to thank Dr. Alan Geater and Ms. Walailuk Jitphiboon for their valuable assistance regarding the statistics used in this project. We also would like to thank Ms. Parichat Damthongsuk for her assistance in collecting the data.

Funding

Faculty of Medicine, Prince of Songkla University.

Authors' contributions

Study concept and design: OA and PP; Acquisition of data: OA, PP, CH, OH, and PS; Analysis and interpretation of data: OA, PP, CH, OH, and PS; Drafting the manuscript: OA and PS; Revising the manuscript critically for important intellectual content: OA, PP, CH, OH, and PS; Study supervision: OA and PP. All authors had full access to all of the data in this study and take responsibility for the integrity of the data and the accuracy of the data analysis. All authors read and approved the final manuscript.

Competing interests

The authors declare that they have no competing interests.

References

1. Goldberg RA, Kim JW, Shorr N. Orbital exenteration: results of an individualized approach. Ophthal Plast Reconstr Surg. 2003;19:229–36.
2. Ben Simon GJ, Schwarcz RM, Douglas R, Fiaschetti D, McCann JD, Goldberg RA. Orbital exenteration: one size does not fit all. Am J Ophthalmol. 2005;139:11–7.
3. Wong JC, Thampy R, Cook A. Life expectancy following orbital exenteration. Br J Ophthalmol. 2015;99:1–4.
4. Gerring RC, Ott CT, Curry JM, Sargi ZB, Wester ST. Orbital exenteration for advanced periorbital non-melanoma skin cancer: prognostic factors and survival. Eye (Lond). 2017;31:379–88.
5. Limawararut V, Leibovitch I, Sullivan T, Selva D. Periocular squamous cell carcinoma. Clin Exp Ophthalmol. 2007;35:174–85.
6. World Health Organization. Change the definition of blindness, 2008. Accessed 2017 July 15. Available from: http://www.who.int/blindness/Change%20the%20Definition%20of%20Blindness.pdf
7. Nilforushan N, Askari S, Karimi N. A common pitfall in glaucoma treatment success assessment. J Glaucoma. 2017;26:195–6.
8. Rahman I, Cook AE, Leatherbarrow B. Orbital exenteration: a 13 year Manchester experience. Br J Ophthalmol. 2005;89:1335–40.
9. Bartley GB, Garrity JA, Waller RR, Henderson JW, Ilstrup DM. Orbital exenteration at the Mayo Clinic. 1967-1986. Ophthalmology. 1989;96:468–73.
10. Levin PS, Dutton JJ. A 20-year series of orbital exenteration. Am J Ophthalmol. 1991;112:496–501.
11. Mohr C, Esser J. Orbital exenteration: surgical and reconstructive strategies. Graefes Arch Clin Exp Ophthalmol. 1997;235:288–95.
12. Rathbun JE, Beard C, Quickert MH. Evaluation of 48 cases of orbital exenteration. Am J Ophthalmol. 1971;72:191–9.
13. Simons JN, Robinson DW, Masters FW. Malignant tumours of the orbit and periorbital structures treated by exenteration. Plast Reconstr Surg. 1966;37:100–4.
14. de Conciliis C, Bonavolonta G. Incidence and treatment of dural exposure and CSF leak during orbital exenteration. Ophthal Plast Reconstr Surg. 1987;3:61–4.
15. Mouriaux F, Martinot V, Pellerin P, Patenotre P, Rouland JF, Constantinides G. Survival after malignant tumours of the orbit and periorbit treated by exenteration. Acta Ophthalmol. 1999;77:326–30.
16. Pushker N, Kashyap S, Balasubramanya R, Bajaj MS, Sen S, Betharia SM, et al. Pattern of orbital exenteration in a tertiary eye care Centre in India. Clin Exp Ophthalmol. 2004;32:51–4.
17. Ali MJ, Pujari A, Dave TV, Kaliki S, Naik MN. Clinicopathological profile of orbital exenteration: 14 years of experience from a tertiary eye care center in South India. Int Ophthalmol. 2016;36:253–8.
18. Lee GA, Williams G, Hirst LW, Green AC. Risk factors in the development of ocular surface epithelial dysplasia. Ophthalmology. 1994;101:360–4.
19. Gichuhi S, Ohnuma S, Sagoo MS, Burton MJ. Pathophysiology of ocular surface squamous neoplasia. Exp Eye Res. 2014;129:172–82.
20. Sepulveda R, Pe'er J, Midena E, Seregard S, Dua HS, Singh AD. Topical chemotherapy for ocular surface squamous neoplasia: current status. Br J Ophthalmology. 2010;94:532–5.
21. Karabekmez FE, Selimoglu MN, Duymaz A, Karamese MS, Keskin M, Savaci N. Management of neglected periorbital squamous cell carcinoma requiring orbital exenteration. J Craniofac Surg. 2014;25:729–34.
22. Kersten RC, Tse DT, Anderson RL, Blodi FC. The role of orbital exenteration in choroidal melanoma with extrascleral extension. Ophthalmology. 1985;92:436–43.
23. Pach JM, Robertson DM, Taney BS, Martin JA, Campbell RJ, O'Brien PC. Prognostic factors in choroidal and ciliary body melanomas with extrascleral extension. Am J Ophthalmol. 1986;101:325–31.
24. Bergman L, Nilsson B, Lundell G, Lundell M, Seregard S. Ruthenium brachytherapy for uveal melanoma, 1979-2003: survival and functional outcomes in the Swedish population. Ophthalmology. 2005;112:834–40.
25. Radhakrishnan V, Kashyap S, Pushker N, Sharma S, Pathy S, Mohanti BK, et al. Outcome, pathologic findings, and compliance in orbital retinoblastoma (international retinoblastoma staging system stage III) treated with neoadjuvant chemotherapy: a prospective study. Ophthalmology. 2012;119:1470–7.
26. Shields JA, Shields CL, Freire JE, Brady LW, Komarnicky L. Plaque radiotherapy for selected orbital malignancies: preliminary observations: the 2002 Montgomery lecture, part 2. Ophthal Plast Reconstr Surg. 2003;19:91–5.
27. Tyers AG. Orbital exenteration for invasive skin tumours. Eye (Lond). 2006;20:1165–70.

31

Repeatability, reproducibility and interocular difference in the assessments of optic nerve OCT in children– a Swedish population-based study

Eva Larsson*[ID], Anna Molnar and Gerd Holmström

Abstract

Background: The aim was, first, to collect normative data of the optic nerve head and the peripapillary retinal nerve fibre layer (RNFL) thickness assessed with Cirrus SD-OCT, in healthy children in a population-based study; second, using these data, to examine repeatability, reproducibility and the interocular difference.

Methods: One-hundred and ten eyes from 57 children aged 6–15 born at term, were examined. Best-corrected visual acuity and refraction were assessed. Both eyes were examined and the interocular difference was calculated. Repeatability was calculated by one examiner performing three assessments. Thereafter, a second examiner repeated the assessments to calculate reproducibility.

Results: Mean RNFL thickness was 99.2 (SD 8.8) µm, mean disc area 1.89 (SD 0.37) mm^2 and mean rim area 1.52 (SD 0.26) mm^2. No significant correlations with age, gender or refraction were found. Repeatability and reproducibility were good overall. There was interocular symmetry between the eyes.

Conclusions: Normal values for optic nerve head and RNFL thickness assessed with Cirrus SD-OCT were gathered to obtain a normal material in children. High repeatability and reproducibility indicated reliability of assessments performed by different examiners on different occasions. Overall, good correlation between right and left eyes was found.

Keywords: Optical coherence tomography (OCT), Children, Normal values, Repeatability, Reproducibility, Interocular difference

Background

Optical coherence tomography (OCT) was first introduced in 1995 [1]. This fast, non-invasive technique has been found to be useful in the investigation of children with various macular pathologies [2, 3]. It has also become an important tool for diagnosing and monitoring optic nerve diseases, such as optic nerve tumours, idiopathic intracranial hypertension and glaucoma [4]. Normal values are necessary to interpret the findings, but for children they are not provided by the OCT software. To date, several OCT studies have been performed regarding normal values in children [5–8], but

only a few authors have studied repeatability and reproducibility in children [9]. Similarly, there are few studies of interocular differences in the RNFL thickness and optic nerve head in children [8, 10, 11], although these are important in evaluation of monocular diseases.

The primary aim of this study was to collect normative data on optic nerve head and peripapillary retinal nerve fibre (RNFL) thickness, assessed with Cirrus SD-OCT, in a population-based cohort of full-term healthy children. A second aim was to examine intra- and inter-observer variability and the interocular difference in the Cirrus OCT assessments.

* Correspondence: eva.larsson@neuro.uu.se
Department of Neuroscience/Ophthalmology, Uppsala University, SE-751 85 Uppsala, Sweden

Methods

Children aged 6–15 years, born at term (≥ 37 weeks of gestation), at normal birth weights (≥ 2500 g), living in Uppsala County were randomly chosen from the birth register of the Swedish National Board of Health and Social Welfare. Ethical approval for the study was obtained from the Regional Ethical Review Board in Uppsala, Sweden. Where applicable, both caregivers of each participating child had to provide written consent.

Assessments were performed at the Department of Ophthalmology, Uppsala University Hospital, Sweden, between September 2012 and December 2013. The inclusion criteria were normal health and no eye disease, best-corrected visual acuity of at least 0.1 logMar, spherical equivalent between + 3.0 and – 3.0 dioptres (D) and astigmatism less than 2.0 D.

Monocular visual acuity (VA) was assessed using linear logMAR charts. If the child was unable to read, an HVOT chart read at 3 m was used [12]. Autorefraction during cycloplegia was performed after dilating the pupils with a mixture of phenylephrine 1.5% and cyclopentholate 0.85%. The fundus was then examined.

The optic disc and the peripapillary retinal nerve fibre layer were measured with spectral domain Cirrus, version 6.0.2.81 (Carl Zeiss Meditec Inc., Dublin, CA) by using the optic disc cube 200 × 200 protocol. The scans were performed through dilated pupils by two examiners. Internal fixation was used. First, three assessments of the optic disc were performed by one of the authors (AM) and the assessments were then repeated by another experienced examiner. The right eye was assessed first by both examiners. The disc size measurements were automatically done by the OCT machine. Peripapillary RNFL thickness was recorded in four sectors (superior, temporal, inferior and nasal) around the optic disc and as an average value. Disc area, rim area, average disc/cup ratio, vertical disc/cup ratio and cup volume were also assessed. The inclusion criteria for the scans were a signal strength of 7 or more and the image being centred on the optic disc. There had to be no eye movement and no blink over the measured area and the thickness boarders automatically drawn by the algorithm of the Cirrus machine were visually validated.

Statistical methods

Statistical analyses were performed using SPSS version 21. Two examiners performed three measurements on each child. The mean values of the three measurements for each examiner were calculated. The descriptive values were based on the assessments of one of the examiners (AM). The Kolmogorov–Smirnov test was used for analysing normal distributions. Correlations between optic nerve parameters and VA, age and refraction were performed using Pearson's correlation test. The independent

sample T-test was used for analysing differences between boys and girls. To avoid overestimation one eye of each child was randomly chosen when comparing the optic nerve with age and gender. The randomisation was performed with the Excel, Microsoft Software. Repeatability (intra-observer variability) was calculated using the three measurements performed by the first examiner. Reproducibility (inter-observer variability) was calculated by comparing the mean values of the two examiners. Repeatability and reproducibility were expressed as a coefficient of variance (CV), i.e. the standard deviation divided by the mean, and an intraclass correlation (ICC). A CV close to 0 and an ICC close to 1.0 are regarded as perfect. Repeatability and reproducibility were also illustrated by Bland–Altman plots [13]. Interocular difference was analysed in children in whom both eyes could be examined. The difference was analysed using Wilcoxon signed rank test. and the correlation using Pearson's correlation test. The mean difference between the eyes was calculated and the limits of agreement (±1.96 SD) noted.

Results

Fifty-seven children, all Caucasian, of those who accepted the invitation (58) were able to complete the assessments in at least one eye. No child was excluded due to low vision or high refractive errors. Of the 57 children, 28 were girls. The mean age of the children was 10.7 years (SD 2.8, range 6–15). In four children, only one eye could be assessed and consequently 110 eyes were analysed. The mean value of VA in the right eyes (RE) was – 0.04 logMAR (SD 0.09, range – 0.2–0.1) and in the left eyes (LE) – 0.05 logMAR (SD 0.07, range – 0.2–0.1) and the mean spherical equivalents were 0.95 (SD 0.63, range – 0.5–2.75) and 0.93 (SD 0.71, range – 0.75–3.0) in the RE and LE respectively. No statistical difference was found between RE and LE regarding VA and spherical equivalent.

Mean values of the optic disc measurements, average RNFL thickness and the RNFL thickness in the superior, temporal, inferior and nasal sectors are given in Table 1. All values, except cup volume, were normally distributed.

No statistically significant correlations were found between age and the optic disc parameters, including peripapillary RNFL thickness. Nor were any correlations found between refraction and the optic disc and RNFL. No statistically significant difference in terms of gender was found either.

A weak correlation between VA and average RNFL thickness ($r = 0.24$, $p = 0.01$) was found, but not with the other disc parameters.

Intra-observer measurement variability (repeatability) and inter-observer variability (reproducibility) expressed as CV and ICC, are presented in Table 1. In five eyes, assessed by the first examiner, only one of three examinations was performed and in two eyes the examination of the second

Table 1 Mean values (SD) and ranges of optic nerve head and peripapillary retinal nerve fibre layer (RNFL) assessed with Cirrus OCT, with intra- and inter-examiner variation

	First examiner (n = 110)		Intra-examiner variation (n = 105)		Inter-examiner variation (n = 108)	
	Mean (SD)	Range	CV mean (SD)	ICC (CI)	CV mean (SD)	ICC (CI)
Average RFNL thickness (µm)	99.2 (8.8)	75.3–122.5	1.6% (1.2)	0.943 (0.920–0.961)	1.5% (1.4)	0.940 (0.914–0.959)
Inferior	130.8 (15.1)	91.3–168.5	2.9% (2.1)	0.916 (0.882–0.942)	2.8% (2.4)	0.889 (0.841–0.923)
Superior	123.2 (14.8)	66.0–167.0	3.0% (2.6)	0.848 (0.791–0.893)	2.8% (4.1)	0.851 (0.790–0.896)
Nasal	74.4 (11.5)	47.0–102.3	3.3% (2.4)	0.925 (0.895–0.948)	3.1% (2.6)	0.925 (0.892–0.948)
Temporal	67.8 (8.2)	47.3–84.0	3.9% (11)	0.894 (0.853–0.926)	3.2% (4.8)	0.767 (0.677–0.835)
Disc area (mm²)	1.89 (0.37)	1.09–3.02	4.2% (5.4)	0.919 (0.887–0.944)	2.9% (4.1)	0.949 (0.926–0.965)
Rim area (mm²)	1.52 (0.26)	1.10–2.29	3.8% (5.0)	0.902 (0.864–0.932)	2.8% (3.6)	0.929 (0.897–0.951)
Average C/D ratio	0.40 (0.15)	0.07–0.66	4.5% (8.4)	0.975 (0.964–0.983)	3.2% (4.8)	0.990 (0.985–0.993)
Vertical C/D ratio	0.39 (0.14)	0.06–0.63	7.5% (12)	0.942 (0.918–0.960)	4.6% (6.6)	0.977 (0.966–0.984)
Cup volume (mm³)	0.10 (0.10)	0.0–0.42	11.0% (23)	0.987 (0.982–0.991)	8.1% (12.4)	0.993 (0.990–0.995)

C/D ratio cup disc ratio, CI confidence interval, CV coefficient of variance, ICC intraclass correlation, n number of eyes

examiner could not be performed. Consequently, the repeatability was analysed in 105 eyes and the reproducibility in 108 eyes. Figures 1 and 2 illustrate the repeatability and reproducibility of average RNFL thickness values as Bland–Altman plots.

In 53 children, both eyes were compared. Mean values for the right and left eyes in these children are given in Table 2, together with the correlation between the eyes and the interocular difference. Values from the right and left eyes correlated significantly ($p < 0.01$). There were no statistical differences between the eyes, except in RNFL thickness in the superior (p < 0.01), nasal (p < 0.01) and temporal ($p < 0.05$) sectors; see Table 2.

Discussion

In the present population-based study, we report normative data for the peripapillary RNFL thickness and optic disc parameters in healthy children aged 6–15. Repeatability (intra-observer) and reproducibility (inter-observer) were good overall, with high intraclass correlations and low coefficients of variances. There were no significant correlations with age, refraction or gender in this age group. The correlations between right and left eyes were good, and differences between the eyes were small.

Use of OCT has been widespread for assessments of the optic nerve, and knowledge of normal values in children is important. Different OCT devices can differ regarding the optic nerve parameters [14, 15]. In the present study, we used the Cirrus OCT, optic disc cube 200 × 200 protocol, as in the studies by Elia et al. [16], Altemir et al. [9, 17], Rao et al. [11], Barrio-Barrio et al. [5], Al-Haddad et al. [6] and, most recently, Pawar et al. [8] and Güragaç et al. [18]. The mean value of the RNFL thickness in our study (99 µm) resembled those found in

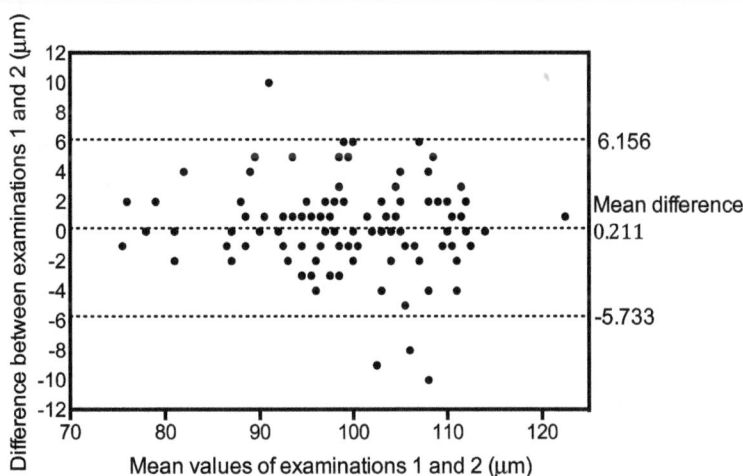

Fig. 1 Bland–Altman plot of repeatability (intra-observer variability) in assessments of average RNFL thickness. The plot shows the differences between examinations 1 and 2

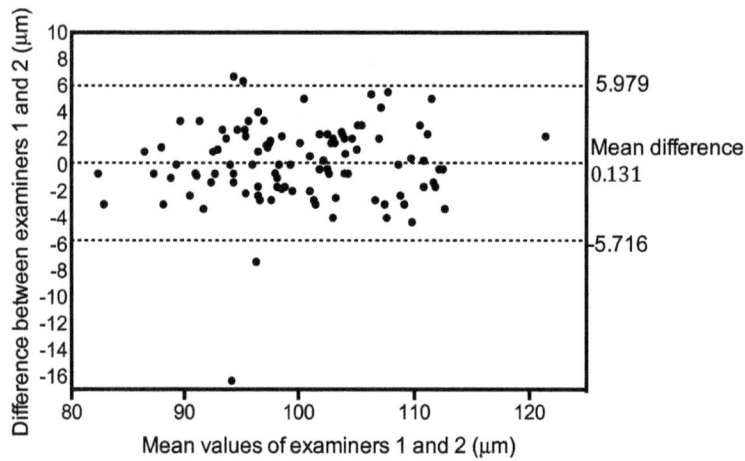

Fig. 2 Bland–Altman plot of reproducibility (inter-observer variability) in assessments of average RNFL thickness. The plot shows the differences between examiners 1 and 2

the other studies, in which the average thickness was between 93 and 98 μm, the two Indian studies [8, 11] having the lower values (93–94 μm). It can be suspected that the lower values depend on ethnicity, since a difference in RNFL thickness among ethnic groups has been found in adults [19]. As in the other studies, the "ISNT rule" was followed, i.e. the RNFL was thickest in the inferior sector, followed by the superior, nasal and temporal sectors. The higher values in the superior and inferior sectors are probably caused by the larger number of fibres converging from the arcuate bundles into the optic nerve.

Regarding disc and rim sizes and cup/disc ratio our values resembled those found by Elia et al. [16], whereas Pawar et al. [8] reported larger disc size and smaller rim size and thus, a higher cup/disc ratio.

In adults, a thinning of the RNFL thickness with age has been reported [20]. However, the present study revealed no correlation between RNFL thickness and age, in accordance with other studies in children [5, 6, 8, 11, 16, 18]. The child's age in this age range therefore need not be considered in interpretation of the results. Regarding refraction, no correlation was found in our study, in contrast to Al-Haddad et al. [6] who had a larger range of myopia and hypermetropia in their group and found a positive correlation between RNFL thickness and spherical equivalent. A positive correlation with refraction was also reported by Barrio-Barrio et al. [5], Güragaç et al. [18], and Rao et al. [11]. The lack of correlation in the present study might be explained by the narrow range of refractive error in the children. Finally, regarding gender, similar values were found in boys and girls, in accordance with the studies by Al-Haddad et al. [6], Barrio-Barrio et al. [5], Elia et al. [16] and Pawar et al. [8], but in contrast to the study by Rao et al. [11], who found thinner RNFL thickness in females.

Repeatability and reproducibility were good in the present study. Chung et al. [21] have compared adults and children using Spectralis OCT and found intra-observer

Table 2 Measures of symmetry between right and left in 53 pair of eyes assessed with Cirrus OCT

	Right eye	Left eye	Correlation RE-LE	Interocular difference RE-LE	
	Mean (SD)	Mean (SD)		Mean difference	95% limits of agreement
Average RFNL thickness (μm)	98.7 (8.4)	98.8 (8.9)	0.881**	−0.126	−8.402–8.150
Inferior	130.1 (15.3)	129.7 (13.6)	0.706**	0.519	−21.45–22.49
Superior	120.1 (14.1)	125.3 (14.7)	0.584**	−5.226	−31.05–20.6
Nasal	75.8 (11.5)	72.9 (11.2)	0.734**	2.909	−13.39–19.21
Temporal	68.8 (8.7)	66.5 (7.6)	0.684**	2.230	−11.36–15.82
Disc area (mm²)	1.85 (0.39)	1.90 (0.32)	0.780**	−0.044	−0.529–0.441
Rim area (mm²)	1.49 (0.26)	1.52 (0.26)	0.810**	−0.035	−0.344–0.274
Average C/D ratio	0.39 (0.16)	0.41 (0.14)	0.989**	−0.014	−0.210–0.181
Vertical C/D ratio	0.38 (0.16)	0.40 (0.13)	0.713**	−0.022	−0.242–0.197
Cup volume (mm³)	0.10 (0.10)	0.09 (0.08)	0.832**	0.005	−0.106–0.117

**p < 0.01 *RE* right eye, *LE* left eye, *SD* standard deviation

Repeatability, reproducibility and interocular difference in the assessments of optic nerve OCT...

225

variability to be almost as good in children as in adults. In a previous study, we found better repeatability regarding RNFL thickness using TD-OCT (Stratus) than when the Heidelberg Retina Tomograph (HRT) was used [22]. In this study, using SD-OCT, we found even better CVs and ICCs. In addition, regarding reproducibility the values were good, in accordance to one previous study in children using Cirrus-OCT [9]. The ICC was lowest in the temporal sector in the present study, in contrast to Altemir et al. who found the lowest ICC in the nasal sector. The differences between the studies could not be fully explained since both studies used Cirrus OCT and the same method [9]. Because of the good intra- and inter-observer correlations, we believe that measurements performed on different occasions and by different examiners, using Cirrus OCT, are reliable. One has to remember that the variability might be different in eyes with diseases. In adults, the effect of disease severity in glaucoma on reproducibility has been contradictory. Studies using Cirrus OCT on normal and glaucoma eyes have shown both similar [23] and worse [24] reproducibility in the affected eyes. Whether, the intra-and inter variations are affected in children with optic nerve diseases has to be further explored.

Knowledge of interocular differences in the measurements of normal eyes is important in evaluation of optic diseases. Regarding RNFL thickness and optic disc size, this has previously been reported in a few studies in children [8, 10, 11, 17]. The present study revealed a good correlation between RE and LE regarding the optic disc and RNFL thickness, and the mean differences were small; see Table 2. Statistically, however, there was a difference in the RNFL in the superior (thinner in REs), inferior and nasal (thinner in LEs) sectors, in accordance with Altemir et al. [17]. Interestingly, Al-Haddad et al. [10] and Pawar et al. [8] also found that the superior sector was thinner in the REs and the temporal sector in the LEs. In the superior sector in the present study, the interval of the 95% limits of agreement was − 31 to 20 μm. This must be considered in evaluation of monocular optic diseases.

Strengths and limitations
The strength of the present study was that it was strictly population-based and that the same two experienced examiners performed all the examinations. The major limitation was the relatively small sample size, especially since the age range was rather broad. However, also in larger studies no correlation with age in this age span has been found. The narrow inclusion criteria of refractive error in the present study could also have been a bias. Finally, information of other morphometric data, such as ocular axial length and the child's height and weight could have added further information to the study,

Conclusion
In this population-based study normative data for optic nerve head and peripapillary RNFL thickness assessed with Cirrus OCT in 57 full-term, healthy children, aged 6–15 were reported. Repeatability (intra-observer) and reproducibility (inter-observer) were good. The interocular correlations were high although a difference between the right and left eyes in three sectors of the peripapillary RNFL was found. There were no correlations with age, refraction or gender in this age group.

Abbreviations
C/D: Cup disc; CI: Confidence interval; CV: Coefficient of variance; D: Dioptres; HRT: Heidelberg retina tomograph; ICC: Intraclass correlation; ISNT: Inferior superior nasal temporal; LE: Left eye; N: Number; OCT: Optical coherence tomography; RE: Right eye; RNFL: Retinal nerve fibre layer; SD: Standard deviation; SD-OCT: Spectral domain optical coherence tomography; VA: Visual acuity

Acknowledgements
We thank research nurse Eva Nuija for her help and her skilful participation in the study. The study was supported by the Crown Princess Margareta's Foundation for the Visually Impaired and the Swedish Society of Medicine.

Funding
The Crown Princess Margareta's Foundation for the Visually Impaired and the Swedish Society of Medicine provided financial support in the form of financial funding.
The sponsor had no role in the design or conduct of this research.

Authors' contributions
EL and GH planned the study. EL wrote the applications to the Ethical Review Board and to the Swedish National Board of Health and Social Welfare. AM contacted the participating families. AM examined the participating children together with EL and GH. EL, AM and GH did the data analyses. EL was the main contributor in writing the manuscript, and GH and AM participated. All authors read and approved the final manuscript.

Competing interests
The authors declare that they have no competing interests.

References
1. Hee MR, Izatt JA, Swanson EA, Huang D, Schuman JS, Lin CP, Puliafito CA, Fujimoto JG. Optical coherence tomography of the human retina. Arch Ophthalmol. 1995;113(3):325–32.

2. Eriksson U, Larsson E, Holmstrom G. Optical coherence tomography in the diagnosis of juvenile X-linked retinoschisis. Acta Ophthalmol Scand. 2004;82(2):218–23.

3. Holmstrom G, Eriksson U, Hellgren K, Larsson E. Optical coherence tomography is helpful in the diagnosis of foveal hypoplasia. Acta Ophthalmol. 2010;88(4):439–42.

4. Gospe SM, Bhatti MT, El-Dairi MA. Emerging applications of optical coherence tomography in pediatric optic neuropathies. Semin Pediatr Neurol. 2017;24(2):135–42.

5. Barrio-Barrio J, Noval S, Galdos M, Ruiz-Canela M, Bonet E, Capote M, Lopez M. Multicenter Spanish study of spectral-domain optical coherence tomography in normal children. Acta Ophthalmol. 2013;91(1):e56–63.

6. Al-Haddad C, Barikian A, Jaroudi M, Massoud V, Tamim H, Noureddin B. Spectral domain optical coherence tomography in children: normative data and biometric correlations. BMC Ophthalmol. 2014;14(1):53.

7. Ayala M, Ntoula E. Retinal fibre layer thickness measurement in normal paediatric population in Sweden using Optical Coherence Tomography. J Ophthalmol. 2016;2016:4160568. Epub Nov 17. https://doi.org/10.1155/2016/4160568.

8. Pawar N, Maheshwari D, Ravindran M, Ramakrishnan R. Interocular symmetry of retinal nerve fiber layer and optic nerve head parameters measured by cirrus high-definition optical tomography in a normal pediatric population. Indian J Ophthalmol. 2017;65:955–62.

9. Altemir I, Pueyo V, Elia N, Polo V, Larrosa JM, Oros D. Reproducibility of optical coherence tomography measurements in children. Am J Ophthalmol. 2013;155(1):171–76 e1.

10. Al-Haddad C, Antonios R, Tamim H, Noureddin B. Interocular symmetry in retinal and optic nerve parameters in children as measured by spectral domain optical coherence tomography. Br J Ophthalmol. 2014;98(4):502–6.

11. Rao A, Sahoo B, Kumar M, Varshney G, Kumar R. Retinal nerve fiber layer thickness in children 5-18 years by spectral-domain optical coherence tomography. Semin Ophthalmol. 2013;28(2):97–102.

12. Hedin A, Olsson K. Letter legibility and the construction of a new visual acuity chart. Ophthalmologica. 1984;189(3):147–56.

13. Bland JG, Altman DG. Statistical methods for assessing agreement between two methods of clinical measurement. Lancet. 1986;1:307–10.

14. Knight O, Chang R, Feuer W, Budenz D. Comparison of retinal nerve fiber layer measurements using time domain and spectral domain optical coherence tomography. Ophthalmol. 2009;116(7):1271–7.

15. Giambene B, Virgili G, Menchini U. Retinal nerve fiber layer thickness by stratus and cirrus OCT in retrobulbar optic neuritis and nonarteritic ischemic optic neuropathy. Eur J Ophthalmol. 2017;27(1):80–5.

16. Elia N, Pueyo V, Altemir I, Oros D, Pablo L. Normal reference ranges of optical coherence tomography parameters in childhood. Br J Ophthalmol. 2012;96:665–70.

17. Altemir I, Oros D, Elia N, Polo V, Larrosa JM, Pueyo V. Retinal asymmetry in children measured with optical coherence tomography. Am J Ophthalmol. 2013;156:1238–43.

18. Güragaç FB, Totan Y, Güler E, Tenlik A, Ertugrul IG. Normaltive spectral domain optical coherence tomography data in healthy Turkish children. Semin Opthalmol. 2017;32(2):216–22.

19. Knight O, Girkin C, Budenz D, Durbin M, Feuer W. For the cirrus OCT normative database study group. Effect of race, age, and axial length on optic nerve head parameters and retinal nerve fiber layer thickness measured by cirrus HD-OCT. Arch Ophthalmol. 2012;130(3):312–8.

20. Wu Z, Saunders L, Zangwill L, Daga F, Crowston J, Medeiros F. Impact of normal aging and progression definitions on the specificity of detecting retinal nerve fiber layer thinning. Am J Ophthalmol. 2017;181:106–13.

21. Chung HK, Han YK, Oh S, Kim SH. Comparison of optical coherence tomography measurement reproducibility between children and adults. PLoS One. 2016;11(1):e0147448.

22. Larsson E, Eriksson U, Alm A. Retinal nerve fibre layer thickness in full-term children assessed with Heidelberg retinal tomography and optical coherence tomography: normal values and interocular difference. Acta Ophthalmol. 2011;89(2):151–8.

23. Vazirabi J, Kaushik S, Sing Pandav S, Gupta P. Reproducability of retinal nerve fiber layer measurements acrss the glaucoma spectrum using optical coherence tomography. Indian J Ophthalmol. 2015;63(4):300–5.

24. Suh MH, Yoo BW, Park KH, Kim H, Kim HC. Reproducibility of spectral-domain optical coherence tomography RNFL map for glaucomatous and fellow normal eyes in unilateral glaucoma. J Glaucoma. 2015;24(3):238–44.

32

Area of the cone interdigitation zone in healthy Chinese adults and its correlation with macular volume

Ruiping Gu[1†], Guohua Deng[2†], Yi Jiang[2], Chunhui Jiang[1,3*] and Gezhi Xu[1]

Abstract

Background: Numerous studies have suggested that the integrity of the cone interdigitation zone (IZ) could be considered to be a marker of photoreceptor damage and its recovery. However, little is known about the IZ in healthy eyes. Our present study was to measure the cone IZ area by optical coherence tomography (OCT), and determine its distribution in healthy adults.

Methods: This was a cross-sectional non-interventional study. We involved a group of 158 emmetropic or low myopic (from −3D to + 0.5D) eyes in 97 healthy adult volunteers. All subjects underwent thorough ophthalmologic examinations and the posterior pole was scanned by OCT. The cone IZ area in healthy adults and its correlation with macular volume and other factors was analyzed.

Results: The cone IZ was visible and clear in all 158 eyes, and the IZ area was successfully measured by 6 radical scans centered on the fovea. The mean IZ area was 30.22 ± 12.70 mm^2, and ranged from 5.91 to 57.47 mm^2. The IZ area exhibited a normal distribution ($P = 0.635$) with 95% confidence interval of 28.06–32.29 mm^2. The IZ area was significantly correlated with the retinal and outer nuclear layer (ONL) volumes within the macula.

Conclusions: The cone IZ area could be measured using a commercially available OCT system. The IZ area showed high variability among healthy adults, and this might be related to the variability in the photoreceptor distribution in healthy adults.

Keywords: Optical coherence tomography (OCT), Cone interdigitation zone (IZ), Ellipsoid zone (EZ), The cone interdigitation zone area, Outer nuclear layer (ONL), Healthy Chinese adult

Background

Optical coherence tomography (OCT), a noninvasive imaging technology, is able to provide detailed images and quantitative information about the retina's structure and has become a standard diagnostic technique in ophthalmology [1–3]. With the spectral domain technique, the single highly reflective band at the outer retina that was observed using the original OCT devices [1–3] was resolved as three separate bands, corresponding to the photoreceptor Ellipsoid zone (EZ), the cone interdigitation zone (IZ), and the retinal pigment epithelium (RPE)-Bruch membrane (BM) compound [4]. The middle band, the IZ, represents the covering of the cone outer segments by apical processes of the RPE in a structure known as the contact cylinder [4–6]. Many studies have suggested that the integrity of the IZ could be considered to be a marker of photoreceptor damage and its recovery [7–11]. However, little is known about the IZ in healthy eyes. To date, only Rii et al. have examined this line, and reported that it was visible in 95% of healthy subjects [12]. Therefore; we performed the present study to improve our knowledge about the features of the IZ in healthy eyes, including the boundary of this line, its variability, and its correlation with other clinical factors.

---

* Correspondence: chhjiang70@163.com
†Ruiping Gu and Guohua Deng contributed equally to this work.
[1]Department of Ophthalmology, Eye and ENT Hospital and Shanghai Key Laboratory of Visual Impairment and Restoration, Shanghai Medical College, Fudan University, Shanghai 200031, China
[3]Department of Ophthalmology, No. 5 People's Hospital of Shanghai, Shanghai 200240, China
Full list of author information is available at the end of the article

Methods

Ethics

This study was approved by the Institutional Review Board of the Eye and ENT Hospital of Fudan University, and was performed in accordance with the principles of the Declaration of Helsinki. All of the subjects signed informed consent forms.

Study participants

Health volunteers were recruited from the Department of Ophthalmology, Eye and ENT Hospital, Fudan University, between January 2016 and June 2016. All of the subjects signed an informed consent form. The study conformed to the tenets of the Declaration of Helsinki, and was approved by the Institutional Review Board of the Eye and ENT Hospital of Fudan University. All subjects underwent thorough ophthalmologic examinations, which included measurement of best-corrected visual acuity (BCVA), refraction measurement, intraocular pressure (IOP) measurement using a non-contact tonometer, measurement of axial lengths (AL) using an IOL master (IOLMaster500, Version 7.7, Carl Zeiss AG, Oberkochen, Germany), slit lamp microscopy, and an undilated fundus examination by direct ophthalmoscopy. The subjects' medical and family histories were also collected. Inclusion criteria were as follows: BCVA ≥0.8, refractive index between − 3 diopters (D) and + 1 D, IOP < 21 mmHg, and AL < 25 mm. Exclusion criteria were prior history of ocular surgery or trauma, BCVA < 0.8, IOP ≥ 21 mmHg, AL ≥ 25 mm, presence of other ophthalmic abnormalities, family history of glaucoma in a first-degree relative, or a systemic disease that might have ocular involvement (e.g. diabetes mellitus or hypertension).

OCT imaging

All OCT images were obtained by a spectral domain system (Spectralis, ver. 1.5.12.0; Heidelberg Engineering, Heidelberg, Germany) with a normal pupil. Two scanning procedures were used: (1) a radial scanning pattern with 6 scan lines centered on the fovea and covered a 30 degree round area (1042 A-scans per line, each line comprising 100 averaged scans obtained using eye tracking); (2) a posterior pole volume scan using 97 raster lines, each line comprising 30 averaged scans, covering an area of 30×25 °. Only scans with good signal strength (signal-to-noise ratio, ≥ 20 dB) were saved for analysis.

Measurement of the cone IZ area

Scans from the radial pattern were used to measure the IZ area. The boundaries of the IZ were defined as the ends of the continuous and smooth highly reflective line between the EZ and the RPE-BM compound on each of the 6 radical scans, with 12 markers for each eye. Then, the IZ area was automatically calculated by the built-in software. The length of the IZ (the distance between the center of the fovea and the boundary of IZ in all 12 directions) was measured manually (Fig. 1). The IZ was measured by one experienced ophthalmologist, who was masked to the subjects' characteristics.

Macular volumes

The results of the posterior pole volume scan were processed according to the macular thickness protocol [13]. The entire macula was divided into 9 regions with 3 concentric rings measuring 1, 3, and 6 mm in diameter centered on the fovea according to the Early Treatment Diabetic Retinopathy Study protocol [14]. The RPE-BM compound was defined as the region from its inner border to its outer border. The full retina was defined as the region from the inner internal limiting membrane (ILM) to the outer border of the RPE-BM compound. The outer nuclear layer (ONL) was defined as the region from the outer border of the outer plexiform layer (OPL) to the external limiting membrane (ELM). The ELM-BM was defined as the region from the ELM to the outer border of the RPE-BM compound. The volumes of these retinal layers within the foveal and para/perifoveal areas were automatically calculated using the built-in software. The photoreceptor layer volume was calculated as the ELM-BM volume minus the RPE-BM compound volume. The volumes of the different layers of the macula were calculated by adding the volumes of the specified layer in the fovea, parafovea, and perifovea.

Repeatability and reproducibility

The first 20 eyes were included to test the repeatability and reproducibility of the method. Two series of radial patterns were taken by OCT in a single visit to determine the repeatability of the IZ area measurements. The intra-observer repeatability of the IZ area was evaluated by measuring the IZ area twice from the same set of radical scans. For inter-observer reproducibility, two observers each measured the same set of scans separately. Intraclass correlation (ICC) and Bland–Altman plots were used to assess the repeatability and reproducibility of the measurements.

Statistical analysis

All analyses were performed using SPSS for Windows, ver. 17.0 (SPSS, Inc., Chicago, IL, USA). The IZ areas were plotted on a frequency histogram. The Kolmogorov–Smirnov test was used to assess the distribution of the IZ area. Analysis of covariance was used to test the correlation between the IZ area and the volumes of each retinal layer and other clinical variables. The differences in the IZ area and lengths in all 12 directions between the right and

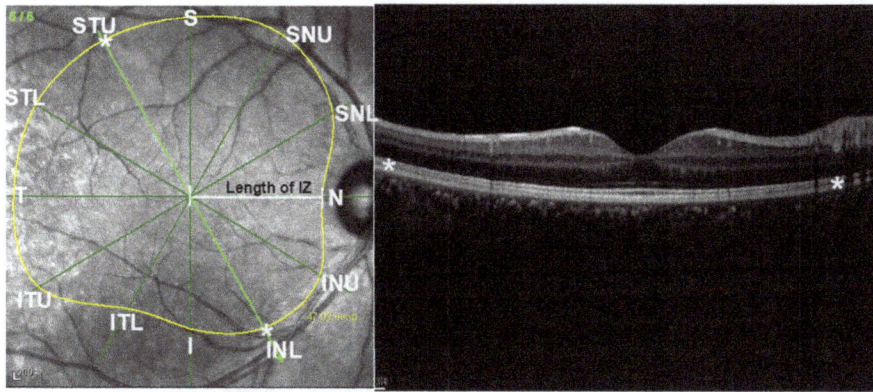

Fig. 1 Measurement of the IZ area and IZ length in 12 directions. The boundary of IZ was defined as the ends (*) of the continuous and smooth, highly reflective line between the ellipsoid zone and the retinal pigment epithelium-Bruch membrane (RPE-BM) compound. The length of the IZ was measured in each direction from the central fovea to the end of the IZ. IZ = interdigitation zone; INL = inferior nasal lower; INU = inferior nasal upper; ITL = inferior temporal lower, ITU: inferior temporal upper, I: inferior, N: nasal, S = superior; SNL: superior nasal lower; SNU = superior nasal upper; STL = superior temporal lower, STU: superior temporal upper; T = temporal

left eyes were tested using Student's t test. The binocular symmetry of them was tested by paired t tests.

Results

A total of 158 eyes in 97 healthy volunteers met the inclusion criteria, including 48 (49.48%) males and 49 (50.52%) females. The mean ± standard deviation age was 32.13 ± 12.08 years (range, 20–61 years), IOP was 14.41 ± 2.89 mmHg, axial length was 23.54 ± 0.79 mm, BCVA was 0.01 ± 0.05 (logarithms of the minimum angle of resolution), and the spherical equivalent was 0.80 ± 1.04 D (Additional file 1: Table S1).

The cone IZ area

The IZ was visible and clear in all the radial scans in all 158 eyes. The mean ± standard deviation IZ area was 30.22 ± 12.70 mm^2 (range 5.91–57.47 mm^2). Kolmogorov–Smirnov test indicated that the IZ area exhibited a normal distribution ($P = 0.635$) (Fig. 2) with a 95% confidence interval of 28.06–32.29 mm^2. The IZ area and the IZ lengths in all 12 directions were similar in the left and right eyes (all $P > 0.05$) (Additional file 1: Table S2). The IZ area and the IZ lengths in most of the 12 directions showed good inter-ocular symmetry (Additional file 1: Figure S1, Table S3). And the cone IZ area showed good symmetry (29.74 ± 13.61 vs. 29.79 ± 12.39 mm^2, $p = 0.981$) (Additional file 1: Table S3) and significant correlation on binoculus ($r = 0.916$, $p < 0.0001$).

Correlation between the IZ area and other variables

The IZ area on OCT measurement was correlated with the volume of full retina ($r = 0.274$, $P = 0.01$), ONL ($r = 0.351$, $P < 0.0001$), as well as the volumes of ELM-BM ($r = 0.324$, $P < 0.0001$), and photoreceptor ($r = 0.351$,

$P < 0.0001$) of the macula, but not with age, gender, SE, IOP, or AL (Table 1).

Repeatability and reproducibility of the IZ area measurements

The mean ICCs for intra-observer repeatability and inter-observer reproducibility of the IZ area were 0.982 and 0.974, respectively. The mean ICC for the repeatability of the IZ area was 0.981. The Bland–Altman plots also showed good repeatability and reproducibility of the method (Additional file 1: Figure S2).

Discussion

OCT was introduced into the field of ophthalmology many years ago [1]. More than 18 anatomic landmarks can be discerned by OCT [6], including the IZ. The IZ is a cylinder joining the RPE apical processes to the external portion of the cone outer segment [4, 5]. To our knowledge, our study was the first to measure the IZ area in a group of healthy adults. The repeatability and reproducibility tests showed good reliability of the measurement method. The mean IZ area was 30.22 ± 12.70 mm^2 (range, 5.91–57.47 mm^2). Although the IZ area showed a normal distribution, it was highly variable. The area was also closely correlated to the full retina and ONL volumes.

Considering the IZ area was successfully measured in all subjects with good repeatability and reproducibility, the methods used here could be reliable for evaluating the state of photoreceptors, mainly cones, in macular studies. The IZ could still be observed when using just one OCT scan line, but the two-dimensional area is probably more clinically relevant than the one-dimensional length. Xu et al. conducted a study of patients with a macular hole and found that the preoperative base area of

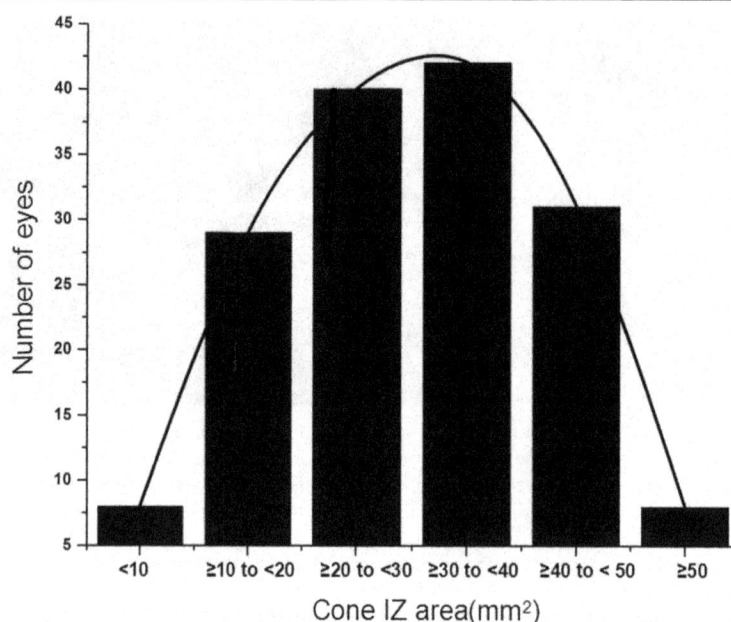

Fig. 2 Frequency distribution of the cone IZ area in healthy adults. The Kolmogorov–Smirnov indicated that the IZ area exhibited a normal distribution ($P = 0.635$). IZ = interdigitation zone

the hole ($P < 0.0001$), but not the minimum diameter of the hole, was a predictor of postoperative BCVA [15]. Additionally, Oh et al. reported that the preoperative EZ defect area, but not the EZ defect diameter, was correlated with the visual improvement in patients with a macular hole [16]. Therefore, the IZ area should be more closely related to the visual function of these patients than its length acquired by a single scan.

Table 1 Correlations between the interdigitation area and other clinical or OCT variables

	r	P
Sex	−0.068	0.393
Age (years)	0.006	0.94
AL (mm)	0.076	0.341
SE (D)	−0.158	0.148
IOP (mmHg)	0.006	0.94
BCVA (LogMAR)	0.075	0.351
Volume of the macular area		
Retina volume	0.265	0.01
ONL volume	0.384	< 0.0001
ELM-BM volume	0.324	< 0.0001
Photoreceptor volume	0.357	< 0.0001
RPE-BM volume	0.111	0.233

AL axial length, *BCVA* best-corrected visual acuity, *BM* Bruch membrane, *D* diopters, *ELM* external limiting membrane, *IOP* intraocular pressure, *LogMAR* logarithms of the minimum angle of resolution, *ONL* outer nuclear layer, *RPE* retinal pigment epithelium, *SE* spherical equivalent. Analysis of covariance was used to determine the correlations between the interdigitation area and the volumes of each retinal layer and other clinical variables

The IZ was visible in all 158 eyes. Rii et al. reported that the IZ was visible in 43/45 healthy eyes, and fragmentation of the IZ was apparent in the fovea [12]. In our study, however, the IZ was observed as a smooth continuous line in all 158 eyes. The difference might be due to the different OCT systems used in each study. Each radical scan taken by Spectrails in our study comprised 100 averaged scans obtained using eye tracking, while Rii et al. used a different OCT system and probably other technique. In addition, they included some moderate and high myopic eyes (− 8.0 D to + 3.25 D), whereas the eyes in our study had a refraction of − 3 D to + 1 D [12]. However, we found a rather large variation in the IZ area, which ranged from 5.91 to − 57.47 mm². Curcio et al. previously reported that the number of cones varied among healthy subjects [17], and our findings are in agreement with theirs. These results are important for clinical research and for daily clinical practice because ophthalmologists should remember that a small IZ area may be normal. In some patients, the IZ might not be able to continue growing after a certain point. This is not necessarily an indication that the patient is not responding well to the prescribed treatment. Instead, the continuity and smoothness of the IZ might be more informative in clinical settings. But apart from the large range of the IZ area, the 95% confidence interval was 28.06–32.29 mm², which was rather small. As a result, the IZ area might be able to provide some useful information in clinic work. On the other hand, the measurement of area could also serve as a baseline in the follow-up of patients with photoreceptor damage, the change of IZ area might be considered as a sign of change in photoreceptor. Moreover, as the symmetry between the two eyes ($r = 0.916$, $p < 0.0001$), the status or area of the contralateral eye could provide as reference.

The IZ area was also correlated with the volumes of the full retina, ONL, and possibly the ELM-BM and photoreceptors. These correlations were still observed after adjusting for age, gender, and AL. These results suggested that eyes with a large IZ area might contain more photoreceptors, probably cones, in the macula. This is particularly relevant to clinical practice because it was reported that the age-related accumulation of lipofuscin was related to the development of age-related macular degeneration [18], and a photoreceptor density might increase the vulnerability of the eye to such diseases.

In this study, only healthy Chinese subjects were enrolled and only one OCT system was used. Therefore, our findings need to be verified by others, and the possible correlation between IZ area and vision in patients with macular diseases should also be evaluated.

Conclusion

In our present research, we successfully measured the IZ area in healthy adults using a commercially available OCT system for the first time. The IZ area showed large variability, and eyes with a large IZ area seemed to contain more photoreceptors, probably cones, in the macula.

Acknowledgements
Publication of this article was supported in part by research grants from the National Major Scientific Equipment Program (2012YQ12008003), the National Natural Science Foundation of China (grant no. 81570854), the national key research & development plan (2017YFC0108200) and the Shanghai Committee of Science and Technology (16140901000, 13430710500 and 15DZ1942204). The authors thank the subjects and our colleagues who helped perform this study.

Funding
The National Major Scientific Equipment Program (2012YQ12008003), the National Natural Science Foundation of China (grant no. 81570854), the national key research & development plan (2017YFC0108200) and the Shanghai Committee of Science and Technology (16140901000, 13430710500 and 15DZ1942204).

Authors' contributions
RG and GD collected and analyzed the data, wrote the paper; RG analyzed the data and draft the paper; YJ did the OCT scan acquisition; CJ designed the study and modified the paper; GX aided the technical support; CJ supervised the study and supported funding. All authors read and approved the final manuscript.

Competing interests
The authors declare that they have no competing interests.

Author details
[1]Department of Ophthalmology, Eye and ENT Hospital and Shanghai Key Laboratory of Visual Impairment and Restoration, Shanghai Medical College, Fudan University, Shanghai 200031, China. [2]Department of Ophthalmology, The Third People's Hospital of Changzhou, Changzhou 213000, China. [3]Department of Ophthalmology, No. 5 People's Hospital of Shanghai, Shanghai 200240, China.

References
1. Huang D, Swanson EA, Lin CP, et al. Optical coherence tomography. Science. 1991;254(5035):1178–81.
2. Puliafito CA, Hee MR, Lin CP, et al. Imaging of macular diseases with optical coherence tomography. Ophthalmology. 1995;102(2):217–29.
3. Huang Y, Cideciyan AV, Papastergiou GI, et al. Relation of optical coherence tomography to microanatomy in normal and rd chickens. Invest Ophthalmol Vis Sci. 1998;39(12):2405–16.
4. Spaide RF, Curcio CA. Anatomical correlates to the bands seen in the outer retina by optical coherence tomography: literature review and model. Retina. 2011;31(8):1609–19.
5. Srinivasan VJ, Monson BK, Wojtkowski M, et al. Characterization of outer retinal morphology with high-speed, ultrahigh-resolution optical coherence tomography. Invest Ophthalmol Vis Sci. 2008;49(4):1571–9.
6. Staurenghi G, Sadda S, Chakravarthy U, Spaide RF. Proposed lexicon for anatomic landmarks in normal posterior segment spectral-domain optical coherence tomography: the IN*OCT consensus. Ophthalmology. 2014; 121(8):1572–8.
7. Park SJ, Woo SJ, Park KH, et al. Morphologic photoreceptor abnormality in occult macular dystrophy on spectral-domain optical coherence tomography. Invest Ophthalmol Vis Sci. 2010;51(7):3673–9.
8. Puche N, Querques G, Benhamou N, et al. High-resolution spectral domain optical coherence tomography features in adult onset foveomacular vitelliform dystrophy. Br J Ophthalmol. 2010;94(9):1190–6.
9. Ooto S, Hangai M, Takayama K, et al. High-resolution imaging of the photoreceptor layer in epiretinal membrane using adaptive optics scanning laser ophthalmoscopy. Ophthalmology. 2011;118(5):873–81.
10. Itoh Y, Inoue M, Rii T, et al. Significant correlation between visual acuity and recovery of foveal cone microstructures after macular hole surgery. Am J Ophthalmol. 2012;153(1):111–9.
11. Itoh Y, Inoue M, Rii T, et al. Correlation between length of foveal cone outer segment tips line defect and visual acuity after macular hole closure. Ophthalmology. 2012;119(7):1438–46.
12. Rii T, Itoh Y, Inoue M, Hirakata A. Foveal cone outer segment tips line and disruption artifacts in spectral-domain optical coherence tomographic images of normal eyes. Am J Ophthalmol. 2012;153(3):524–9.
13. Jacobsen AG, Bendtsen MD, Vorum H, et al. Normal value ranges for central retinal thickness asymmetry in healthy Caucasian adults measured by SPECTRALIS SD-OCT posterior pole asymmetry analysis. Invest Ophthalmol Vis Sci. 2015;56(6):3875–82.
14. Grover S, Murthy RK, Brar VS, Chalam KV. Normative data for macular thickness by high-definition spectral-domain optical coherence tomography (spectralis). Am J Ophthalmol. 2009;148(2):266–71.
15. Xu D, Yuan A, Kaiser PK, et al. A novel segmentation algorithm for volumetric analysis of macular hole boundaries identified with optical coherence tomography. Invest Ophthalmol Vis Sci. 2013;54(1):163–9.
16. Oh J, Smiddy WE, Flynn HJ, et al. Photoreceptor inner/outer segment defect imaging by spectral domain OCT and visual prognosis after macular hole surgery. Invest Ophthalmol Vis Sci. 2010;51(3):1651–8.
17. Curcio CA, Sloan KR, Kalina RE, Hendrickson AE. Human photoreceptor topography. J Comp Neurol. 1990;292(4):497–523.
18. Dorey CK, Wu G, Ebenstein D, et al. Cell loss in the aging retina. Relationship to lipofuscin accumulation and macular degeneration. Invest Ophthalmol Vis Sci. 1989;30(8):1691–9.

33

Factors related to amblyopia in congenital ptosis after frontalis sling surgery

Youn-Shen Bee[1,2,3]* ⓘ, Pei-Jhen Tsai[1], Muh-Chiou Lin[1] and Ming-Ying Chu[1]

Abstract

Background: Amblyopia is a main concern in children undergoing frontalis sling surgery for repairing congenital ptosis. This study aimed to evaluate factors related to amblyopia in children undergoing frontalis sling surgery.

Methods: IRB-approved retrospective review of children under the age of 12 who received frontalis sling surgery. Preoperative demographic data, strabismus, margin reflex distance 1 (MRD1), lid fissure height, sling type, refraction errors, surgical outcome and amblyopia were evaluated.

Results: This study included 48 eyelid procedures performed in 38 patients. Median age was 4.0 years. Etiology was congenital ptosis in 42 eyes (87.5%) and blepharophimosis in 6 eyes (12.5%). Mersilene mesh was the sling material used in 36 eyes (75%), silicone in 6 eyes (12.5%), and polytetrafluoroethylene (PTFE) in 6 eyes (12.5%). Mean duration of follow-up was 27.8 ± 25.0 months (range, 3 to 128 months). Amblyopia was observed in 17 eyes (35.4%) at the final follow-up. Factors significantly associated with final amblyopia included blepharophimosis ($p = 0.017$), preoperative MRD1 ≤ -1.0 mm ($p = 0.038$), preoperative lid fissure ≤ 4.5 mm ($p = 0.035$), preoperative anisometropia (spherical equivalent) ($p = 0.011$), and postoperative astigmatism ($p = 0.026$).

Conclusions: Study results suggest that blepharophimosis, preoperative MRD1 ≤ -1.0 mm, preoperative lid fissure ≤ 4.5 mm, preoperative anisometropia (spherical equivalent), and postoperative astigmatism are associated with amblyopia after frontalis sling surgery in patients with congenital ptosis.

Keywords: Congenital ptosis, Frontalis sling suspension, Amblyopia, Mersilene mesh, Silicone rode, Polytetrafluoroethylene

Background

The incidence of amblyopia has been reported to be higher among patients with childhood ptosis than in the general population [1–3]. This is likely the result of increased prevalence of eyelid occlusion of the visual axis, strabismus, and significant refractive error [4–7]. Mersilene mesh, silicone, and polytetrafluoroethylene (PTFE, Gore-Tex) have been successfully used in frontalis sling surgery for congenital ptosis [8–13]. This study was undertaken to evaluate factors related to amblyopia in children undergoing frontalis suspension surgery utilizing Mersilene mesh, silicone, or PTFE as the sling material.

Methods

Ethics

The study was approved by the Institutional Review Board of Kaohsiung Veterans General Hospital, allowing retrieval of patient charts and review of medical information. A waiver of consent was granted given the retrospective nature of the project and anonymous analysis of the data.

Participants and procedures

Data from 48 eyelid procedures in 38 patients under the age of 12 who underwent frontalis sling surgery to correct congenital ptosis with poor levator function at Kaohsiung Veterans General Hospital between January 2005 and July 2014 were analyzed. Patients who had simple congenital ptosis or blepharophimosis without neurologic or traumatic pathology were included in this

* Correspondence: ysbee@vghks.gov.tw
[1]Department of Ophthalmology, Kaohsiung Veterans General Hospital, 386 Ta-Chung 1st RD, Kaohsiung 81346, Taiwan
[2]Yuh-Ing Junior College of Health Care and Management, Kaohsiung, Taiwan
Full list of author information is available at the end of the article

study. Patients with less than 3 months of follow-up were excluded.

All patients underwent an ophthalmic examination including orthoptic evaluation and cycloplegic refraction; however, preoperative refraction data were missing for some younger patients due to poor cooperation. Visual acuity was measured with age-appropriate methods, including the Snellen chart and Allen symbols. Anisometropia was defined as difference between the eyes in spherical equivalent or astigmatism in any meridian on cycloplegic refraction. Amblyopia was defined as best-corrected visual acuity within two Snellen lines compared with age-matched normal children and more than two Snellen lines of difference between eyes [7]. Patients diagnosed with amblyopia were treated according to individual patient condition. Frontalis sling surgery was performed with a pentagon incision and sling procedure. A sling suture was passed in a closed cerclage-type fashion through skin entry by way of a supra-lash or eyebrow incision. Mersilene mesh, silicone, or PTFE was used as the sling material. In cases using Mersilene mesh or PTFE of the single-loop design, two stab incision sites approximately 10–12 mm apart were marked above the lash line centered over the area of desired maximal elevation. In cases using silicone rod, one additional stab incision was made in the middle of the two previous incisions with double pentagon technique [14]. Another two stab incision sites were marked above the eyebrow, approximately in line with lateral and medial canthus; an additional stab incision site was made above the eyebrow in the middle of the previous eyebrow incisions. Sling material was tied together beneath the frontalis muscle layer in the middle incision site in all cases.

Data collected and analyzed included age, gender, diagnosis, presence of strabismus, presence of chin-up sign, margin reflex distance 1 (MRD1), lid fissure height, sling type, refraction error, MRD1 elevation, lid fissure elevation, surgical outcome, follow-up duration, and presence of amblyopia at the last visit. During follow-up, outcomes were categorized as good, moderate, or poor. A good outcome was defined as postoperative MRD1 ≥ 2 mm or bilateral nonsymmetric lid fissure ≤1 mm. A moderate outcome was defined as postoperative MRD1 < 2 mm or > 1 mm or bilateral non-symmetric lid fissure > 1 mm. A poor outcome was defined as postoperative MRD1 ≤ 1 mm or bilateral nonsymmetric ≥2 mm. Preoperative and postoperative photographs of each surgery were obtained using a digital camera (Nikon Inc., Tokyo, Japan) in examination rooms with equivalent lighting. Postoperative follow-up records and photographs were reviewed.

Statistical analysis

Statistical analysis was performed using SPSS version 18.0 (SPSS Inc., Chicago, IL). Basic descriptive statistics were calculated using the data gathered and are reported as mean ± standard deviation or n (%) as appropriate. Differences between continuous outcome variables were established and putative factors were sought using the Mann-Whitney U-test and Student's t-test as appropriate. Categorical data were examined using Pearson's chi-square and Fisher's exact test. All tests were two-tailed and a p-value ≤0.05 was considered statistically significant.

Results

In total, data from 48 eyelid procedures in 38 patients were collected. Of the 38 patients, 27 had unilateral procedures and 11 had bilateral procedures. One female patient with bilateral ptosis experienced left ocular trauma with sling rupture 1 week after frontalis sling surgery, and this procedure was excluded. Twenty-four procedures were performed on the right side and 24 were on the left side. Age ranged from 1 to 12 years, with a mean age of 4.3 ± 2.4 years and median age of 4.0 years. Postoperative follow-up time ranged from 3 to 128 months, with a mean of 27.8 ± 25.0 months. Etiology was congenital ptosis in 42 eyes (87.5%) and blepharophimosis in 6 eyes (12.5%). Mersilene mesh was used as the sling material in 36 eyes (75%), silicone in 6 eyes (12.5%), and PTFE in 6 eyes (12.5%). Amblyopia was found in 23 eyes (47.9%) preoperatively. In 14 of these eyes, amblyopia was attributed to occlusion of the visual axis only, 9 eyes had high astigmatism or anisometropia, and 6 eyes exhibited a combined refractive and occlusive mechanism. Preoperative visual acuity (log MAR) was 0.28 ± 0.22 and postoperative visual acuity (log MAR) was 0.19 ± 0.21. Preoperative and postoperative refraction data are listed in Table 1. Due to poor cooperation of very young patients who were aged 1–2 years, preoperative refraction data were missing for 4 eyes. The demographics of the patients grouped by sling material used in surgery are shown in Table 1.

Amblyopia was found in 17 eyes (35.4%) at the final follow-up. Eight eyes diagnosed with amblyopia preoperatively had normal visual acuity at final follow-up, and absence of both significant refraction error and strabismus besides lid drooping were common characteristics of these eyes. There was no significant association between age at operation and incidence of final amblyopia. At the final follow-up, 12 of 48 eyes (25%) with congenital ptosis and 5 of 6 eyes (83%) with blepharophimosis had amblyopia. Factors significantly associated with final amblyopia included blepharophimosis (p = 0.017), preoperative MRD1 (p = 0.018), preoperative MRD1 ≤ – 1.0 mm (p = 0.038), preoperative lid fissure (p < 0.001), preoperative lid fissure ≤4.5 mm (p = 0.035), and preoperative anisometropia (spherical equivalent) (p = 0.011) (Table 2). Presence of preoperative chin-up sign, strabismus, and preoperative amblyopia were not related to amblyopia at the final visit.

Table 1 Demographic data in total eyelids with different sling material

Factor	Total	Mersilene mesh	Silicone	PTFE (Gore-Tex)
	$n = 48$	$n = 36$	$n = 6$	$n = 6$
Age,years (mean ± SD)	4.28 ± 2.38	4.56 ± 2.49	3.15 ± 2.38	3.73 ± 1.42
Gender (male/female)	30/18 (62.5%/37.5%)	26/10 (72.2%/27.8%)	2/4 (33.3%/66.7%)	2/4 (33.3%/66.7%)
Side (Right/Left)	24/24 (50.0%/50.0%)	18/18 (50.0%/50.0%)	3/3 (50.0%/50.0%)	3/3 (50.0%/50.0%)
Lateral (uni/bil)	27/21 (56.2%/43.8%)	22/14 (61.1%/38.9%)	2/4 (33.3%/66.7%)	3/3 (50.0%/50.0%)
Diagnosis				
congenital	42 (87.5%)	33 (91.7%)	6 (100%)	3 (50.0%)
blepharophemosis	6 (12.5%)	3 (8.3%)	0 (0%)	3 (50.0%)
Follow period (months)	27.77 ± 24.99	28.61 ± 27.78	30.17 ± 8.70	20.33 ± 17.67
Pre-op MRD1[a] (mm)	− 0.61 ± 1.37	− 0.68 ± 1.47	0.00 ± 0.95	− 0.83 ± 0.98
Pre-op Lid fissure (mm)	3.89 ± 1.06	3.86 ± 1.14	4.25 ± 0.76	3.67 ± 0.82
Pre-op chin up				
yes	31 (64.6%)	23 (63.9%)	4 (66.7%)	4 (66.7%)
no	17 (35.4%)	13 (36.1%)	2 (33.3%)	2 (33.3%)
Pre-op strabismus				
yes	10 (20.8%)	8 (22.2%)	2 (33.3%)	0 (0%)
no	38 (79.2%)	28 (77.8%)	4 (66.7%)	6 (100%)
Pre-op amblyopia				
yes	23 (47.92%)	17 (47.22%)	5 (83.33%)	1 (16.67%)
no	25 (52.08%)	19 (52.78%)	1 (16.67%)	5 (83.33%)
Pre-op log MAR	0.28 ± 0.22	0.28 ± 0.23	0.29 ± 0.15	0.28 ± 0.22
Post-op log MAR	0.19 ± 0.21	0.18 ± 0.20	0.21 ± 0.29	0.22 ± 0.23
Pre-op sphere[b]	−0.22 ± 2.01	0.01 ± 1.69	−0.79 ± 3.26	−1.05 ± 2.37
Post-op sphere[b]	0.35 ± 1.55	0.49 ± 1.70	−0.42 ± 0.74	0.25 ± 0.89
Pre-op astigmatism[b]	−1.47 ± 1.17	− 1.50 ± 1.29	−1.38 ± 0.80	−1.40 ± 0.76
Post-op astigmatism[b]	− 1.44 ± 1.32	−1.53 ± 1.32	−0.54 ± 0.68	−1.79 ± 1.62
Pre-op spherical equivalent[b]	−0.96 ± 1.97	−0.74 ± 1.56	−1.48 ± 3.45	−1.75 ± 2.41
Post-op spherical equivalent[b]	−0.37 ± 1.48	−0.27 ± 1.66	−0.69 ± 0.68	−0.65 ± 0.74
Pre-op anisometropia (astigmatism)[b]	1.03 ± 1.15	1.14 ± 1.27	0.79 ± 0.60	0.50 ± 0.47
Post-op anisometropia (astigmatism)[b]	0.94 ± 0.92	1.05 ± 1.03	0.75 ± 0.39	0.50 ± 0.16
Pre-op anisometropia (spherical equivalent)[b]	0.94 ± 0.92	0.68 ± 0.73	2.02 ± 0.98	1.35 ± 1.07
Post-op anisometropia (spherical equivalent)[b]	1.01 ± 1.10	1.07 ± 1.21	0.46 ± 0.06	1.25 ± 0.88

[a]marginal reflex distance 1
[b]Refraction unit = Diopter

Table 3 lists the various factors related to amblyopia at the final visit after surgery. At the final follow-up, postoperative astigmatism was significantly associated with final amblyopia ($p = 0.037$), whereas postoperative spherical equivalent and postoperative anisometropia were not associated with final amblyopia. MRD1 elevation > 3 mm and lid fissure elevation > 3.5 mm were associated with final amblyopia ($p = 0.032$ and $p = 0.039$, respectively). The results may be related to preoperative lid height. In order to achieve the desired postoperative lid height, patients with smaller preoperative MRD1 underwent greater MDR1 elevation, and those with lower preoperative lid fissure height underwent greater lid fissure height elevation. There was no correlation between type of sling used in surgery and final amblyopia. Of the 48 eyes, 39 (81.3%) had a good outcome, 8 (16.7%) had a moderate outcome, and 1 (2.0%) had a poor outcome. The above numbers were the sum of those with or without amblyopia. The cosmetic score was not associated with final amblyopia (Table 3).

Table 4 lists the complications of surgery, which included sling exposure without infection in 1 Mersilene mesh case and exposure keratitis after 3 months in 4 Mersilene mesh cases and 1 polytetrafluoroethylene case. None of the cases

Table 2 Preoperative factors related to amblyopia in the final visit

Factor	No amblyopia[1]	Amblyopia[2]	P valve
	n = 31	n = 17	
Age, years (mean ± SD)	4.66 ± 2.41 (1–9)	3.57 ± 2.23 (1–8)	0.131
Gender (male/female)	22/9 (71.0%/29.0%)	8/9 (47.1%/52.9%)	0.093
Side (Right/Left)	17/14 (54.8%/45.2%)	7/10 (41.2%/58.8%)	0.547
Lateral (uni/bil)	20/11 (64.5%/35.5%)	7/10 (41.2%/58.8%)	0.140
Diagnosis			
congenital	30 (96.8%)	12 (70.6%)	0.017[a]
blepharophemosis	1 (3.2%)	5 (29.4%)	
Follow period (months)	28.68 ± 27.57 (3–128)	26.12 ± 20.12 (3–63)	0.738
Pre-op sphere[3]	−0.16 ± 1.79	−0.33 ± 2.42	0.426
Pre-op astigmatism[3]	− 1.27 ± 1.11	−1.83 ± 1.21	0.963
Pre-op spherical equivalent[3]	− 0.80 ± 1.87	−1.24 ± 2.16	0.457
Pre-op anisometropia (astigmatism)[3]	0.92 ± 0.83	1.20 ± 1.58	0.449
Pre-op anisometropia (spherical equivalent)[3]	0.68 ± 0.79	1.40 ± 0.98	0.001 [b]
Pre-op MRD1 (mm)	−0.27 ± 1.21	− 1.24 ± 1.46	0.018[b]
pre-op MRD1 (mm) ≤ − 0.5	12 (38.7%)	11 (64.7%)	0.131
pre-op MRD1 (mm) ≤ −1.00	10 (32.3%)	11 (64.7%)	0.038[a]
Pre-op Lid fissure (mm)	4.27 ± 0.94 (2.50–6.00)	3.18 ± 0.90 (1.50–5.00)	< 0.001[b]
pre-op Lid fissure (mm) ≤5.00	28 (90.3%)	17 (100%)	0.543
pre-op Lid fissure (mm) ≤4.50	20 (64.5%)	16 (94.1%)	0.035[a]
Pre-op chin up			
yes	17 (54.8%)	14 (82.4%)	0.068
no	14 (45.2%)	3 (17.6%)	
Pre-op strabismus			
yes	5 (16.1%)	5 (29.4%)	0.295
no	26 (83.9%)	12 (70.6%)	
Prep-op amblyopia			
yes	14 (45.2%)	9 (52.9%)	0.766
no	17 (54.8%)	8 (47.1%)	

[1]No amblyopia in the final follow up
[2]Amblyopia in the final follow up
[3]Refraction unit = Diopter
[a]The P value was estimated by Fisher's exact test
[b]The P value was estimated by student t test

developed sling infection. The incidence of sling exposure was 2.8%, and the incidence of exposure keratitis after 3 months was 10.4%. All cases of exposure keratitis were managed with lubricant medication without the need for revision surgery.

Discussion

Congenital ptosis with poor levator function of less than 4 mm is usually corrected with frontalis suspension surgery. Frontalis suspension surgery can be performed using various techniques and different sling materials [13–15]. Materials used can be autogenous or banked fascia and alloplastic materials including silicone, Mersilene mesh, braided polyester, polypropylene, nylon, silk, collagen, stainless steel, and PTFE [13, 16–21]. Prior research has suggested that double slings to Crawford allow better results than thinner single slings [22]. Ben Simon and Goldberg reported no statistically significant difference in results between different suture materials or loop shape used in frontalis suspension surgery. In recent years, many studies have evaluated the functional success of various sling materials used in frontalis sling surgery [13, 23–25]. In the current study, frontalis suspension surgery was performed using Mersilene mesh, silicone rod, or PTFT, and no significant difference in surgical outcome or presence of amblyopia at the final

Table 3 Factors related to the amblyopia in the final visit after surgery

Factor	No amblyopia [1] n = 31	Amblyopia [2] n = 17	P valve
Sling type			
mersilene mesh	24 (77.4%)	12 (70.6%)	0.878
silicone	4 (12.9%)	2 (11.8%)	
PTFE (Gore-Tex)	3 (9.7%)	3 (17.6%)	
Post-op sphere[3]	0.17 ± 1.21	0.66 ± 2.03	0.378
Post-op astigmatism[3]	− 1.15 ± 1.14	−1.97 ± 1.49	0.037[b]
Post-op spherical equivalent[3]	− 0.40 ± 1.35	−0.32 ± 1.73	0.874
Post-op anisometropia (astigmatism)[3]	1.01 ± 0.94	0.82 ± 0.88	0.511
Post-op anisometropia (spherical equivalent)[3]	0.96 ± 1.11	1.10 ± 1.12	0.680
Post-op MRD1 (mm)	2.21 ± 0.76	2.26 ± 0.69	0.806
MRD1 elevation (mm)	2.48 ± 1.14	3.50 ± 1.85	0.023[b]
MRD1 elevation (mm) > 2.5	12 (38.7%)	10 (58.8%)	0.232
MRD1 elevation (mm) > 3.0	8 (25.8%)	10 (58.8%)	0.032[a]
MRD1 elevation (mm) > 3.5	5 (16.1%)	10 (58.8%)	0.004[a]
Post-op Lid fissure (mm)	7.05 ± 0.86	6.74 ± 0.95	0.252
Lid fissure elevation (mm)	2.77 ± 1.03	3.56 ± 1.17	0.020[b]
lid fissure elevation (mm) > 2.5	15 (48.4%)	12 (70.6%)	0.224
lid fissure elevation (mm) > 3.0	11 (35.5%)	10 (58.8%)	0.140
lid fissure elevation (mm) > 3.5	5 (16.1%)	8 (47.1%)	0.039[a]
Post-op lago (mm)	1.31 ± 0.64	1.29 ± 0.53	0.946
Cosmetic score			
good[4]	25 (80.6%)	14 (82.4%)	1.000
Moderate[5]	5 (16.1%)	3 (17.6%)	
Poor[6]	1 (3.2%)	0 (0%)	

[1]No amblyopia in the final follow up
[2]Amblyopia in the final follow up
[3]Refraction unit = Diopter
[4]Post op MRD1 ≥ 2 mm or bilateral nonsymteric ≤1 mm
[5]Post op 2 mm > MRD1 > 1 mm or bilateral nonsymetric > 1 mm
[6]Post op MRD1 ≤ 1 mm or bilateral nonsymetric ≥2 mm
[a]The P value was estimated by Fisher's exact test
[b]The P value was estimated by student t test

follow-up was observed, further indicating that sling material is not related to final amblyopia.

Amblyopia has an estimated prevalence of 3.0 to 3.2% in the general population. Among patients with childhood ptosis, the incidence of amblyopia has been reported to be higher than that in the general population. [1, 2] Amblyopia with any form of childhood ptosis occurred in 14.9% of a cohort of 107 patients [7]. Of 96 patients in this cohort, 14% who were diagnosed with a congenital form of ptosis demonstrated amblyopia. These rates are at the low end of the range of previous non-population-based estimates, which were reported to be between 14 and 48% [1–3]. In our study, twenty three eyes (47.9%) were diagnosed with amblyopia prior

Table 4 Complications of surgery

Factor	Mersilene mesh n = 36	Silicone n = 6	PTFE (Gore-Tex) n = 6	Total n = 48
Sling exposure	1 (2.8%)	0 (0%)	0 (0%)	1 (2.8%)
Sling infection	0 (0%)	0 (0%)	0 (0%)	0 (0%)
Exposure keratitis after 3 months	4 (11.1%)	0 (0%)	1 (16.7%)	5 (10.4%)

to surgery, and 17 eyes (35.4%) had amblyopia at the final visit, suggesting that 6 eyes (12.5%) improved after undergoing both ptosis surgery and occlusion with or without refractive treatment. The incidence of amblyopia at the final follow-up was 35.4%, and this higher rate of amblyopia might be attributed to the greater severity in these cases due to the need for frontalis sling surgery.

The prevalence of amblyopia may correlate with the severity of ptosis [1, 5, 26]. The cause of the increased prevalence of amblyopia among patients with congenital ptosis remains debatable. Occlusion of the visual axis was found to be the leading cause of amblyopia in patients with congenital ptosis in prior research [7]. Subsequent studies have demonstrated that 1.6 to 12.3% of patients with congenital ptosis will have amblyopia due to occlusion of the pupil [1, 4, 5]. Prevalence of amblyopia has been previously reported to be as high as 56.4% in patients with blepharophimosis [27]. Hornblass et al. found a statistically significant correlation between severe nonocclusive ptosis (≥ 4 mm) and the development of amblyopia [26]. In this study, factors significantly associated with final amblyopia were blepharophimosis, preoperative MRD1 < − 1 mm, and preoperative lid fissure < 4.5 mm, all of which were related to severity of visual axis occlusion. Moreover, patients with smaller preoperative lid fissure were more likely to have amblyopia at the final visit. All patients diagnosed with amblyopia were treated with occlusion therapy and refraction error correction. Although patients with a poor or moderate cosmetic score experienced more lid drooping than those with a good cosmetic score during the follow-up period, cosmetic score was not related to amblyopia at the final visit. Final MRD1 and lid fissure showed no relation with amblyopia at the last visit, whereas preoperative MRD1 and lid fissure were indeed related to the incidence. Preoperative but not postoperative occlusion of the visual axis was a factor related to final amblyopia, even after frontalis sling surgery and amblyopia treatment.

Several large retrospective studies evaluating congenital ptosis revealed that the leading causes of amblyopia are strabismus and refractive errors [2–5]. Srinagesh et al. reported that almost all cases of congenital ptosis with amblyopia occur in the context of coexisting anisometropia or strabismus [3]. Harrad et al. also found that of 216 cases of simple congenital ptosis, 17% developed amblyopia, among which 21% had anisometropic amblyopia [4]. Stark et al. reported a 40% incidence of refractive errors causing amblyopia in congenital ptosis patients [28]. Oral et al. observed that the overall incidence of refractive errors causing amblyopia was much higher, with 71% of patients having congenital ptosis [2]. Schneider et al. reported that the incidence of astigmatism causing amblyopia was 28% in unilateral ptosis and 46% in bilateral ptosis [29]. In the present study, preoperative anisometropia (spherical equivalent) and postoperative astigmatism were significantly related to amblyopia at the final visit.

While the incidence of strabismus ranges between 1 and 5% in the general population, it has been reported to be 12 to 76% in patients with congenital ptosis [1, 2, 4, 5, 30]. Schneider et al. reported that amblyopia was related to strabismus in only 6% of patients; the rate of amblyopic refractive errors combined with strabismus was higher in eyes with severe ptosis [29]. In this study, preoperative strabismus was found in 16.1% of eyes without final amblyopia and in 29.4% of eyes with final amblyopia, implying that strabismus may be associated with amblyopia. However, further analysis of our data revealed that strabismus was not a significant factor related to amblyopia at the final visit after frontalis sling surgery.

This study has some limitations. First, the sample size was relatively small. In addition, the study was retrospective in design and preoperative refraction data were missing for 4 eyes of very young patients. To better elucidate the factors related to amblyopia in children with congenital ptosis after frontalis sling surgery, a study of larger scale involving a greater number of patients would be required. In particular, the numbers of cases using silicone rod and PTFT were small, and more cases for analysis would be desirable. Although the age at which the patients underwent frontalis sling surgery was not a factor related to amblyopia, the children with amblyopia at the last visit tended to receive the procedure at an earlier age in this study, which might be related to smaller preoperative lid fissure height. Those with smaller lid fissure height usually would undergo earlier frontalis sling surgery.

Despite these limitations, this study successfully identified factors related to amblyopia at the final visit through a review of cases of children with congenital ptosis undergoing frontalis sling surgery. All of the included patients underwent corrective surgery due to poor levator muscle function. This study found that Mersilene mesh, silicone rod, and PTFT can be safely and effectively used in frontalis sling surgery in children with no significant difference in incidence of final amblyopia among the materials used. Blepharophimosis, preoperative MRD1 ≤ − 1 mm, preoperative lid fissure ≤4.5 mm, preoperative anisometropia (spherical equivalent), and postoperative astigmatism were associated with amblyopia at the final visit. Results suggest that children with smaller lid fissure, higher preoperative anisometropia, and postoperative astigmatism may have a greater risk of amblyopia even after frontalis sling surgery. Furthermore, in the management of children with ptosis, amblyopia treatment for improving vision should not be overlooked, even after frontalis sling surgery.

Abbreviations

logMAR: Logarithm of the minimum angle of resolution; MRD1: Margin reflex distance 1; PTFE: Polytetrafluoroethylene

Acknowledgments

The authors thank Professor Luo-Ping Ger of the Department of Medical Education and Research, Kaohsiung Veterans General Hospital, Taiwan for his assistance in statistical analyses.

Funding

The authors have no financial interest in any of the materials used in this study.

Authors' contributions

YSB and MCL conceived of and designed the experiments. YSB, PJT, and MYC carried out data acquisition and coordinated the statistical analysis. YSB drafted the manuscript. All authors read and approved the final manuscript.

Competing interests

The authors declare no competing interest and have nothing to disclose.

Author details

[1]Department of Ophthalmology, Kaohsiung Veterans General Hospital, 386 Ta-Chung 1st RD, Kaohsiung 81346, Taiwan. [2]Yuh-Ing Junior College of Health Care and Management, Kaohsiung, Taiwan. [3]National Defense Medical Center, Taipei, Taiwan.

References

1. Anderson RL, Baumgartner SA. Amblyopia in ptosis. Arch Ophthalmol. 1980; 98(6):1068–9.
2. Oral Y, Ozgur OR, Akcay L, Ozbas M, Dogan OK. Congenital ptosis and amblyopia. J Pediatr Ophthalmol Strabismus. 2010;47(2):101–4.
3. Srinagesh V, Simon JW, Meyer DR, Zobal-Ratner J. The association of refractive error, strabismus, and amblyopia with congenital ptosis. J AAPOS. 2011;15(6):541–4.
4. Harrad RA, Graham CM, Collin JR. Amblyopia and strabismus in congenital ptosis. Eye (Lond). 1988;2(Pt 6):625–7.
5. Dray JP, Leibovitch I. Congenital ptosis and amblyopia: a retrospective study of 130 cases. J Pediatr Ophthalmol Strabismus. 2002;39(4):222–5.
6. Lin LK, Uzcategui N, Chang EL. Effect of surgical correction of congenital ptosis on amblyopia. Ophthal Plast Reconstr Surg. 2008;24(6):434–6.
7. Griepentrog GJ, Diehl N, Mohney BG. Amblyopia in childhood eyelid ptosis. Am J Ophthalmol. 2013;155(6):1125.
8. Hintschich CR, Zurcher M, Collin JR. Mersilene mesh brow suspension: efficiency and complications. Br J Ophthalmol. 1995;79(4):358–61.
9. Chong KK, Fan DS, Lai CH, Rao SK, Lam PT, Lam DS. Unilateral ptosis correction with mersilene mesh frontalis sling in infants: thirteen-year follow-up report. Eye (Lond). 2010;24(1):44–9.
10. Carter SR, Meecham WJ, Seiff SR. Silicone frontalis slings for the correction of blepharoptosis: indications and efficacy. Ophthalmology. 1996;103(4):623–30.
11. Friedhofer H, Nigro MV, Sturtz G, Ferreira MC. Correction of severe ptosis with a silicone implant suspensor: 22 years of experience. Plast Reconstr Surg. 2012;129(3):453e–60e.
12. Hayashi K, Katori N, Kasai K, Kamisasanuki T, Kokubo K, Ohno-Matsui K. Comparison of nylon monofilament suture and polytetrafluoroethylene sheet for frontalis suspension surgery in eyes with congenital ptosis. Am J Ophthalmol. 2013;155(4):654–63 e651.
13. Ben Simon GJ, Macedo AA, Schwarcz RM, Wang DY, McCann JD, Goldberg RA. Frontalis suspension for upper eyelid ptosis: evaluation of different surgical designs and suture material. Am J Ophthalmol. 2005;140(5):877–85.
14. Goldberger S, Conn H, Lemor M. Double rhomboid silicone rod frontalis suspension. Ophthal Plast Reconstr Surg. 1991;7(1):48–53.
15. Dailey RA, Wilson DJ, Wobig JL. Transconjunctival frontalis suspension (TCFS). Ophthal Plast Reconstr Surg. 1991;7(4):289 97.
16. Leone CR Jr, Rylander G. A modified silicone frontalis sling for the correction of blepharoptosis. Am J Ophthalmol. 1978;85(6):802–5.
17. Zweep HP, Spauwen PH. Evaluation of expanded polytetrafluoroethylene (e-PTFE) and autogenous fascia lata in frontalis suspension. A comparative clinical study. Acta Chir Plast. 1992;34(3):129–37.
18. Lam DS, Gandhi SR, Ng JS, Chen IN, Kwok PS, Chan GH. Early correction of severe unilateral infant ptosis with the Mersilene mesh sling. Eye (Lond). 1997;11(Pt 6):806–9.
19. Esmaeli B, Chung H, Pashby RC. Long-term results of frontalis suspension using irradiated, banked fascia lata. Ophthal Plast Reconstr Surg. 1998;14(3):159–63.
20. Wasserman BN, Sprunger DT, Helveston EM. Comparison of materials used in frontalis suspension. Arch Ophthalmol. 2001;119(5):687–91.
21. Mehta P, Patel P, Olver JM. Functional results and complications of Mersilene mesh use for frontalis suspension ptosis surgery. Br J Ophthalmol. 2004;88(3):361–4.
22. Bruun D, Hatt M. Ptosis operations with silicone suspension at the eyebrow. Klin Monatsbl Augenheilkd. 1991;199(6):457–60.
23. Steinkogler FJ. A new material for frontal sling operation in congenital ptosis. Klin Monatsbl Augenheilkd. 1987;191(5):361–3.
24. Downes RN, Collin JR. The Mersilene mesh sling--a new concept in ptosis surgery. Br J Ophthalmol. 1989;73(7):498–501.
25. Nakauchi K, Mito H, Mimura O. Frontal suspension for congenital ptosis using an expanded polytetrafluoroethylene (Gore-Tex((R))) sheet: one-year follow-up. Clin Ophthalmol. 2013;7:131–6.
26. Hornblass A, Kass LG, Ziffer AJ. Amblyopia in congenital ptosis. Ophthalmic Surg. 1995;26(4):334–7.
27. Beaconsfield M, Walker JW, Collin JR. Visual development in the blepharophimosis syndrome. Br J Ophthalmol. 1991;75(12):746–8.
28. Stark N, Walther C. Refractive errors, amblyopia and strabismus in congenital ptosis. Klin Monatsbl Augenheilkd. 1984;184(1):37–9.
29. Gusek-Schneider GC, Martus P. Stimulus deprivation amblyopia in human congenital ptosis: a study of 100 patients. Strabismus. 2000;8(4):261–70.
30. Multi-ethnic Pediatric Eye Disease Study G. Prevalence of amblyopia and strabismus in African American and Hispanic children ages 6 to 72 months the multi-ethnic pediatric eye disease study. Ophthalmology. 2008;115(7): 1229–36 e1221.

34

The treatment and risk factors of retinopathy of prematurity in neonatal intensive care units

Yunxia Leng[1,2], Wenzhi Huang[1], Guoliang Ren[1], Cheng Cai[1], Qingbiao Tan[1], Yuqin Liang[1], Weizhong Yang[1] and Zongyin Gao[1,2]* (iD)

Abstract

Background: Retinopathy of prematurity (ROP) is a vascular proliferative disorder of the developing retina and a significant cause of childhood blindness around the world. The incidence of ROP is affected by many factors, and the incidence rate varies from country to country. The purpose of this study is to report the incidence and risk factors of ROP in neonatal intensive care unit (NICU) of Guangzhou First People's Hospital in China.

Methods: A retrospective review was performed on 436 premature infants who were consecutive ROP screened in the NICU of Guangzhou First People's Hospital from March 2013 to October 2017. The single-factor analysis and the logistic multivariate regression analysis were used to detect risk factors of ROP.

Results: Total 436 premature infants were consecutive ROP screened, 138 (31.65%) were found ROP, and 61(13.99%) were treated. The single-factor analysis revealed that the incidence of ROP was associated with multiple births, gestational age, birth weight, mechanical ventilation, intravascular hemolysis, the number of operations and blood culture results. The logistic multivariate regression analysis revealed that gestational age; birth weight, mechanical ventilation, minimum SaO2 and daily weight gain were independent risk factors for ROP onset. Forty-nine patients underwent retinal laser photocoagulation with recurrence 20 patients. Twelve patients underwent anti-VEGF drug (Ranibizumab) via intraocular injection with 5 patients of recurrence.

Conclusions: The incidence of ROP in NICU of Guangzhou China will match those in middle-income countries, but higher than high-income countries. Anti-VEGF drugs could be preferred as a good treatment method for zone 1 ROP and aggressive posterior ROP.

Keywords: Anti-VEGF, Neonatal intensive care unit/NICU, Retinopathy of prematurity/ROP

Introduction

Retinopathy of prematurity (ROP) is one of the major causes of blindness in children and is the most common cause of retinal vasculopathy in premature or low-birth-weight infants [1]. The physiological process by which the retina is vascularized in human embryos is divided into two stages: vasculogenesis and angiogenesis. Vasculogenesis is the process that occurs during the early stage of retinal vascularization in which endothelial

progenitor cells differentiate into endothelial cells to form blood vessels. This process begins at 12 weeks and finishes at 21 weeks of gestational age. Angiogenesis is a process that occurs in the advanced stage of retinal vascularization, during which the superficial plexuses that are responsible for the central hemal arch form. The blood vessels gradually grow and develop to surround the retina from the optic disk beginning at 16 weeks of gestational age, reaching the nasal retina at 32 weeks and the temporal retina at 36 to 40 weeks [2–4]. However, in premature babies the retinal blood vessels it is incomplete. With many factors, the vessels maybe grow and branch abnormally, and then ROP would develop. These abnormal blood vessels may grow up from

* Correspondence: eylengyx@scut.edu.cn
[1]Guangzhou First People's Hospital, Guangzhou city, China
[2]Second Affiliated Hospital of South China University of Technology, Guangzhou city, China

the plane of the retina and may bleed inside the eye. When the blood and abnormal vessels are reabsorbed, it may give rise to multiple bands like membranes, which can pull, up the retina, causing detachment of the retina and eventually blindness before 6 months.

In recent years, with the development of neonatal medical technology, an increasing number of severe premature infants have survived, including cases of prematurity associated with in vitro fertilization (IVF), multiple births and infants with very low birth weight, very low gestational age, congenital dysplasia, immaturity, septicemia, severe infections and multiple surgeries after birth. The survival rates of extremely immature premature infants < 26 weeks and < 1000 g worldwide have continuously increased, and the incidence of ROP has been increasing in parallel [5–8].

This study retrospectively analyzed the screening and treatment of ROP in severe premature infants who were admitted to the Neonatal Intensive Care Unit (NICU) of Guangzhou First People's Hospital from March 2013 to October 2017. The results revealed that ROP was common in severe premature infants with risk factors and that anti-VEGF treatment of ROP produced a curative effect. Guangzhou First People's Hospital is a comprehensive Grade 3A hospital in economically developed regions of China with advanced neonatal care. The purpose of this study was to analyze the prevalence and risk factors of ROP in advanced neonatal care hospitals in a single centre of China.

Subjects and methods

Ethical approval

The medical ethics committee of Guangzhou First People's Hospital approved this study. The patient-related data collected in this study include the following: name, age, and clinical diagnosis. The names were replaced by numbers, and the relevant data of the patient was encrypted and stored in the main study. We had obtained the written informed consent of the parents of the children.

Research subjects

A retrospective analysis was performed on premature infants who underwent ROP screening in the NICU of Guangzhou First People's Hospital from March 2013 to October 2017.

Screening criteria

According to the 2004 and 2014 China ROP screening guidelines [9], ROP screening was performed on premature and low birth weight infants with a gestational age < 32 weeks or birth weight < 2000 g. For infants with severe illness or a clear history of oxygen intake over a long period of time, ROP screening standards were appropriately relaxed.

Screening methods

The first fundus examination was performed at 4 to 6 weeks after birth or at 32 weeks of postmenstrual age (PMA). The following methods and procedures were used: (1) the primary screening was performed by binocular indirect ophthalmoscopy with appropriate mydriasis. Infants with suspected ROP were examined with Retcam (retina camera). (2) The surgeon determined the use and method of treatment based on the results and images got from the Retcam examination. (3) Examination results and treatment recommendations were recorded in detailed electronic medical records. They are location of the disease into zones (1, 2, and 3), the circumferential extent of the disease based on the clock hours (1–12), the severity of the disease (stage 1–5) and the presence or absence of "Plus Disease". And screen or treatment information, which included follow-up, treatment methods. (4) Follow-up treatments and condition progression were recorded in detailed electronic medical records according to the international staging and classification standard for ROP [10]. They are location of the disease into zones (1, 2, and 3), the circumferential extent of the disease based on the clock hours (1–12), the severity of the disease (stage 1–5) and the presence or absence of "Plus Disease".

Treatment methods

Laser photocoagulation and anti-VEGF drug (Ranibizumab) were used in 61 premature infants with ROP who reached the therapeutic threshold. Forty-nine with ROP in zone 2 or zone 3 underwent retinal laser photocoagulation, and 12 with ROP in zone 1 or aggressive posterior ROP (AP-ROP) were given anti-VEGF drug (Ranibizumab 0.25 mg) via intraocular injections. All patients with ROP recurrence were retreated with laser photocoagulation. Infants with ROP were monitored until 54 weeks of PMA as the study endpoint.

Data collection

Data related to the objectives were collected from the electronic medical record. Data included the following: (1) birth data (gestational age, single/multiple pregnancy, gender, body weight, head circumference, body length, etc.), (2) relevant data obtained within 30 days after birth (average daily weight gain, blood oxygen saturation, mechanical ventilation, intravascular hemolysis (IVH) and congenital dysplasia, etc.), (3) long-term follow-up data for infants with ROP (treatment regimen, number of treatments and curative effect).

Statistical analysis

SPSS 17.0 (SPSS Inc. Chicago, IL) was used for all statistical analyses. A single-factor analysis was used to analyze correlations with ROP and identify a normal fundus (ROP (−) or ROP (+). All measurement data are presented as percentages (%) and were measured with the χ^2 test. A multivariate logistic regression analysis was used to determine independent risk factors for ROP. $P < 0.05$ was defined as the threshold for a statistically significant difference.

Results

Baseline clinical information

The total number of newborns was 11,275 in Guangzhou First People's Hospital from March 2013 to October 2017. Four hundred thirty-six severely premature infants met the ROP screening criteria and completed a first ROP ophthalmological examination at which their general condition was recorded. Among these patients, 256 (58.72%) were boys, and 180 (41.28%) were girls. The incidence of all stages ROP was 31.25% (80) girls and 32.22% (58) boys. The treatment of ROP was 12.89% (33) girls and 15.56% (28) boys. There are 286 (65.60%) were single births, 116 (26.60%) were twin births, and 34 (7.80%) were gestations births. The incidence of ROP was 33.57% (96) in single births, 23.28%(27) in twin births, and 44.12%(15) in gestations births. The treatment of ROP was 12.24%(35) in single births, 13.79%(16) in twin births, and 44.12%(29.41) in gestations births. The average gestational age was 33.84 weeks (min 26 max 39 weeks). Overall, 342 of the patients (78.44%) had a gestational age ≤ 32 weeks, and 94 patients (21.56%) had a gestation age > 32 weeks. The incidence of ROP were 31.56% (117) in gestational age < 32 weeks and 22.34% (21) in gestational age > 32 weeks. The treatment of ROP were 16.4%(56) in gestational age < 32 weeks and 5.3%(5) in gestational age > 32 weeks. The mean birth weight was 2160.23 g (min 1015 max 3690 g). Birth weights ≤1500 g were recorded in 251 cases (57.57%), weights 1501–2000 g were recorded in 109 cases (25%), and weights > 2000 g were recorded in 76 cases (17.43%). The incidence of ROP were 46.61% (117) in birth weights ≤1500 g, 16.51% (18) in birth weights 1501-2000 g, and 3.95% (3) in birth weights > 2000 g. The treatment of ROP was 21.51%(54) in birth weights ≤1500 g, 6.42% (7) in birth weights 1501-2000 g, and 0 in birth weights > 2000 g. One hundred forty-two of the patients (32.57%) were mechanical ventilation > 96 h group, and 294 patients (67.43%) were mechanical ventilation < 96 h group. The incidence of ROP were 54.22% (77) in mechanical ventilation > 96 h group, and 20.75%(61) in mechanical ventilation < 96 h group. The treatment of ROP were 28.17% (40) in mechanical

ventilation > 96 h group, and 7.87%(21) in mechanical ventilation < 96 h group.

Analysis of ROP pathogenesis

Single-factor correlation analysis

According to the screening results and treatment, all children were divided into two groups: ROP (−) and ROP(+). Four hundred thirty-six severely premature infants, 298 patients (68.35%) were ROP (−), and 138 patients (31.65%) were ROP (+). In ROP(+) group, 61 patients (44.20%) received treatment (12 patients reviewed anti-VEGF drug treatment and 49 patients received laser treatment). The ROP (+) and ROP (−) groups were included in a univariate analysis. The results showed that the incidence of ROP was correlated with many factors including multiple birth, gestational age, birth weight, mechanical ventilation, IVH, number of operations, and positive blood culture (Table 1)

Multifactor nonconditional logistic regression analysis

Independent variables found to be highly related to ROP in previous publications and significantly related to ROP in the single-factor analysis of variance performed in the present study ($P < 0.05$), which were introduced into a logistic regression equation for a multi-factor unconditional logistic regression analysis. The independent risk factors that were introduced into the logistic regression model included gestational age, birth weight, mechanical ventilation, oxygen saturation, and average daily weight gain (Table 2).

Selection and effect analysis of ROP treatments

Selection of ROP treatments

Among the 138 included premature infants with ROP, 61 achieved the treatment threshold, including 49 patients with ROP in zone 2 or zone 3 who underwent retinal laser photocoagulation and 12 with ROP in zone 1 or AP-ROP who were given anti-VEGF drug (Ranibizumab) via intraocular injections. Ranibizumab was injected into the vitreous with 0.25 mg per dose. In the laser photocoagulation treatment group, 21 patients (42.86%) exhibited recurrence of ROP. In the Ranibizumab treatment group, 5 patients (41.67%) had recurrence of ROP. All infants with ROP recurrence were retreated with laser photocoagulation. The conditions of all infants were controlled after retreatment until 54 weeks of PMA. No serious complications such as retinal detachment occurred in any patient in our study. The results of the analysis showed that both the number of gestational weeks and birth weight were significantly lower in the Ranibizumab treatment group than in the laser photocoagulation treatment group and the untreated ROP (+) group (Table 3).

Table 1 Single factor correlation analysis

Items	No.	ROP (+)/case (%)	ROP(−) /case (%)	OR (95%CI)	χ2	P
Gender				0.956(0.635~ 1.440)	0.046	0.830
F	256	80 (31.25)	176 (68.75)			
M	180	58 (32.22)	122 (67.78)			
Number of fetuses				(not a 2 × 2 table, could not calculate)	6.689	0.035
Single birth	286	96 (33.57)	190 (66.43)			
Twin birth	116	27 (23.28)	89 (76.72)			
Multiple birth	34	15 (44.12)	19 (55.88)			
Gestational age				1.808(1.059~ 3.084)	4.802	0.028
≤ 32 w	342	117 (34.21)	225 (65.79)			
>32 w	94	21 (22.34)	73 (77.66)			
Birth weight				(not a 2 × 2 table, could not calculate)	74.550	0.000
≤ 1000 g		0	0			
~ 1500 g	251	117 (46.61)	134 (53.39)			
~ 2000 g	109	18 (16.51)	91 (83.49)			
> 2000 g	76	3 (3.95)	73 (96.05)			
Mechanical ventilation > 96 h				4.525(2.931~ 6.994)	49.605	0.000
Y	142	77 (54.22)	65 (45.78)			
N	294	61 (20.75)	233 (79.25)			
Intravascular hemolysis				3.095(2.037~ 4.701)	29.064	0.000
Y	169	79 (46.75)	90 (53.25)			
N	267	59 (22.09)	208 (77.91)			
Number of operation				(not a 2 × 2 table, could not calculate)	22.246	0.000
≥ 2	30	13 (43.33)	17 (56.67)			
1	111	54 (48.64)	57 (51.35)			
0	295	74 (25.08)	221 (74.92)			
Blood culture				2.299(1.260~ 4.194)	7.662	0.006
Positive	49	24 (48.98)	25 (51.02)			
Negative	387	114 (29.46)	273 (70.54)			

Discussion

The proportion of blindness as a result of ROP varies greatly among countries and is influenced by both the level of neonatal care and the availability of effective screening and treatment programs [11, 12]. A global perspective of the epidemiological studies of ROP showed that ROP has exhibited three epidemics since it was first described in the 1940s [13, 14]. The "first epidemic" occurred in the 1940s and 1950s and principally affected premature infants in the USA and Western Europe. At that time unmonitored supplemental oxygen was the principal risk factor [15]. The "second epidemic" began in the 1970s, as a result of the increased survival rates of extremely premature infants in industrialized countries [16, 17]. Data from Canada, the USA and the UK show that the low birth weight and low gestational age of infants are risk factors for The "third epidemic" of ROP began in the 2000s due to the increased survival rates of

Table 2 Multifactor non-conditional logistic regression analysis

Variables in the equation	Regression coefficient	Standard deviation	Wald	P	OR	95% CI of EXP (B)
Gestational age	−0.338	0.103	10.682	0.001	0.713	0.582–0.873
Birth weight	−0.002	0.001	6.771	0.009	0.998	0.996–0.999
Mechanical ventilation	−0.046	0.392	0.014	0.006	0.955	0.443–2.060
Minimum SaO2	−0.058	0.025	5.532	0.019	0.944	0.899–0.990
Average daily weight gain	−1.843	0.938	3.858	0.050	0.158	0.25–0.996

Table 3 Comparison of gestational age and birth weight with different treatment groups

Treatment	Cases (N)	Gestational age (weeks)	Birth weight (g)
Anti-VEGF	12	28.76 ± 3.16	1074 ± 204
Laser treatment	49	31.37 ± 2.58	1566 ± 229
Non treatment	77	33.88 ± 2.24	2272.79 ± 338
Total	138	$P < 0.01$	$P < 0.01$

premature infants in middle income countries including Eastern Europe, Latin America, India and China [18–22]. According to China's population growth data [23], the number of newborns were extremely large in China before 1980. But the survival rate of premature infants is very low with the poor medical care. So the ROP incidence was low in that period. To 2000, China implemented the family planning policy to control the population. Although the level of neonatal care has improved significant, most families choose eugenics, and many premature babies were abandoned for treatment and rescue. The incidence of ROP was still low in that period. After 2000, China's medical care has developed greatly, ROP screening got attention. The Chinese medical association formulated and improved the unified ROP screening guidelines twice in 2004 and 2014 [9]. According to the ROP screening guideline of China, the incidence of ROP in different regions of China is 6–18% [24, 25].

In this study, all subjects were severely premature infants who underwent ROP screening in the NICU of at Guangzhou First People's Hospital from March 2013 to October 2017. There was a high incidence rate of ROP in multiple births, low birth weight, low gestational age, congenital dysplasia, developmental immaturity, sepsis, mechanical ventilation, and severe infection. The overall incidence of ROP was 31.65% (138 cases), and 13.99% (61 cases) of premature infants with ROP required treatment. These values are similar to those in many Chinese reports (from 10.8 to 17.6%) [26–28]; However, they are different from the values of Northwest China ROP report (5.5%) [29]. The incidence of ROP in China is lower than that in African countries, such as Kenya, Burundi, and Ethiopia [30]. The incidence of ROP in Kenya was 41.7, and 20.9% of premature infants with ROP required treatment [31]. However, the incidence of ROP in our study is higher than that in European countries, such as Switzerland and Sweden [32, 33]. The incidence of ROP in Switzerland was 9.3, and 1.2% of premature infants with ROP required treatment [32]. We assumed that the differences in ROP incidence were primarily related to the following factors: (1) some pregnant women did not receive regular antenatal care, and they're maybe a significant error in the calculation of gestational age. (2) The survival rate of premature infants of very low birth weight and low gestational age was lower than that in developed countries. (3) The ROP screening guideline and the medical care of neonates in China were different to developed countries.

ROP is a disease involving multiple factors, and its exact etiology is not known. According to many reports, gestational age and birth weight are currently recognized as the primary risk factors for ROP [31]. Our results indicate that infants with a low birth weight or small gestational age or who require extended oxygen inhalation treatment have an increased incidence of ROP. This result is consistent with many other reports [34–36].

We also analyzed the correlation between ROP and individual factors in this study; the results showed that the factors significantly associated with the incidence of ROP include IVH, invasive examinations, and positive blood culture. However, the mechanisms by which these factors cause ROP are not clear. We speculate that these factors may lead to vital signs instability, and long-term, high-flow oxygen absorption is usually given as a treatment method.

In a logistic regression analysis, gestational age, birth weight and unmonitored supplemental oxygen were indicated as the primary risk factors for ROP [26]. Our study identified these three risk factors too. We also found two other independent risk factors, including minimum oxygen saturation, and average daily weight gain. We suspect that low oxygen saturation will prolong the duration of oxygen inhalation treatment, thereby increasing the incidence of ROP. The average daily weight gain is affected by a variety of disease factors such as growth factor secretion, which is associated with an increased incidence of ROP [37, 38].

With the rapid development of perinatal medicine and continuous improvements in treatment facilities, the survival rate for premature and low-birth weight infants has substantially improved, and the incidence of ROP has also significantly increased in China. Many studies have suggested that the up-regulated expression of VEGF plays an important role in the development of ROP [39], and anti-VEGF drugs can inhibit the over-expression of VEGF and thereby control intraocular angiogenesis and provide a good drug treatment for ROP [7, 40–42].

In report of the developed countries, the ROP that need treatment includes zone 1, any stage with plus disease; zone 1, stage 3, with or without plus disease; and zone 2, stage 2 or 3, with plus disease. The ROP that need watch and wait includes zone 1, stage 1 or 2 without plus disease and zone 2, stage 3 without plus disease. However, there is no uniform treatment threshold for ROP in China [9, 43]. Due to the special condition of China medical, many children will leave the NICU before the 54 weeks endpoint of the corrected gestational age. The ROP review should be performed at the outpatient clinic until the 54 weeks endpoint of the corrected gestational age. However, sometimes the ROP outpatient review cannot be carried out in time, furthermore some infants would lost control once leave hospital. In order to prevent the rapid progress of ROP, we would like to do retinal photocoagulation for some infants with ROP of zone3, stage3, and > 1 quadrant range. So there are little bit different in our report about the standard of treatment on ROP. In addition, the extremely severe premature infants born in our hospital, such as the extremely low born weight (< 1000 g), the extremely low gestational age (<26w) and systemic serious complications, would be transferred to the more specialized children's hospital (Guangzhou Women and Children's Medical Center) NICU. ROP incidence for those infants were not included in our study.

Retinal laser photocoagulation is a standard treatment for ROP. However, it can result in many problems, such as a wide range of retinal damage and the loss of vision in the photocoagulation area, and is not suitable for some patients, such as those with ROP in zone 1 or AP-ROP [44–46]. Anti-VEGF drugs may reduce complications when treating ROP. At the same time, anti-VEGF drugs can maintain the balance of VEGF and promote the continued development of retinal blood vessels in children with ROP [7, 40–42]. Many studies are currently ongoing to evaluate the use of anti-VEGF drugs in children with ROP [47, 48]. Anti-VEGF drugs for ROP treatment include Bevacizumab and Ranibizumab. Bevacizumab was used to treat ROP at first in 2006 [49, 50]. Bevacizumab is cheap and lasts long in ROP treatment, but it may have unknown systemic effects. Ranibizumab is a new anti-VEGF drug with a half-life of only 30 days and less systemic effects [51, 52]. In China, Bevacizumab couldn't be used to treat ocular diseases, so we used Ranibizumab to treat ROP in this study.

In our study, children with ROP in zone 2 or 3 were treated with traditional retinal laser photocoagulation, whereas children with ROP in zone 1 and posterior polar invasion ROP were given Ranibizumab via intraocular injections. The recurrence of ROP in the laser treatment and anti-VEGF treatment groups were 42.86 and 41.67%, respectively. Because anti-VEGF drugs may induce systemic risks in premature infants, all infants who had ROP recurrence were retreated with laser photocoagulation.

The conditions of all children were controlled after retreatment was given until 54 weeks of PMA. No serious complications such as retinal detachment occurred in any patients in our study. We speculate that may be related to the fact that children with a very low birth weight (< 1000 g) and gestational age (< 26 weeks) were not included in this study. An analysis of the two groups showed that the gestational age and birth weight were significantly lower in the anti-VEGF treatment group than that in the laser treatment group. This result is similar to other reports [8, 44, 53–57].

In conclusion, in this study, we systemically analyzed the incidence of and risk factors for ROP in severely premature infants treated in the NICU at Guangzhou First People's Hospital. The results of our study suggest that the incidence of ROP is 31.65% which will match those in middle-income countries, but higher than high-income countries. Anti-VEGF drugs could be preferred as a good treatment method for zone 1 ROP and aggressive posterior ROP.

Abbreviations
anti-VEGF: Anti-vascular endothelial growth factor; AP-ROP: Aggressive posterior ROP; IVF: In vitro fertilization; IVH: Intravascular hemolysis; NICU: Neonatal intensive care unit; PDA: Patent ductus arteriosus; ROP: Retinopathy of prematurity

Acknowledgements
Not applicable.

Funding
This research was supported by the Science and Technology Program of Guangzhou (No. 11C33150706) and the Natural Science Foundation of Guangdong Province (No. 2018A030313761).

Declarations
The human body was not subjected any adverse effects.

Authors' contributions
Study conception and design: YL, WY and ZG; collection, management and interpretation of data: WH, GR, CC, QT and YL; data analysis and writing of the article: YL; preparation, review, and approval of the manuscript: WH, WY and ZG. YL contributed to the manuscript as the first author; ZG contributed to the manuscript as the corresponding author. All authors read and approved the final manuscript.

Competing interests
The authors declare that they have no competing interests.

References
1. Castro Conde JR, et al. Retinopathy of prematurity. Prevention, screening and treatment guidelines. An Pediatr (Barc). 2009;71(6):514–23.

2. Hartnett ME, Penn JS. Mechanisms and management of retinopathy of prematurity. N Engl J Med. 2013;368(12):1162–3.

3. Jasani B, Nanavati R, Kabra N. Mechanisms and management of retinopathy of prematurity. N Engl J Med. 2013;368(12):1161–2.

4. Rao RC, Dlouhy BJ. Mechanisms and management of retinopathy of prematurity. N Engl J Med. 2013;368(12):1161.

5. Celebi AR, et al. The incidence and risk factors of severe retinopathy of prematurity in extremely low birth weight infants in Turkey. Med Sci Monit. 2014;20:1647–53.

6. Sukgen EA, Kocluk Y. The vascularization process after intravitreal ranibizumab injections for aggressive posterior retinopathy of prematurity. Arq Bras Oftalmol. 2017;80(1):30–4.

7. Lundgren P, et al. Aggressive posterior retinopathy of prematurity is associated with multiple infectious episodes and thrombocytopenia. Neonatology. 2017;111(1):79–85.

8. Lundgren P, et al. Duration of anaemia during the first week of life is an independent risk factor for retinopathy of prematurity. Acta Paediatr. 2018; 107(5):759–66.

9. Group., C.M.A.o. Screening guide for retinopathy of premature infants in China. Chin J Ophthalmol. 2014;50(0412–4081.2014.12.017):933–5.

10. International Committee for the Classification of Retinopathy of, P. The International Classification of Retinopathy of Prematurity revisited. Arch Ophthalmol. 2005;123(7):991–9.

11. Gilbert C, et al. Characteristics of infants with severe retinopathy of prematurity in countries with low, moderate, and high levels of development: implications for screening programs. Pediatrics. 2005;115(5): e518–25.

12. Gilbert C, et al. Retinopathy of prematurity in middle-income countries. Lancet. 1997;350(9070):12–4.

13. Skalet AH, et al. Telemedicine screening for retinopathy of prematurity in developing countries using digital retinal images: a feasibility project. J AAPOS. 2008;12(3):252–8.

14. Gilbert C. Retinopathy of prematurity: a global perspective of the epidemics, population of babies at risk and implications for control. Early Hum Dev. 2008;84(2):77–82.

15. King MJ. Retrolental fibroplasia; a clinical study of 238 cases. Arch Ophthal. 1950;43(4):694–711.

16. Clemett R, Darlow B. Results of screening low-birth-weight infants for retinopathy of prematurity. Curr Opin Ophthalmol. 1999;10(3):155–63.

17. Lee SK, et al. Evidence for changing guidelines for routine screening for retinopathy of prematurity. Arch Pediatr Adolesc Med. 2001;155(3):387–95.

18. Trinavarat A, Atchaneeyasakul LO, Udompunturak S. Applicability of American and British criteria for screening of the retinopathy of prematurity in Thailand. Jpn J Ophthalmol. 2004;48(1):50–3.

19. Astasheva IB, Sidorenko EI. Fulminant retinopathy of prematurity ("plus-disease"): incidence, risk factors, diagnostic criteria, and variations in course. Vestn oftalmol. 2002;118(6):5–9.

20. Chen Y, Li X. Characteristics of severe retinopathy of prematurity patients in China: a repeat of the first epidemic? Br J Ophthalmol. 2006;90(3):268–71.

21. Dutta S, et al. Risk factors of threshold retinopathy of prematurity. Indian Pediatr. 2004;41(7):665–71.

22. Varughese S, et al. Magnitude of the problem of retinopathy of prematurity. Experience in a large maternity unit with a medium size level-3 nursery. Indian J Ophthalmol. 2001;49(3):187–8.

23. Zhaoliang H. Review and recognition on urban size of Beijing. J Urban Reg Plann. 2011;2:18.

24. Xu Y, et al. Screening for retinopathy of prematurity in China: a neonatal units-based prospective study. Invest Ophthalmol Vis Sci. 2013;54(13): 8229–36.

25. Jin J, et al. Analysis on the result of retinopathy of prematurity screening in 1225 premature infants. Zhonghua Er Ke Za Zhi. 2010;48(11):829–33.

26. Chen Y, et al. Risk factors for retinopathy of prematurity in six neonatal intensive care units in Beijing. China Br J Ophthalmol. 2008;92(3):326–30.

27. Chen Y, et al. Analysis of changes in characteristics of severe retinopathy of prematurity patients after screening guidelines were issued in China. Retina. 2015;35(8):1674–9.

28. Shao XM Y, Qiu XS. Retionopathy of prematurity. Practicalneonatology. 4th ed. Beijing: People's Medical Publishing House; 2011. p. 887–92.

29. Ma Xue-ren ZQ, Hong K, Xue-Ping LI, Zhen-Juan Z, Juan W. Screening results and risk factors of 310 cases of retinopathy of prematurity in Qinghai Province. Chinese J Fundus Dis. 2017;33:631–2.

30. Varughese S, et al. Retinopathy of prematurity in South Africa: an assessment of needs, resources and requirements for screening programmes. Br J Ophthalmol. 2008;92(7):879–82.

31. Onyango O, et al. Retinopathy of prematurity in Kenya: prevalence and risk factors in a hospital with advanced neonatal care. Pan Afr Med J. 2018;29: 152.

32. Gerull R, et al. Incidence of retinopathy of prematurity (ROP) and ROP treatment in Switzerland 2006-2015: a population-based analysis. Arch Dis Child Fetal Neonatal Ed. 2018;103(4):F337–42.

33. Holmstrom G, et al. Increased frequency of retinopathy of prematurity over the last decade and significant regional differences. Acta Ophthalmol. 2018; 96(2):142–8.

34. Ali NA, et al. Prevalence of retinopathy of prematurity in Brunei Darussalam. Int J Ophthalmol. 2013;6(3):381–4.

35. Ludwig CA, et al. The epidemiology of retinopathy of prematurity in the United States. Ophthalmic Surg Lasers Imaging Retina. 2017;48(7):553–62.

36. Ugurbas SC, et al. Comparison of UK and US screening criteria for detection of retinopathy of prematurity in a developing nation. J AAPOS. 2010;14(6): 506–10.

37. Hard AL, Smith LE, Hellstrom A. Nutrition, insulin-like growth factor-1 and retinopathy of prematurity. Semin Fetal Neonatal Med. 2013;S1744-165X(13)00007-3.

38. Can E, et al. Early aggressive parenteral nutrition induced high insulin-like growth factor 1 (IGF-1) and insulin-like growth factor binding protein 3 (IGFBP3) levels can prevent risk of retinopathy of prematurity. Iran J Pediatr. 2013;23(4):403–10.

39. Hartnett ME, Penn JS. Mechanisms and management of retinopathy of prematurity. N Engl J Med. 2012;367(26):2515–26.

40. Feng J, et al. Vascular endothelial growth factor and apelin in plasma of patients with retinopathy of prematurity. Acta Ophthalmol. 2017; 95(6):e514–5.

41. VanderVeen DK, et al. Anti-vascular endothelial growth factor therapy for primary treatment of type 1 retinopathy of prematurity: a report by the American Academy of ophthalmology. Ophthalmology. 2017;124(5):619–33.

42. Fernandez MP, et al. Histopathologic characterization of the expression of vascular endothelial growth factor in a case of retinopathy of prematurity treated with Ranibizumab. Am J Ophthalmol. 2017;176:134–40.

43. Chuang LJ, et al. A modified developmental care bundle reduces pain and stress in preterm infants undergoing examinations for retinopathy of prematurity (ROP): a randomized controlled trial. J Clin Nurs. 2018.

44. Kabatas EU, et al. Comparison of intravitreal bevacizumab, intravitreal Ranibizumab and laser photocoagulation for treatment of type 1 retinopathy of prematurity in Turkish preterm children. Curr Eye Res. 2017; 42(7):1054–8.

45. Mota A, et al. Combination of intravitreal ranibizumab and laser photocoagulation for aggressive posterior retinopathy of prematurity. Case Rep Ophthalmol. 2012;3(1):136–41.

46. Gotz-Wieckowska A, et al. Ranibizumab after laser photocoagulation failure in retinopathy of prematurity (ROP) treatment. Sci Rep. 2017;7(1):11894.

47. Zhao M, et al. Expression of Total vascular endothelial growth factor and the anti-angiogenic VEGF 165 b isoform in the vitreous of patients with retinopathy of prematurity. Chin Med J. 2015;128(18):2505–9.

48. Sonmez K, et al. Vitreous levels of stromal cell-derived factor 1 and vascular endothelial growth factor in patients with retinopathy of prematurity. Ophthalmology. 2008;115(6):1065–70 e1.

49. Raizada S, Kandari JA, Sabti KA. Will the BEAT-ROP study results really beat ROP? Invest Ophthalmol Vis Sci. 2011;52(12):9288–9.

50. Moshfeghi DM, Berrocal AM. Retinopathy of prematurity in the time of bevacizumab: incorporating the BEAT-ROP results into clinical practice. Ophthalmology. 2011;118(7):1227–8.

51. Wallace DK. Retinopathy of prematurity: anti-VEGF treatment for ROP: which drug and what dose? J AAPOS. 2016;20(6):476–8.

52. Gonzalez Viejo I, Ferrer Novella C, Pueyo Royo V. Use of anti-VEGF (anti-vascular endothelial growth factor) in retinopathy of prematurity (ROP). Arch Soc Esp Oftalmol. 2011;86(7):207–8.

53. Wu WC, et al. Serum vascular endothelial growth factor after bevacizumab or Ranibizumab treatment for retinopathy of prematurity. Retina. 2017;37(4): 694–701.

54. Shah N, Gupta MP, Chan RVP. Persistent angiographic abnormalities after intravitreal anti-vascular endothelial growth factor therapy for retinopathy of prematurity. JAMA Ophthalmol. 2018;136(4):436-7.

Permissions

The contributors of this book come from diverse backgrounds, making this book a truly international effort. This book will bring forth new frontiers with its revolutionizing research information and detailed analysis of the nascent developments around the world.

We would like to thank all the contributing authors for lending their expertise to make the book truly unique. They have played a crucial role in the development of this book. Without their invaluable contributions this book wouldn't have been possible. They have made vital efforts to compile up to date information on the varied aspects of this subject to make this book a valuable addition to the collection of many professionals and students.

This book was conceptualized with the vision of imparting up-to-date information and advanced data in this field. To ensure the same, a matchless editorial board was set up. Every individual on the board went through rigorous rounds of assessment to prove their worth. After which they invested a large part of their time researching and compiling the most relevant data for our readers.

The editorial board has been involved in producing this book since its inception. They have spent rigorous hours researching and exploring the diverse topics which have resulted in the successful publishing of this book. They have passed on their knowledge of decades through this book. To expedite this challenging task, the publisher supported the team at every step. A small team of assistant editors was also appointed to further simplify the editing procedure and attain best results for the readers.

Apart from the editorial board, the designing team has also invested a significant amount of their time in understanding the subject and creating the most relevant covers. They scrutinized every image to scout for the most suitable representation of the subject and create an appropriate cover for the book.

The publishing team has been an ardent support to the editorial, designing and production team. Their endless efforts to recruit the best for this project, has resulted in the accomplishment of this book. They are a veteran in the field of academics and their pool of knowledge is as vast as their experience in printing. Their expertise and guidance has proved useful at every step. Their uncompromising quality standards have made this book an exceptional effort. Their encouragement from time to time has been an inspiration for everyone.

The publisher and the editorial board hope that this book will prove to be a valuable piece of knowledge for researchers, students, practitioners and scholars across the globe.

List of Contributors

Ahmed N. Sedky
Eye Subspecialty Center, Cairo, Egypt, 18 Elkhalifa Elmamoun Street, Heliopolis, Cairo, Egypt

Sherine S. Wahba and Maged M. Roshdy
Ain Shams University, Al Watany Eye Hospital and Watany Research and Development Center (WRDC), Cairo, Egypt

Nermeen R. Ayaad
Eye Subspecialty Center, Cairo, Egypt

Maged Alnawaiseh and Nicole Eter
Department of Ophthalmology, University of Muenster Medical Center, Albert-Schweitzer Campus 1, Building D15, 48149 Muenster, Germany

Cristin Brand
Centre of Reproductive Medicine and Andrology, University of Muenster, Muenster, Germany

Eike Bormann and Cristina Sauerland
Institute of Biostatistics and Clinical Research, University of Muenster, Muenster, Germany

Wenyi Tang, Ruiping Gu and Ting Zhang
Department of Ophthalmology, Eye and ENT Hospital of Fudan University, 83 Fenyang Road, Shanghai 200031, China

Gezhi Xu
Department of Ophthalmology, Eye and ENT Hospital of Fudan University, 83 Fenyang Road, Shanghai 200031, China
Shanghai Key Laboratory of Visual Impairment and Restoration, Fudan University, Shanghai 200031, China

Stephan Tobalem and James S. Schutz
Department of Ophthalmology, University Hospitals and School of Medicine, Geneva, Switzerland

Argyrios Chronopoulos
Department of Ophthalmology, Addenbrooke's Hospital, Cambridge University Hospital NHS Foundation Trust, Box 41, Hills Road, Cambridge CB2 0QQ, UK

Xinrong Zou
Shanghai General Hospital, Nanjing Medical University, No. 100, Haining Road, Hongkou District, Shanghai 200080, China
Department of Ophthalmology, Fengcheng Hospital, No.9983, Chuannanfeng Road, Fengxian District, Shanghai 201411, China

Lina Lu, Yi Xu, Jianfeng Zhu, Jiangnan He and Bo Zhang
Department of Preventative Ophthalmology, Shanghai Eye Disease Prevention and Treatment Center, No. 380, Kangding Road, Jingan, Shanghai 200040, China

Haidong Zou
Shanghai General Hospital, Nanjing Medical University, No. 100, Haining Road, Hongkou District, Shanghai 200080, China
Department of Preventative Ophthalmology, Shanghai Eye Disease Prevention and Treatment Center, No. 380, Kangding Road, Jingan, Shanghai 200040, China
Department of Ophthalmology, Shanghai General Hospital, Shanghai Jiao Tong University, Shanghai, China
Shanghai Key Laboratory of Fundus Disease, Shanghai, China

Peirong Lu
Department of Ophthalmology, The First Affiliated Hospital of Soochow University, Suzhou 215006, China

Jianyan Hu, Shufeng Li and Qiang Wu
Department of Ophthalmology, Shanghai Jiaotong University Affiliated Sixth People's Hospital, Shanghai 200233, China

Ming-Hui Zhao
Department of Ophthalmology, The First Affiliated Hospital of Soochow University, Suzhou 215006, China
Department of Ophthalmology, Shanghai Jiaotong University Affiliated Sixth People's Hospital, Shanghai 200233, China

Juan Cao, Minglan Cui, Songtao Yuan, Qinghuai Liu and Wen Fan
Department of Ophthalmology, The First Affiliated Hospital with Nanjing Medical University, Nanjing, China

Min Zhuang
Department of Ophthalmology, The First Affiliated Hospital with Nanjing Medical University, Nanjing, China
Department of Ophthalmology, The Fourth Affiliated Hospital of Nantong University, Yancheng, China

Huimin Hu, Weiling Zhang, YizhuoWang, Dongsheng Huang, Yi Zhang and Yan Zhou
Department of Pediatrics, Beijing Tongren Hospital, West South road 2, Yizhuang Economic and Technological Development Zone, Daxing District, Beijing 100176, China

Jitong Shi and Bin Li
Department of Ophthalmology, Beijing Tongren Hospital, Capital Medical University, Beijing 100176, China

Jiangnan He, Qiuying Chen, Haidong Zou and Xun Xu
Shanghai Eye Disease Prevention and Treatment Center, Shanghai, China

Jianfeng Zhu and Shanshan Li
Shanghai General Hospital, Shanghai, China

Dong Ju Kim, Joo-Hee Park and Minwook Chang
Department of Ophthalmology, Dongguk University, Ilsan Hospital, 814, Siksadong, Ilsan-dong-gu, Goyang, Gyeonggido 410-773, South Korea

Ke Zheng, Tian Han, Yinan Han and Xiaomei Qu
Department of Ophthalmology, Eye and ENT Hospital of Fudan University and Myopia Key Laboratory of Ministry of Health, Shanghai, China

J. Rezapour, S. Nickels, A. K. Schuster and N. Pfeiffer
Department of Ophthalmology, University Medical Center Mainz, Mainz, Germany

M. Michal and M. E. Beutel
Department of Psychosomatic Medicine and Psychotherapy, University Medical Center Mainz, Mainz, Germany

T. Münzel
Center for Cardiology I, University Medical Center Mainz, Mainz, Germany

A. Schulz
Center for Thrombosis and Hemostasis (CTH), University Medical Center Mainz, Mainz, Germany

P. S. Wild
Preventive Cardiology and Preventive Medicine / Center for Cardiology, University Medical Center Mainz, Mainz, Germany
Center for Thrombosis and Hemostasis (CTH), University Medical Center Mainz, Mainz, Germany
German Center for Cardiovascular Research (DZHK), partner site Rhine-Main, Mainz, Germany

I. Schmidtmann
Institute for Medical Biostatistics, Epidemiology and Informatics, University Medical Center Mainz, Mainz, Germany

K. Lackner
Institute for Clinical Chemistry and Laboratory Medicine, University Medical Center Mainz, Mainz, Germany

Yi Xu, Jiangnan He, Senlin Lin, Bo Zhang, Jianfeng Zhu, Lina Lu and Haidong Zou
Shanghai Eye Disease Prevention and Treatment Center / Shanghai Eye Hospital; Shanghai Key Laboratory of Ocular Fundus Diseases; Shanghai General Hospital; Shanghai Engineering Center for Visual Science and Photomedicine, 380 Kangding Road, Shanghai 200040, China

Serge Resnikoff
Brien Holden Vision Institute and SOVS, University of New South Wales, Sydney, NSW, Australia

Chan Min Yang, Sungsoon Hwang, and Tae-Young Chung
Department of Ophthalmology, Samsung Medical Center, Sungkyunkwan University School of Medicine, #81 Irwon-ro, Gangnam-gu, Seoul 06351, South Korea

Dong Hui Lim
Department of Ophthalmology, Samsung Medical Center, Sungkyunkwan University School of Medicine, #81 Irwon-ro, Gangnam-gu, Seoul 06351, South Korea
Department of Preventive Medicine, Catholic University School of Medicine, Seoul, South Korea

Joo Hyun
Department of Ophthalmology, Saevit Eye Hospital, Goyang, South Korea

Aiwu Fang, Peijuan Wang, Rui He and Jia Qu
Wenzhou Medical University Eye Hospital, Wenzhou 325027, China

Jingli Guo, WenYi Tang, Xiaofeng Ye, Haixiang Wu, Gezhi Xu, Wei Liu and Yongjin Zhang
Department of Ophthalmology, Eye and ENT Hospital of Fudan University, Shanghai Key Laboratory of Visual Impairment and Restoration, Shanghai 200031, China

Hun Lee
Department of Ophthalmology, International St. Mary's Hospital, Catholic
Kwandong University College of Medicine, Incheon, South Korea
The Institute of Vision Research, Department of Ophthalmology, Yonsei University
College of Medicine, Seoul, South Korea

Kyoung Yul Seo and Tae-im Kim
The Institute of Vision Research, Department of Ophthalmology, Yonsei University
College of Medicine, Seoul, South Korea

David Sung Yong Kang, Jin Young Choi and Byoung Jin Ha
Eyereum Eye Clinic, Seoul, South Korea

Eung Kweon Kim
The Institute of Vision Research, Department of Ophthalmology, Yonsei University
College of Medicine, Seoul, South Korea
Corneal Dystrophy Research Institute, Department of Ophthalmology, Yonsei University College of Medicine, Seoul, South Korea

Je-Hyun Baek
R&D Center for Clinical Mass Spectrometry, Seegene Medical Foundation, Seoul 04805, South Korea

Daehan Lim, Jae-Byoung Chae, Hyoik Jang and Hyewon Chung
Department of Ophthalmology, Konkuk University School of Medicine, Konkuk University Medical Center, 120-1 Neungdong-ro, Gwangjin-gu, Seoul, Republic of Korea

Kyu Hyung Park
Department of Ophthalmology, Seoul National University College of Medicine, Seoul National University Bundang Hospital, Seongnam 13620, South Korea

Jonghyun Lee
Department of Ophthalmology, Ilsan Paik Hospital, Inje University College of Medicine, Goyang 10380, South Korea

Wei Xu, Weijing Cheng, Hua Zhuang, Jian Guo and Guoxing Xu
Department of Ophthalmology, First Affiliated Hospital of Fujian Medical University, No. 20 Chazhong Road, Fuzhou 350005, China

Fashe Markos Cherinet, Sophia Yoseph Tekalign, Dereje Hayilu Anbesse and Zewdu Yenegeta Bizuneh
Department of Ophthalmology, St. Paul's Hospital Millennium Medical College, Addis Ababa, Ethiopia

Choul Yong Park
Department of Ophthalmology, Dongguk University, Ilsan Hospital, Goyang, South Korea

Jimmy K. Lee and Roy S. Chuck
Department of Ophthalmology and Visual Sciences, Montefiore Medical Center, Albert Einstein College of Medicine, Bronx, NY, USA

Keiichiro Minami, Tadatoshi Tokunaga and Kazunori Miyata
Miyata Eye Hospital, 6-3 Kurahara-cho, Miyakonojo, Miyazaki 885-0051, Japan

Keiichiro Okamoto
Tomey Corporation, Nishi-ku, Nagoya, Aichi, Japan

Tetsuro Oshika
Department of Ophthalmology, Faculty of Medicine, University of Tsukuba, Tsukuba, Ibaraki, Japan

Shu-Ya Wu and Elizabeth P. Shen
Department of Ophthalmology, Taipei Tzu Chi Hospital, Buddhist Tzu Chi Medical Foundation, No. 289, Jianguo Rd., Xindian Dist., New Taipei City 231, Taipei, Taiwan (R.O.C.)

Chien-Yi Pan
Wu Chou Animal Hospital, Taipei, Taiwan

I-Shiang Tzeng
Department of Research, Taipei Tzu Chi Hospital, Buddhist Tzu Chi Medical
Foundation, Taipei, Taiwan

Wei-Cherng Hsu
Department of Ophthalmology, Taipei Tzu Chi Hospital, Buddhist Tzu Chi Medical Foundation, No. 289, Jianguo Rd., Xindian Dist., New Taipei City 231, Taipei, Taiwan (R.O.C.)
Tzu Chi University College of Medicine, Hualien, Taiwan

Ke Xu, Hong Qi, Rongmei Peng, Gege Xiao, Jing Hong, Yansheng Hao and Boping Ma
Department of Ophthalmology, Beijing Key Laboratory of Restoration of Damaged Ocular Nerve, Peking University Third Hospital, 49 North Garden RoadHaidian District, Beijing 100191, People's Republic of China

Florence Hoogewoud, Pauline Butori and Antoine P. Brézin
Department of Ophthalmology, National Referral Center for rare Ocular Diseases, Hôpital Cochin, APHP, Université Paris Descartes, Paris, France

Philippe Blanche
Department of Internal Medicine, National Referral Center for Rare Systemic Autoimmune Diseases, Hôpital Cochin, APHP, Paris, France

Chan Ho Cho and Sang-Bumm Lee
Department of Ophthalmology, Yeungnam University College of Medicine, 170, Hyunchung-ro, Nam-gu, Daegu 705-717 (42415), South Korea

Lan Li
Department of Ophthalmology, the First People's Hospital of Kunming City,
Kunming, China

Hua Zhong
Department of Ophthalmology, the First Affiliated Hospital of Kunming Medical University, Kunming, China

Jun Li
Department of Ophthalmology, the Second People's Hospital of Yunnan Province, Kunming, China

Cai-Rui Li
Department of Ophthalmology, the First Affiliated Hospital of Dali University, 32 Mangyong Road, Dali 671003, China

Chen-Wei Pan
5School of Public Health, Medical College of Soochow University, 199 Ren Ai Road, Suzhou 215123, China

Taku Toyama, Masato Yoshitani, Rei Sakata and Jiro Numaga
Department of Ophthalmology, Tokyo Metropolitan Geriatric Hospital and Institute of Gerontology, 35-2, Sakae-cho, Itabashi-ku, Tokyo 173-0015, Japan

Takashi Ueta
Department of Ophthalmology, Graduate School of Medicine and Faculty of Medicine, The University of Tokyo, 7-3-1, Hongo, Bunkyo-ku, Tokyo 113-8655, Japan
Department of Ophthalmology, Center Hospital of the National Center for Global Health and Medicine, 1-21-1 Toyama Shinjyuku-ku, Tokyo 162-8655, Japan

Lei Xi
Department of Ophthalmology, Peking University International Hospital,
Beijing, China

Chen Zhang
Tianjin Medical University Eye hospital, Tianjin Medical University Eye Institute, School of Optometry and Ophthalmology, Tianjin, China

Yanling He
Department of Ophthalmology, Peking University People's Hospital, Xizhimen South Street 11, Xi Cheng District, Beijing 100044, China

Orapan Aryasit, Passorn Preechawai, Chakree Hirunpat, Orasa Horatanaruang and Penny Singha
Department of Ophthalmology, Faculty of Medicine, Prince of Songkla University, 15, Kanjanavanich Rd, Kohong, Hat Yai, Songkhla 90110, Thailand

Eva Larsson, Anna Molnar and Gerd Holmström
Department of Neuroscience/Ophthalmology, Uppsala University, SE-751 85 Uppsala, Sweden

Ruiping Gu and Gezhi Xu
Department of Ophthalmology, Eye and ENT Hospital and Shanghai Key Laboratory of Visual Impairment and Restoration, Shanghai Medical College, Fudan University, Shanghai 200031, China

Guohua Deng and Yi Jiang
Department of Ophthalmology, The Third People's Hospital of Changzhou, Changzhou 213000, China

Chunhui Jiang
Department of Ophthalmology, Eye and ENT Hospital and Shanghai Key Laboratory of Visual Impairment and Restoration, Shanghai Medical College, Fudan University, Shanghai 200031, China
Department of Ophthalmology, No. 5 People's Hospital of Shanghai, Shanghai 200240, China

Youn-Shen Bee
Department of Ophthalmology, Kaohsiung Veterans General Hospital, 386 Ta-Chung 1st RD, Kaohsiung 81346, Taiwan

Yuh-Ing Junior College of Health Care and Management, Kaohsiung, Taiwan
National Defense Medical Center, Taipei, Taiwan

Pei-Jhen Tsai, Muh-Chiou Lin and Ming-Ying Chu
Department of Ophthalmology, Kaohsiung Veterans General Hospital, 386 Ta-Chung 1st RD, Kaohsiung 81346, Taiwan

Wenzhi Huang, Guoliang Ren, Cheng Cai, Qingbiao Tan, Yuqin Liang and Weizhong Yang
Guangzhou First People's Hospital, Guangzhou city, China

Yunxia Leng and Zongyin Gao
Guangzhou First People's Hospital, Guangzhou city, China
Second Affiliated Hospital of South China University of Technology, Guangzhou city, China

Index

www.ingramcontent.com/pod-product-compliance
Lightning Source LLC
Chambersburg PA
CBHW061305190326
41458CB00011B/3767